ACUTE CARE SURGERY

Notice

Medicine is an ever-changing science. As new research and clinical experience broaden our knowledge, changes in treatment and drug therapy are required. The authors and the publisher of this work have checked with sources believed to be reliable in their efforts to provide information that is complete and generally in accord with the standards accepted at the time of publication. However, in view of the possibility of human error or changes in medical sciences, neither the authors nor the publisher nor any other party who has been involved in the preparation or publication of this work warrants that the information contained herein is in every respect accurate or complete, and they disclaim all responsibility for any errors or omissions or for the results obtained from use of the information contained in this work. Readers are encouraged to confirm the information contained herein with other sources. For example and in particular, readers are advised to check the product information sheet included in the package of each drug they plan to administer to be certain that the information contained in this work is accurate and that changes have not been made in the recommended dose or in the contraindications for administration. This recommendation is of particular importance in connection with new or infrequently used drugs.

ACUTE CARE SURGERY
A Guide for General Surgeons

Editors

Vicente H. Gracias, MD
Associate Professor of Surgery
Chief, Surgical Critical Care
Medical Director Critical Care
University of Pennsylvania School of Medicine
Philadelphia, Pennsylvania

Mark G. McKenney, MD
Professor of Surgery
Chief of Surgery, University of Miami Hospital
Chief, Trauma and Surgical Critical Care
University of Miami Miller School of Medicine
Co-Director, Ryder Trauma Center
Jackson Memorial Hospital
Miami, Florida

Patrick M. Reilly, MD
Associate Professor of Surgery
Trauma and Surgical Critical Care
University of Pennsylvania School of Medicine
Philadelphia, Pennsylvania

George C. Velmahos, MD, PhD, MSEd
John F. Burke Professor of Surgery
Harvard Medical School
Chief, Division of Trauma, Emergency Surgery, and Surgical Critical Care
Massachusetts General Hospital
Boston, Massachusetts

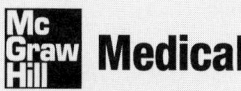 **Medical**

New York Chicago San Francisco Lisbon London Madrid Mexico City Milan
New Delhi San Juan Seoul Singapore Sydney Toronto

Acute Care Surgery: A Guide for General Surgeons

Copyright © 2009 by the McGraw-Hill Companies, Inc. All rights reserved. Printed in the United States of America. Except as permitted under the United States Copyright Act of 1976, no part of this publication may be reproduced or distributed in any form or by any means, or stored in a database or retrieval system, without the prior written permission of the publisher.

1 2 3 4 5 6 7 8 9 0   CCW/CCW   12 11 10 9 8

ISBN 978-0-07-147290-6
MHID 0-07-147290-8

This book was set in Stone Serif by International Typesetting and Composition, Inc.
The editors were Marsha Loeb and Peter J. Boyle.
The production supervisor was Catherine H. Saggese.
The designer was Edward Drewery.
Project management was provided by Gita Raman, International Typesetting
and Composition, Inc.
Courier Westford was printer and binder.

This book is printed on acid-free paper.

Library of Congress Cataloging-in-Publication Data

Acute care surgery : a guide for general surgeons / editors, Vicente H.
   Gracias ... [et al.].
      p. ; cm.
   Includes bibliographical references and index.
   ISBN-13: 978-0-07-147290-6 (hardcover : alk. paper)
   ISBN-10: 0-07-147290-8 (hardcover : alk. paper)
   1. Surgical intensive care.   2. Surgical emergencies.   3. Wounds and injuries—Surgery.
 I. Gracias, Vicente H.
   [DNLM: 1. Emergency Treatment—methods.   2. Surgical Procedures, Operative—
methods.   3. Critical Care—methods.   4. Wounds and Injuries—surgery.
WO 700 A187 2009]
RD51.5.A28 2009
617′.026—dc22

                                                                    2008037024

*To my family: my mother and father who taught me to care, my brothers
and sister who taught me to strive,
my wife (Wendy) and children who taught me to love,
my partners and fellows who taught me to listen,
and my patients who teach me every day.*

*To those who follow, remember: above all else the patient comes first—
be valiant in this charge.*

—VHG

*To my wife Kim, I still cannot believe that you married me.
To our children Kyle, Kelly, and Katie, each day is joy because of you.
To my parents, Al and Betty, I still look up to you for who you are,
what you have done. Thank you and I love you.*

—MGM

*For Luke, Jack, Grace, and Tim.
May you have access to expert emergency surgical care
wherever your lives take you.*

—PMR

*To the two persons who made me and I love, my parents—
the three persons that I made and I love, my children—
and the one person that I made and was made of and I love, my wife.*

—GCV

CONTENTS

PART III TRAUMA

CONTRIBUTORS

J. M. Kofi Abbensetts, MD
Assistant Professor of Surgery
Assistant Professor of Traumatology and Emergency
Medicine
University of Connecticut School of Medicine
Trauma Attending
Trauma Program, Hartford Hospital
Hartford, Connecticut
Chapter 3

Thomas Abbruzzese, MD
Division of Vascular and Endovascular Surgery
Massachusetts General Hospital
Harvard Medical School
Boston, Massachusetts
Chapter 15

Scott B. Armen, MD
Assistant Professor of Surgery
Ohio State University
Columbus, Ohio
Chapter 21

Juan A. Asensio, MD
Professor and Chief
Division of Clinical Research in Trauma Surgery
Department of Surgery, Division of Trauma
Senior Trauma Attending
University Hospital
University of Medicine and Dentistry of New Jersey at
Newark
Newark, New Jersey
Chapter 28

Chirag Badami, MD
Resident in General Surgery
Department of Surgery
New Jersey Medical School
Newark, New Jersey
Chapter 6

Philip S. Barie, MD, MBA
Professor
Division of Critical Care and Trauma
Department of Surgery
Division of Medical Ethics
Department of Public Health
Weill Cornell Medical College
Chief, Trauma Services
Director, Ann and Max A. Cohen Surgical Intensive
Care Unit
New York–Presbyterian Hospital/Weill Cornell
Medical Center
New York, New York
Chapter 23

Aaron Bransky, MS, MD
Private Practice
Presbyterian Hospital of Plano
Plano, Texas
Chapter 17

Benjamin Braslow, MD
Assistant Professor
Department of Surgery
University of Pennsylvania School of Medicine
Division of Traumatology and Surgical Critical Care
Hospital of the University of Pennsylvania
Philadelphia, Pennsylvania
Chapter 10

Susan I. Brundage, MD, MPH
Associate Professor
Department of Surgery
Stanford University Medical Center
Stanford, California
Chapter 5

Karen A. Chojnacki, MD
Assistant Professor
Department of Surgery
Thomas Jefferson University
Surgery Residency Director
Thomas Jefferson University Hospital
Philadelphia, Pennsylvania
Chapter 10

Nikunj K. Chokshi, MD
Research Fellow, Pediatric Surgery
Childrens Hospital Los Angeles
Los Angeles, California
Resident, Department of Surgery
Medical College of Wisconsin
Milwaukee, Wisconsin
Chapter 18

Edward E. Cornwell III, MD
Professor of Surgery
Associate Professor of Anesthesia and Critical Care
Medicine
Adult Trauma
Department of Surgery
Johns Hopkins School of Medicine
Baltimore, Maryland
Chapter 9

Bryan A. Cotton, MD
Assistant Professor of Surgery
Division of Trauma, Emergency Surgery, and Surgical
Critical Care
Department of Surgery
Vanderbilt University School of Medicine
Nashville, Tennessee
Chapter 25

Michael D. Crittenden, MD
Staff Cardiac Surgeon
Division of Cardiac Surgery
Department of Surgical Service
VA Boston Health
West Roxbury, Massachusetts
Chapter 2

Demetrios Demetriades, MD, Ph.D
Professor of Surgery
Director, Division of Trauma Surgery and Surgical
Critical Care
Department of Surgery
Keck School of Medicine and the Los Angeles County
University of Southern California Medical Center
Los Angeles, California
Chapter 20

Marc de Moya, MD
Instructor in Surgery
Trauma, Emergency Surgery and Surgical Critical Care
Department of Surgery
Massachusetts General Hospital
Boston, Massachusetts
Chapter 11

Sharmila Dissanaike, MD
Critical Care Fellow
Trauma & Surgical Critical Care
Department of Surgery
University of Washington
Seattle, Washington
Chapter 30

Lisa S. Dresner, MD
Associate Professor of Surgery
Division of Trauma and Surgical Critical Care
Department of Surgery
State University of New York–Downstate Medical
Center
Brooklyn, New York
Chapter 24

Scott A. Dulchavsky, MD, PhD
Roy D. McClure Chair, Department of Surgery
Henry Ford Health System
Professor of Surgery, Molecular Biology, and Genetics
Wayne State University School of Medicine
Detroit, Michigan
Chapter 8

Soumitra R. Eachempati, MD
Associate Professor
Division of Critical Care and Trauma
Department of Surgery
Division of Medical Ethics
Department of Public Health
Weill Cornell Medical College
Director, Quality Assurance, Trauma Services
New York–Presbyterian Hospital/Weill Cornell
Medical Center
New York, New York
Chapter 23

David T. Efron, MD
Assistant Professor of Surgery
Chief, Division of Trauma and Surgical Critical Care
Johns Hopkins School of Medicine
Baltimore, Maryland
Chapter 9

Frederick W. Endorf, MD
Staff Surgeon
Division of Burns
Department of Surgery
Regions Hospital
Saint Paul, Minnesota
Chapter 32

Timothy C. Fabian, MD
Harwell Wilson Alumni Professor and Chairman
Department of Surgery
University of Tennessee Health Science Center
Memphis, Tennessee
Chapter 7

David V. Feliciano, MD
Professor and Surgeon-in-Chief
Department of Surgery
Grady Memorial Hospital
Atlanta, Georgia
Chapter 12

Henri R. Ford, MD
Vice President and Surgeon-in-Chief
Childrens Hospital Los Angeles
Professor and Vice-Chairman
Department of Surgery
Keck School of Medicine
University of Southern California
Los Angeles, California
Chapter 18

Heidi Frankel, MD
Professor of Surgery
Division of Burn Trauma Critical Care
Department of Surgery
University of Texas Southwestern Medical Center
Dallas, Texas
Chapter 17

David F. Gaieski, MD, FACEP
Assistant Professor
Co-Director, Center for Resuscitation Science
Department of Emergency Medicine
University of Pennsylvania School of Medicine
Philadelphia, Pennsylvania
Chapter 1

Stephen C. Gale, MD
Assistant Professor of Surgery
Acute Care Surgery
Department of Surgery
University of Texas Medical School
Houston, Texas
Chapter 27

Richard L. Gamelli, MD
Robert J. Freeark, MD, Professor of Trauma Surgery
Surgery, Trauma, Surgical Critical Care and Burns
Pediatrics, General Pediatrics
Department Chairman, Surgery
Director, Burn and Shock Trauma Institute
Medical Director, Burn Unit
Loyola University Medical Center
Maywood, Illinois
Chapter 32

George D. Garcia, MD
Trauma Surgery & Surgical Critical Care Fellow
Division of Trauma Surgery and Surgical Critical Care
DeWitt Daughtry Department of Surgery
University of Miami
Miller School of Medicine
Miami, Florida
Chapter 28

Larry Gentilello, MD
Professor of Surgery
Burns, Trauma, Critical Care
Department of Surgery
University of Texas Southwestern Medical School
Dallas, Texas
Chapter 17

Claudia E. Goettler, MD
Assistant Professor
Trauma and Surgical Critical Care
Department of Surgery
Brody School of Medicine, East Carolina University
Greenville, North Carolina
Chapter 4

Munish Goyal, MD, FACEP
Assistant Professor
Emergency Medicine
University of Pennsylvania School of Medicine
Philadelphia, Pennsylvania
Chapter 1

Vicente H. Gracias, MD
Associate Professor of Surgery
Chief, Surgical Critical Care
Medical Director Critical Care
University of Pennsylvania School of Medicine
Philadelphia, Pennsylvania
Chapter 13

Elliot R. Haut, MD
Assistant Professor, Director of the Trauma/Acute Care
Surgery Fellowship
Division of Trauma and Surgical Critical Care
Department of Surgery and Anesthesiology and
Critical Care Medicine
Johns Hopkins University, School of Medicine
Baltimore, Maryland
Chapter 9

Sharon Henry, MD
Associate Professor of Surgery
Surgical Critical Care
Department of Surgery
University of Maryland School of Medicine
Chief, Wound Healing and Metabolism
Wound and Soft Tissue Department
University of Maryland Medical Center/R.A. Cowley
Shock Trauma
Baltimore, Maryland
Chapter 14

James H. Holmes IV, MD
Assistant Professor of Surgery
Trauma and Burns
Department of Surgery
Wake Forest University School of Medicine
Winston-Salem, North Carolina
Chapter 22

David B. Hoyt, MD
Chairman, Department of Surgery
The John E. Connolly Professor of Surgery
Division of Trauma and Critical Care
Department of Surgery
University of California, Irvine Medical Center
Orange, California
Chapter 29

Kenji Inaba, BS, MS, MD
Assistant Professor of Surgery
Trauma Surgery and Surgical Critical Care
Department of Surgery
Keck School of Medicine and the Los Angeles County
University of Southern California Medical Center
Los Angeles, California
Chapter 20

Nabil Issa, MD
Critical Care Surgery Fellow
Acute Care Surgery
Department of Surgery
University of Michigan
Ann Arbor, Michigan
Chapter 26

Benjamin M. Jackson, MD
Instructor in Surgery
Vascular Surgery
Department of Surgery
University of Pennsylvania
Philadelphia, Pennsylvania
Chapter 16

Lenworth M. Jacobs, MD, MPH
Professor of Surgery
Professor and Chairman
Department of Traumatology and Emergency
Medicine
University of Connecticut School of Medicine
Director, Trauma Program, Hartford Hospital
Hartford, Connecticut
Chapter 3

Jay S. Jenoff, MD
Instructor of Surgery
Traumatology and Surgical Critical Care
Department of Surgery
University of Pennsylvania School of Medicine
Philadelphia, Pennsylvania
Chapter 13

Ronald Jou, MD
General Surgery Resident
Department of Surgery
Stanford University
Stanford, California
Chapter 5

Gregory J. Jurkovich, MD
Chief of Trauma and Professor of Surgery
Trauma and Surgical Critical Care
Department of Surgery
University of Washington
Seattle, Washington
Chapter 30

Sadaf Khan, MBBS
Staff Surgeon
Henry Ford Health System
Detroit, Michigan
Chapter 8

Shukri F. Khuri, MD
Chief of Cardiothoracic Surgery
Cardiac Surgery
Surgical Service
VA Boston Healthcare System
West Roxbury, Massachusetts
Chapter 2

Christopher J. Kwolek, MD
Assistant Professor of Surgery, Harvard Medical School
Division of Vascular and Endovascular Surgery
Massachusetts General Hospital
Harvard Medical School
Boston, Massachusetts
Chapter 15

Michael E. Lekawa, MD
Associate Professor of Surgery
Chief, Division of Trauma and Critical Care
Department of Surgery
University of California, Irvine
Orange, California
Chapter 29

Peter Letarte, MD
Chief, Section of Neurological Surgery
Department of Surgery
Edward G. Hines Veterans Hospital
Maywood, Illinois
Chapter 31

David H. Livingston, MD
Professor and Chief of Trauma Surgery
Department of Surgery
New Jersey Medical School
Newark, New Jersey
Chapter 6

Frederick A. Luchette, MD, MS
The Ambrose and Gladys Bowyer Professor of Surgery
Division of General Surgery
Department of Surgery
Stritch School of Medicine,
Loyola University of Chicago
Maywood, Illinois
Chapter 32

Larry C. Martin, MD
Professor of Surgery
University of Florida
General Evaluation and Resuscitation
Columbus, Ohio
Chapter 21

Kenneth L. Mattox, MD
Professor and Vice Chair
Michael E. DeBakey Department of Surgery
Baylor College of Medicine
Houston, Texas
Chapter 27

Kimball I. Maull, MD
Director, Trauma Service
The Trauma Center at Hamad
Hamad General Hospital
Doha, Qatar
Chapter 31

Addison K. May, MD
Associate Professor of Surgery and Anesthesiology
Trauma and Surgical Critical Care
Department of Surgery
Vanderbilt University Medical Center
Nashville, Tennessee
Chapter 25

Bruce A. McKinley, PhD
Department of Surgery
Medical School
University of Texas–Health Science Center at Houston
Houston, Texas
Chapter 19

Frederick A. Moore, MD
Head, Division of Surgical Critical Care & Acute Surgery
Department of Surgery
The Methodist Hospital
Houston, Texas
Chapter 19

Lena M. Napolitano, MD
Professor of Surgery, Division Chief
Acute Care Surgery
Trauma, Burns, Critical Care, Emergency Surgery
Associate Chair, Department of Surgery
University of Michigan
Ann Arbor, Michigan
Chapter 26

Patricia A. O'Neill, MD
Associate Professor of Surgery
Division of Trauma and Surgical Critical Care
Department of Surgery
State University of New York – Downstate Medical Center
Brooklyn, New York
Chapter 24

Craig A. Reickert, MD
Senior Staff Surgeon
Division of Colon and Rectal Surgery
Department of Surgery
Henry Ford Health System
Detroit, Michigan
Chapter 8

Ernest L. Rosato, MD
Associate Professor
Department of Surgery
Thomas Jefferson University
Chief, Division of Gastrointestinal Surgery
Thomas Jefferson University Hospital
Philadelphia, Pennsylvania
Chapter 10

Michael F. Rotondo, MD
Professor and Chair
Chief, Trauma and Surgical Critical Care
Department of Surgery
Brody School of Medicine, East Carolina University
Greenville, North Carolina
Chapter 4

Thomas M. Scalea, MD
Physician and Chief
R. Adam Crowley Shock Trauma Center
Baltimore, Maryland
Chapter 14

Thomas J. Schroeppel, MD
Instructor of Surgery
Department of Surgery
University of Tennessee Health Science Center
Memphis, Tennessee
Chapter 7

Robert W. Schulze, MD
Assistant Professor of Surgery
Division of Trauma and Surgical Critical Care
Department of Surgery
State University of New York–Downstate Medical Center
Brooklyn, New York
Chapter 24

Jason W. Smith, MD
Ohio State University
Resident in Surgery
Ohio State University Medical Center
General Evaluation and Resuscitation
Columbus, Ohio
Chapter 21

David A. Spain, MD
Professor of Surgery
Chief of Trauma
Critical Care and Emergency Surgery
Division of General Surgery
Department of Surgery
Stanford University
Stanford, California
Chapter 5

Jeffrey S. Upperman, MD
Director, Trauma Program
Attending Pediatric Surgeon
Associate Professor of Surgery
Department of Pediatric Surgery
Childrens Hospital Los Angeles
Keck School of Medicine
University of Southern California
Los Angeles, California
Chapter 18

Gary A. Vercruysse, MD
Assistant Professor
Department of Surgery
Emory University
Co-Director, Burn Unit
Grady Memorial Hospital
Atlanta, Georgia
Chapter 12

Andrew L. Warshaw, MD
W. Gerald Austen Professor of Surgery
Department of Surgery
Harvard Medical School
Surgeon-in-Chief and Chairman
Department of Surgery
Massachusetts General Hospital
Boston, Massachusetts
Chapter 11

Michael T. Watkins, MD
Associate Professor of Surgery, Harvard Medical
School
Director, Vascular Surgery Research Laboratory
Division of Vascular and Endovascular Surgery
Massachusetts General Hospital
Harvard Medical School
Boston, Massachusetts
Chapter 15

Edward Y. Woo, MD
Assistant Professor
Vascular Surgery
Department of Surgery
University of Pennsylvania
Philadelphia, Pennsylvania
Chapter 16

FOREWORD

The acute care surgery (ACS) concept is sweeping the globe as many countries struggle with providing emergency surgical care to an increasing population of people who present to emergency rooms and trauma centers with life- and limb-threatening surgical disease. Founded in the trauma surgery world, ACS is rapidly taking on the huge deficit of care created by specialty surgeons. The surgical arena is replete with specialized practices and elder surgeons who no longer cover the "emergency room call." Throughout the United States these in-house ACS surgeons are being recognized for their availability, expertise, and improved outcomes for urgent surgical problems.

Though contemporary in name, the ACS concept of a surgeon being knowledgeable, well trained, experienced, and willing to provide expert care for a wide breadth of surgical emergencies is not new; in fact, it was the core of all general surgical training and practice until the latter part of the twentieth century. General surgeons have always been the key group to respond to emergency rooms (and later departments) and care for the acute abdomen, the ischemic leg, soft tissue infection, trauma, and a multitude of critical problems. In addition, they have always been the hospitals' doctors for the "sick patients."

Long before critical care was a recognized specialty, general surgeons provided intensive care to their patients. Acute care surgery recaptures this type of practice but focuses on an all-emergency environment. Its training curriculum, developed and published by the American Association for the Surgery of Trauma (AAST) assures that the ACS surgeon is expert at trauma, critical care, burn management, and the vast majority of surgical emergencies. In addition, the ACS concept capitalizes on the trauma system design that has been so successful, where a surgeon is available, willing, and able to resuscitate, manage, operate, and treat in all phases of major surgical diseases. It employs contemporary evidence-based guidelines and strong performance improvement methods to assure optimal outcomes.

By broadening the responsibility of the trauma and critical care surgeon to include all emergency surgery and by employing the same requirements of optimal outcomes through evidence-based decisions and continual analysis and improvement, a new type of surgeon has emerged. The reported experience thus far is extremely favorable and many centers are reporting increased efficiency, patient satisfaction, cost effectiveness, and improved clinical outcomes.

What has been lacking until now is a contemporary textbook that provides the physician with a comprehensive view of the practice of an ACS surgeon and emphasizes the emergency management of surgical disease by making "emergency" the principal focus. In *Acute Care Surgery: A Guide for General Surgeons* by Gracias, McKenney, Reilly, and Velmahos, the editors embrace these concepts and deliver chapter after chapter on the diagnosis, resuscitation, and management of a very broad base of surgical emergencies. *This is unique!* The three sections: Emergency Surgery, Critical Care, and Trauma provide not only an overview of the breadth of ACS but also succinct and organized chapters that are easy to read and filled with useful tables and "pearls."

The authors, in general, are all well-known surgeons who are senior clinicians and bring their years of experience at the bedside, in the operating room, and in the intensive care unit to their writing. In addition, the editors have selected some of the country's leading gastrointestinal, thoracic, and vascular surgeons to be "partner authors" on key chapters. Even more provocative for a surgical text is the initial section, "The Interface with Emergency Medicine" by Goyal and Gaieski, which provides insight into the practice, needs and concerns of the emergency physician and department of emergency care and how important prompt and expert surgical consultation is for them and their emergency patients.

Finally, this "first of its kind" textbook on acute care surgery is exactly what the title says it is: a guide for any general surgeon who has a practice based on critical patients and requires a quick and reliable reference for decision making and emergency treatment. It will serve all who have adopted the emergency surgical patient as our own and now seek to train the following generations of emergency surgeons.

C. William Schwab, MD
Professor of Surgery
Chief, Division of Traumatology and
Surgical Critical Care
University of Pennsylvania School of Medicine
Philadelphia, Pennsylvania

PREFACE

The discipline of acute care surgery is both an approach to the future of trauma surgery and a return to the fundamental principles that created the wide-ranging world of specialized surgery we now see around us. The overall reaction among those who practice general surgery today is wonderment regarding what all the fuss is about. A more pragmatic view, shared by many current trauma and surgical critical care practitioners, is how best to establish a surgical practice serving those whose lives are immediately threatened by surgical disease. This imperative requires the delivery of rapid resuscitation and urgent surgical intervention.

Acute Care Surgery: A Guide for General Surgeons was conceived as a means of doing exactly that: guiding surgeons and trainees through the myriad categories of knowledge and possible responses to acute surgical problems. The editors hope that this book can distill the complexity of acute surgical options into a manageable tool for clinicians to employ during the treatment of the most common challenges they face. This work was conceived as a rapid reference for the "heat of battle," to better arm clinicians during the early and most crucial phases of surgical resuscitation and decision making. When possible and when supported by literature, algorithms and an evidence-based approach are used to enhance the reader's ability to make sound surgical decisions and improve judgment. It is not intended to be an all-inclusive reference but, that being said, contains an enormous amount of practical information which should prove useful to all who struggle with these patients, from the emergency department and trauma bay, through the OR, and into the ICU. The book is organized into the three main foci of acute care surgery: emergency surgery, surgical critical care, and trauma surgery.

The authors were selected based on their experience in practicing various aspects of acute care surgery and, more importantly, because of their participation in national training programs and their dedication to preparing the future representatives of our specialty. We hope all who read and use this book become enamored by this brave new world we have rediscovered.

VHG
MGM
PMR
GCV

Part I

EMERGENCY SURGERY

Chapter 1

THE INTERFACE WITH EMERGENCY MEDICINE

Munish Goyal, MD, FACEP, and David F. Gaieski, MD, FACEP

INTRODUCTION

Acute care surgeons frequently interact with emergency physicians (EPs) by the nature of their practice. Both professions involve around-the-clock care of patients who require time-sensitive interventions. Patients with surgical emergencies are often referred or go directly to a proximal emergency department (ED). EDs represent the common portal of entry to the U.S. health care system. More than half of the admissions to U.S. community hospitals for conditions other than pregnancy, childbirth, and neonatal care originate in EDs.[1] In 2004, there were an estimated 110 million ED visits. Many of these patients were critically ill, with over 1 million visits requiring immediate attention and approximately 12% resulting in hospital admission. Abdominal pain was the leading patient complaint and illness-related diagnosis.[2] Socioeconomic diversity exists in most EDs; however, patients without insurance are more likely to use the ED as their usual source of health care compared with insured patients.[3] EDs are often the only access to health care for the 44 million uninsured Americans.

Unlike surgery or internal medicine, emergency medicine (EM) is a young specialty, with the first board exam administered in 1980. Although only 63.5% of EPs are board-certified, board certification in EM requires training in the initial evaluation, management, and disposition of surgical emergencies, including early surgical consultation in patients who may require operative intervention.[4] Very little information about the interaction between EM and Surgery exists in the medical literature.[5] Like EM, Acute Care Surgery (ACS) is a fusion of practices still in its infancy. As EM and ACS continue to grow, a mutual understanding of the scope of practice, objectives, strengths, and limitations of each specialty will define realistic expectations and enhance patient care. In this chapter, we will discuss the history of EM, its role in the modern health care system, current barriers to care in the ED, the relationship between EM and ACS, and some of the dynamic issues of this relationship, including pain management, consultation, trauma care, and preoperative hemodynamic optimization.

EPIDEMIOLOGY

Over the last four decades, the hospital ED has transformed into an effective setting for urgent and lifesaving care. An extraordinary range of capabilities converge in the ED: highly trained emergency providers, the latest imaging and therapeutic technologies, and highly trained on-call specialists in almost any field—often available 24/7.[6] EPs are expected to triage, evaluate, initiate treatment, resuscitate, stabilize, and attain disposition of undifferentiated patients. The EP must consider and evaluate all life-threatening causes of a patient's complaints, both medical and surgical.[7,8] Patients may present in an undifferentiated early stage of illness, starting to show classic signs of disease, or at an obvious stage of presentation when they are triaged. Depending on the time course of the specific disease, they can remain statically in one of these stages during their ED period or progress from one stage to the other during the course of their evaluation and may appear very different to the consultant at the time of their evaluation than they did to the EP at the time of his or her evaluation. This variability in disease course presentation necessitates the EP's understanding of the natural history, not just the beginning stages, of most illnesses. In addition to evaluating the patients in the ED, EPs must consider the potential pathology in the waiting room. Maintaining flow in the ED minimizes time from triage to initial patient-physician interaction.[9,10] With the recent recognition of illness time-sensitivity, EPs face increased pressure to maintain flow as a prerequisite to life-saving interventions such as early antibiotics, thrombolytics, and early goal-directed therapy.[11-14]

Although EPs care for the acutely ill and injured, one-third of ED visits are deemed semi- or nonurgent.[2]

Emergency departments are a core provider of routine health care, particularly to lower socioeconomic communities. They serve as a "safety net" provider, as defined by the Institute of Medicine (IOM), which serves uninsured or otherwise vulnerable populations.[15] They differ, however, from other safety net providers by offering access to specialty care within the hospital at any hour, prompting ED visits specifically to see specialists, including surgeons. Furthermore, the Emergency Medical Treatment and Labor Act (EMTALA) states that ED patients cannot be turned away, regardless of payer status. As a result, over 17 million patients without insurance were treated in U.S. EDs in 2004, further increasing the burden placed on overwhelmed EDs.[2] The percentage of uninsured patients can approach 75% of the patients triaged in urban EDs in impoverished neighborhoods.[16]

In many smaller institutions, EPs are tasked with responding to various in-hospital (out-of-ED) situations demanding rapid response (ie, cardiac arrest, respiratory arrest, etc). This is especially true during nights, weekends, and holidays, when the only attending physician available to manage unstable patients is the EP working in the ED.[17] In those institutions with single EP coverage, responding to such situations leaves the ED without direct physician coverage. This prevents the flow of ED patients, the emergent management of new, potentially ill ED patients, and continuity of other ancillary tasks (ie, prehospital medical command, etc).

A constant, dynamic balance between completeness of evaluation, treatment, and disposition of the individual patient *and* the potential pathology of patients in the waiting room and the prehospital setting must be maintained. One of the fundamental decisions in this balance is that of, "sick versus not sick," a decision that is made on an individual patient at several levels and points-in-time in any ED visit. This decision is at the center of the interface between ACS and EM and influences the interaction between the specialties

BARRIERS TO CARE IN THE EMERGENCY DEPARTMENT

Increasing demands have escalated emergency care to a tipping point. A number of issues including increasing patient visits, decreasing hospital beds, an aging patient population, and increasingly complex medical and technological interventions impede patient flow and can endanger patient welfare. The decline in emergency care capacity and quality is only visible to those outside the system when EDs are forced to go on divert, patients complain about ED care, or various performance measure goals are missed. Recognition of these issues will help the consultant understand the emphasis placed on throughput by the EP.

ED overcrowding has reached epidemic proportions. Numerous reports have questioned the ability of EDs to handle the current demand for emergency services.[15] From 1994 through 2004, the number of ED visits increased by 18%. This represents an average increase of more than 1.5 million visits per year. The number of hospital EDs in the United States decreased by about 12.4% during the same period.[2] Emergency departments are visited by a disproportionate percentage of older adults. Over the last 11 years, visit rates of patients $\geq$ 65 years of age have increased by 8%.[2] Public awareness of EM as a medical specialty, consumer expectations of rapid and comprehensive emergency care, difficulty accessing primary care, lack of medical insurance, the evolution of our 24/7 culture and workplace, and other factors are contributing to this increase in utilization. Emergency departments are viewed by some consumers as "one-stop shopping" that bypasses many of the inconveniences of modern medical care. As our population ages and the treatment of previously terminal conditions expand, EDs can only expect to get busier.

On June 14, 2006, the IOM released its report on the state of emergency medical care in the United States titled, *Hospital-Based Emergency Care: At the Breaking Point*. The report describes the extreme overcrowding in EDs, the frequency of ambulance diversions, and the impact these factors have on the ability to deliver quality care, especially in truly emergent situations. The report went as far as to describe the situation as an epidemic of overcrowding in EDs and trauma centers, and asserts that overcrowding is at the root of the majority of problems facing the delivery of emergency care in the United States.[6] This epidemic impacts on the quality of care that patients receive and the interactions between various disciplines attempting to manage critically ill patients under stressful, overburdened, and resource-depleted conditions. Several recent studies support this assertion. For example, Hollander et al found that activation of the trauma system at a large, academic Level I Trauma Center negatively impacted time to important benchmarks of care in patients with acute chest pain and potential acute coronary syndrome. They also found statistically significant negative impact on 30-day outcomes of recurrent angina, readmission, and myocardial infarction.[18] When resources are stretched too thin, providing one form of critical care (trauma management) has implications about the ability to simultaneously or sequentially perform other critical care (acute coronary syndrome management). These concerns are particularly relevant to the delivery of emergency surgical care as the vast majority of diseases and conditions requiring emergent surgical intervention are time-sensitive. Outcomes in penetrating trauma, ruptured abdominal aortic aneurysm (AAA), perforated viscous, and appendicitis are, in all likelihood, improved by decreased time to definitive surgical interventions. The IOM specifically noted that overcrowding can produce unnecessary delays, which can contribute to suboptimal outcomes; that patients are dissatisfied if they have to wait for an extended period to receive care; that malpractice claims escalate in an overcrowded environment; and that workforce stress is accentuated within disciplines and between disciplines when overcrowding becomes the norm. All of these issues have direct implications for the interface between EPs and acute care surgeons and must be considered when trying to make the consultation process function in a way most beneficial to the patient. Requesting a computed tomography (CT) scan in the ED for a nonemergent indication may seem like "just one imaging study," but every impediment to patient throughput is a potential bottleneck to that patient's and subsequent patients' dispositions.

SURGICAL CONSULTATION—EMERGENCY MEDICINE PERSPECTIVE

A number of issues, including crowding, impede patient flow and endanger patient welfare. Working with the EPs to accelerate patient flow through the ED with prearrival notification of referred patients, prompt consultation, and minimization of nonemergent tests are important steps to removing obstacles to patient flow.

PRENOTIFICATION

Prenotification serves many purposes and can help expedite ED care. For example, a properly designed trauma system allows ED and trauma care providers to assign space, prepare airway and resuscitation equipment, summon ancillary staff (ie, respiratory therapist, x-ray technician, etc), and secure an operating room before the patient's arrival. Prenotification of referrals from clinics and of patients coming to the ED from home also serves several purposes. In addition to the aforementioned resource allocation and preparation of necessary equipment, prenotification by the primary surgeon assists with appropriate patient triage. Communicating concern of hemodynamic instability or other need for rapid evaluation will minimize patient time at triage or in the waiting room. It also allows for prenotification of the in-house surgeon, if necessary. By contrast, communication of a specific concern allows evaluation of a discrete medical problem rather than an undifferentiated patient, which usually requires more resources. Furthermore, the best source of recent medical information is the patient's primary physician. Receiving this information minimizes the amount of duplicated efforts, shifting time wasted on rediagnosis to the management of the acute problem. Prenotification of a surgical patient being sent to the ED for urgent admission helps to define the triage priorities, necessary laboratory and imaging studies, and required in-patient level-of-care. It must be noted that although ED referral of potentially unstable patients for probable admission should be encouraged, stable patients with no acute problems should not be sent to the ED to arrange routine admission if a direct admission can be arranged through the hospital's admissions center. Using the ED as the portal of entry for routine admissions leads to delays in care for undifferentiated patients and can impact negatively on the care delivered to patients with time-sensitive, critical illness.

CONSULTATION

Consultation—derived from the Latin *consulere*, "to deliberate, consider,"—represents one of the unique dynamics in medicine. In a consultation, a physician with one body of expertise requests the input of a physician with a different body of expertise to solve a problem. This request occurs within the social norms of the house of medicine—in one sense, a request for consultation can be defined as a polite cry for help. This interaction can occur in a professional, collegial fashion or be tainted by condescension about the lack of knowledge of the person or the specialty requesting the consultation. There is very little published on the rules of consultation and even less on the art and science of surgical consultation in the ED. Medical consultation before surgery—"preoperative medical clearance"—is one of the most thoroughly researched aspects of medical consultation. Goldman has developed and validated predictive rules—taking into consideration known coronary artery disease, cardiac functional status, cardiac risk factors—that help classify patients with regard to their preoperative cardiovascular risk and make recommendations for further preoperative evaluation.[19] These criteria are widely used by medical consultation services. However, despite studies demonstrating the validity of the Goldman criteria, other studies have demonstrated disagreement about the usefulness of preoperative medical clearance and their perceived utility by anesthesiologists and surgeons. In one study, although 80.2% of surgeons "felt obligated" to follow the medical consultant's recommendations, only 16.6% of the anesthesiologists felt obliged.[20] No such body of literature exists examining surgical consultations to the ED.

Surgical consultation should occur when a high likelihood of a surgical emergency exists; it should, in general, not occur when a patient with a benign physical exam, unremarkable laboratory values and a normal CT scan has ongoing, unexplained abdominal pain. Early SBO and missed appendicitis are common serious etiologies misdiagnosed as nonspecific abdominal pain on initial ED presentation. Abdominal pain represents approximately 10% of closed malpractice claims filed against EPs, which may prompt liberal surgical consultation.[21] Consultation to spread out the medicolegal responsibility of unclear or difficult cases is inappropriate. However, just as a certain percentage of appendices removed during emergent appendectomy will reveal normal tissue on pathologic sectioning, a certain percentage of surgical consultations to the ED will end with no findings of acute pathology and a high likelihood of the patient's being discharged to home. This is not necessarily a reflection of inappropriate consultation; rather, it is inherent in one of the key tasks of EM: triage. Triage—derived from Latin, meaning "to sort"—involves the separating of patients into categories based on the severity and acuity of their chief complaint. The decision about whether a patient is "sick" or "not sick" is based on a brief encounter between triage nurse or physician and the patient and is a semiscientific sorting that is a summation of the complaint, its possible complications, the appearance of the patient, their basic vital signs, and a truncated physical examination.[22]

After initial triage, patients are repeatedly recategorized throughout their ED stay in relation to their clinical condition. Surgical consultation should occur when a certain threshold is crossed, denoting sufficient suspicion of the presence of a pathologic process requiring surgical intervention or in-patient surgical management. Activating a trauma team after prehospital notification is an example of early mobilization of surgical resources—the trauma team is assembled before the patient's arrival—based on the probability of the patient requiring surgical intervention or in-patient trauma team management. This probability is determined by the prehospital health care providers based on recognized trauma criteria—findings associated with a high likelihood of morbidity and mortality. These factors include vital sign abnormalities such as systolic blood pressure < 90 mm Hg; mental status assessments including Glasgow Coma Scale < 13; and mechanisms of injury associated with a high likelihood of morbidity and mortality including the amount of intrusion into the vehicle, being thrown from a vehicle, or being in a vehicle involved in a collision in which another occupant was killed.[23] This process is labor-intensive, time-dependent, and overly sensitive, but it is an effective means of reducing morbidity and mortality by having potentially critically injured patients evaluated systematically during the most proximal period of their illness, the "Golden Hour" of trauma care.[24]

Inevitably, there are numerous false positive activations of the trauma system—patients who are not severely injured and could have been successfully managed by the regular ED staff. To have sufficient sensitivity for capturing critically ill patients, some specificity is sacrificed. The same principle applies to surgical consultation. The appropriateness of a surgical consultation is not dependent on the presence of pathology at the end of the evaluation; it is dependent on a reasonable possibility of the presence of surgical pathology at the time when the consultation is requested. Effective consultation involves the ED staff

weeding out unnecessary consultations through the algorithmic evaluation of patients based on history, physical examination, vital signs, laboratory studies, and imaging techniques combined with the timely input and thoughtful recommendations of the surgical consultant. A well-functioning ED will efficiently filter out the vast majority of nonsurgical cases; a well-functioning surgical consultation system will efficiently assess the remainder, sorting them into obviously surgical, undifferentiated, and obviously nonsurgical cases and providing organized recommendations for the resolution of the undifferentiated cases. Additional logistical issues arise when the private patient of an attending surgeon is referred to the ED for evaluation; these patients may receive surgical consultation even though the EP has a low suspicion of acute surgical pathology requiring operative intervention or in-patient surgical management.

Furthermore, the logistics of obtaining a consultation vary from institution to institution. The process may be very different at a small community hospital versus a regional referral center with some residency programs versus a large tertiary care academic center with a surgical residency and multiple surgical subspecialty fellowship programs. At community hospitals, request for consultation is often made from the ED attending to the surgical attending, who may develop a friendship over time and acquire a mutual understanding of each other's practice style. At a regional referral center, a resident in the ED may call the on-call surgeon's nurse practitioner or physician's assistant to obtain a surgical consultation. At a large academic medical center, a surgical resident may be assigned to ED consultations; consultations will systematically proceed from this resident through a hierarchy extending to the senior resident, the chief resident, and the attending surgeon. Each of these paradigms has advantages and disadvantages in relation to the expertise of the consultant and the efficiency of the process. In turn, these variables will influence the nature of the consultation. The consultation may be as brief as a phone call between colleagues, "I've got a 45-year-old woman with cholecystitis who needs admission." "Is she stable?" "Yes, blood pressure and heart rate are good, she's been given antibiotics, fluids, and pain medication. Her ultrasound shows a dilated common bile duct and pericholecystic fluid." "All right, keep her NPO, put her on my service, I'll see her when I get to the hospital in a few hours. Can you put the nurse on so I can give some holding orders?" In a different setting, the consultation may evolve over several hours, as the patient is seen by the surgeon on duty (SOD), presented to the senior resident, who discusses the case with the attending physician. Regardless of institutional process, mutual respect is the essence of any functional relationship and must form the foundation of the interaction between professionals. Jokes about "all they know how to do is triage," or "would you like the next suture cut too short or too long," undermine the development of a working relationship.

The EP requesting a surgical consultation should know the patient and should be able to describe the patient's presenting complaint, history, pertinent examination findings, laboratory results, and radiographic results succinctly, and clearly state the reason for the consultation: the question the surgical consultant is being asked to answer. A majority of the time, these questions revolve around the central concern: "Does this patient require emergent surgical intervention?" In return for an organized, reasonable, and thoughtful request for a surgical consultation, the EP should expect the consultant to act professionally, respond in a timely fashion—both to pages and to the request to see the patient in the ED, evaluate the patient thoroughly, clearly communicate his or her thoughts about the patient's condition, diagnosis, and recommendations for further evaluation and treatment. Because patients present at various stages of illness and may progress during their stay in the ED, they may appear very different to the consultant at the time of their evaluation than they did to the EP at the time of his or her initial evaluation. The disease in question may be much more obvious at the time of the consultant's evaluation than it was at the time of the request for consultation. Frequent reevaluation by the EP can minimize these "surprises," but the realities of progression of disease combined with constraints on optimal care in a crowded ED may negate this possibility.

Protocolized consultation has the potential to improve care by standardizing interventions and hastening the process of transition from prehospital to ED triage, initial ED evaluation, hemodynamic stabilization, and definitive operative management. For example, some EDs have protocols for the management of ruptured AAA, which attempt to streamline care from the prehospital setting to operative intervention. These protocols include standardized orders for large bore IVs, controlled volume resuscitation, typing, cross-matching, and transfusion of blood, STAT vascular surgery consultation, along with emergent ultrasound or CT as appropriate, with all steps facilitating the identification of ruptured AAAs amenable to operative intervention and shorting time to operation room (OR). So-called aorta codes have been implemented at some institutions and the rationale behind their implementation appears irrefutable; however, no data are available at this time to suggest a mortality benefit. Creation of such institutional protocols between EM and ACS require cooperation and mutual respect, and have the potential of improving patient care.

COMMUNICATION

According to estimates from the IOM, 44,000 to 98,000 patients die in U.S. hospitals annually because of medical errors.[25] The nature of these errors ranges from gross incompetence to medication errors to poor communication. Breakdowns in communication often result in errors, many of which are preventable. An Australian study involving 28 hospitals reviewed the causes of adverse events and found that communication errors were the leading underlying cause, associated with twice as many deaths as was clinical inadequacy.[26] Poor communication has been implicated as a major causal element for incorrect identification of recipients of invasive procedures.[27] By nature, communication between EPs and acute care surgeons involves critically ill patients potentially requiring emergent surgical intervention. The urgency involved with caring for these patients often leads to brief transfers of information between stressed providers. For example, a disorganized request for a consultation may make addressing the central problem more difficult; similarly, impatient interruptions of a well-organized request for consultation may lead to delays in appropriate care because of lack of awareness of essential data. Interventions to improve communication and reduce medical errors such as computerized physician order entry systems are not foolproof and can produce a new set of problems and potential errors.[28] In our ED, the implementation of computerized emergency medical records (Emtrac 2000, Hospital of the University of Pennsylvania) produced the unwanted consequence of more frequently misplaced consultation notes. For surgical consultations, this problem was addressed by training the consultants in Emtrac and having them use templated, computerized consultation forms.

IMAGING STUDIES

Imaging studies serve many purposes in the emergent evaluation of possible surgical patients. These can include functioning as an adjunct to a properly performed physical examination, as a delay to consultation, as a confirmatory study in equivocal cases. A balance must exist between too aggressive and too conservative use of imaging studies during the evaluation of acute abdominal pain. Suspected appendicitis can serve as an illustrative example. In 1999, approximately 7% (250,000) of the 3.4 million patients with abdominal pain seeking medical attention in U.S. EDs had appendicitis and required emergent appendectomy.[29,30] An aggressive surgical approach favoring early laparotomy can have as high as a 20% false positive rate, with pathology revealing normal appendix on frozen section; this percentage can soar to 40% in women and older adults. A more conservative surgical approach suggests imaging studies should be performed in equivocal cases. Spiral CT scan has a sensitivity of 90 to 100% and a specificity of 91 to 97% for patients with suspected appendicitis.[30] As Karnath and Luh pointed out in a letter to the editors of the *New England Journal of Medicine*, "The recommendation of diagnostic imaging for 'equivocal cases' must bear in mind that the determination of what is equivocal lies in the hands of the examiner."[31]

They supported their argument with data from Ozuah et al's 2001 *Journal of the American Medical Association* article on the declining physical examination skills of U.S. and international medical graduates.[32] Additionally, the use of imaging studies must be tempered by emerging data on increased lifetime cancer risk in patients receiving CT scans. These concerns are especially important in the pediatric population and women of childbearing age.[33] At the interface of EM and ACS lies a responsibility to develop shared protocols that maximize diagnostic accuracy, minimize complications resulting from delays in care, lower mortality, and decrease radiation exposure. The ideal algorithm will weave expert EP evaluation, early analgesia, early surgical consultation, expert physical examination skills, understanding of the predictive value of different laboratory tests, and judicious use of imaging studies with the unique needs of individual institutions to rapidly diagnose the majority of emergent patients.

PAIN CONTROL

The issue of administering or withholding analgesia for acute abdominal pain patients being evaluated in the ED was, for years, a metaphor for the relationship between EPs and surgical consultants: disbelief at the others' perspective. The idea of withholding analgesia until a firm diagnosis is established has been attributed to Sir Zachary Cope, who, more than 75 years ago, in an early addition of his classic text, *Cope's Early Diagnosis of the Acute Abdomen,* asserted that early provision of analgesic medications might obscure the correct diagnosis. This perspective persisted until the 1990s; the 19th edition, edited by William Silan, included the following statement: "The realization that narcotics can obscure the clinical picture has given rise to the unfortunate dictum that these drugs should never be given until a diagnosis has been firmly established. With the numerous layers of triage nurses, medical students, residents, and attending physicians in modern emergency units, and with the addition of time-consuming tests often done before an adequate history and physical examination, the suffering patient is sometimes forced to wait hours before any relief is offered. This cruel practice is to be condemned, but I suspect that it will take many generations to eliminate it because the rule has become so firmly ingrained in the minds of physicians."[34] The text goes on to propose that the best solution is early examination of the patient by a "responsible surgeon." Despite the change in heart about whether analgesia should be withheld, Silen's perspective perpetuates many misconceptions about analgesia administration and the relationship between EPs and surgical consultants. The solution of a responsible surgeon examining the patient early ignores the fact that EPs are also experts in the examination of patients with acute abdominal pain and, one could argue, *the most accessible*

experts in the initial evaluation of the undifferentiated acute abdomen. The most recent National Hospital Ambulatory Medical Care Survey showed that abdominal pain was the most common chief complaint of patients triaged in U.S. EDs, over 7 million annual visits; there is no data on what percentage of these visits has surgical consultation as part of the ED evaluation; what percentage gets admitted; or what percentage requires emergency surgery; however, it is clear that the expert evaluation by EPs safely weeds out the vast majority of patients who do not require surgical intervention.[2]

Multiple studies have demonstrated the safety of early, judicious administration of narcotic analgesics to patients with acute abdominal pain. In 1992, Attard et al published a classic study on the safety of early pain relief for acute abdominal pain. They prospectively randomized 100 patients admitted to a surgical service with acute, undifferentiated abdominal pain to receive either papaveretum (a standardized preparation of mixed opioids) or saline injection and then followed their hospital course examining the outcome measures of pain score, tenderness score, and incorrect diagnosis.[35] Their results demonstrated statistically significant improvements in pain score and tenderness scores with opioid administration; these improvements were coupled with a *decrease* in incorrect diagnoses from nine in the saline group to two in the papaveretum group. Other papers provide similar results.[36,37] More recently, in 2003 in the *Journal of the American College of Surgeons,* Thomas et al published the results of a prospective, randomized, double-blind trial in which 72 patients with undifferentiated abdominal pain were randomized to receive either placebo or morphine sulfate. Their results demonstrated no difference between the two groups in terms of likelihood of change in the severity of tenderness, change in pain location, diagnostic accuracy, clinical course, and masking of final diagnosis. They concluded that their results supported the early, adequate provision of analgesia to patients with acute, undifferentiated abdominal pain.[38] Despite the convincing data from multiple randomized controlled trials, in 1999 Graber et al published the results of a survey of general surgeon's attitudes toward the use of pain medications in patients with acute abdominal pain and found that 67% of responding surgeons felt that administration of pain medication would interfere with diagnostic accuracy and 82% considered the issue of diagnostic accuracy when deciding to withhold pain medication.[39] Furthermore, in 2000, Wolfe et al published the results of a 1997 survey of American College of Emergency Physicians' members examining their practice patterns in regard to analgesic administration in patients with acute abdominal pain. The survey found that although a vast majority (85%) of EPs felt that judicious use of analgesia did not alter important physical examination findings, more than three-fourths (76%) of the same physicians withheld opiate analgesia until the patient was examined by a surgeon.[36]

In a 2004 review article on pain management in *Annals of Emergency Medicine*, Timothy Rupp and Kathleen Delaney analyzed factors in medical culture that influence the provision of adequate analgesia to patients with acute abdominal pain, and summarized this disconnect between study results and practice standards: "Although some emergency physicians may simply dread conflict with surgical consultants, they may also have learned pain management techniques from other disciplines, such as general surgery, in which prejudice toward withholding analgesics remains firmly entrenched."[40] We suspect that day-to-day practice realities have changed significantly over the past decade and that Rupp and Delaney's article is several years behind the actual practice of EPs and surgeons caring for patients with acute abdominal pain. At our institution, EPs and surgeons alike support the policy of early, adequate opiate analgesia for patients with acute, differentiated or undifferentiated, abdominal pain, given either concurrent with or immediately following initial evaluation by the ED staff.

RESUSCITATION

Acutely ill surgical patients in the ED are often in need of hemodynamic resuscitation. These patients frequently present volume depleted, with some degree of cardiovascular dysfunction. Although the data are limited, it is logical to apply lessons learned from cardiac, trauma, and high-risk general surgery to ED patients destined for the OR. Initial work by Shoemaker et al suggested that hemodynamic optimization of high-risk elective surgical patients dramatically improved postoperative morbidity and mortality.[41] Preoperative optimization included intravascular euvolemia measured by pulmonary capillary wedge pressure, normal mean arterial pressure (MAP), cardiac output, and urine output. Subsequent work has validated the concept of preoperative optimization in various subsets of high-risk patients.[42-47] Patients at risk include those with organ dysfunction, shock, multitrauma, old age, and sepsis. A significant percentage of surgical emergencies are caused by infection including necrotizing fasciitis, abscess, appendicitis, diverticulitis, cholecystitis, and many others.[48] These infectious processes produce local inflammation and, with uninterrupted progression, can lead to a systemic inflammatory process. Arguably, the majority of patients that are taken to the OR from the ED can be classified as "high-risk."

Rivers et al adapted Shoemaker's concepts in a single center, prospective, randomized trial of hemodynamic optimization in the ED of patients with either severe sepsis and a lactate level $\geq$ 4 mmol/L or septic shock, defined as ongoing hypotension after adequate fluid challenge.[11] In the most proximate phase of their hospital course, patients were randomized to receive either standard therapy (central venous pressure [CVP] 8-12 mm Hg; MAP > 65 mm Hg; urine output > 0.5 mL/kg/h) or goal-directed resuscitation (in which the hemodynamic abnormalities were addressed in an algorithmic fashion and the goal of central venous oxygen saturation $\geq$ 70% was added). Both groups received central venous access, arterial lines, and urinary catheters. A total of 263 patients were randomized; 133 to standard therapy; 130 to early goal-directed therapy (EGDT). In-house mortality was reduced from 46.5% in the standard therapy group to 30.5% in the EGDT group. Much of this reduction was related to a decrease in sudden cardiovascular collapse in the EGDT group.

Although "a requirement for immediate surgery" was an exclusion criterion for enrollment in the study, the necessity of emergent surgical intervention was not obvious at the time of enrollment in some patients. Rather, reflecting the dynamic process of infection, 7 patients did not complete the 6-hour study period because it became apparent that they required emergent surgical intervention. An additional 4 patients were deemed to require immediate surgery during the 6-hour enrollment period, but a decision to discontinue "aggressive surgical treatment" was made and no further hemodynamic optimization occurred. In all, 21 patients (16.1%) were classified primarily as having a "surgical condition." Because the inflammatory, anti-inflammatory, and hemodynamic perturbations of medical (pneumonia, urosepsis, meningitis, cellulitis) and surgical sepsis are similar, if not the same, it follows that the hemodynamic optimization principles forming the foundation of EGDT should apply equally in this population.

A number of delays impair patient transit once the surgical consultant decides that a patient in the ED needs to go to the operating room.[49] Although institutions must work to minimize these delays, this also represents an opportunity for preoperative optimization. Ideally, an algorithm should be created between services, considering available resources, which targets specific preoperative goals, including obtaining adequate venous access, initiating volume resuscitation, administering appropriate antibiotics, sending preoperative labs, and achieving hemodynamic goals. Which goal (ie, central venous oxygen saturation, urine output, cardiac index, etc) is not as important as predefining the division of labor that fits best with the individual institution. This may range from preoperative admission to the intensive care unit to EP directed resuscitation in the ED. Preoperative resuscitation efforts must be balanced with minimizing time to source control and appropriate utilization of finite resources.[50,51]

TRAUMA CARE

Trauma care is as old as medicine itself, dating back to the ancient Egyptians.[52] Lessons learned on the battlefields, such as the appreciation of brevity between the infliction of wounds and adequate shock treatment, have been translated to civilian care. The organized approach to caring for trauma patients was introduced into the civilian setting by R. Adams Cowley in Baltimore, MD, while EM was in its infancy in the early 1970s.[53] Dr. Cowley introduced the concept of the "golden hour" and stressed the importance of early interventions.

With the growth of EM as a discipline, EPs have become the initial care providers of most patients that are critically injured, particularly in community hospitals. The "golden hour" of most patients is spent under the supervision of an EP. Many trauma centers have developed a multidisciplinary approach to optimize patient care that incorporates EPs and acute care surgeons. Although it is difficult to study the impact of EPs on trauma care, Taylor et al demonstrated improved survival, decreased complication rate, and decreased hospital length of stay in Level I trauma centers with EM residency programs versus those without EM residency programs.[54] Specific provider roles and responsibilities are variable and often are based on local culture and institution history. The American College of Surgeons recognizes the importance of EPs in trauma care and has included the presence and participation of EPs as an essential component of the trauma teams of all Level 1, 2, and 3 trauma centers.[55] As trauma care continues to shift toward nonoperative management, EPs may play an expanded role in the future.[55-57] Regardless of the division of labor, EPs and acute care surgeons must understand the principles of trauma management and continue to work together.

In addition to the general roles of the trauma team, EPs increasingly are becoming responsible for airway management. Residency training in EM includes extensive experience with intubation, use of neuromuscular blocking agents, and management of the difficult airway. Although still debated in some hospitals with readily available anesthesiology personnel, a number of studies demonstrate no significant differences in overall success and immediate complication rates between EM and anesthesiology providers.[58-61] Furthermore, EPs are immediately available to attend to patients who arrive with no or short notification. As such, the American College of Surgeons Task Force for Level I trauma centers recommends that airway control fall under the auspices of Surgery, Anesthesiology, or EM[59]. At our institution, over a 3-year period, Levitan et al demonstrated no significant differences in intubation success or cricothyrotomy rate in 648 trauma airways managed on an every-other-day basis by EM versus Anesthesiology residents.[60] These results led to EM assuming primary responsibility of trauma airway management.

SUMMARY

Like Acute Care Surgery, Emergency Medicine is a fusion of practices still in its infancy, with many of its roots in general surgery. Providing around-the-clock care to patients who require time-sensitive interventions is the common thread that brings these two specialties together. Many institutions already enjoy fruitful relationships between EM and Trauma Surgery. Expanding the role of the trauma surgeon to include ACS takes advantage of the in-house coverage provided by the trauma service, and emphasizes the importance of the relationship between EM and ACS. As the leading portal of entry to the U.S. health care system, EDs represent a frequent source of ACS patients.

Protocols that weave expert EP evaluation, early surgical consultation, goal-directed resuscitation, understanding of the predictive value of different laboratory tests, and judicious use of imaging studies with the unique needs of individual institutions can improve the care of the sickest surgical patients and optimize the use of inherent delays in modern medical practice.

Realizing the dangers of overcrowding, the significance of maintaining patient flow, the importance of prenotification, and need for effective communication will help the ACS consultant appreciate the EPs perspective. As EM and ACS continue to grow, a mutual understanding of the scope of practice, objectives, strengths, and limitations of each specialty will define realistic expectations and enhance patient care.

REFERENCES

1. Owens P EA. *Hospital Admissions That Began in the Emergency Department, 2003. Statistical Brief #1.* Rockville, MD: Agency for Healthcare Research and Quality, http://wwwhcup-usahrqgov/reports/statbriefs/sb1pdf 2006.

2. McCaig LF, Nawar EW. National Hospital Ambulatory Medical Care Survey: 2004 emergency department summary. *Adv Data* 2006;372:1-30.

3. Walls CA, Rhodes KV, Kennedy JJ. The emergency department as usual source of medical care: estimates from the 1998 National Health Interview Survey. *Acad Emerg Med* 2002;9(11):1140-1145.

4. Hockberger RS, Binder LS, Graber MA, et al. The model of the clinical practice of emergency medicine. *Ann Emerg Med* 2001;37(6):745-770.

5. Rhodes RS, Levine BA, Miller TA, et al. The impact of emergency medicine on surgical care in the emergency ward. *J Surg Res* 1982;33(6):457-462.

6. IOM. *Hospital-Based Emergency Care: At the Breaking Point.* Washington, DC: The National Academies Press; 2006.

7. Zink BJ. *Anyone, Anything, Anytime: A History of Emergency Medicine.* 1st ed. Philadelphia, PA: Elsevier Mosby; 2006.

8. Hockberger RS, Binder LS, Chisholm CD, et al. The model of the clinical practice of emergency medicine: a 2-year update. *Ann Emerg Med* 2005;45(6):659-674.

9. Moorhead JC, Gallery ME, Hirshkorn C, et al. A study of the workforce in emergency medicine: 1999. *Ann Emerg Med* 2002;40(1):3-15.

10. Branney SW, Pons PT, Markovchick VJ, Thomasson GO. Malpractice occurrence in emergency medicine: does residency training make a difference? *J Emerg Med* 2000;19(2):99-105.

11. Rivers E, Nguyen B, Havstad S, et al. Early goal-directed therapy in the treatment of severe sepsis and septic shock. *New England Journal of Medicine* 2001;345(19): 1368-1377.

12. Kumar A, Roberts D, Wood KE, et al. Duration of hypotension before initiation of effective antimicrobial therapy is the critical determinant of survival in human septic shock. *Crit Care Med* 2006;34(6): 1589-1596.

13. Houck PM, Bratzler DW, Nsa W, Ma A, Bartlett JG. Timing of antibiotic administration and outcomes for Medicare patients hospitalized with community-acquired pneumonia. *Arch Intern Med* 2004;164(6): 637-644.

14. Menon V, Harrington RA, Hochman JS, et al. Thrombolysis and adjunctive therapy in acute myocardial infarction: the Seventh ACCP Conference on Antithrombotic and Thrombolytic Therapy. *Chest* 2004;126(suppl 3):549S-575S.

15. Trzeciak S, Rivers EP. Emergency department overcrowding in the United States: an emerging threat to patient safety and public health. *Emerg Med J* 2003;20(5):402-405.

16. Bindman AB, Grumbach K, Keane D, Rauch L, Luce JM. Consequences of queuing for care at a public hospital emergency department. *JAMA* 1991;266(8):1091-1096.

17. Skrifvars MB, Castren M, Kurola J, Rosenberg PH. In-hospital cardiopulmonary resuscitation: organization, management and training in hospitals of different levels of care. *Acta Anaesthesiol Scand* 2002;46(4):458-463.

18. Fishman P. *Ann Emerg Med* 2006.

19. Mangano DT, Goldman L. Preoperative assessment of patients with known or suspected coronary disease. *N Engl J Med* 1995;333(26):1750-1756.

20. Katz RI, Barnhart JM, Ho G, Hersch D, Dayan SS, Keehn L. A survey on the intended purposes and perceived utility of preoperative cardiology consultations. *Anesth Analg* 1998;87(4):830-836.

21. Karcz A, Korn R, Burke MC, et al. Malpractice claims against emergency physicians in Massachusetts: 1975-1993. *Am J Emerg Med* 1996;14(4):341-345.

22. Kennedy K, Aghababian RV, Gans L, Lewis CP. Triage: techniques and applications in decision making. *Ann Emerg Med* 1996;28(2):136-144.

23. Surgeons Committee on Trauma–American College of Surgeons, *Resources for Optimal Care of the Injured Patient*, American College of Surgeons, Chicago, IL (1998).

24. MacKenzie EJ, Rivara FP, Jurkovich GJ, et al. A national evaluation of the effect of trauma-center care on mortality. *New Engl J Med* 2006;354(4):366-378.

25. Kohn LT CJ, Donaldson MS, McKenzie D. *To Err Is Human: Building a Safer Healthcare System, in Committee on Quality and Healthcare in America*. Institute of Medicine Washington, DC: National Academy Press; 2000.

26. Wilson RM, Runciman WB, Gibberd RW, Harrison BT, Newby L, Hamilton JD. The quality in Australian health care study. *Med J Aust* 1995;163(9):458-471.

27. Chassin MR, Becher EC. The wrong patient. *Ann Intern Med* 2002;136(11):826-833.

28. Koppel R, Metlay JP, Cohen A, et al. Role of computerized physician order entry systems in facilitating medication errors. *JAMA* 2005;293(10):1197-1203.

29. Owings MF, Kozak LJ. Ambulatory and inpatient procedures in the United States, 1996. *Vital Health Stat* [13] 1998(139):1-119.

30. Paulson EK, Kalady MF, Pappas TN. Clinical practice. Suspected appendicitis. *N Engl J Med* 2003;348(3): 236-242.

31. Karnath BM, Luh JY. Suspected appendicitis. [comment]. *N Engl J Med* 2003;349(3):305-306; author reply 306.

32. Ozuah PO, Curtis J, Dinkevich E. Physical examination skills of US and international medical graduates. *JAMA* 2001;286(9):1021.

33. Nickoloff EL, Alderson PO. Radiation exposures to patients from CT: reality, public perception, and policy. [comment]. *AJR Am J Roentgenol* 2001;177(2):285-287.

34. Cope Z. *Cope's Early Diagnosis of the Acute Abdomen.* 19th ed. New York: Oxford University Press; 1996.

35. Attard AR, Corlett MJ, Kidner NJ, Leslie AP, Fraser IA. Safety of early pain relief for acute abdominal pain. *BMJ* 1992;305(6853):554-556.

36. Wolfe JM, Lein DY, Lenkoski K, Smithline HA. Analgesic administration to patients with an acute abdomen: a survey of emergency medicine physicians. *Am J Emerg Med* 2000;18(3):250-253.

37. Pace S, Burke TF. Intravenous morphine for early pain relief in patients with acute abdominal pain. *Acad Emerg Med* 1996;3(12):1086-1092.

38. Thomas SH, Silen W, Cheema F, et al. Effects of morphine analgesia on diagnostic accuracy in Emergency Department patients with abdominal pain: a prospective, randomized trial. *J Am Coll Surg* 2003;196(1):18-31.

39. Graber MA, Ely JW, Clarke S, Kurtz S, Weir R. Informed consent and general surgeons' attitudes toward the use of pain medication in the acute abdomen. *Am J Emerg Med* 1999;17(2):113-116.

40. Rupp T, Delaney KA. Inadequate analgesia in emergency medicine. *Ann Emerg Med* 2004;43(4):494-503.

41. Shoemaker WC, Appel PL, Kram HB, Waxman K, Lee TS. Prospective trial of supranormal values of survivors as therapeutic goals in high-risk surgical patients. *Chest* 1988;94(6):1176-1186.

42. Boyd O, Grounds RM, Bennett ED. A randomized clinical trial of the effect of deliberate perioperative increase of oxygen delivery on mortality in high-risk surgical patients. *JAMA* 1993;270(22):2699-2707.

43. Berlauk JF, Abrams JH, Gilmour IJ, O'Connor SR, Knighton DR, Cerra FB. Preoperative optimization of cardiovascular hemodynamics improves outcome in peripheral vascular surgery: a prospective, randomized clinical trial. *Ann Surg* 1991;214(3):289-297; discussion 298-299.

44. Boyd O, Bennett ED. Enhancement of perioperative tissue perfusion as a therapeutic strategy for major surgery. *New Horiz* 1996;4(4):453-465.

45. Scalea TM, Simon HM, Duncan AO, et al. Geriatric blunt multiple trauma: improved survival with early invasive monitoring. *J Trauma* 1990;30(2):129-134; discussion 134-136.

46. Tote SP, Grounds RM. Performing perioperative optimization of the high-risk surgical patient. *Br J Anaesth* 2006;97(1):4-11.

47. Wilson J, Woods I, Fawcett J, et al. Reducing the risk of major elective surgery: randomised controlled trial of preoperative optimisation of oxygen delivery. *BMJ* 1999;318(7191):1099-1103.

48. Ciesla DJ, Moore EE, Moore JB, Johnson JL, Cothren CC, Burch JM. The academic trauma center is a model for the future trauma and acute care surgeon. *J Trauma* 2005;58(4):657-661; discussion 661-662.

49. Wyatt MG, Houghton PW, Brodribb AJ. Theatre delay for emergency general surgical patients: a cause for concern?. *Ann R Coll Surg Engl* 1990;72(4):236-238.

50. Marshall JC, Maier RV, Jimenez M, Dellinger EP. Source control in the management of severe sepsis and septic shock: an evidence-based review. *Crit Care Med* 2004;32(suppl 11):S513-S526.

51. Jimenez MF, Marshall JC, International Sepsis F. Source control in the management of sepsis. *Intensive Care Med* 2001;27(suppl 1):S49-S62.

52. Breasted JH (editor). The Edwin Smith Surgical Papyrus: Hieroglyphic Transliteration, Translation and Commentary. V1. Kessinger Publishing, LLC. 2006.

53. Edlich RF, Wish JR, Britt LD, Long WB. An organized approach to trauma care: legacy of R Adams Cowley. *J Long Term Eff Med Implants* 2004;14(6):481-511.

54. Taylor SF, Gerhardt RT, Simpson MP. An association between Emergency Medicine residencies and improved trauma patient outcome. *J Emerg Med* 2005;29(2):123-127.

55. Bozeman WP, Gaasch WR, Barish RA, Scalea TM. Trauma resuscitation/critical care fellowship for emergency physicians: a necessary step for the future of academic emergency medicine. *Acad Emerg Med* 1999;6(4):331-333.

56. Santucci RA, Fisher MB. The literature increasingly supports expectant (conservative) management of renal trauma—a systematic review. *J Trauma* 2005;59(2):493-503.

57. Britt LD, Cole FJ. "Alternative" surgery in trauma management. *Arch Surg* 1998;133(11):1177-1181.

58. Omert L, Yeaney W, Mizikowski S, Protetch J. Role of the emergency medicine physician in airway management of the trauma patient. *J Trauma* 2001;51(6):1065-1068.

59. Levitan RM, Rosenblatt B, Meiner EM, Reilly PM, Hollander JE. Alternating day emergency medicine and anesthesia resident responsibility for management of the trauma airway: a study of laryngoscopy performance and intubation success. *Ann Emerg Med* 2004;43(1):48-53.

60. Bushra JS, McNeil B, Wald DA, Schwell A, Karras DJ. A comparison of trauma intubations managed by anesthesiologists and emergency physicians. *Acad Emerg Med* 2004;11(1):66-70.

61. Chang RS, Hamilton RJ, Carter WA. Declining rate of cricothyrotomy in trauma patients with an emergency medicine residency: implications for skills training. *Acad Emerg Med* 1998;5(3):247-251.

Chapter 2

PATIENT SAFETY

Michael D. Crittenden, MD, and Shukri F. Khuri, MD

INTRODUCTION

Patient safety is of universal concern that is equally applicable to all facets of surgery. This chapter addresses patient safety as part and parcel of the overall quality of surgical care, sharing with it the same metric and the same determinants. It emphasizes the importance of coordination and communication within systems of care in determining patient safety and the overall quality of surgical care, and underscores the need for increased diligence in assuring the quality of processes and systems of care under emergent conditions.

PATIENT SAFETY AND QUALITY IN SURGICAL CARE

Two happenings over the past decade have shaped our contemporary thoughts with regard to patient safety in surgery. The first was the publication in 1999 of the Institute of Medicine (IOM) report *To Err is Human*,[1] which was considered by some as the most influential health care publication in two decades.[2] The second was the development of the Veterans Administration (VA) National Surgical Improvement Program (NSQIP)[3] and its migration in 1994 to the private sector, through the efforts of the American College of Surgeons (ACS-NSQIP) (http://www.acsnsqip.org).

THE IOM REPORT, TO ERR IS HUMAN

The IOM report focused the attention on preventable provider errors and cast patient safety in terms of safety from iatrogenic injury.[1] It estimated that as many as 98,000 people die in any given year from medical errors that occur in hospitals. For surgeons, such errors would include surgery on the wrong site or side, retained foreign materials, transfusion mismatch, medication errors, mishaps in the operating room, and accidents in care, in and outside the operating room. The IOM report emphasized that errors also occurred, much more frequently than previously anticipated, in health care environments outside the hospital, such as doctors'

offices, day surgical centers, and outpatient care facilities. Understandably, this publication created a major national concern about patient safety, and prompted a wide variety of constituencies in health care to engage in efforts to improve patient safety. Laudable efforts have been expended by anesthesia and surgery to achieve this goal.[4] The anesthesia community was ahead of its times in establishing in 1985 the Anesthesia Patient Safety Foundation,[5,6] the activities of which were markedly accelerated by the IOM report.[4] Following the publication of the IOM report, the Department of Veterans Affairs established the National Center for Patient Safety, which has developed new safety guidelines that have been implemented in all Veterans Health Administration operating rooms.[7] The Joint Commission has developed and published on its website new guidelines for the enhancement of patient safety.[8] The American College of Surgeons designated safety and quality as its primary objectives[9] and published a useful manual covering all aspects of patient safety in surgery.[10] Various surgical specialty societies, such as the American College of Obstetricians and Gynecologists, set up new patient quality and safety committees (http://www.acog.org). The Agency for Health Research and Quality and other granting agencies dedicated special funds for the investigation and enhancement of patient safety, resulting in a proliferation of studies and publications on patient safety. A National Patient Safety Foundation was formed, to be an "indispensable resource for individuals and organizations committed to improving the safety of patients" (http://www.npsf.org).

The IOM report set as a goal for these national efforts a 50% reduction in error-related deaths by 2005. Although the report prompted the development of the majority of the safety measures and guidelines in surgery that are described later in this chapter, there is yet no concrete evidence to suggest that the implementation of these measures and guidelines have resulted in an overall reduction in error-related deaths.[11] One possible reason for the failure to properly evaluate the impact and efficacy of all of these patient safety initiatives was the lack of a proper metric for the assessment of patient safety.

THE NATIONAL SURGICAL QUALITY IMPROVEMENT PROGRAM

The National Surgical Quality Improvement Program (NSQIP)[3] was established in the VA in 1994 following the conduction of a 44-center study that demonstrated that proper data collection and risk adjustment of 30-day postoperative morbidity and mortality after major surgery provided a reliable tool for the comparative measurement and enhancement of the quality of surgical care.[12-15] The hallmark of the program is a dedicated nurse at each medical center collecting preoperative, intraoperative, and outcome data in a standardized manner, with periodic assessment of nurse competency and interrater reliability. Predictive models of 30-day morbidity and mortality are developed annually and form the basis for the generation of an observed/expected (O/E) ratio for morbidity and mortality. The O/E ratio is the risk-adjusted measure of outcome used by the NSQIP. It is generated for the totality of operations performed at a hospital and for each of the surgical subspecialties. Continuous quality improvement is achieved through the feedback of comparative risk and outcome data to the providers and through the mining of the rich, prospectively collected, database. (At the time of this writing, the NSQIP database comprises data on more than 1.5 million operations.) In the years following the inception of the program, the 30-day postoperative mortality in the VA fell by 27% and the 30-day postoperative morbidity fell by 45%.[16] A recent multicenter study conducted in large academic surgical centers outside the VA has validated the applicability of the NSQIP to the private sector, and prompted the American College of Surgeons to establish the infrastructure necessary for hospitals outside the VA to partake in the Program.[17] The ACS-NSQIP is rapidly being implemented in the private sector and is becoming the standard for the quantification of risk-adjusted outcomes of surgery nationwide, and for the comparative assessment and improvement of the quality of surgical care.[18]

The experience with the NSQIP over the past decade, and the compendium of the studies performed on its database to date, place patient safety in surgery in a broader context than that of the IOM report.[19] Specifically, three paradigms related to the safety of the surgical patient have been learned from the NSQIP:

1. Patient safety in surgery needs to be defined in terms of safety from all adverse outcomes of surgical care, not only from iatrogenic provider "errors." A complication is an unsafe event and mortality is the ultimate lack in patient safety. There is a wide variation among hospitals in mortality and morbidity O/E ratios,[12,13,16] as exemplified in Fig. 2-1.[17] High O/E ratios also can be reduced significantly through improvement of processes and structures of care (Fig. 2-2).[20] The wide variation in risk-adjusted outcomes between high- and low-outlier hospitals

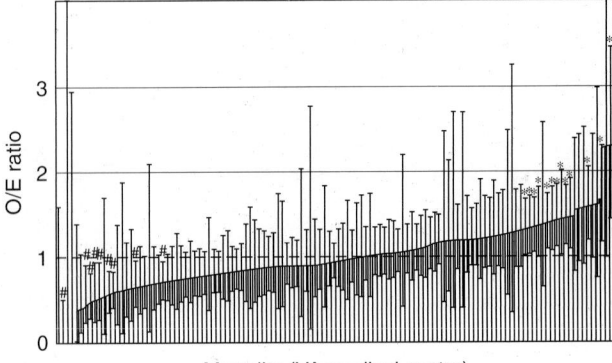

Figure 2-1 *Thirty-day mortality observed/expected (O/E) ratios with 90% confidence intervals for all operations in all hospitals participating in the National Surgical Quality Improvement Program, as they appear in the Chief of Surgery Annual Report. The identity of the hospitals is blinded by code (displayed on the x-axis), with each hospital privy to only its own code.*
VA, Department of Veterans Affairs.
*Statistically significant high outlier hospital: the unadjusted mortality rate is significantly higher *than would be expected based on the severity of illness of its patient population.*
#Statistically low outlier hospital: the unadjusted mortality rate is significantly lower *than would be expected based on the severity of illness of its patient population. (Reprinted from Khuri S. The NSQIP: a new frontier in surgery.* Surgery *2005;138:837-843, with permission from Elsevier.)*

indicates that a low-outlier hospital provides a safer environment to patients than a high-outlier hospital, and that patients at a high-outlier hospital have complications that are preventable through process improvement. In essence, defining patient safety in terms of safety from adverse outcomes makes safety indistinguishable from quality.

2. Because quality in surgery can be measured and compared based on risk-adjusted outcomes, patient safety in surgery, as defined previously, can be quantified and compared by risk-adjusted outcomes as well. The NSQIP thus provides, for the first time, a metric with which (1) patient safety in surgery can be quantified, and (2) the effects of interventions to improve patient safety can be properly assessed.

3. Adverse outcomes in surgery are mostly the result of deficiencies in systems of care, not necessarily provider errors. The provider is important in as much as he or she contributes to the quality of the system. Site visits conducted by the NSQIP to high- and low-outlier hospitals showed that structures and processes of systems of care were more important determinants of the outlier status than individual actions of a single provider.

The NSQIP predictive models have identified emergency surgery as one of the top five predictors of

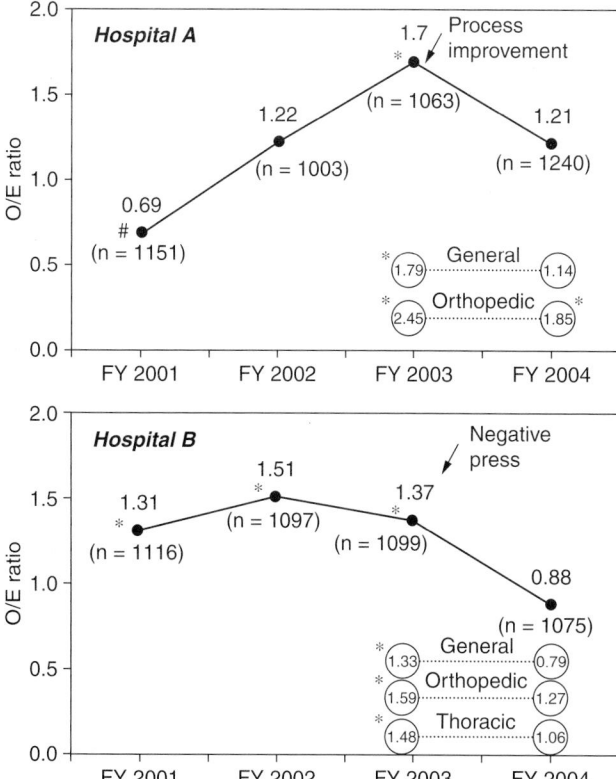

Figure 2-2   *Time course of the observed to expected (O/E) 30-day morbidity ratio in all-operations model over 4 fiscal years in 2 separate Veterans Affairs medical centers. A statistically significant high outlier at the 99% confidence level is indicated by the asterisk (*) and a statistically significance low outlier is indicated by the pound sign (#). (A; Hospital A) This hospital was a low outlier in FY01; the morbidity rate increased over the next 2 years, mostly in general surgery and orthopedics, causing it to become a high outlier in FY 03. Process improvement reversed the overall O/E ratio, but although it ceased to be an outlier in the all operations model and general surgery, it continued to be a high outlier in orthopedics, indicating that additional process improvement needed to be directed toward orthopedic surgery at that hospital. (B; Hospital B) This hospital was a high outlier in morbidity for 3 consecutive years. Negative press about the quality of care at that hospital prompted process improvement that resulted in a marked decrease in morbidity rate from 17.5% to 10.8%. These 2 case studies exemplify the fact that surgical morbidity rates can be reduced effectively though local process improvement. (Reprinted with permission from Khuri SF, et al. Determinants of long-term survival after major surgery and the adverse effect of postoperative complications. Ann Surg 2005;242:326-343.)*

30-day morbidity and mortality after major surgery, probably because the unpredictability and complexity of the emergent state can be more readily disruptive of systems of care. Assurance of quality and patient safety is therefore much more challenging in emergency than in elective surgery, and a systems approach to error prevention is paramount to the assurance of safety in emergency surgery.

A SYSTEMS APPROACH TO PATIENT SAFETY IN SURGERY

Figure 2-3 provides a conceptual framework of patient safety in a system of surgical care.[19] As illustrated in section A, there is an unsafe domain within every system caring for the surgical patient. This domain comprises the totality of the adverse outcomes experienced by patients being cared for within that system. Preventable errors, as conceptualized by the IOM report *To Err is Human* or as described by Joint Commission as "sentinel events," form a very small part of the unsafe domain, which is dominated by the totality of the usual complications and adverse postoperative outcomes. Sentinel events are also not the only preventable adverse outcomes within the system. Preventability in the figure is represented by a spectrum with white on one end, representing preventable adverse outcomes, and black on the other, representing unpreventable adverse outcomes. Potentially, every adverse outcome should be preventable as quality improvement efforts intensify within a system of care and the size of the unsafe domain is reduced (Fig. 2-3 SectionB)). The better the quality, the fewer the adverse outcomes and the smaller the unsafe domain. Hence, the size of the unsafe domain is an inverse measure of the quality of care, making safety an integral part of quality. In a quality and safe system of surgical care (ie, a system that is a statistically low-outlier by NSQIP criteria), the size of the unsafe domain would be small, and the ratio of preventable to unpreventable adverse outcomes would also be small. Conversely, in a poor and unsafe system of surgical care (statistically high outlier by NSQIP criteria), the size of the unsafe domain would be large as would be the ratio of preventable to unpreventable adverse outcomes. Quality improvement within a system of care reduces the unsafe domain by primarily reducing preventable adverse outcomes, thus resulting in a small unsafe domain that is primarily composed of unpreventable adverse outcomes (Fig. 2-3 section B). One can appreciate from this construct the futility of addressing patient safety only in terms of sentinel events, and the error one would be committing by excluding from the definition of patient safety system errors that account for the majority of preventable adverse postoperative outcomes.

COORDINATION AND COMMUNICATION IN SYSTEMS OF SURGICAL CARE

Coordination and communication are important determinants of the quality of systems of surgical care, and hence of the safety of the surgical patient. In a substudy from the VA National Surgical Risk Study, external auditors were able to distinguish between VA surgical programs that had significantly higher than expected operative mortality and morbidity as compared

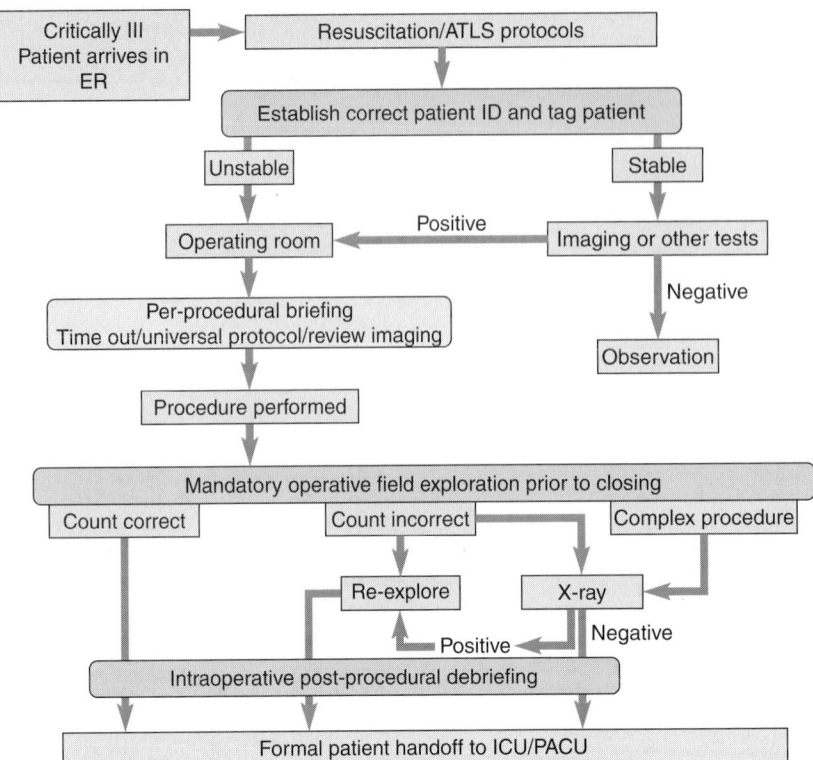

Figure 2-3 *A conceptual schema wherein patient safety in surgery in inseparable from quality of surgical care. Within a surgical system of care, there is an unsafe domain that comprises the totality of the adverse outcomes experienced by patients being cared for by the system. Within this domain, the adverse outcomes vary over a spectrum of preventability. Sentinel events, which have been the focus of numerous national patient safety initiatives since the publication of the IOM report* To Err Is Human,[1] *are preventable errors that comprise a very small fraction of the unsafe domain.*
Effective QI initiatives that reduce the incidence of preventable adverse outcomes (left arrow) should reduce the size of the unsafe domain and, within it, the ratio of preventable to unpreventable adverse outcomes. Conversely, poor quality of care (right arrow) leads to an increase in preventable adverse outcomes, and an expansion of the unsafe domain within a system of surgical care. (Reprinted from: The American Surgeon. *Vol 72. Khuri SF. Safety, quality, and the NSQIP. Am Surg 2006;994-998, with permission from the Editor,* The American Surgeon.*)[19]*

to those surgical programs with lower than expected operative mortality and morbidity, based on their on-site assessment of the degree of coordination and communication between surgeons, nurses, anesthesiologists, and other OR personnel.[13] Surgical programs in the VA with lower than expected operative mortality and morbidity were found to have more effective patterns of coordination and communication among the staff responsible for perioperative care.[21] A systems approach to patient safety with adequate coordination and communication is particularly important in the operating room environment.[22-25] Although it is evident that close coordination between members of the surgical team is essential, direct observation of surgical teams[26] and attitudinal surveys of OR personnel suggest that the level of agreement differs according to team members' role and their position in the OR hierarchy.[27,28] Trained observers monitored the intraoperative patterns of communication between surgical team members (anesthesia, surgery, and nursing) for a

3-month period.[24] There were 421 instances of "procedurally relevant" communication events observed. Communication failure was noted in 129 of the communication events observed, of which one-third of these communication failures jeopardized patient safety. Christian and associates[29] observed nine patients scheduled to undergo complex hepatobiliary or colorectal operations as they progressed from the preanesthetic holding area into the operating room and during their immediate postanesthetic care. The investigators recorded more than 4500 observations over 63 hours. There were two system features that influenced the progression of intraoperative events and patient safety—communication and information flow and coordination of workload and competing auxiliary tasks. Information loss during handoffs was a common feature that contributed to poor communication. Nearly 90% of the instances in which information was lost resulted in delays in case progression, increased workload to recapture lost data, case cancellation, and led to a compromise in patient safety. Faulty communication was a leading root cause of perioperative sentinel events collected by the Joint Commission since 1995.[30] Statistics from the VA's National Center for Patient Safety database reveal that ineffective communication was a critical contributing factor in over 80% of the 3533 adverse events collected by local VA hospitals and analyzed using a formal root cause analysis process.[31]

SURGICAL DECISION MAKING, INFORMATION FLOW, AND PATIENT SAFETY

In theory, the process required to schedule an elective operation is straightforward: (1) evaluate the patient to determine whether a surgical approach is warranted; (2) select an appropriate procedure which is approved by the patient; and (3) arrange for a mutually convenient operative date. The surgeon conveys patient-specific and procedure-specific information to the OR scheduling office in order to obtain a particular day and time for surgery. Before the scheduled date of surgery, the patient undergoes a preoperative risk evaluation by the anesthesiologist, often at a separate location. On the day of surgery, the patient-specific and procedure-specific information provided by the surgeon is reviewed jointly with the preadmission testing data. If the preceding information conforms with the operative site and procedure specified on the operative consent form then the patient is taken into the surgical suite. A "time out" is performed as a last safety check to ensure that everyone present in the surgical suite is confident that the correct patient will undergo the correct procedure at the appropriate site before the operation begins. In practice, this essential sequence of preoperative events is reliant upon the close coordination between the surgeon, the anesthesiologist and the operating room nurses. Failure to execute any part of the sequence properly may place the patient at undue risk for an adverse event. Given that a majority of the preoperative evaluation was performed independently in large part by surrogates of the staff present in the surgical suite, except for the surgeon, expectations about the progression of customary intraoperative events (eg, patient positioning, antibiotic administration, the retrieval of special instrumentation or the time required to perform the planned procedure) may differ depending on the complexity of the procedure, the experience level of the respective OR team, and whether or not the team members present in the OR have worked together previously. Team member experience and familiarity among the surgical staff may minimize these differences, particularly in cases where the progression of intraoperative events is routine (eg, CABG or cataract surgery); however, an incomplete preoperative risk assessment, unexpected pathologic findings at surgery, or emergent operations on critically ill patients may breakdown customary patterns of interaction and lead to poor coordination and communication. Vigilance, technical skill, fund of knowledge, and operative experience may not be enough to mollify certain types of adverse events, particularly in the setting of less than optimal teamwork.[24,32] Carthey and associates[33] found that if surgical teams scored high on behavioral markers of excellence (ie, team leadership, crew communication, situational awareness, teamwork, the ability to plan ahead, and the level of assertiveness of junior staff) they were better able to compensate for in the instance of a major negative event than those who did not score as well. If the occurrence of human error is accepted as a given, then training in methods of error avoidance and error mitigation will allow surgical teams attain resiliency during the conduct of complex surgical procedures in high-risk patients.

LEARNING FROM CREW RESOURCE MANAGEMENT

A lot can be learned in the setting of emergency surgery from high-reliability organizations. High-reliability organizations can be defined simply as organizations that focus on safety as a primary goal and as a result experience fewer accidents than can normally be expected. The nuclear power utilities and the commercial airline industry are two examples of high-reliability organizations. In part, the aviation industry developed its high-reliability designation through the implementation of Crew Resource Management (CRM). In late 1979, a workshop convened by the National Aeronautics and Space Administration (NASA) analyzed data taken from airplane accidents and near misses.[34] The investigation determined that nearly 70% of these mishaps hinged on the failure of interpersonal communications, poor decision making, and flawed leadership among airline crews. Based on these findings, CRM training was developed to address these findings. The Federal Aviation Administration defines CRM as the utilization of all available human, informational, and equipment resources toward the effective performance of a safe and efficient flight.[35] CRM is an active process by crew members to identify significant threats to an operation, communicate them to a person in charge, and to develop, communicate, and carry out a plan to avoid or mitigate each threat.

In recognition of the gains made in commercial aviation based on this type of training, the use of CRM principles was advocated by the 1999 IOM report as a method to improve communication across disciplines in nearly every health care setting. CRM principles that would translate to the operating room setting are preflight (preprocedural) briefings used to establish a "shared mental model" of the flight (operation); the use of assertive communication styles designed to overcome command hierarchies and interpersonal disagreements when appropriate, and the inclusion of active strategies for error avoidance such as reading back requests for a change in altitude or switching instrument settings such that the other members of the flight crew concur with progression of in-flight adjustments. Before boarding an aircraft, the pilot and copilot review the flight plan and then, on entering the cockpit, they review a series of challenge questions and replies that are read from a standard preflight checklist. The checklist is completed in its entirety before moving the aircraft in position for takeoff. Checklists have been used in anesthesia[36] to ensure the safe functioning of the anesthetic gas machine and also by perfusionists to make sure that the fluid level alarms, air embolism alarms, and pump tubing are fitted properly on the heart-lung machine.[37]

Leonard and colleagues[38] describe the implementation of a formalized briefing process by the surgical teams at the Orange County Kaiser Permanente Hospital, which involved the use of a formal checklist. Their team found that this process reduced wrong-site surgery, improved how staff felt about teamwork and communication, and enhanced the OR nurses' perception of how their input was received by other team members.

In 2003, the VA National Center for Patient Safety implemented a pilot project designed to teach a formal CRM program throughout the VA health care system. The program, entitled Medical Team Training (MTT), was implemented to test two hypotheses: (1) CRM training will improve patient outcomes by enhancing communication between providers and (2) improved communication between providers will lead to better job satisfaction. Comparing survey data collected before and after a Medical Team Training course, Awad and associates[23] found that communication between the surgical and anesthesia attending staff was significantly better 2 months later.

A SYSTEMS APPROACH TO THE PREVENTION OF SENTINEL EVENTS IN SURGERY

A sentinel event is an unexpected occurrence involving death or serious physical or psychological injury, or the risk thereof. Serious injury specifically includes loss of limb or function. The phrase or the "risk thereof" includes any process variation for which a recurrence would carry a significant chance of a serious adverse outcome. (http://www.jointcommission. org/SentinelEvents/)

On February 20, 1995, Willie King was taken to the operating room at the University Community Hospital in Tampa, Florida. This 51-year-old diabetic patient with bilateral lower extremity tissue damage signed a consent form giving his surgeon permission to perform a below-knee amputation of his *right* leg. When he left the operating room, his *left* leg had been amputated. Investigation into the incident demonstrated that the operating room schedule incorrectly listed the

procedure as a left below-knee amputation. Following the OR schedule, the operating room team prepped and draped the wrong extremity. The surgeon did not review the consent form and proceeded to perform a left below-knee operation.[39] Following this well-publicized event as well as several others, the Joint Commission initiated a Sentinel Event Policy in order to identify the leading causes of medical errors. The initiative mandated that accredited hospitals: (1) convey certain "reportable" sentinel events to the Joint Commission; (2) thoroughly analyze the inciting factors that led to the sentinel events; (3) develop an action plan to reduce their risk of recurrence; and (4) share their findings with the Joint Commission so that the lessons learned could be shared with other organizations.[40] In 2002, the National Quality Forum (NQF) developed a list of 27 Serious Reportable Events.[41] Five of the 27 events related to surgical adverse events. The four applicable surgical events were wrong-site surgery, wrong-patient surgery, wrong-side surgery, and retained foreign bodies. By June 2005, the Joint Commission had listed wrong-site surgical procedures (eg, those procedures performed on a site that neither the surgeon nor the patient intended) and the unintentional failure to retrieve surgical implements before wound closure as "reportable sentinel events."

WRONG-SITE SURGICAL PROCEDURES

The notoriety of the "Willie King incident" focused our attention on this problem; however, the threat of wrong-site procedures has existed for decades. A survey of 1050 hand surgeons revealed that 16% of them had nearly operated on an incorrect site and 21% reported that they had operated on the incorrect site at least once in their career.[42] The Physician Insurers Association of America (PIAA) reviewed 10 years of closed claims data (1985-1995) in order to determine the number of wrong-site operations.[43] A total of 331 "wrong-site" procedures were identified. In their analysis, the number of wrong-site orthopedic procedures exceeded by a factor of two the number of wrong-site, nonorthopedic procedures. Similarly, the Joint Commission reported on 126 cases of wrong-site procedures voluntarily reported to them with complete fact finding data.[44] Wrong-site orthopedic and podiatry cases comprised 41% of the sample compared with 20% for general surgery, 14% for neurosurgery, and 11% for urology. Predisposing factors included failure of the surgeon to exercise due care; assumption that someone else has confirmed the procedure and site location, left-right discordance as a result of reversed x-rays, multiple procedures, multiple surgeons, incomplete communication among members of the surgical team, and undue pressure to decrease preoperative preparation time. Based on these findings, the Joint Commission developed guidelines in 2001 that were designed to reduce the rate of wrong-site procedures. The guidelines recommended that

(1) the surgeon clearly mark the operative site; (2) an OR checklist be used to compare the intended site with the operative consent and preoperative imaging; (3) verify the site with the patient and surgical team; and (4) the surgical team should pause for a "time out" to verify that the correct patient, procedure, and site are in place. Eliminating wrong-site surgical procedures was one of the initial National Patient Safety Goals listed by the Joint Commission in 2003. Following a Summit on Wrong-Site Surgery later that year, the Joint Commission refined their previous guidelines and issued the "Universal Protocol for Preventing Wrong Site, Wrong Procedure, and Wrong Person Surgery."[45] Since July 1, 2004, the Universal Protocol has been a required process measure for all Joint Commission accredited organizations. The Universal Protocol requires the surgical team to perform three steps before making the surgical incision. First, the team should verify that the preoperative workup, operative consent, and appropriate imaging are all concordant. The surgeon should mark the operative site in order to ensure that the correct site and side are clear to the patient and the team in the OR, and that the mark remains visible throughout the skin preparation and after draping. Finally, the surgical team should pause for a "time out" in order to actively vocalize their consensus that the correct patient will undergo the planned surgical procedure on the correct site using, if applicable, an appropriate implant for that site and side.

A more recent analysis of malpractice claims data taken from the Controlled Risk Insurance Company (CRICO) found wrong-site operative procedures to be exceedingly rare.[46] Out of nearly 3 million surgical procedures performed over two decades, only 25 instances of nonspine wrong-site operations were identified using malpractice claims data. Thirteen of these malpractice cases had sufficient medical records to allow the investigators to determine if these adverse events could have been prevented if the Joint Commission's Universal Protocol had been in effect. The investigators concluded that only 8 of the 13 instances of wrong-site operative procedures could have been prevented through the use of the Universal Protocol. The other five cases would not have been discovered because of mislabeled (same name—different patients) x-ray films from a referring institution, removal of the second rib instead of the first in a thoracic outlet syndrome case, and a case in which neither the surgeon nor the patient could recall which one of the multiple skin lesions they had previously agreed to excise during an earlier preoperative visit. If the Universal Protocol is correctly applied, then wrong-site, wrong-side, or wrong-patient operative events should become extremely rare. In addition to serving as a last safety check before making a surgical incision, the most important contribution of the Universal Protocol will be its role as a forcing function, ie, the surgical team must engage in a focused dialogue, which will improve OR communication.

RETAINED FOREIGN BODIES

Donald Church had undergone an abdominal operation to remove a large tumor. His postoperative recovery was remarkable for persistent flank discomfort, which delayed the resumption of his usual daily activities. Two months following his operation, an abdominal CT scan revealed the presence of a malleable retractor in his abdomen. He underwent a second procedure to remove the object.[47] Pat Skinner's postoperative convalescence following a colon resection left her with persistent abdominal pain. She tolerated this discomfort for nearly 18 months before insisting on having an abdominal x-ray performed. The abdominal plain film showed that a pair of Metzenbaum scissors remained in her pelvis.[48] She underwent a second operation to remove the scissors, which necessitated the removal of adherent bowel. These adverse events understandably received a great deal of attention when the patients and particularly their x-rays were shown on worldwide media outlets. Understandably, the public sympathized with these patients who had been victims of iatrogenic injury and questioned the competence of surgeons who could not keep track of such large instruments during an operation. The counting of sponge, sharp, and instrument counts in tandem between the scrub nurse and circulating nurse is a time-honored tradition that has face validity but little evidence-based corroboration.[49] The operating room is a complicated environment where the concerns of safety, time, sterility, resource utilization, roles, and situation may be interpreted differently by the surgeons, housestaff, anesthesiologists, and nurses.[50] In spite of this complexity, the number of retained foreign bodies is remarkably small, based on recent data from the Minnesota Department of Health. In 2003, the Minnesota state legislature passed an "Adverse Health Event Reporting" Law mandating that each hospital in the state collect adverse event data for each of the 27 Serious Reportable Events as outlined by the NQF. In 2005, the Minnesota Department of Heath published a list of hospital-specific data for all 27 serious reportable events.[51] Data was collected on retained foreign bodies as one of the five reportable (surgical) events. Over a 15-month period, 356,094 operations were performed in Minnesota hospitals with 31 retained foreign body events detected. This amounts to an event rate of $\approx$ 8 events/100,000 operations. This number is probably an underestimate of the true incidence retained foreign bodies; however, unlike malpractice claims, this web-based data repository can easily be verified. A study of 9729 closed malpractice claims compiled over 6 years found 40 patients who filed claims alleging negligence as a result of the discovery of a retained surgical sponge.[52] The group was comprised of 29 patients who had nonvaginal procedures and 11 patients who had vaginal suspended deliveries. No sponge counts were performed during the vaginal deliveries. Falsely correct sponge counts were performed in 22 of the 29 nonvaginal cases. Retained sponges were left behind in three cases as a result of falsely negative x-ray interpretations. There was no sponge count performed in three other cases. The surgeon in the remaining case decided against obtaining an intraoperative x-ray and reexploring the patient to retrieve the missing sponge despite an incorrect count. The authors concluded that sponge counts should be performed whenever a body cavity or space is entered and that surgeons should not be content with a correct count ,but should check the operative field thoroughly before closing the incision. Analysis of malpractice claims data from Massachusetts drawn collected over a 15-year period identified patient and procedure specific factors that raised the risk of retained foreign bodies.[53] Multivariate analysis revealed that emergency operations, an unplanned change in the operative procedure, and operations on larger patients (BMI > 28.2) were all significant "high-risk" factors for the retention of foreign bodies. The lack of sponge and instrument counts did not increase the risk of a retained foreign body; however, the cases most likely not to have a count performed in their analysis were emergency operations or those in which there was an abrupt change in the planned procedure. In these instances, sponge and instrument counts would be extremely useful. However, given that a vast majority of patients found to have retained foreign bodies had a "correct count" in the operating room, certain high-risk procedures (eg, bariatric surgery, emergency operations, or more than one surgical team) should undergo radiographic imaging as an additional safety measure. The Board of Regents of the American College of Surgeons published a statement on the prevention of retained foreign bodies that endorsed the traditional counting protocol, methodic wound exploration before closure, the use of only x-ray detectable items at the surgical site, and x-ray imaging were appropriate.[54] Although these guidelines are consistent with the recommended practices of the Association of Operating Room Nurses,[55] direct observation of surgical teams has found that the counting protocol inadvertently may impede the safe conduct of surgery by taking both the scrub nurse and circulating nurse out of the flow of the operation, particularly when the count is incorrect.[56] Until newer technologies such as bar coding or radiofrequency labeling of sponges, sharps, and instruments become user-friendly, we will continue to rely on manual counting to assist in tracking these implements. Intraoperative radiographic imaging, traditionally used only when the manual count was incorrect, may be a necessary adjunct in complex surgical cases with "high-risk features," even when the manual count is correct.

CONCLUSIONS AND RECOMMENDATIONS

GENERAL MEASURES FOR PATIENT SAFETY DURING EMERGENCY SURGERY

Recognizing that safety from adverse events is not limited to safety from iatrogenic sentinel events, and that the totality of adverse events define, in good part, the quality of surgical care, safety-prevention efforts should be directed toward the prevention of all adverse outcomes through a continuous improvement of the quality of systems of care within the hospital environment. This is achieved first and foremost by assuring adequate coordination, adequate communication, and adequate leadership within surgical systems of care, particularly in the setting of emergency surgery where breakdowns in coordination and communication are more likely to occur. Participation in the National Surgical Quality Improvement Program will provide a comparative metric with which one can assess the efficacy of the measures taken to prevent adverse outcomes of surgical care.

SPECIFIC MEASURES FOR PATIENT SAFETY DURING EMERGENCY SURGERY

By necessity, the diagnosis and treatment of critically ill patients who require emergency surgery is nonlinear and must occur simultaneously. These situations are often chaotic. The temptation to bypass established procedural protocols is enormous; therefore, errors and adverse events are likely to occur despite the vigilance and technical skills found in experienced trauma teams. Rigorous adherence to the principles described in this chapter (Fig. 2-3) will enable teams comprised of differing levels of training and technical expertise to work together toward the shared goal of preserving life.

Authenticating a patient's identification and labeling that patient with some type of a tag is a crucial initial step in the midst of triage and resuscitation. This certification of identity, particularly when multiple victims have suffered similar injuries (eg, gunshot wounds or transit system accidents), will guarantee that every subsequent step of care is patient-specific as each patient passes through different levels of care. The appropriate body part is marked by the operating surgeon ensuring that the site marked is consistent with the physical exam and diagnostic imaging.

On entering the surgical suite, the operating room team should review all relevant data from the prehospital and initial resuscitation phases of care, any pertinent laboratory testing and diagnostic imaging, and the anticipated operative plan. Before the incision is performed, the OR team should all agree that the correct patient is in the operating room; that the correct site has been selected for the planned procedure, which corresponds to the preoperative imaging, and that the site was marked by the surgeon. Even with patients in extremis, a time-efficient preprocedural briefing will facilitate communication and can serve to focus team members on continuing the resuscitation, control of hemorrhage, limitation of intestinal spillage, and the debridement of nonvital tissues.

Once these "damage control principles" have been achieved, then a manual operative field exploration should be performed before closing the chest or abdominal cavity. While the manual exploration of the operative field is being performed, the scrub nurse and the circulating nurse should complete a traditional sponge, instrument, and needle count. If the operative procedure was uncomplicated and the count was correct, then the procedure is completed and the patient is prepared to leave the surgical suite.

If the count is not correct, then the first option is to reopen the surgical field and repeat a manual exploration until the retained surgical item is found. A second option is to obtain an intraoperative x-ray of the chest or abdomen, which can be obtained once the wound is closed. That x-ray should be read by the radiologist who has been informed about the nature of the missing item or by the surgeon who performed the operation. If the x-ray demonstrates the retained surgical item, then the wound is reopened and the item is retrieved. An intraoperative x-ray should also be obtained if a patient has undergone a complex operation that required multiple surgical teams or involved the repair of multisystem injuries. If the intraoperative x-ray does not reveal a retained surgical item, then the procedure is completed and the patient is prepared to leave the surgical suite.

Before leaving the operative room, an intraoperative debriefing should be performed. The surgeon should interrogate the members of the operating room team about the course of the intraoperative events.

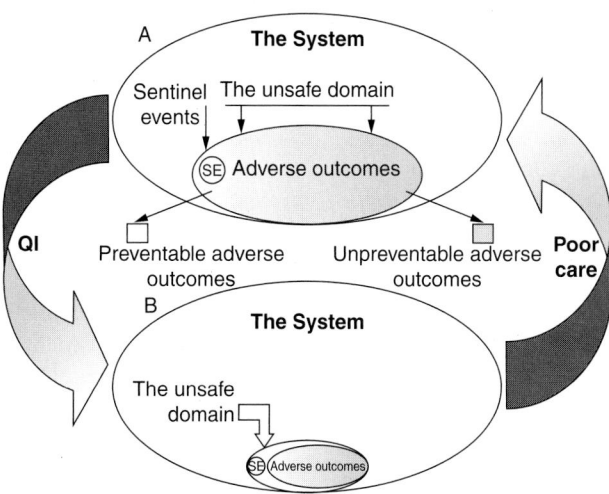

Figure 2-4 *These processes of care should be strictly adhered to in the emergency situation unless the patient's moribund condition makes their application impossible.*

Suggestions that pertain to process improvements, barriers to communication, or resource needs should be collected formally at the time of the debriefing, then conveyed to surgical leadership for quality assurance and process improvement.

At this stage, the patient is taken to a location where there is an appropriate level of postoperative support. A detailed face-to-face handoff should be delivered to those providers who are accepting responsibility for the patient. From thereon, efforts should be expended on the prevention of adverse postoperative outcomes that are much more likely to occur than adverse sentinel events. As shown in Fig. 2-4, the better the quality of systems of care within a surgical environment, the less likely is the occurrence of adverse postoperative outcomes.

REFERENCES

1. Committee on Quality Health Care in America IOM. *To Err is Human: Building a Safer Health Care System.* Kohn L, Corrigan J, Donaldson M, eds. Washington, DC: Washington National Academy Press; 1999.
2. Altman DE, Clancy C, Blendon RJ. Improving patient safety: five years after the IOM report. *N Engl J Med* 2004;351:2041-2043.
3. Khuri SF, Daly J, Henderson WG, et al. The Department of Veterans Affairs NSQIP: the first national validated, outcome-based, risk-adjusted, and peer-controlled program for the measurement and enhancement of the quality of surgical care. *Ann Surg* 1998;228: 491-507.
4. Stoelting RK, Khuri SF. Past accomplishments and future direction: Risk prevention in anesthesia and surgery. In: *Anesthesiology Clinics of North America. Anesthesia and Surgery Risk Prevention.* Philadelphia, PA: Elsevier; 2006:235-253.
5. Pierce EC. The 34th Rovenstine lecture: 40 years behind the mask: safety revisited. *Anesthesiology* 1996;84:965-975.
6. Stoelting RK. A historical review of the origin and contributions of the Anesthesia Patient Safety Foundation. *ASA 100 Newsletter (Special Commemorative Issue 1905-2005)*; 2005. Available at http://www.asahq.org/newsletter/2005/centennial/szabat100.html.
7. Department of Veterans Affairs National Center for Patient Safety. Frequently questions on marking the surgical site. *OR Manager* 2003;19:18-19.
8. American College of Obstetrics and Gynecology. ACOG Committee Opinion #328: Patient Safety in the Surgical Environment. *Obstet Gynecol* 2006;107: 429-433.
9. Russell TR, Jones RS. American College of Surgeons remains committed to patient safety. *Am Surg* 2006;72:1005-1009.

10. Manuel BM, Nora PF, eds. *Surgical Patient Safety: Essential Information for Surgeons in Today's Environment.* Chicago, IL: American College of Surgeons; 2004.

11. Brennan TA, Gawande A, Thomas E, et al. Accidental deaths, saved lives, and improved quality. *N Engl J Med* 2005;353:1405-1409.

12. Khuri SF, Daley J, Henderson W, et al. Risk adjustment of the postoperative mortality rate for the comparative assessment of the quality of surgical care. Results of the National VA Surgical Risk Study. *J Am Coll Surg* 1997;185:315-327.

13. Daley J, Khuri SF, Henderson W, et al. Risk adjustment of the postoperative morbidity rate for the comparative assessment of the quality of surgical care: Results of the National VA Surgical Risk Study. *J Am Coll Surg* 1997;185:328-340.

14. Daley J, Forbes MG, Young GJ, et al. Validating risk-adjusted surgical outcomes: Site visit assessment of process and structure. *J Am Coll Surg* 1997;185: 341-351.

15. Khuri DF, Daley J, Henderson W, et al. The Department of Veteran's Affairs NSQIP: The first national validated, outcome-based, risk-adjusted, and peer-controlled program for the measurement and enhancement of the quality of surgical care. *Ann Surg* 1998;228: 491-507.

16. Khuri S, Daley J, Henderson WG. The comparative assessment and improvement of quality of surgical care in the Department of Veterans Affairs. *Arch Surg* 2002;137:20-27.

17. Khuri SF. The NSQIP: A new frontier in surgery. *Surgery* 2005;138:837-843.

18. Napolitano LM, Bass BL. Risk-adjusted outcomes and perioperative care. In: *Surgical Clinics of North America.* Philadelphia: Elsevier.; 2005:85:1341-1346.

19. Khuri SF. Safety, quality and the National Surgical Quality Improvement Program. *Am Surg* 2006;72: 994-998.

20. Khuri SF, Henderson WG, DePalma RG, et al. Determinants of long-term survival after major surgery and the adverse effect of postoperative complications. *Ann Surg* 2005;242:326-343.

21. Young GJ, Charns MP, Daley J, et al. Best practices for managing surgical services: Role of coordination. *Health Care Manage Rev* 1997;22:72-81.

22. Vincent C, Moorthy K, Sarker SK, et al. Systems approaches to surgical quality and safety: From concept to measurement. *Ann Surg* 2004;239:475-482.

23. Awad SS, Fagan SP, Bellows C, et al. Bridging the communication gap in the operating room with medical team training. *Am J Surg* 2004;239:475-482.

24. Lingard L, Espin S, Whyte S, et al. Communication failures in the operating room: An observational classification of recurrent types and effects. *Qual Saf Health Care* 2004;13:330-334.

25. Lingard L, Espin S, Rubin B, et al. Getting teams to talk: Development and pilot implementation of a checklist to promote interprofessional communication in the OR. *Qual Saf Health Care* 2005;145:340-346.

26. Roth EM, Christian CK, Gustafson M, et al. Using field observations as a toll for discovery: Analyzing cognitive and collaborative demands in the operating room. *Cogn Tech Work* 2004;6:148-157.

27. Sexton JB, Thomas EJ, Helmreich RL. Error, stress, and teamwork in medicine and aviation: cross sectional surveys. *BMJ* 2000;320:745-749.

28. Makary MA, Sexton JB, Freischlag JA, et al. Operating room teamwork among physicians and nurses: teamwork in the eye of the beholder. *J AM Coll Surg* 2006;202:747-752.

29. Christian CK, Gustafson MI, Roth EM, et al. A prospective study of patient safety in the operating room. *Surgery* 2006;139:159-173.

30. Root Causes of Op/Post-Op Events. Available at: http://www.jointcomission.org/NR/rdonlyres/16DD96 17-BFBE-475F-8B5D-F969BD4302FF/0/se_rc_oppost_ opevents.jpg. Accessed June 10, 2006.

31. Topics in Patient Safety Newsletter, Vol 4, Issue 5, November/December 2004. Available at: http://www.va.gov/ncps/TIPS/Docs/TIPS_NovDec04.pdf. Accessed June 10, 2006.

32. Campion EW. A death at Duke. *N Engl J Med* 2003;348: 1083-1084.

33. Carthey J, deLeval MR, Wright DJ, et al. Behavioural markers of surgical excellence. *Saf Sci* 2003;41:409-425.

34. Helmreich RL, Merritt AC, Wilhelm JA. The evolution of crew resource management training in commercial aviation. *Int J of Aviation Psych* 1999;9:19-32.

35. Airport ramp and crew performance. Section II.8.5 Crew resource management. http://www.fda.gov/ other_types/aviation_industry/designees_delegations/ designee_types/ame/media/Section II.8.5 Crew Resource Management.doc - 2005-09-27. Accessed June 10, 2006.

36. Auerbach AD, Murff HJ, Islam SD. Chapter 23: Pre-anesthesia checklists to improve patient safety. In: *Making Health Care Safer: A Critical Analysis of Patient Safety Practices.* Evidence Report/Technology Assessment: Number 43. AHRQ Publication No. 01-E058, July 2001. Rockville, MD: Agency for Healthcare Research and Quality. http://www.ahrq.gov/ clinic/ptsafety/chap23.htm. Accessed June 10, 2006.

37. Polanzo DA. Perfusion safety: defining the problem. *Perfusion* 2005;20: 195-203.

38. Leonard M, Graham S, Bonacum D. The human factor: importance of effective teamwork and communication in providing safe care. *Qual Saf Health Care* 2004;13(Suppl 1):i85-i90.

39. Emergency Care Research Institute. Wrong Site Surgery. In: Healthcare Risk Control. Supplement A. *Surgery and Anesthesia* 2000;4:1-13.

40. Sentinel Event Policy and Procedures. Available at: http://www.jointcommission.org/SentinelEvents/ PolicyandProcedures/. Accessed June 10, 2006.

41. National Quality Forum. *Serious Reportable Events in Healthcare: A Consensus Report.* Washington, DC: National Quality Forum; 2002.

42. Meinberg EG, Stern PJ. Incidence of wrong-site surgery among hand surgeons. *J Bone Joint Surg* 2003;85A: 193-197.

43. Risk Management Tips Preventing Wrong-Site Surgery. Available at: http://www.medicalmutual.com/risk/ tips/HCF/07.htm. Accessed June 10, 2006.

44. A Follow-Up Review of Wrong-Site Surgery. Sentinel Event Alert. Issue 24. December 5, 2001. Available at: http://www.jointcommission.org/SentinelEventsAlert/ sea_24.htm. Accessed June 10, 2006.

45. Universal Protocol For Preventing Wrong Site, Wrong Procedure, Wrong Person Surgery. Available at: http://www.jointcommission.org/PatientSafety/ UniversalProtocol/. Accessed on June 10, 2006.

46. Kwaan MR, Studdert DM, Zinner MJ, et al. Incidence, patterns, and prevention of wrong-site surgery. *Arch Surg* 2006;141:353-358.

47. UW hospital pays $97,000 over retractor left inside patient. Associated Press State & Local Wire. December 3, 2001.

48. New South Wales: Surgical Scissors left in woman for 18 months. Australian Associated Press. April 19, 2004.

49. Gibbs VC. Patient safety practices in the operating room: correct-site surgery and no thing left behind. *Surg Clin N Am* 2005;85:1307-1319.

50. Lingard L, Reznick R, Espin S, et al. Team communications in the operating room: talk patterns, sites of tension, and implications for novices. *Acad Med* 2002;77:232-237.

51. Minnesota Department of Public Health. Adverse Health Events in Minnesota Hospitals. First Annual Public Report. January 2005.

52. Kaiser CW, Friedman S, Spurling KP, et al. The retained surgical sponge. *Ann Surg* 1996;224:79-84.

53. Gawande AA, Studdert DM, Orav EJ, et al. Risk factors for retained instruments and sponges after surgery. *N Engl J Med* 2003;348:229-235.

54. Gibbs VC, McGrath MH, Russell TR. The prevention of retained foreign bodies after surgery. *Bull Am Coll Surg* 2005;90:12-16.

55. AORN Recommended Practices Committee. Recommended practices for sponge, sharps and instrument counts. *AORN J* 2006;83:418-433.

56. Dierks MM, Christian CK, Roth EM, et al. Healthcare safety: the impact of disabling "safety" protocols. *IEEE Trans System Man Cybernetics. Part A: Systems and Humans* 2004;34:693-698.

Chapter 3

EMERGENCY MANAGEMENT OF THE OROPHARYNX AND NECK

Lenworth M. Jacobs, MD, MPH, and J. M. Kofi Abbensetts, MD

INTRODUCTION

Surgical emergencies of the oropharynx and neck represent one of the most difficult and challenging diagnostic and therapeutic dilemmas for the emergency surgeon. The surgeon is faced with an extremely anxious patient in significant distress who may be having difficulty with the airway, drooling, difficulty with speaking, and therefore an inability to communicate the problem accurately.

The surgeon has to make an immediate clinical diagnosis and determine whether this condition is anxiety provoking or if the patient is in iminent danger of airway obstruction. Furthermore, there may be very little time to confirm the diagnosis before having to develop and implement a treatment plan. It is important to have a well-thought-out diagnostic and therapeutic schema to navigate a successful outcome for the patient.

FUNCTIONS

A number of functions occur in the oropharynx. The most essential of these functions is a patent airway to allow the patient to effectively ventilate and oxygenate. The airway has a transnasal and a transoral component. The normal resting patient should be able to ventilate through the nares with the mouth closed. Air should effectively pass into the nares through the inferior middle and superior concha. These structures increase the surface area through which the air has to pass and along with the vibrissae both filter and warm the air. The airflow passes over the hard palate and the soft palate and proceeds through the superior pharynx into the larynx and the trachea. In the event that there is an obstruction to the passage of air either because of trauma, inflammation, abscess formation, or a tumor, the patient will augment their airflow through the oropharynx. Air passage through the oropharynx is dependent on a normal tongue and oral cavity allowing air to pass through the posterior oral cavity into the pharynx and down into the larynx and bronchus.

Trauma to the teeth, the mandible, the floor of the mouth, or the tongue can significantly decrease the volume of the oropharynx. Similarly, a La Forte–type fracture of the maxilla can disrupt the roof of the oral cavity and cause significant airway problems. Inflammatory or infection processes that elevate the floor of the oropharynx or create difficulty in initiating swallowing while not being anatomically constricting can present airway and ventilation problems. The posterior aspect of the tongue or the oral portion of the pharynx also can be partially obstructed by inflammatory conditions of the tonsillar ring. Similarly, peritonsillar abscesses can significantly compromise the oropharyngeal opening.

SPEECH

Any process that compromises the movement of the tongue, the movement of the vocal cords, and the resonating ability of the larynx will change the character, pitch, and volume of phonation. It is important for the surgeon to identify which anatomic structure is compromised with difficulty in phonation. Inability to move the tongue effectively significantly compromises the ability to effectively articulate specific words and sentences. Inadequate or inappropriate motions of the vocal cords compromise the precision of making sounds, particularly high-pitched sounds. There is great difficulty in saying the letter e. Conditions that change the diameter and lamina flow in the larynx change the pitch and timber of the voice. These conditions may be the result of trauma, hematoma, or a fracture of the larynx. Similarly, inflammatory processes leading to edema of the mucosa can have a similar effect. Merely asking the patient to speak and identifying the particular problem with speech or individual letters can anatomically locate the site of the problem and allow for precision in a physical exam and focused diagnostic tests.

MASTICATION

Effective mastication requires dentition to effectively break the food bolus into smaller particles. The tongue creates a bolus, and saliva lubricates the food particles as well as assisting in forming a round bolus for posterior passage into the oropharynx. Any condition that affects any of these functions can present a substantial problem for the patient. Soft tissue infections or dental abscesses can cause significant pain along with difficulty in moving the tongue and accelerating the bolus posteriorly. The classic diagnostic feature is drooling from the mouth. This condition can rapidly become life threatening if there is any difficulty in ventilating through the nasal pharynx. Frequently, the patient can become agitated and develop uncoordinated breathing and swallowing movements resulting in aspiration. Classically, these patients are extremely afraid and agitated and tend to sit upright so that saliva drains anteriorly out of the open mouth rather than posteriorly into the posterior oropharynx and the esophagus.

SWALLOWING

The swallowing mechanism is a posterior pharyngeal phenomenon. Effective swallowing requires the superior, middle, and inferior constrictors to function in a coordinated, integrated manner. The peristaltic process captures liquids and solids that are injected from the oropharynx and then initiates the swallowing mechanism to effectively conduit these materials into the superior esophagus. Any process that disrupts this integrative peristaltic wave is likely to be painful and distressing to the patient. Frequently, a lack of coordination will cause food and liquids to pass anteriorly through the epiglottic opening into the larynx. This process initiates coughing and choking. Any circumstance in which there is an inflammatory process or injury to the constrictors or the posterior pharynx has the potential to initiate vomiting and aspiration. At the lateral aspects of the airway, the carotid sheath contains the carotid arteries along with the jugular veins. The phrenic and vagus nerves are adjacent to the vessels. Similarly, the thyroid and parathyroid glands are immediately adjacent to the trachea in the neck and, therefore, at considerable risk for injury in the event of a blunt or penetrating injury to the neck.

ANATOMY OF THE OROPHARYNX AND NECK

The oral cavity is bounded by the hard palate superiorly to the buccal tissues of the cheek along with the buccinator muscle laterally. The tongue represents the base of the oral cavity. The teeth form the walls of the cavity when the mouth is closed. The floor of the mouth is an important area for the emergency surgeon to understand because infections of this area can rapidly track from one side of the cavity across the midline to the other. The tongue occupies a substantial area of the mouth. The sublingual space beneath the tongue is located posteriorly. The submandibular spaces are lateral and the submental space is found anteriorly in the floor of the mouth. The floor of the submandibular space is formed by the deep cervical fascia, which stretches from the hyoid bone to the mandible. The submandibular space is most commonly affected by primary infections of the mouth, which frequently originate from the periodontoid or dental elements. Infections of the submandibular and sublingual glands can frequently spread across the entire floor of the mouth.

THE NECK

The neck is divided into three zones. These zones contain specific structures and guide the diagnostic and therapeutic management of injuries or emergent conditions in the neck.

ZONE I

Zone I is described as the area between the clavicles and the cricoid cartilage. It is frequently described as the thoracic outlet and contains the carotid arteries, the vertebral arteries, the trachea, esophagus, spinal cord, thoracic duct, and the apicis of the lungs.

ZONE II

Zone II is described as the area between the cricoid cartilage and the angle of the mandible. This area is not protected by bony structures and is at high risk for both penetrating and blunt injuries. The structures contained in Zone II are structures within the carotid sheath, the common carotid artery, the internal and external branches of the carotid, and the jugular veins. The vertebral arteries, the thyroid, and parathyroid glands, as well as the trachea and esophagus, are also located in Zone II. Fortunately, structures that are injured in this area are relatively easily identified and repaired by a wide surgical exposure in the neck.

ZONE III

Zone III is located between the angle of the mandible and the base of the skull. This is the most technically challenging area for the surgeon. The pharynx, the vertebral arteries, and the internal carotid artery, along with the jugular veins, are located in Zone III. Exposure of injured vessels in this area is difficult and may require disarticulation of the mandible to gain adequate exposure of the injured vessel.

SPECIFIC EMERGENT CONDITIONS IN THE OROPHARYNX AND NECK

ANGIOEDEMA OR A HEMATOMA OF THE TONGUE

The patient who presents following an allergic reaction or a bee sting of the tongue is usually agitated, distressed, and drooling from the mouth, as they are unable to initiate swallowing. The tongue is large and swollen. It is difficult for the patient to communicate because movement of the tongue is difficult and phonation is severely compromised. The patient classically is sitting upright and points with the finger to the swollen tongue. This condition may worsen quickly as the swelling from either the anaphylactic reaction or the bee sting continues to occupy more space in the oral cavity. A hematoma at the base of the tongue may also present as an expanding space occupying lesion. As this progresses, the tongue is forced superiorly and protrudes anteriorly out of the mouth.

The diagnosis is usually made clinically and there rarely is time for radiographic evaluation. The mainstay of therapy is 100% oxygen delivered through nasal prongs, gentle communication with the patient, and a rapid determination if, in fact, the airway is eminently compromised. The underlying cause of the problem then needs to be quickly determined. If there is an anaphylactic antigen/antibody reaction, epinephrine and steroids need to be immediately administered. If the situation continues to deteriorate, an awake emergent airway needs to be secured. The patient should be allowed to sit partially upright. Frequently, placing the patient horizontally is extremely poorly tolerated and induces intense anxiety. It is wise to secure the assistance of an experienced anesthesiologist and have appropriate suction and the full range of airway devices immediately available. Local anesthesia is then used and a vertical incision made in the midline over the cricoid membrane and extended inferiorly. Either a cricothyroidotomy or a tracheostomy is then performed taking care to use adequate volumes of local anesthetic. Once the emergent airway is secured, the patient is ventilated with 100% oxygen. The definitive management of the problem can then be undertaken. In the event of a hematoma at the base of the tongue, frequently this is a self-limiting condition that does not require operative intervention.

LUDWIG ANGINA

Ludwig angina can be a substantial clinical challenge for the surgeon. The typical presentation is that of a young man who presents with pain and swelling in the floor of the mouth and neck. The patient usually has poor dentition with obvious dental or periodontal infection. The initial symptoms are usually localized to the area of the involved premolar tooth. There is associated pain, tenderness, and fever. The patient complains of increasing swelling, tenderness, and rigidity of the affected area. This usually progresses to the floor of the mouth and crosses the midline resulting in bilateral mouth and jaw symptoms. As the cellulitis progresses with increasing edema or abscess formation, the swelling at the base of the tongue pushes it superiorly. The edema rapidly increases to cause the tongue to fill the buccal cavity. The swelling at the base of the tongue causes extreme pain on any movement. The patient quickly has difficulty in swallowing and there is significant drooling and progressive difficulty in breathing.

As this condition progresses, the patient refuses to sit and tends to remain erect with the head held forward so that secretions can drain out of the mouth. This condition needs to be identified rapidly and recognized as a potential airway disaster.

A physical examination of the oropharynx is difficult as the submandibular and submental tissues are tense and tender. There is considerable induration of the structures at the base of the tongue. The tongue begins to protrude through the teeth and there is trismus. Examination of the larynx is very difficult as any instrumentation of the oropharynx is poorly tolerated. Fortunately, the periglottic and laryngeal tissues are usually not involved in this process.

Ludwig angina is defined as progressive cellulitis, which can occasionally progress to abscess formation. The structures of the floor of the mouth have a typical brawny induration, which do not pit on digital pressure.

TREATMENT

The most important treatment modality is to be sure that there is a patent airway for adequate ventilation. Once the airway is secured, the appropriate antibiotic, specific to the infected organism, should be administered. Organisms that are common are those that frequent the oral cavity. Classically, this is a mixed group of organisms involving anaerobes and aerobes. Alpha hemolytic streptococci and staphylococci are frequently identified. A number of oral bacteria including *Peptococcus* and bacteroides also have been identified. High doses of intravenous antibiotics are initiated immediately. If the patient's condition does not improve rapidly, the abscessed tooth should be extracted. In a case with more extensive disease, the soft tissues at the floor of the mouth should be palpated. If there is fluctuance, the patient should be taken to the operating room for an incision and drainage. The incision should be made over the area of fluctuance. The area should be opened widely and care should be taken to be sure that all of the fascial compartments are opened so that any contained infections can be adequately drained. The abscess usually originates laterally at the peri premolar area of the mandible. The length of the incision depends on the size and number of loculations within the abscess. The infection generally tracks across the midline to the other side of the floor of the mouth. The mylohyoid muscle is split in the midline and drainage of both sides of the floor of the mouth is affected by opening the tissue plains. This is often performed by digital exploration. Suction drains should be placed widely in this area. Frequently, the tissues are indurated and edematous. Following decompression, the floor of the mouth may continue to drain for a number of days. It is wise to follow the patient closely for signs of continuing sepsis. A CT scan of the oropharynx and neck with contrast should be obtained to be sure that all residual collections of pus are adequately drained. Once the swelling has resolved and all signs of sepsis have resolved, the surgical airway can be removed electively.[1]

PERITONSILLAR ABSCESS

Peritonsillar abscess is the most common severe deep infection of the head and neck.[2,3] The disease classically begins as relatively benign tonsillar cellulitis. As this disease progresses, the tonsils become swollen, inflamed, and tender. If the process does not resolve, it progresses to become a peritonsillar abscess. The consequences of untreated peritonsillar abscesses are significant. They include expanding peritonsillar and pharyngeal infections, airway compromise, and extreme difficulty in swallowing.

Peritonsillar abscess is most common in the adult population ranging between 20 and 40 years of age. It is equally distributed between men and women. Young children frequently have bouts of tonsillitis, but it is unusual for this to progress to abscess formation. The exception to this is those children who are immunocompromised.

ANATOMY

The palatine tonsils are part of a lymphoid ring which is found at the posterior aspect of the oropharynx. The palatine tonsils are located between two tonsillar pillars. The anterior border is the palatoglossal arch and the posterior boundary is the palatopharyngeal arch. The tonsils arise from the second pharyngeal pouch and are nestled between the anterior and posterior pillars.[4] The blood supply and the nerves that innovate the tonsils pass from laterally to medially in the depression formed between the anterior and posterior arches. The tonsil has a number of irregular indentations, which are known as tonsillar crypts. In any inflammatory condition, the lymphoid tissue becomes edematous and can swell so that it moves to the midline. In very severe infections of both sides of the

mouth, the tonsillar masses can approximate in the midline.

The natural progression of the disease moves from cellulitis to abscess formation. As pus collects in the tonsillar fossa, the tonsils are rotated inferiorly and medially. The surrounding anatomy, which can include the pterygoid muscles, the superior constrictors, and ultimately the masseter muscles, can have a profound effect on swallowing and mastication. This process can progress to trismus, drooling, and nasal breathing. On rare occasions, the infection can progress laterally to the carotid sheath.

ETIOLOGY

There are many organisms that are associated with peritonsillar abscess. The most common is Group A, *beta hemolytic streptococcus* (*S pyogenes*). Anaerobic organisms are also incriminated in this process. The most common is Fusobacterium. Frequently, multiple organisms of both aerobic and anaerobic type are identified in the pus aspirated from a peritonsillar abscess.

CLINICAL MANIFESTATIONS

The diagnosis of peritonsillar abscess is most effectively made by a clinical history and physical examination. There will usually be a history of pharyngitis for a number of days, which may have been treated with antibiotics. Classically, these symptoms will have started on one side but will frequently have progressed over time to involve both sides of the oropharynx. The patient will complain of significant pain in the throat, which is aggravated by swallowing, chewing, or speaking. For this reason, the patient usually has difficulty in speaking. The classic auditory signs are described as if the patient has a "hot potato" in his or her mouth. There is usually drooling from an open mouth, and the patient will avoid initiating swallowing. There is significant halitosis and the odor is described as rancid.

On physical examination, the patient will demonstrate great difficulty in opening the mouth. The medial pterygoid muscle, which is in lateral proximity to the inflamed tonsil, is usually in spasm. This will prevent opening of the mouth. Because it is difficult to eat or drink, the patient frequently is dehydrated. If one is able to inspect the oropharynx, a tongue depressor should be placed as far back on the tongue as possible. The uvula is usually deviated away from the side of the lesion and the enlarged tonsil is identified just posterior to the anterior palatine arch. If the disease is confined to one side of the tonsillar bed, the uvula can frequently be deviated almost to the other side of the posterior oropharynx. The tonsil is noted to be inflamed and there may be areas of pus identified on the surface. Palpation of the neck at the angle of the mandible is exquisitely tender. There are frequently enlarged lymph nodes in this area. Palpation of the floor of the mouth will also induce spasm and is exquisitely tender.

It is important to conduct a thorough physical examination of the oral cavity at this time to inspect the teeth, the salivary glands, and to palpate the carotid artery.

Inspection of the edematous gland, the position of the uvula, and the visual inspection of pus on the gland are usually sufficient to confirm the diagnosis of peritonsillar abscess.

ADJUNCTIVE DIAGNOSTIC MEASURES

Recently the use of intraoral ultrasound has been added to the armamentarium of the clinician. One of the problems of using the ultrasound probe is that it requires a cooperative patient who can open his or her mouth wide enough to accept the probe.[5] Once the probe is in place, the patient needs to cooperate enough to have the probe placed on the tonsil. The architecture of the tonsil, the palatine arches, and the posterior aspect of the gland can be identified with ultrasound. The presence of solitary or multiocular abscesses in the tonsil can then be identified. The posterior and lateral extent of these abscesses can be quantified. This data can be extremely helpful in guiding needle aspiration of the uni- or multiocular abscess. The abscess is identified as an echo-free cavity with a well-defined circumference. If the patient will not cooperate sufficiently to have the probe placed in the oral cavity, ultrasound may be performed by placing the probe over the submandibular gland. The advantage of this technique is that it is more effectively tolerated by the patient. The disadvantage is that there is considerable tissue between the end of the probe and the tonsillar abscess. This can frequently lead to inaccurate or missed diagnoses of peritonsillar abscess.

The advent of fine-cut CT scanning has also aided the diagnosis of peritonsillar abscess. The scan should be performed with contrast and abscesses are usually well-defined. Although this confirms the diagnosis, it does not give a useful aid to the exact location of the abscess, and, therefore, needle drainage has to be performed based on the clinical acumen of the operator.

NEEDLE ASPIRATION

The clinical diagnosis of peritonsillar abscess is best confirmed by the direct aspiration of pus from the tonsillar gland. This procedure requires a cooperative patient who is able to open the mouth wide enough to allow Cetacaine spray 0.5% benzalkonium to be sprayed into the posterior oropharynx. This spray should be applied liberally and a period of time

allowed for adequate anesthesia to be obtained. It is critical to establish a cooperative and calm relationship with the patient, as it is absolutely essential that the patient does not move as the needle is introduced into the oral cavity. Once the area is anesthetized with Cetacaine, lidocaine and epinephrine gargle should be performed. This furthers the anesthetic process and also allows the operator to see that the patient has some control over the tongue and the musculature within the oropharynx.

An 18-g needle attached to a 10-ml syringe is then introduced into the oral cavity and passed directly into the peritonsillar abscess. The syringe is aspirated as the needle is advanced. Special care should be taken not to advance the needle past the lateralmost aspect of the tonsil. The operator should be aware that the carotid artery is in proximity to this area. Once pus is obtained from the abscess, it should be sent for Gram stain and culture so that the appropriate antibiotic can be used to treat the infection.

There are reports of ultrasound-assisted needle-guided aspiration that have been successful.[5] However, there are also reports in the same series of negative aspirations from what were thought to be abscessed cavities. The final diagnosis was cellulitis, raising the issue of whether the needle-guided aspiration was necessary at all.

TREATMENT

Severe tonsillitis and peritonsillar abscesses represent a thoughtful dilemma for the treating surgeon. The choice of antibiotics is an important decision at this time. Previously, penicillin was the antibiotic of choice since the majority of bacteria were exquisitely sensitive to penicillin. Beta lactamase–producing bacteria have changed the treatment regime. Clindamycin and a second- or third-generation oral cephalosporin is now frequently the antibiotic of choice. Although the antibiotics must be given as soon as the diagnosis is made, it is important to obtain material for culture and sensitivity. As soon as the specific bacteria for the identified organism are available, the appropriate antibiotic should be instituted. Frequently, antibiotic therapy alone is sufficient to resolve the disease process.

There is now considerable controversy over the role of an immediate tonsillectomy. This is described as a hot quinsy tonsillectomy. A significant problem with this procedure is that the tonsil is significantly hyperemic and bleeding can be a major problem.[6] This is particularly true in patients who have had anticoagulation. There are a number of isolated reports in the literature of patients who have died from complications when a tonsillectomy has been performed in an anticoagulated patient. The current recommendation is not to perform an immediate tonsillectomy. Patients should be reevaluated 3 to 6 months after the abscess has been either excised and drained or treated with antibiotics. If there are recurrent episodes of tonsillitis, cellulites, or peritonsillar abscess, then a tonsillectomy should be considered. It is appropriate to solicit otolaryngological consultation in this circumstance.

STEROIDS

There has been considerable discussion as to the role of steroids in the management of peritonsillar abscess. There is a report of management of peritonsillar abscess in the native American population who were treated on an outpatient basis with antibiotics and dexamethasone and methylprednisolone followed by prednisone for 10 days. The report stated that 96% of the patients did well and 4% required posttreatment needle aspiration or incision and drainage.[7] There is no other documented series in the literature to support the use of steroids in the management of peritonsillar abscess.

Peritonsillar abscess is a common and vexing clinical problem, which can present emergently to the surgeon. It is critical to understand the pathophysiology and anatomy of this disease process. The diagnosis can be easily made with clinical history and physical examination. The role of adjunctive studies such as intraoral and transcutaneous ultrasound as well as CT scanning is an important adjunct for diagnostic and therapeutic guidance. Needle aspiration and incision and drainage along with antibiotics are extremely beneficial. The role of immediate tonsillectomy for the management of peritonsillar abscess is controversial and is rarely indicated.

CRICOTHYROIDOTOMY

The cricothyroidotomy is a surgical otomy via the skin and cricothyroid membrane into the trachea with the placement of an endotracheal tube. The procedure is performed to create an emergent airway in a patient who is unable to be intubated by the endotracheal or nasotracheal route.

Indications for the cricothyroidotomy are

■ Airway obstruction in which a foreign body in the upper airway precludes the safe passage of an endotracheal or nasotracheal tube. A surgical airway distal to the obstruction is required. Possible causes of airway obstruction include
  ■ facial and oropharyngeal edema from inhalation injuries.
  ■ facial and oropharyngeal edema from anaphylaxis.
  ■ facial and oropharyngeal edema or swelling from various infectious processes.
  ■ foreign objects.

■ Congenital deformities of the oropharynx or nasopharynx, which prevent nasotracheal or orotracheal intubation.
■ Trauma to the head and neck, which would preclude the use of an Ambu-bag, oropharyngeal airway, nasopharyngeal airway, or endotracheal tube insertion.
  ■ facial and oropharyngeal edema from severe trauma
  ■ facial fractures, such as severe comminuted mandibular fractures
■ Cervical spine fractures in patients who require an airway but in whom nasotracheal or endotracheal intubation is unsuccessful or contraindicated. For example:
  ■ nasal bone fractures
  ■ cribriform fractures
■ In situations where the healthcare provider is unable to establish an airway by any other means and this is the last resort.

ANATOMY

The cricothyroid membrane is the easiest portal into the trachea because the only overlying structure to the cricothyroid membrane is skin and subcutaneous tissue. The cricothyroid membrane is located in the anterior neck, inferior to the thyroid cartilage and superior to the cricoid cartilage. It is the small palpable indentation on the anterior aspect of the midneck just inferior to the lower edge of the thyroid cartilage.

The cricothyroid membrane is a dense fibroelastic trapezoidal membrane, bordered laterally by the cricothyroid muscles. The membrane may be pierced by small blood vessels that are situated at its attachment to the thyroid and cricoid cartilages inferiorly and superiorly. The size of the cricothyroid membrane varies in adults; it tends to be smaller in females than in males. The cricothyroid membrane in adults measures between 22 and 33 mm wide and 9 and 10 mm in height.[8] Eight millimeters is the maximum allowable diameter of endotracheal tube used in the procedure of a cricothyroidotomy. Larger tubes may cause injury to the thyroid cartilage and vocal cords, which are located superiorly and anteriorly to the cricothyroid membrane.

There are no nerves in the area of the cricothyroid membrane. The cricothyroid artery arises from the superior laryngeal artery, a branch of the superior thyroid artery. The right and left cricothyroid arteries traverse the superior portion of the cricothyroid membrane and have not been found to be clinically significant for the procedure. The artery is noted to cross the superior border of the cricothyroid membrane. This may account for some of the reports of postcricothyroidotomy bleeding that have been reported in the literature. Because of the normal path of the artery along the superior border of the cricothyroid membrane, it is recommended that incisions through the membrane be made in the lower half of the cricothyroid membrane. This will avoid damage to the vocal cords and injury to the cricothyroid artery.[9]

The vocal cords are attached to the internal anterior surface of the thyroid cartilage. They are situated superiorly approximately 1 cm above the site of the incision. Therefore, the endotracheal tube should be inserted caudally. Any cephalad passage of the tube during a cricothyroidotomy could result in significant damage to the vocal cords.

Bennett et al demonstrated in a cadaver study that the mean distance from the upper border of the cricothyroid membrane to the vocal cords was 9.0 mm in adults.[10]

CRICOID CARTILAGE

The cricoid cartilage is made up of an arch anteriorly and a lamina posteriorly and is situated at the level of C6. The cricothyroid ring is a complete cartilaginous ring. It serves as a stent and maintains a patent airway after cricothyroidotomy. This factor is important because an inadvertent laceration of the cricoid cartilage can result in instability of the trachea as a result of loss of the stenting effect of the cricoid cartilage.

PROCEDURE

In order to be successful in performing a cricothyroidotomy, one must be thoroughly familiar with the anatomy of the anterior neck. Palpation of the thyroid cartilage should be performed and the cricoid cartilage identified. An incision should be made in the skin directly over the cricothyroid membrane. The incision can be transverse or longitudinal. Controversies surrounding the type of incision for an emergency cricothyroidotomy are minor. Some surgeons believe that transverse incisions may result in more bleeding as a result of lacerations to the branches of the anterior jugular veins, whereas a longitudinal incision has less chance of inadvertent injury to blood vessels. The use of a local anesthesia is preferred. Once the skin incision is made, a transverse incision is made in the underlying cricothyroid membrane at its inferior border along the cricoid cartilage. Care should be taken when making the incision to not insert the blade deeply into the trachea as it may create a laceration of the posterior wall of the trachea. A clamp is then used to spread open the membrane. The endotracheal or tracheostomy tube can then be passed through the opening in the cricothyroid membrane and into the trachea inferiorly. The balloon is then inflated and the patient ventilated. The patient should be in a supine position to maximize exposure of the neck. The nondominant hand should be used to stabilize the thyroid cartilage. Tension should be placed on the thyroid cartilage and the overlying skin to facilitate the incision over the cricothyroid membrane.

In clinical situations of distorted neck anatomy, such as infectious processes causing significant swelling of the anterior neck or the presence of a Combitube with the large balloon inflated in the hypopharynx causing distortion of the anterior neck, a cricothyroidotomy can be a challenging procedure. The distortion of the landmarks may make it difficult for the palpation and identification of the cricothyroid membrane.

CONTRAINDICATIONS

Contraindications to cricothyroidotomy include inflammatory laryngeal pathology, trauma to the larynx and translaryngeal intubation. The procedure is also contraindicated in children; only a needle cricothyroidotomy is indicated for children less than 12 years of age. Anatomically in children, the narrowest section of the airway, especially in infants, is the cricoid cartilage. It is the only completely circumferential supporting structure. The risk of injury to the cricoid cartilage in children with subsequent subglottic stenosis is significant. As a result, the procedure should be avoided in children under 12 years old.

COMPLICATIONS

Complications include intraoperative and postoperative bleeding at the site of the incision. This is of special concern in patients who may be on anticoagulation therapy. The most significant complication associated with the procedure is subglottic stenosis. The incidence of subglottic stenosis ranges anywhere from 1.5% to 1.9%.[11,12]

Changes in voice have also been noted as a complication. The causative factor is possible injury to the vocal cords as a result of forcing an oversized endotracheal tube placed through the otomy. Laryngeal damage has also been described. Aspiration and pneumonia are also complications associated with this procedure. Perforation of the esophagus is possible. Recurrent laryngeal nerve injury is also another possible injury.

Lim et al noted significant changes in swallowing in patients with intact cricothyroidotomies. The tube minimizes base of the tongue movement and laryngeal elevation impairing epiglottic displacement. This can result in loss of the airway protective function of the epiglottis.[13]

SUMMARY

The surgeon faced with emergencies in the oropharynx and neck needs to understand fully the clinical features that constitute a pending crisis. A sound understanding of the anatomy and the pathophysiology of the disease processes in this anatomic area is essential. Rapid diagnosis and a carefully thought-out plan for intervention are critical in order to achieve a successful outcome.

REFERENCES

1. Maksimovich P. Ludwig's angina. *Mpilo Medical Journal* 1999;1(3).
2. Steyer TE. Peritonsillar abscess: diagnosis and treatment. *Am Fam Physician* 2002;65:93-96.
3. Epperly TD, Wood TC. New trends in the management of peritonsillar abscess. *Am Fam Physician* 1990;42:102-111.
4. Kahary W, Taepke J. Management of peritonsillar abscess: needle aspiration versus incision and drainage versus tonsillectomy. *Amer J of Therapeutics* 2005;12:344-350.
5. Blaivas M, Theodoro D, Duggal S. Ultrasound-guided drainage of peritonsillar abscess by the emergency physician. *Amer J of Emerg Med* 2003;21(2):1-7.
6. Dunne AA, Granger O, Folz BJ, Sesterhenn A, Werner JA. Peritonsillar abscess—critical analysis of abscess tonsillectomy. *Clin Otolarynog* 2003;28:420-424.
7. Lamkin RH, Portt J. An outpatient medical treatment protocol for peritonsillar abscess. *Ear Nose Throat J* 2006;85(10):658-660.
8. Kress TD, Balasubramaniam S. Cricothyroidotomy. *Ann Emerg Med* 1982;111:197-201.
9. Dover K, Howdieshell TR, Colborn GL. The dimensions and vascular anatomy of the cricothyroid membrane: relevance to emergent surgical airway access. *Clin Anat* 1996;9:291-295.
10. Bennett JDC, Guha SC, Sankar AB. Cricothyrotomy the anatomical basis. *J R Coll Surg Edinb* 1996;41:57-60.
11. Brautigan. Subglottic stenosis after cricothyroidotomy. *Surgery* 1982;91:217.
12. Schroeder. Cricothyroidotomy: when, why and why not? *Am J Otol* 2000;21(3):195-201.
13. Lim J. Epiglottic position after cricothyroidotomy. *Ann Otol Rhinol Laryngol* 1997;106.

Chapter 4

EMERGENCY CHEST SURGERY

Claudia E. Goettler, MD, and
Michael F. Rotondo, MD

INTRODUCTION

Although uncommon, nontraumatic chest diseases requiring emergency surgery may be complex to diagnose and manage. The majority of thoracic emergency procedures remain the domain of the cardiothoracic surgeon, particularly aortic dissection and acute coronary ischemia. Other conditions, however, must be recognized, understood, and treated by the emergency surgeon. In this chapter, these relatively rare but rapidly life-threatening conditions will be discussed. We assume that rapid and aggressive resuscitation for all conditions is understood and discuss specific management of these disorders.

BRONCHI/LUNGS

UPPER AIRWAY OBSTRUCTION
Epidemiology
Causes of upper airway obstruction are legion, and hence demographics depend on the specific disease process. The majority of lesions are chronic in nature and as they enlarge gradually cause symptoms of stridor, dyspnea, and cough. These rarely require emergent intervention, and when they do, are all managed similarly regardless of initial pathology. Airflow is related to the fourth power of the diameter of the airway, hence patients with a critical lesion may decompensate rapidly with only a minimal change in the size of the lesion.[1]

The most common cause of acute upper airway obstruction is aspiration of foreign bodies and this will be the main focus of the following discussion. These result in about 3000 deaths per year in the United States.[1-3] Peanuts are the most commonly aspirated item in children (34-38%), and dental and medical appliances are most common in adults. Risks include dental procedures, neurologic disorders, and substance use.[3,4]

Obstructing airway foreign bodies are usually managed before arrival to the hospital by Heimlich maneuver. Otherwise, these patients typically die at the scene. Patients present with sudden choking (89%), (the most sensitive and specific symptom), cough (81-83%), wheezing (11%), stridor (4%), and cyanosis (25%). Physical exam may show decreased breath sounds (61%), tachypnea (53%), or retractions (20%) and is normal in 15%.[3] Generally, choking, cough, and stridor is seen with objects in the trachea, whereas bronchial objects typically have few symptoms and only wheezing on exam.[4] From 40 to 70% of objects go to the right side, most commonly in the right lower lobe bronchus, 30-44% to left side, and 6-20% remain in the trachea.[3,4]

Preoperative Management
Initial airway assessment is critical. If there is complete or impending obstruction, the airway must be cleared without delay. If this is not possible, immediate airway control is necessary. A single trial of intubation is warranted by the most experienced personnel available.

Failure of intubation is usually as a result of edema, secretions, or obstructing lesions and requires a rapid surgical airway. Generally, cricothyroidotomy is the optimal management for ease, speed, and requirement of few supplies. Exceptions to this are children less than 8 years of age and patients with laryngeal pathology. These patients require emergency tracheostomy. Under emergency conditions, it may be impossible to determine the level of obstruction. In these cases, cricothyroidotomy should be done. Foreign bodies may be dislodged through this incision.

Racemic epinephrine by inhalation, corticosteroids, histamine blockers, and antibiotics are appropriate, depending on the disease process. They may result in reversal of symptoms, but waiting for medical therapies to work should not delay securing the airway as needed.[2] Heliox therapy has been utilized to temporarily manage airway obstruction until medical or surgical therapy can be undertaken. The flow characteristics of the gas allow oxygenation beyond the obstructive lesion.[5]

In more stable patients, history, exam, and further workup are helpful. Plain radiographs can be helpful of the chest and neck for inflammatory diagnoses and aspirated foreign bodies, but these should not precede or preclude airway management and hence should be performed portably. Computed tomography rarely adds to the diagnosis and should be undertaken only in patients with a secure airway.[2]

With aspirated foreign bodies, radiographs are helpful in 72-86% of patients. They may show a radiopaque foreign body (13%), atelectasis caused by obstruction (35%), pneumonia or bronchiectasis (11%), whereas partial obstruction may result in hyperinflation (27%). Delay in diagnosis is common, with complications including recurrent pneumonia, bronchial injury, hemoptysis, pleural effusion, and empyema.[4]

Operative Management

Treatment of foreign body aspiration is via rigid or flexible bronchoscopy. Although there is argument about which method is optimal, it is clear that flexible bronchoscopy can be done by more physicians and is becoming the more common method of management.[3,4] If the patient's history is consistent with aspiration, diagnostic bronchoscopy should be completed even if the remainder of the evaluation is negative to be sure there is not a radiolucent object present.

Organic aspirated material or pills can cause mucosal reaction and increase in size as it hydrates. Because of the irritation and swelling, these should be removed urgently.[3,4] Inert, partially obstructing items are managed on a semiurgent basis, usually by pulmonary specialists, although acute care surgeons also may be called on to do this work, particularly when airway compromise is present or imminent. Airway should either be controlled or preparations for emergency control must be in place. Conscious sedation can assist in removal by preserving the cough reflex.[4]

If possible, the aspirated object should be duplicated so that various instruments can be tried extracorporeally to determine the best method for control of the object prior to attempting removal from the patient. Grasping forceps, snares, and various baskets can be utilized. Balloon catheters are used to dislodge distal impacted objects. Cryotherapy is helpful with soft or friable objects and magnetic probes are useful for metallic objects. Laser is sometimes necessary to coagulate or remove granulation tissue. Once an object is controlled, the bronchoscope, grasping instrument, and the foreign body should be removed together.[4]

Loss of the object in the nasal passages is a difficult problem; hence, approach should be via the mouth. Risk with flexible bronchoscopy removal is loss of control of the item in the subglottic area with complete airway obstruction. If this occurs, the item can be pushed into a mainstem bronchus and the patient ventilated before repeat removal attempt.[3,4]

Postoperative Management

Postbronchoscopy complications occur in 5-8% of cases, consisting of stridor as a result of bronchospasm, laryngospasm, or laryngeal edema, and pneumonia, pneumothorax, pneumomediastinum, or hemoptysis. Bronchoscopy (rigid or flexible) is successful in 86-100% of cases. The remainder required tracheotomy or thoracotomy. Location or length of time in the airway did not predict complications or success.[3,4] In-hospital mortality rates are now less than 1%.[3]

Special Topics

Malignant tumors frequently can be debulked by laser or cautery, with or without stenting, with improvement in airway size and symptoms in 75-89% of patients. Extrinsic malignancies can be managed with airway stenting, either for palliation or as a bridge to treatment with chemotherapy or radiation. Success in weaning off mechanical ventilation after stenting occurs in 72-94% of patients. These methods also have been used to treat benign masses and inflammatory conditions.[6]

Acute epiglottitis is most common in children but also seen in adults. Patients present with stridor, drooling, and sit with their head forward. Cough is not present and this is highly predictive of epiglottitis rather than other upper airway infection. Initial evaluation is a portable lateral neck radiograph for soft tissue swelling. Rapid securing of the airway should be undertaken, either by intubation or surgically. Early intubation has reduced mortality of this disease. Laryngoscopy should not be undertaken without preparations for intubation and surgical equipment and personnel standing by. Although *peritonsillar/retropharyngeal abscesses and Ludwig angina* also have potential for airway compromise, they can usually be drained and treated without emergent airway management. Generally tracheostomy should be avoided in these patients as the field is typically infected, particularly with Ludwig angina. Extremely rarely, vocal cord paralysis, hematoma from anticoagulation, sarcoid, erythema nodosum, or Wegener granulomatosis result in significant obstruction. Internal airway injury, either from intubation, inhalation injury, or aspiration may result in edema, vocal cord paralysis, and increased secretion production. *Edematous conditions* such diphtheria, laryngitis, angioedema, and anaphylaxis need airway management as indicated by the degree of respiratory compromise. Angioedema requires airway management in about 20% of patients. Mortality remains 25% in this population, usually because of inability to secure the airway early enough.[1,2]

Smoke, caustic, and chemical inhalations should have fiberoptic laryngoscopy for diagnostic purposes with an endotracheal tube loaded on the bronchoscope for immediate intubation if indicated. These injuries can progress over several hours to complete obstruction and, hence, injured airways require intubation early to prevent subsequent loss of the airway. In minimal injury, repeat examination can be considered, although there is little risk to empiric intubation early.

Tracheotomy is rarely needed for burn injury but is common for caustic aspiration.[1,2]

PNEUMOTHORAX

Epidemiology

Pneumothoraces may be spontaneous, traumatic, iatrogenic, or a result of barotrauma. Primary spontaneous pneumothorax (SP) occurs without underlying lung disease. There is a male predominance, usually tall, thin young patients. It is strongly associated with smoking. The primary pathology of primary SP is unclear. Many patients have small subpleural blebs, whereas others have visibly normal lung tissue. Nonspecific collagen-vascular disorders also may contribute.[7,8]

Secondary spontaneous pneumothorax is associated with lung disease and is more typically seen in older patients (60-65 yrs peak incidence). The most commonly associated lung disorders are chronic obstructive pulmonary disease and *Pneumocystis carinii* pneumonia, although tuberculosis should also be considered. These tend to be more dangerous than primary SP, as patients with underlying disease have less cardiopulmonary reserve. Secondary SP patients nearly always have blebs or bullae as a cause for the pneumothorax.[7,8]

Preoperative Management

Management depends first on physiology. Any patient with a known or suspected pneumothorax with either hemodynamic or respiratory compromise should undergo thoracostomy tube insertion without delay. Needle decompression can be used if equipment is delayed and the patient is in extremis. Outside of these situations, decisions on therapy are based on chest radiograph findings and underlying pathology. Determination of the size of pneumothorax on plain radiograph is difficult, however, if there is separation of the entire lung along the lateral chest wall, or greater than a 2 cm drop from the apex, the pneumothorax should be considered large. Diagnosis may be complicated in secondary SP by the presence of large bullae on radiographs that make visualization of the pneumothorax difficult. Computed tomography, in a stable patient, may be needed for differentiation and is helpful for planning later surgical intervention.[7]

Patients with primary SP are usually only minimally symptomatic. Pneumothorax of less than 15-20% without symptoms may be managed by observation and a repeat radiograph. Larger pneumothoraces requires aspiration or thoracostomy tube insertion. Aspiration is successful in 70%, and some authors advocate discharge home after a repeat radiograph in 6 hrs. Several small, poorly randomized studies show no significant difference in success, hospital stay or recurrence between aspiration (sometimes repeated) and tube thoracostomy. If tube thoracostomy is chosen, a small caliber tube is sufficient and suction does not improve resolution over water-seal or Heimlich valve. A thoracostomy tube alone will treat 85-100% of first primary SPs, but success decreases with subsequent recurrences. Overall, the risk of recurrence ranges from 16 to 52%.[7-9]

Secondary SP is more difficult to manage, as reexpansion may be limited by poor lung compliance. Aspiration is only successful in about 37%; hence, all secondary SPs should be treated with thoracostomy tube drainage. Suction is needed only for failure to expand. The recurrence rate is high (39-47%).[7-9]

Operative Management

Definitive management of primary SP remains controversial, as the pathophysiology is poorly understood. Surgery is recommended for prolonged air leak (4-7 days) or for a secondary occurrence. With minimally invasive procedures such as video assisted thoracoscopy (VATS) and axillary thoracotomy, many patients are being offered surgery after the first pneumothorax, especially patients involved in high-risk activities such as diving and flying.[7,8] VATS and resection of apical blebs decreases the risk of recurrence to 1.5%. Mechanical pleurodesis or pleurectomy shows similar reduction. Pleurodesis via chest tube is also an option. Talc has a small inherent risk of lung injury or respiratory failure.[7-9] The choice to perform pleurodesis must take into account that future surgery will be difficult and dangerous caused by pleural scaring. Most experts support apical pleurectomy and mechanical pleurodesis of the remainder of the thoracic wall (Fig. 4-1).[9]

With secondary SP, surgery is recommended in all patients who are able to tolerate anesthesia. VATS with resection of bullae (recurrence 2-14%) is sufficient in most, though more extensive thoracotomy (recurrence 0-7%) is needed in patients with extensive bullous disease or those unable to tolerate single lung ventilation (Fig. 4-2).[7]

Special Topics

Catamenial pneumothorax is found in women of childbearing years, usually 30-40 years old. Although all menses are not associated with the development of a pneumothorax, all pneumothoraces occurs within 72 hrs of onset of menses. These patients may or may not have history or symptoms of pelvic endometriosis. Frequently, patients will have multiple pneumothorax recurrences before diagnosis and definitive therapy. The pneumothorax is right-sided in 92% of cases. The cause is felt to be thoracic endometriosis, although the exact mechanism is not known. Many patients have small perforations in the right tendinous diaphragm (26%) with endometrial implants of the pleura (13%) or diaphragm (40%).

Because of the high rate of recurrence, surgical therapy, either by VATS or thoracotomy is recommended. Some patients (23%) will have bullae or blebs, which should be resected. It is critical to inspect

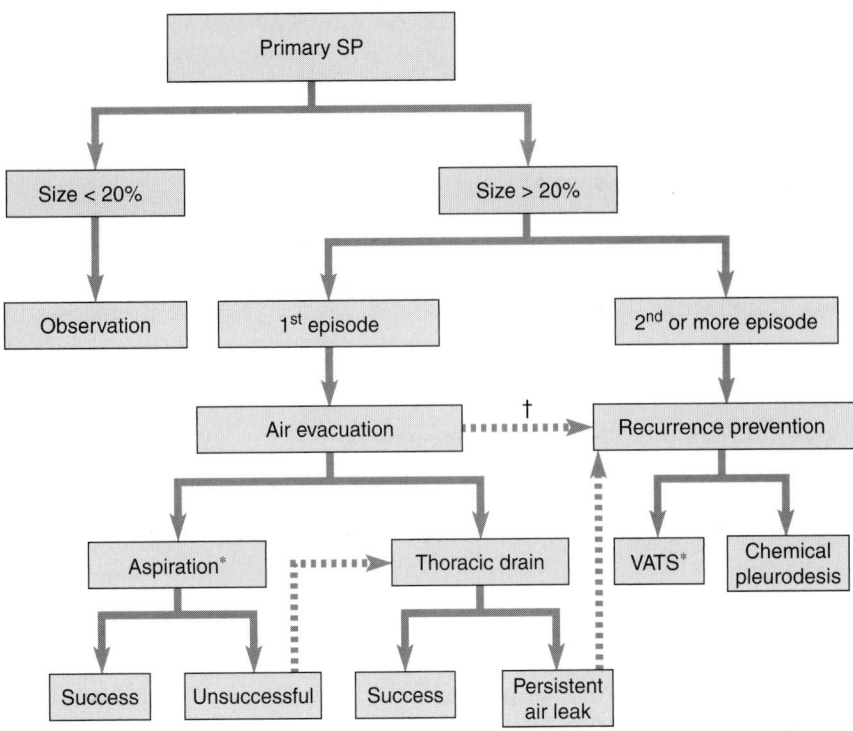

Figure 4-1 *Management of primary spontaneous pneumothorax. Reproduced with permission from Van Schil PE, Hendriks JM, De Maeseneer MG, Lauwers PR. Current management of spontaneous pneumothorax. Monaldi Arch Chest Dis 2005;63(4):204-212.*

the diaphragmatic surface during surgery, with removal of visible implants. The best therapy seems to be closing diaphragm defects and pleurodesis. Chemical suppression should be considered with luteinizing hormone-releasing hormone analog therapy. This also has been used successfully without surgical intervention.[10]

Tension pneumothorax occurs with increased pressure collapsing the affected lung, compressing the contralateral lung, and compressing the mediastinum. It occurs rarely with spontaneous pneumothorax, is most commonly a result of trauma, but also associated with iatrogenic and barotraumas pneumothoraces especially with positive pressure ventilation. The diagnosis should be made clinically, by decreased ipsilateral breath sounds, contralateral tracheal deviation, and evidence of hemodynamic compromise. The patient should not undergo chest radiography if suspected but should immediately be decompressed. A rush of air followed by normalization of the physical exam confirms the diagnosis. In cases where the diagnosis is in question, it is much safer to place a tube thoracostomy, than wait for radiographic evidence and risk death of the patient. Needle decompression in the second intercostal space, midclavicular line, can be used as a temporizing measure before tube thoracostomy but may not be effective up to 30% of the time because of a thick chest wall or occlusion of the needle.

Reexpansion pulmonary edema is a rare complication of draining air or fluid from the thorax. The expansion of the lung results in shear stress to the alveoli and reperfusion with resultant cytokine release. This causes severe ipsilateral and occasionally bilateral pulmonary edema. The incidence has been reported to be as high

as 14% in spontaneous pneumothorax patients and has a mortality approaching 20%. Patients develop respiratory distress unresponsive to oxygen as a result of

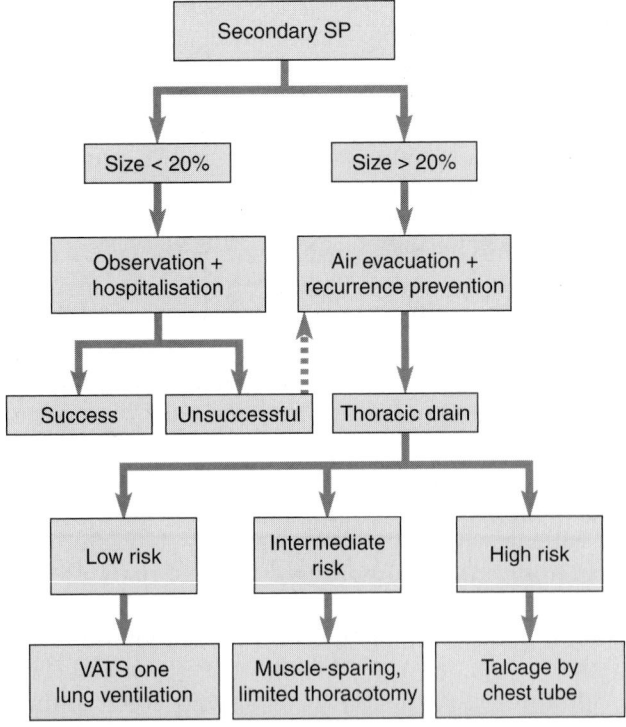

Figure 4-2 *Management of secondary spontaneous pneumothorax. Reproduced with permission from Van Schil PE, Hendriks JM, De Maeseneer MG, Lauwers PR. Current management of spontaneous pneumothorax. Monaldi Arch Chest Dis 2005;63(4):204-212.*

shunting within the lung. Severe coughing typically heralds the decline. Up to 64% of patients who developed reexpansion pulmonary edema do so within 1 hour and all within 24 hours.

Patients at increased risk are those of young age (20-39 yrs), prolonged lung collapse, and large pneumothorax (0% for less than 30% collapse, 17% in total collapse, and 44% in tension pneumothorax). Additionally, rapid reexpansion seems to contribute; in an animal study, edema occurred in all on negative pressure and none on water seal alone. Therapy is intubation and ventilator support. Symptoms usually resolve in 24 to 72 hours.[11]

HEMOPTYSIS
Epidemiology
Although hemoptysis is relatively common, it is considered massive in only 1.5% of cases. The amount considered massive is variable but generally is more than 600 cc/24 hrs. The amount of bleeding is difficult to quantitate as some blood is retained in the lungs and some is coughed up and swallowed. As a general rule, any amount of hemoptysis that is life-threatening should be considered massive. This may be as little as 400 cc, which is the estimated amount to cause oxygenation failure. The majority of patients have critical oxygenation and ventilation failure rather than hemodynamically significant bleeding.[12]

Pathophysiology
The majority of bleeding is from bronchial arteries (90%) and may result in life-threatening hemorrhage as a result of systemic pressures, whereas pulmonary arterial bleeding occurs in only 5% and is less threatening because of lower pressures. There are many causes of massive hemoptysis, which include infections, especially tuberculosis, bronchiectasis, fungal balls, necrotizing pneumonia, and lung abscess. Other causes include carcinoma, coagulopathy, bronchovascular communication, including thoracic aneurysm, trauma, and AV malformations. Less common medical causes include Goodpasture syndrome, Behcet disease, and lymphangioleiomyomatosis. A careful history will help pinpoint diagnosis but should not delay emergent management of life-threatening bleeding.[12]

Preoperative Management
Airway control is necessary in any patient with severe bleeding, hypoxemia, or hypercarbia. The largest possible endotracheal tube possible should be used to allow therapeutic bronchoscopy. Increased positive end expiratory pressure may assist with bleeding control as well as enhancing oxygenation. Cough suppression is recommended by some authors but is controversial.

The most critical initial maneuver, even in lesser bleeding, is to protect the contralateral lung from flooding with blood. To this end, the patient should be placed in lateral decubitus position with the bleeding side down. Physical exam alone provides localization in 50%, whereas chest radiograph provides localization in 54-80% of cases.[12,13]

With brisk bleeding from a single lung, mainstem intubation, either blind on the right or bronchoscopically guided on the left into the nonbleeding lung is a rapid protective mechanism, but then precludes local measures of bleeding control. The second option is double lumen intubation, which will allow each lung to be examined separately. This has the benefit of protecting the nonbleeding lung, but requires facility with insertion and limits therapeutic bronchoscopy because of the smaller size of the lumens.[12-14]

Bronchoscopy should be performed next. This allows removal of blood from the airways as well as localization of the bleeding source. Optimally, the bleeding site can be narrowed down to a specific lobar segment, although, depending on the amount of blood loss, may allow only determination of which lung is involved. With severe bleeding, no visualization may be possible. There are two options in this situation. Lavage of the lung with iced saline or dilute epinephrine solution (1:20,000) may decrease bleeding enough for visualization. Iced saline can cause hypothermia as a result of central cooling of large volumes of blood and epinephrine absorption may result in tachyarrhythmias. Both may worsen hypoxemia as a result of alveolar flooding.[12-14]

Endobronchial tamponade is then attempted as a temporizing measure. A rigid bronchoscope is optimal; however, this instrument is rarely used and requires an experienced practitioner, hence flexible bronchoscopy is the norm. Optimally, a bronchial blocker is used to occlude the bleeding bronchus, allowing ventilation of the remaining lung. This is accomplished by passing a Fogarty catheter through the instrument channel of the bronchoscope into the effected bronchus under direct vision. The end of the Fogarty must be cut off to allow removal of the bronchoscope, but the balloon can then be inflated with a blunt catheter inserted into the end of the Fogarty. A size 8 Fogarty is appropriate for the main bronchi and a size 4 for smaller airways. Additionally, a specific double lumen catheter has been developed but is not available in all centers. It has a balloon with a detachable filling port and a second lumen for vasoactive products. Alternatively, a small guide wire may be passed through the instrument channel and a balloon catheter from angiography passed over this with the bronchoscope inserted separately for visualization.[12,13]

Tamponade of the bleeding segment with adequate oxygenation and ventilation will typically allow adequate patient stabilization and planning for definitive therapy. During this time, or if the diagnosis of the hemorrhage source is in question, upper gastrointestinal and nasopharyngeal sources should be ruled out by endoscopy. Computed tomography is helpful in patients of adequate stability either to localize the bleeding source or help determine the cause.[12] Frequently, it is more specifically diagnostic than bronchoscopy, although unstable patient should not be taken for imaging. The combination of bronchoscopy and computed tomography maximizes the overall diagnostic yield and hence allows for optimal therapeutic planning.[13,14]

Operative Management

Endobronchial tamponade as described above is generally a temporizing procedure. The tamponade catheter should be left in place with specific measures such as embolization or surgery.[12] In 10% of cases, bronchoscopy alone is definitive if the bleeding source can be visualized. Topical epinephrine or thrombin may be sufficient for minimal lesions. Electrocautery, cryotherapy, and laser via bronchoscope have also been successful on occasion.[13,14]

Medical therapy alone is frequently sufficient for blood dyscrasias, anticoagulation and Goodpasture disease.[12] Steroid therapy for immune diseases and hormonal therapy of catamenial hemoptysis will control bleeding for these disorders. After 24 hrs, the endobronchial balloon can be taken down under direct vision. If there is no bleeding, the catheter should be left in place, deflated, for an additional 24 hrs before removal.[13]

Angiographic embolization is the method of choice for control of hemorrhage. It is generally safe and usually will convert an emergency to a stable situation that allows evaluation and planning of potential surgical management. The bronchial artery should be evaluated first; then, if no source is found, pulmonary angiography is imaged (8% of bleeding sources). The major but rare contraindication is risk of embolization to a spinal cord artery branching from the bronchial system. Small areas of pulmonary ischemia are usually not clinically significant but may result in transient pleuritic pain. Additionally, transient odynophagia occurs as a result of minor interruption in esophageal blood supply. Embolization is initially effective in 91-98% of cases, but up to 16-21% will rebleed. Failure of embolization is usually a result of nonbronchial collateral vessels. Lesions with high risk of rebleed include cavitary lesions and lung necrosis and should have resection when stabilized (Fig. 4-3).[13,14]

Surgery is considered both the therapy of last resort and the most definitive therapy. It is indicated for bleeding despite embolization, if embolization is not possible, or if the patient rebleeds or has high likelihood of rebleeding.[13] Surgery in emergent circumstances is a thoracotomy on the side of bleeding with attempts to locate the lobe affected intraoperatively. Lobectomy or pneumonectomy is usually necessary. Other methods to control bleeding, as described earlier, allow surgery to be planned. In these cases, the type of resection is dependant on disease type. In the past, surgery was done most frequently for high-pressure bronchial

bleeding associated with tuberculosis-induced aneurysm. With medical therapy for tuberculosis, surgery has become less common, although with the resurgence of multi-drug-resistant tuberculosis, rates may again increase. Surgery is still considered the treatment of choice for thoracic vascular injury, arteriovenous malformation, leaking thoracic aneurysm, and any other conditions in which there is a localized respectable source in which vascular control alone is not curative (malignancy, cavitary disease).[12,13] Surgery is contraindicated in advanced carcinoma, bilateral disease, and limited pulmonary reserve.[12-14]

Radiation therapy may be helpful with malignancy or aspergilloma if surgery or embolization is not possible. It is believed that localized vascular necrosis results in definitive hemorrhage control. Clearly this is not a useful therapy in aggressively bleeding lesions.[13,14] Vasopressin has been used systemically, as with gastrointestinal bleeding. It can reduce bleeding but causes bronchial artery constriction, which may limit embolization.[13]

Postoperative Management

Overall surgical mortality is 50%, which is lower than medical management (86%), likely caused by selection bias.[13] Embolization alone, if definitive, has a much lower mortality, although few meaningful numbers are available. Surgery after control with embolization has a lower mortality than emergency surgery.[12,13]

Mortality depends greatly on the underlying cause and the degree of bleeding. Mortality is 59% with malignancy, 58% with bleeding of greater than 1 l/24 hrs, and only 9% with lesser degrees of bleeding. Malignancy together with bleeding of greater 1 l/24hrs has a mortality of 80%.[12]

Special Topics

Pulmonary artery (PA) rupture caused by PA catheterization is uncommon but may result in massive hemorrhage. Patients at highest risk are those with pulmonary hypertension, anticoagulation, and older age (greater than 60-70 years). The risk during cardiac bypass is associated with manipulation of the heart and hypothermia, but these cases can be managed operatively at the time.

The majority of patients (69%) presents with massive hemoptysis and should be managed as all other causes of massive hemoptysis, with the following caveats. The majority of these bleeds occur on the right side, so the patient should be placed in right lateral decubitus position. The PA catheter should not be removed, but only withdrawn about 3 cm and the balloon reinflated to decrease flow to the injured vessel. Increasing positive end expiratory pressure on the ventilator has been described; although no trials exist to support this, it is unlikely to be harmful and may provide some tamponade. In extreme cases, injection of clotted patient blood through the distal PA catheter

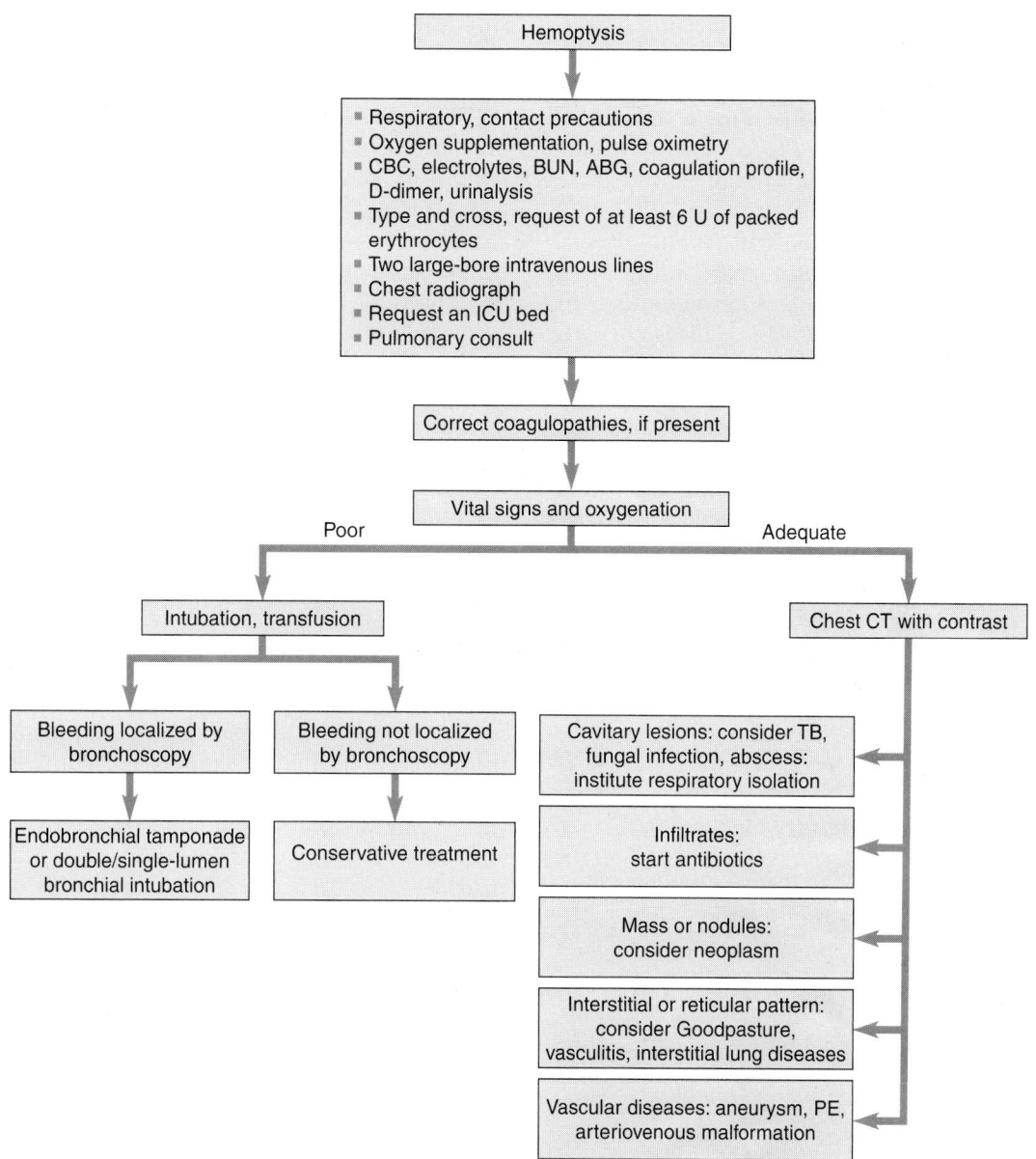

Figure 4-3 *Management of massive hemoptysis.Reproduced with permission from Jean-Baptiste E. Clinical assessment and management of massive hemoptysis.* Crit Care Med *2001;29(5):1098.*

port to induce flow directed embolization has also been described.[15-17]

Unfortunately, blind mainstem intubation is not helpful in these cases as a result of right-sided bleeding. Turning the existing endotracheal tube 180 degrees and turning the head to the right has been reported to improve success with left mainstem intubation. Additionally, if available, fluoroscopy may be used for guidance.[18]

Many patients have a sentinel bleed. These stop spontaneously in 45%, but have a high rate of recurrence; hence, angiographic evaluation for a pseudoaneurysm should be undertaken, even if the initial bleeding was not copious.[15-17] Embolization is the therapy of choice in patients of adequate stability.[17]

Those who are unstable or have evidence of free rupture (hemothorax) will require operative intervention. This is best accomplished via a posterolateral thoracotomy in fifth interspace.[15] Occasionally, direct arterial repair is possible; however, when the lung or lobe has already filled with blood, lobectomy or pneumonectomy is required.[15,17] Temporary occlusion of the pulmonary artery with a loop has been described in two cases, without need for lung resection. This method could be used as a bridge to angiography with potential for lung salvage. Extracorporal support also has been used to decrease pulmonary pressures and result in salvage without resection.[17]

Mortality is of PA catheter induced rupture is 50%. Death typically is caused by hypoxia resulting from blood aspiration, rather than from exsanguination.[15-17]

Tracheo-innominate fistula is a classic cause of massive postsurgical airway bleeding. Similar bleeding can occur after lung resection and lung transplants. Additionally, it has rarely been described with expandable bronchial stents and after thoracic vascular graft erosion.

This condition is very rare, occurring in 0.5 to 5% of tracheostomies. Up to 50% of patients will have a sentinel bleed, which should prompt bronchoscopy. The fistula opening is usually small and located under the anterior tip of the tracheostomy. Hence, the tracheostomy should be backed up over the bronchoscope to evaluate the mucosa.

Initial management of active bleeding is to hyperinflate the tracheostomy cuff and pull anteriorly. If this fails to control bleeding adequately, the patient can be orally intubated and a finger inserted in the tracheostomy stoma can be used to apply pressure to the posterior sternum and compress the innominate artery. The patient will require rapid transportation to the operating room for sternotomy and ligation of the innominate artery. This is the one indication in hemoptysis for sternotomy rather than thoracotomy. Reconstruction of the artery should not be attempted as these repairs invariably become infected. Risk of major neurologic injury with ligation is 10%. Covered stent grafts have been used in very high-risk patients.[13]

LUNG ABSCESS
Epidemiology
Lung abscess is a rare complication seen typically in association with risk of aspiration and periodontal disease. These patients usually present with a prolonged indolent course with cough, fever, malaise, and night sweats. The infection is usually caused by anaerobic bacteria as predicted by the risk factors. The majority of abscess cavities will communicate with the bronchi as evidenced by air/fluid levels in the cavity, and hence will drain spontaneously. Other causes of abscess include necrotizing pneumonia, septic emboli, and cavitation of cancer or tuberculosis.[19]

Preoperative Management
Sputum analysis should be performed to rule out other infections, such as tuberculosis. Usually, a mixture of bacteria will grow, with poor anaerobic culture reliability. Bronchoscopy should be performed for diagnostic purposes as necessary, but not for drainage, as this risks flooding the lung with infected secretions. Prolonged antibiotics, for at least 2 months, will result in successful treatment in 85-90% of patients. Chest radiographs are slow to normalize and should not be considered treatment failure. Failure is more likely in elderly or immunocompromised patients, and for large cavities (> 6 cm), necrotizing pneumonia, and bronchial obstruction.[19]

Operative Management
Failure of antibiotics alone requires improved drainage. Percutaneous drainage rarely causes empyema, bleeding, or bronchopleural fistula, and is the initial method of choice. Percutaneous drainage will be definitive therapy in 70% of antibiotic treatment failures, and can be used to stabilize an ill patient for surgery. Surgery is required in fewer than 10% of patients. It is utilized for failure of medical management and external drainage, for rupture of the abscess with pyothorax, or for concern for bronchogenic cancer-causing obstruction. A double lumen tube is mandatory to prevent spillage of infectious material into the remaining lung. Because of infection at time of resection, there is increased risk of bronchial stump breakdown and bronchopleural fistula; hence, the bronchial stump should be covered with viable tissue, such as a pleural flap. Survival is dependant on the underlying disease.[19]

EMPYEMA THORACIS
Epidemiology
Between 20% and 60% of patients with pneumonia develop pleural effusions. Although these rarely become superinfected, rapid treatment is paramount to prevent complications of empyema. Pleuritic chest pain and fever are common, although steroids may mask these symptoms. Anaerobic infections tend to present with malaise and weight loss and are typically recognized late.[19-21]

Pathophysiology
Empyema most commonly develops as a result of infection of pleural effusions associated with pneumonia, and hence typically has the same bacteriology. Other sources include ruptured lung abscess and mediastinal, esophageal, abdominal, or paravertebral infections with extension of infection. Infection may be introduced by trauma or thoracentesis, or may follow thoracic surgery, particularly if a bronchopleural fistula develops. Subclinical aspiration may present as "spontaneous" empyema. *Staphylococci, Streptococci,* and oral anaerobes are the most common bacterial pathogens.[19-21]

Preoperative Management
Chest radiographs show pleural effusion but give no indication as to whether there is infection. Lateral decubitus films indicate presence of loculations and are more sensitive for small amounts of fluid (< 250 cc). Thoracic ultrasound is helpful for determining loculations and optimal drainage location. The best imaging modality is computed tomography as it allows delineation of the amount of fluid, loculations, underlying pathology, and may indicate infection by enhancement of the pleura.

Small effusions (less than 1 cm thick on decubitus film) typically resolve with only antibiotic therapy of the underlying disease. Larger effusions should be

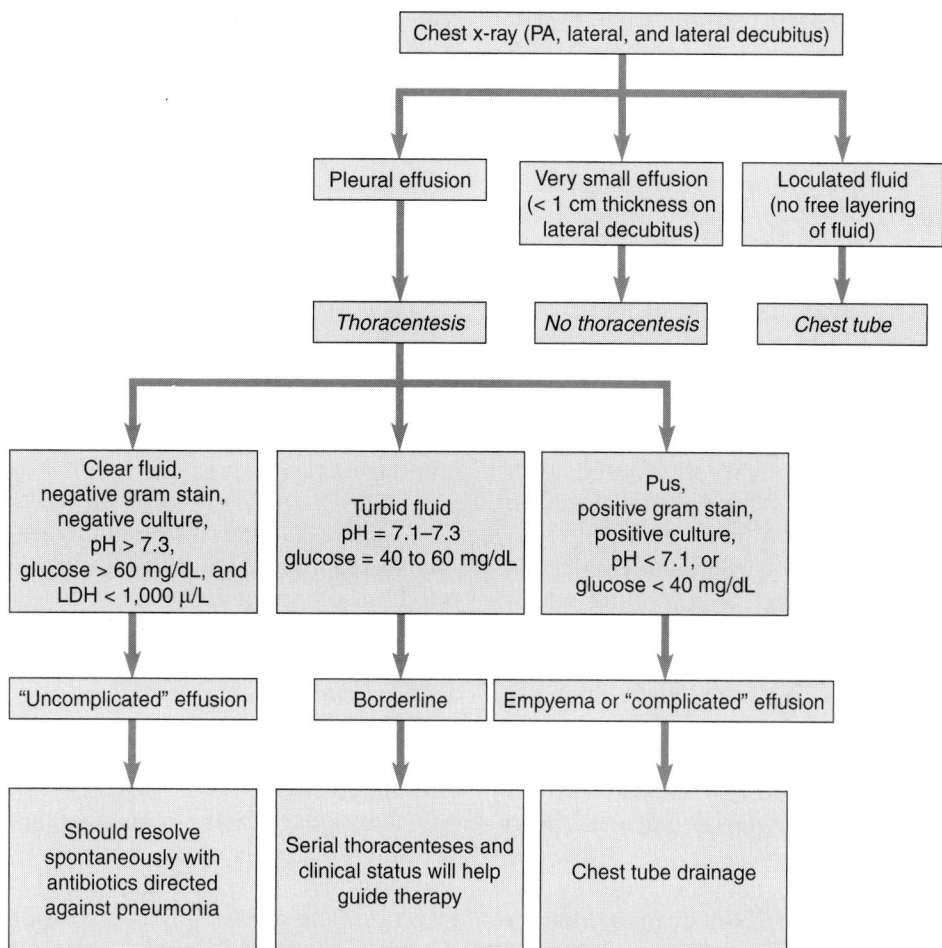

Figure 4-4 *Laboratory data and management of simple and infected pleural effusions. Reproduced with permission from Wiedemann HP, Rice TW.* Lung Abscess and Empyema. Semin Thorac Cardiovasc Surg *1995;7(2):119-128.*

aspirated, both for diagnostic purposes and to remove the potential infection developing or progressing, which can occur rapidly. Fluid obtained should be examined for infection. Purulent fluid or positive Gram stain/culture necessitates adequate drainage. Otherwise, fluid is sent for pH, lactic dehydrogenase and glucose (Fig. 4-4) to determine likelihood of infection.[19,20]

Operative Management

Management of empyema requires drainage of the purulent fluid and expansion of the lung. Antibiotic coverage for the underlying disease and nutritional support are important adjuncts. The optimal method of thoracic control depends on the stage of the empyema.

Early empyema, or exudative phase, is characterized by thin, free-flowing fluid. This is easily drained by thoracostomy tube, or occasionally by repeated thoracentesis. At this point, the lung readily expands to fill the thoracic cavity. Even thick pus can usually be drained completely, sometimes assisted with irrigation through the thoracostomy tube.

In the fibrino-purulent phase, the empyema fluid becomes thick and loculations begin to form. Drainage is more difficult by thoracostomy tube as a result of loculations, and multiple radiographically directed catheters may be needed. If more than two drainage catheters are required, success of complete drainage is unlikely and surgery should be considered. Closed suction drainage should be used whenever possible to assist with lung reexpansion to obliterate the empyema cavity and prevent reaccumulation. Closed suction drainage in the exudative and fibrino-purulent phase is successful in about 75% of patients. Prolonged drainage may be necessary to prevent reaccumulation. As the lung becomes adherent to the thoracic wall, the tube can be converted to open drainage ("empyema tube") and gradually backed out. This can be done on an outpatient basis if the patient is otherwise well.[19-21]

Lytic agents (particularly streptokinase) have shown up to an 80% success rates in assisting in the drainage of loculated collections. These can be injected into the thoracostomy tube and left in place for 6-8 hrs, repeated daily for up to 1 week. Systemic fevers and chest pain may be associated with streptokinase administration. Failure of rapid complete drainage necessitates surgical intervention, as discussed later, before development of a fibrous peel.[19,20]

The final phase of empyema, organization, develops over 4-6 weeks. Uniformly, surgical management is required, as the fibrous pleural peel prevents lung reexpansion. Hence, decortication with removal of the infected material and the fibrous rind is necessary. This can be done with VATS in about 60% of patients. VATS tends to be more successful earlier in the course and is being used more often in the fibrino-proliferative phase to completely evacuate the chest and remove loculations. Other patients will require a thoracotomy for full removal of the empyema peel. Careful technique is needed for both VATS and thoracotomy to minimized bleeding and lung injury which will result in air leak. In areas of thin, densely adherent peel, cross-hatch cuts may be sufficient to allow lung expansion without removal of the fibrous tissue. The lung must be fully decorticated to allow lung expansion, as well as diaphragm and mediastinal mobility. Inability to fully obliterate the cavity will result in reaccumulation. In these rare cases, thoracoplasty, muscle flap rotation, or Eloesser flap (inferiorly-based flap with the skin marsupialized to the parietal pleura) with open drainage may become necessary.

In patients unable to tolerate thoracotomy, rib resection with dependant open drainage or Eloesser flap creation should be considered, at least as a method to stabilize sepsis and permit future definitive operation. These procedures are possible only for chronic mature empyema with thick well-developed cavities and adherent lung; otherwise, an open pneumothorax is created. Local anesthetic only may be used in rib resection if the patient is sufficiently ill to prevent general anesthetic.[19-21]

Outcome
Mortality of patients with empyema has decreased dramatically with antibiotic therapy, and is usually related to the underlying disease and degree of disability. Overall, mortality is about 4.3%.[21]

Special Topics
Empyema necessitans is a thoracic empyema that drains spontaneously to the skin. These cases require management of the intrathoracic component, as well as soft tissue infection present. Rib resection is typically necessary and may require serial debridement of necrotic soft tissue as well as ribs involved with osteomyelitis. Formal decortication is usually not necessary, or should be delayed until the patient's overall condition is stabilized.

Tuberculous empyema has become uncommon with the declining rates of tuberculosis; however, it may still be seen in immigrants from other countries and in immunocompromised patients. These patients usually present with chronic illness rather than septic complications. Drainage is contraindicated as failure of healing is the norm and a chronic draining wound will develop. Additionally, because of calcification associated with this disease process, decortication is extremely difficult and fraught with complications. Long-term antimicrobial therapy is the treatment of choice.[20]

ESOPHAGUS

ESOPHAGEAL PERFORATION
Epidemiology
Although diagnostic endoscopy has a very low risk of esophageal perforation (0.03%), it is such a common procedure that it has become the most common cause of esophageal perforation (33-75%). The risk is increased with therapeutic maneuvers such as dilation, injection, and stenting (0.9-6%). Foreign bodies (7-14%), trauma, and pill ulcers may result in perforation. Operative procedures in the neck, mediastinum, and at the diaphragmatic hiatus may also result in iatrogenic perforation.[22-24]

Pathophysiology
As the esophagus has no enveloping serosal layer, it perforates relatively easily. Additionally, the loose surrounding alveolar tissues allow rapid dissemination of infection, and a relatively poor blood supply worsens the sequelae of injury.

Patients typically present with immediate pain localized to the area of the perforation. Fever and subcutaneous and/or mediastinal air follow commonly. As symptoms are nonspecific, delays in diagnosis are common. Air is palpable in 60% and radiographically visible in 95% from cervical perforations and palpable in 30% and radiographically visible in 40% of thoracic perforations. Occasionally, mediastinal air can be heard via stethoscope as "Hamman crunch." Pleural effusions are seen in 50% of patients with thoracic perforations. These will have high amylase content and lead to respiratory symptoms and empyema.[22-24]

Preoperative Management
History and physical exam is usually nonspecific, but imaging is diagnostic. Chest radiograph shows nonspecific signs in 90% of patients, usually mediastinal air (60%) or pleural effusion (50%). Water-soluble contrast swallow is the initial study of choice (barium will deposit in the mediastinum), but negative studies should be followed with a barium swallow as it provides better coating and is more sensitive for smaller leaks. In cases of suspected tracheo-esophageal fistula, barium should be used as water-soluble contrast causes severe pneumonitis.[22,23] Swallow studies have a 10% false negative rate.[23] Computed tomography studies can provide additional data if a leak has already sealed, is difficult to locate, or if a swallow study is not possible.[22,24]

In cases with very high index of suspicion, endoscopy can be performed if other tests are negative, but must be done with extreme care and minimal insufflation. Thoracentesis is sometimes diagnostic if low pH, high amylase, or food particles are found.[23,24]

Definitive Management

Therapy is controversial and depends on the initial pathology, time to diagnosis, and the degree of injury and leak. Regardless, delays in diagnosis and treatment result in great increases in morbidity and mortality.[22,24]

Nonoperative management can be considered in patients with minimal symptoms, no septic findings, and partial thickness or small contained tears. Patients with perforated malignancy, intra-abdominal perforation or obstruction distal to the perforation are not candidates for nonoperative management. Generally, cervical injuries are better tolerated than thoracic injuries as infection is more contained and easier to drain. Patients should receive broad-spectrum antibiotics, parenteral nutrition, and oral and nasoesophageal suction. This management should continue until follow-up contrast studies show resolution of the injury—usually about 2 weeks. At this time, liquid diet can begin. Contained ruptures that drain well into the esophagus are also able to have liquids, but should not have solids until this cavity resolves. Clinical deterioration or failure to improve will require surgical intervention and occurs in about 20% of nonoperatively managed patients.[22,24]

Operative Managment

Surgery remains the gold standard of therapy and should be used for any patient with large or uncontained perforations and any patients with sepsis or shock. Cervical perforations are managed via a left sternocleidomastoid incision. Upper and mid-esophageal perforations are managed via a 4th-5th interspace posterolateral right thoracotomy and distal perforations via a 6th-7th interspace posterolateral left thoracotomy.[22,24]

Occasionally, perforation is recognized immediately, as may be the case with endoscopic injury. These patients can be taken immediately to the operating room. If no contamination is found, a primary repair can be carried out over a large bougie. This requires a longitudinal myotomy to expose the entire mucosal defect. Mucosa should be closed carefully. The muscle layer is then closed and the repair buttressed with healthy surrounding tissue, such as a pleural or thoracic muscle flap. Despite careful repair, leak rates range from 25 to 50%; hence, drainage with closed suction drains or chest tubes must be provided (Fig. 4-5).[24]

Patients with preexisting esophageal pathology must have this managed concurrently or the repair is certain to fail. Resection of distal malignancy, treatment of strictures, or antireflux procedures may be necessary. Esophagectomy with primary reconstruction may be undertaken if early diagnosis of the perforation and minimal contamination has occurred. Transhiatal esophagectomy is preferred for cases of

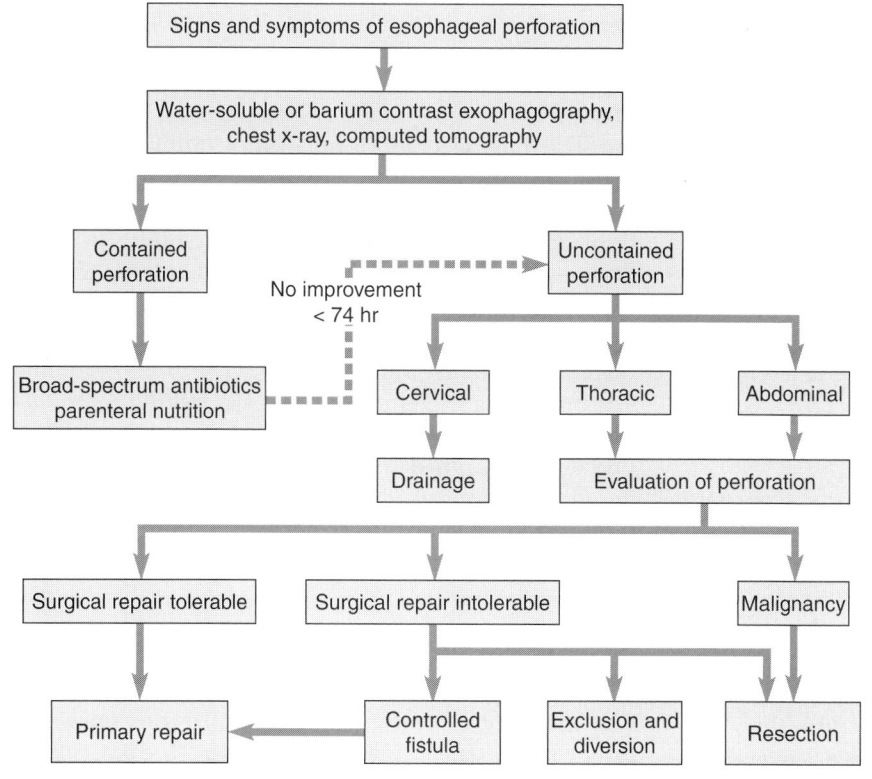

Figure 4-5 *Management of esophageal perforation. Reproduced with permission from Brinster CJ, Singhal S, Lee L, Marshall MB, Kaiser LR, Kucharczuk JC. Evolving options in the management of esophageal perforation.* Ann Thorac Surg *2004;77(4): 1475-1483.*

minimal thoracic contamination or in cervical perforations, as this allows the anastomosis to be cervical and, hence, clear of a potentially infected thoracic region. Transthoracic esophagectomy is preferred if decortication or additional drainage of the thoracic space is needed. Primary intrathoracic anastomosis has been successful in a small series of such patients. All patients should not be fed by mouth until a swallow study in 5-7 days confirms success of the repair.[22-24]

With extensive contamination and inflammation, repair is not safe and frequently not technically feasible. Repair and drainage will be adequate for cervical perforations if there is no mediastinal extension of infection. Thoracic perforations have a high risk of sepsis and hence are managed with esophageal control and drainage. Closure of the perforation with proximal and distal division, a proximal cervical or thoracic esophagostomy, wide drainage, and a gastrostomy is the most conservative method. The excluded segment of the esophagus must be drained or resected. Use of absorbable ligature to close the distal esophagus has been described to allow automatic future recannulation. Future reconstruction is required, either by reversal of the esophagostomy if there is distal continuity, or by resection and interposition of some type. Placement of a large T-tube in the defect to create a controlled fistula is also an option if the opening is small and there is not extensive contamination.[22,24]

Covered esophageal stents and esophageal closure with endoscopic clips have been described in patients who were not surgical candidates as a result of comorbidities. Although some successes have been reported, these new technologies have not been evaluated in any extensive fashion and cannot be currently recommended as optimal management.[23]

Postoperative Management

Outcome is dependant on the initial disease and presenting physiology. Patients managed nonoperatively have a mortality of 0-33%, although this is clearly a highly select group of patients. Those with iatrogenic perforations have 5-26% mortality. Cervical perforations have a 0-14% mortality compared to 13-59% for thoracic perforations.[23] Mortality for surgically managed patients ranges from 0 to 30% when treatment was within 24 hours to 26-64% for treatment later than 24 hours.[23,24]

Special Topics

Caustic ingestion represents an important subcategory of esophageal perforation. Acid and alkali ingestions are treated similarly, although alkali typically causes deeper injury as a result of coagulative necrosis. Attempts at neutralization are contraindicated as a result of heat production, and induction of emesis should not be undertaken, as it will increase the exposure. Nasogastric drainage is also contraindicated, as it may induce emesis or aspiration. The airway should be evaluated early, as edema is common and rapidly progressive. If edema is present, there should be strong consideration for urgent tracheostomy. A history of the amount and type of ingestant will help guide therapy.

Chest and abdominal radiographs should be obtained to look for free air indicating perforation, as well as consideration for computed tomography as it is more sensitive. Patients with free air, shock, or peritonitis require immediate operative intervention. The remainder should undergo careful, gentle endoscopic evaluation with a small caliber endoscope.

Ingestion injury is graded like surface burns. Patients with first and superficial second-degree burns will be unlikely to have complications and can start diet in 24 hours. Deep second-degree burns develop strictures in 70% and should be monitored for about 48 hours before starting diet. Third-degree burns progress to perforation in 25% and stricture in 90%. All high-grade burns should have serial barium swallows after discharge. There are no known techniques for preventing stricture. Operative management is as previously described, although nearly all patients will require resection of a large portion of the esophagus as a result of liquefactive necrosis. The stomach is often also affected and requires partial or total resection. Feeding access should be provided and a second look should be planned to assess for progression of necrosis (Fig. 4-6).[23,25]

Achalasia dilation perforation is usually recognized quickly. Primary repair of these tears should be performed, but the patient will also require a myotomy of the contralateral side of the esophagus, both to treat the disease process and prevent strain on the repair.[22]

Boerhaave syndrome, or postemetic rupture of the esophagus, has become a rare cause of esophageal perforation (7-19%). It is usually seen after severe retching (75%) or sudden severe increase in intra-abdominal pressure. It is most often associated with alcohol use but also has been reported in any number of other conditions including pregnancy. Up to 25% are in shock at presentation. Diagnosis is often delayed as the signs and symptoms frequently mimic multiple other diseases, such as pancreatitis, peptic ulcer disease, myocardial infarction, and aortic dissection.

The majority of Boerhaave ruptures occur in the distal esophagus and present with pneumomediastinum and left pleural effusion. Computed tomography is frequently needed to eliminate other disease processes. Surgical management is as previously described; however, contamination is usually extensive caused by high intra-abdominal pressure driving gastric contents into the chest and delay in presentation and diagnosis.[22,23]

ESOPHAGEAL FOREIGN BODIES
Epidemiology

The majority of swallowed material passes uneventfully through the upper digestive tract. Even so, nearly

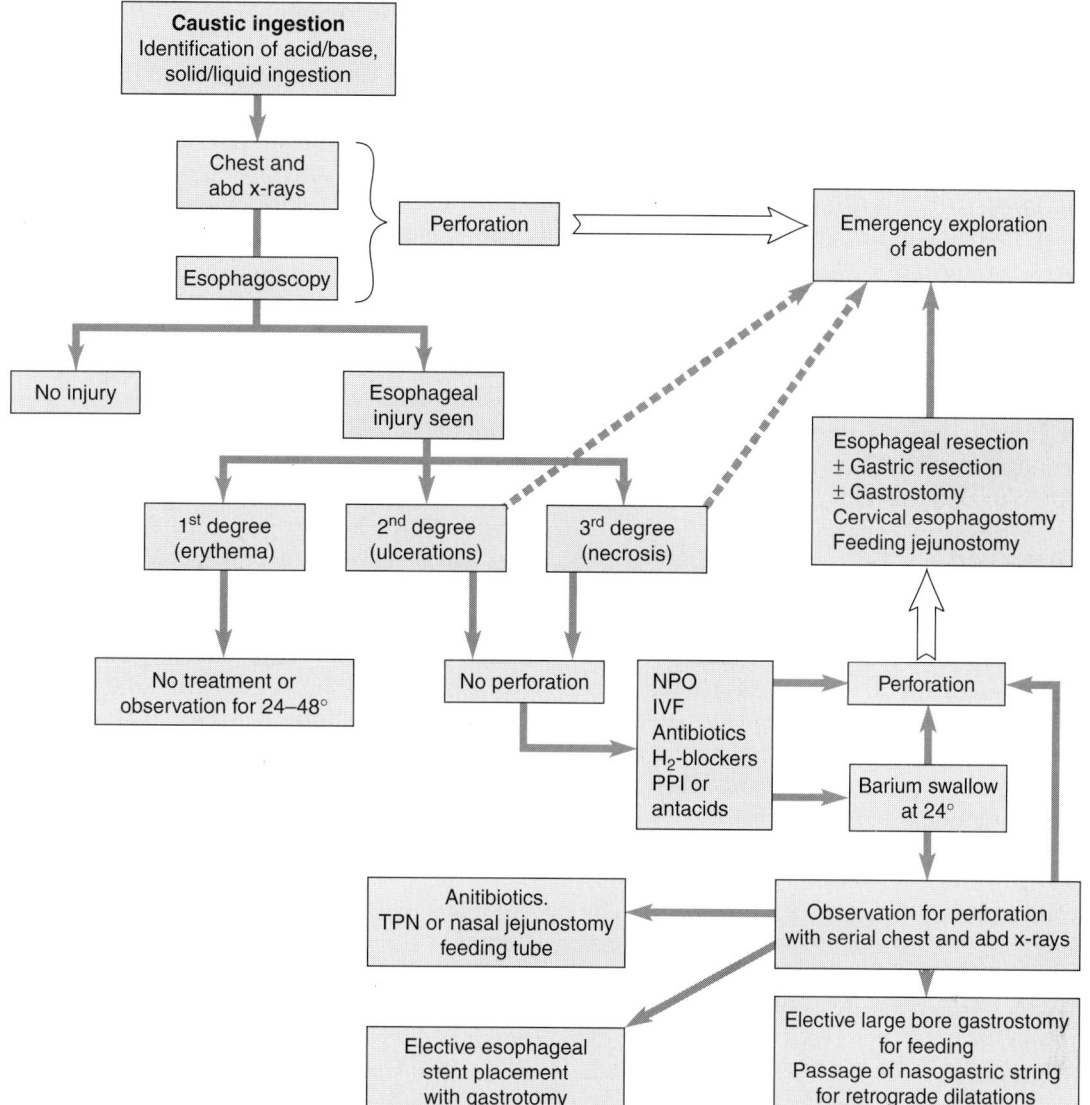

Figure 4-6 *Management of caustic ingestion. Reproduced with permission from Zwischenberger JB, Savage C, Bidani A. Surgical aspects of esophageal disease: perforation and caustic injury.* Am J Respir Crit Care Med *2002;165(8):1037-1040.*

1500 patients die yearly from GI foreign bodies. Risk factors are young age (3 mo to 6 yrs), psychiatric disease, esophageal pathology and dental abnormalities (dentures, bridges, or edentulousness). The common obstruction items are food (34-59%) and bones (16-18%). Other items such as coins (66% of childhood foreign bodies), pills, dental plates, and batteries account for most of the remainder.[23]

Impaction of items usually occurs at areas of esophageal narrowing. These normally occur at the cricopharyngeus muscle (23-36% of impactions) and at the aortic arch, left mainstem bronchus, and lower esophageal sphincter (38-53%). Patients with cardiac enlargement from congestive heart failure will also have esophageal narrowing at the left atrium.[23,26]

Patients present with dysphagia, odynophagia, and chest pain. With complete obstruction, patients will spit or drool because of an inability to swallow saliva.

Associated airway obstruction occurs in 5% resulting in stridor and cough.[23]

Preoperative Management
Localization of the object requires lateral and antero-posterior radiographs of the neck or chest. Usually the foreign body is radio-opaque and is easily located. Computed tomography scanning is helpful in delineating nonopaque items. Patients with symptoms but no findings on imaging should undergo endoscopy. Swallow studies are generally not indicated, as there is significant risk of aspiration and barium obscures endoscopic visualization.[23]

All sharp or obstruction objects should be removed promptly to avoid risk of perforation (15-35%). Retrieval is usually possible with a flexible endoscope, using care to avoid injury to the esophagus while pulling out the object. Baskets, overtubes, and vacuum adapters have been used to protect the esophageal wall. A rare but catastrophic complication is the erosion or penetration of a foreign body into the aorta if lodged at the aortic arch. This frequently presents with a herald bleed and required rapid diagnosis and operative intervention.[23] Button batteries should also be removed promptly, as they can cause alkaline injury to the esophagus. If already in the stomach, they may be allowed to pass if they do not contain mercury.

Administration of glucagon has been demonstrated to relax the lower esophageal sphincter which may allow passage of the object into the stomach. Failure to pass within 12 hrs necessitates endoscopy for removal to prevent ischemic pressure necrosis of the mucosa. Surgery is required in only about 1% of patients, either for failure of removal of the item or for perforation.[23,26]

ESOPHAGEAL BLEEDING
Epidemiology
Upper gastrointestinal (UGI) bleeding is quite common but bleeding as a result of esophageal causes much less so. Esophageal varices and Mallory-Weiss tears are the third and fourth most common causes of UGI bleeding.

Esophageal varices are found in patients with portal hypertension, especially cirrhotics. Hence, this population is usually of middle age with a history of hepatitis or alcohol use. This bleeding is typically brisk and melena or hematochezia is common. Dilated portosystemic vessels are present in many areas of the body in portal hypertension, but those in the distal esophagus are the most prone to bleeding.

Mallory-Weiss tears are usually seen in men (3-6 times male predominance) in the third to fifth decade. Alcohol (31-80%) and aspirin use are common. Hiatal hernia is also commonly seen in this population (17-52%). Classic presentation is hematemesis following vomiting or retching, but may occur in any process causing rapid increases in intraabdominal pressure. Mucosal tears occur at the GE junction or gastric cardia, most within 2 cm of the GE junction. Melena is the chief complaint in 4-10% and shock from massive bleeding is present in 5-10%. Other concurrent lesions are frequently seen, and the Mallory-Weiss tear is felt to be responsible for the bleeding in 50%.[22,27]

Preoperative Management
Resuscitation, correction of coagulopathy, and maintenance of normothermia are critical to the management of any bleeding. H_2 blockers are effective with reduction of rebleeding by 10%, decreasing the need for emergency surgery by 20% and reduction of the death rate by 30%. Nasogastric lavage can confirm a source proximal to the duodenum and allow clearance of blood.

Endoscopy is diagnostic in 90% of UGI bleeding, and may be therapeutic. If no bleeding source is found, nasal or pulmonary bleeding should be evaluated. Also, angiography or nuclear bleeding scans can be helpful.[28]

Definitive Management
Esophageal Varices
Management of esophageal varices and Mallory-Weis tear vary considerably. Several modalities exist to control variceal bleeding; all have been shown to have the same long-term outcome. Up to 72% of esophageal varices will stop bleeding spontaneously with resuscitation and transfusion of plasma. Vasopressin has been utilized to decrease portal pressures. It has the same efficacy and fewer side effects when given intravenously rather than by catheter-directed infusion into the celiac or superior mesenteric artery. Control of bleeding with vasopressin occurs in 44-71% of cases, with decreased bleeding in additional patients. Addition of nitroglycerine results in decreased coronary vasoconstriction, and also causes decreased portal flow. Terlipressin (vasopressin analogue with long half-life) and somatostatin have been used successfully in several studies as well.

Balloon tamponade with a Minnesota or Sengstaken-Blakemore tube has equivalent efficacy to vasopressin and either may be used with failure of the other. Severe complications of balloon tamponade include esophageal perforation, aspiration, and airway obstruction. Intubation is recommended for all of these patients. Additionally, rebleeding occurs on deflation in 27-45% of cases.

Percutaneous portal access and embolization of coronary or short gastric veins is successful in up to 80%, but has a rebleeding rate of 35-65% and a morbidity of 21-52% as a result of portal vein thrombosis. Hence, it not often used and is a temporizing measure but may be considered in concert with percutaneous portocaval shunting.

As these methods tend to have a high failure rate, they are considered temporizing and endoscopic control is the treatment of choice. Endoscopic sclerotherapy seems to have the best success, especially for advanced cirrhosis. A single intervention stops bleeding in 70% and, with rebleeding, a second intervention stops 90%. Repeat sclerotherapy is recommended for any subsequent bleeding episodes as well. Sclerotherapy has been shown to have equal short- and long-term efficacy to portacaval shunting. Risks include stricture (0-12%), perforation (0-5%), and aspiration (2-14%.)

Operative Management
Surgical therapy for variceal bleeding has extremely poor outcomes. Portacaval shunting is optimally performed by interventional radiology as it is considerably less invasive. When done as a surgical emergency, survival is dismal, as it is for Child C cirrhosis. It should be reserved for lesser degrees of cirrhosis and done in stable patients. Regardless of the approach, morbidity, particularly encephalopathy, is high. Lastly, a salvage operative technique of esophageal devascularization can be carried out utilizing an end-to-end anastomosis (EEA) stapler. The EEA, with the anvil

attached, is introduced via a small gastrotomy and the esophagus is cinched around the stem of the anvil. When the stapler is fired, a small segmental resection of the distal esophagus results in interruption of the variceal vessels. Pyloric drainage procedures must be considered because of interruption of the vagal nerves. Although the success for bleeding control is high (87-100%), mortality is nearly as high (73-100%) and, therefore, this procedure is not generally recommended.[28]

Mallory-Weis Tear

Therapy for patients with Mallory-Weis tear is supportive initially, as 90% will stop bleeding without specific therapy. Those bleeding at time of endoscopy are less likely to stop spontaneously and should have endoscopic therapy. Patients with portal hypertension are more likely to have ongoing bleeding (88% vs 27%) and 38% will develop a second tear over the next 17-month period. Injection or cautery by endoscopy will control most active bleeding. Angiographic vasopressin or embolization are options as well, particularly in patients who are poor surgical candidates. Use of a Sengstaken-Blakemore tube is contraindicated because of the association of Mallory-Weiss tears with hiatal hernia. Pressure necrosis or extension of the tear could result. The rebleeding rate is low if no active bleeding is seen at endoscopy (0-2% vs. 8-15% with active bleeding). Lesions typically heal in 2-3 days. Surgery, when needed, requires oversewing of the bleeding tear via gastrotomy.[22,27]

Outcome

The overall mortality for UGI bleed is low (10%), but it is based on initial disease, general medical condition, and age. Mortality increases with risk factors including age (13.4% for age greater than 60 years vs 8.7% for younger patients), cirrhosis, organ failure, shock, rebleeding, and development of bleeding while hospitalized for other reasons (4-5 times increased mortality, 23-64%). Because of these factors, and because surgery is reserved for failure of medical management, mortality for surgical intervention ranges from 14 to 45%.

Survival from variceal bleeding is based on the degree of liver disease (Child's A 53%, B 38%, C 21% over 1 yr). Up to 42% will die in 6 months, as a result of bleeding in the majority (60%). Morality during the hospitalization is 30-50%.[28]

Special Topics

Intramural tears of the esophagus are long, submucosal hematomas associated with increased intraluminal pressure, usually caused by vomiting. These present with hematemesis and chest pain. Management is supportive; these spontaneously stop bleeding and heal well.[22]

Esophagitis is a rare cause of UGI bleeding. Surgery is almost never needed, but, if so, an antireflux procedure is usually adequate to control bleeding.[22,27]

HEART

Cardiac emergencies are mostly the domain of the cardiothoracic surgeon and require bypass for management. Cardiac trauma is also not discussed in this chapter. One cardiac disease process that can be managed by emergency general surgeons is pericardial effusion.

PERICARDIAL EFFUSION
Epidemiology

The pericardium normally contains a small amount of fluid that acts as a lubricant. It is drained by the right lymphatic and thoracic ducts. Any injury to the pericardium results in production of more pericardial exudative fluid as well as fibrin deposition. Causes of this response are numerous, including myocardial infarction, malignancy, infection, renal or heart failure, inflammatory and autoimmune disorders, and infection.[29] Congestive heart failure or profoundly low serum albumin may result in a transudative pericardial effusion with a low protein content. Bloody effusions are seen with trauma, malignancy, and coagulopathies.[30]

Slow accumulation of an effusion usually does not result in any symptoms as there is gradual stretching of the pericardium. If symptoms are experienced, they are usually related to compression of surrounding structures. Rapid accumulation may lead to tamponade physiology even with only small additional volumes.[29] Thickening of the pericardium results in constrictive pericarditis or obliteration of the pericardial space. In these cases, very small amounts of fluid may cause tamponade physiology due to indistensibility of the pericardium.[30]

Echocardiography is the best technique for diagnosis and evaluation of pericardial effusion. It is portable and hence can be used at bedside, as it is very sensitive and specific and can determine early signs of tamponade physiology. Computed tomography can show small effusions (50 cc) and can help determine etiology based on fluid density. It is a relatively poor modality for determination of hemopericardium because of the high density of the fluid. MRI is also highly sensitive and specific, but it is limited to the acuity of patients who can be evaluated. Neither radiographic test provides information about cardiac physiology.[29]

Preoperative Management

For stable patients, management of the underlying disease is the priority. Drainage is only undertaken if the cause is in question. Pericardiocentesis is a generally safe procedure and provides excellent drainage if there is not clotted blood in the pericardium. The pericardium is approached at a 45-degree angle toward the right shoulder via a subxiphoid puncture with ultrasound or ECG monitoring. Risks include ventricular puncture, arrhythmia, and pneumothorax. The fluid can be evaluated for malignancy by cytology, which is diagnostic in 87%. Recurrence after drainage is about 50%, which then requires a more aggressive approach. Catheter placement with intermittent drainage can act as a temporizing procedure and may be accomplished with a standard central line kit. Sclerosants can be instilled into the pericardial cavity, similar to pleurodesis. Many different agents have been utilized, usually with tumoricidal activity. Success rate varies but is about 80% overall.[29]

Definitive pericardial drainage can be obtained by pericardial window, either percutaneously or by surgery. Percutaneous balloon pericardotomy is performed in the catheterization lab and utilizes a balloon catheter passed under fluoroscopic guidance. A hole is created in the pericardium allowing decompression into the thorax. Success for this procedure is 92% with few complications, although mortality is high, likely because of associated malignancy and debility precluding an operative approach. [29]

Operative Management

Surgery is clearly more invasive and, hence, associated with increased morbidity. Additionally, not all patients can tolerate anesthesia. Surgical drainage has the advantage of allowing pericardial biopsy, which is sometimes needed for diagnosis. Failure of other methods of control also necessitates surgical drainage. Subxiphoid pericardial window is sufficient in 90% of surgical patients, and may be done with local anesthesia if necessary. Continuing drainage utilizing a soft mediastinal tube is optimal, while treating the underlying cause. Drainage into the abdomen by incision of the central tendon of the diaphragm is also an option, but it should not be done in the presence of a malignancy, and usually will seal over time. Left fourth interspace anterolateral thoracotomy is can also be utilized with creation of a pericardial window into the pleural cavity. Intraoperative mortality is 1.7% and recurrence is low (4-11%). Pericardectomy is necessary for failure of regular pericardial window drainage.[29,30]

Special Topics

Pericardial tamponade occurs when accumulated pericardial fluid is under sufficient pressure to inhibit cardiac function. This most often occurs with rapid collection of small amounts of fluid, usually a result of trauma or postoperatively. Pressures rise in the pericardium resulting in left atrial or ventricular compression and lack of filling. This can be seen during hemodynamic monitoring when the central venous pressure approaches the pulmonary artery wedge pressure. Clinically, patients have tachycardia, hypotension, distended jugular veins, and pulsus paradoxus. The full Beck triad of muffled heart sounds, hypotension, and jugular venous distension is rare (15-30%). On echocardiogram, chamber collapse is an indicator of tamponade, although this may also be seen with hypovolemia.

Aggressive volume resuscitation can support these patients until emergent drainage is undertaken.[29]

CHEST WALL

Chest wall emergencies are mainly caused by infection and traumatic injury, which will not be discussed in this chapter. In general, infections of the chest wall are managed no differently than anywhere else on the body. Empyema necessitans is mentioned specifically previously. Additional comments are necessary regarding breast abscess.

EPIDEMIOLOGY

Puerperal Breast Abscess

Puerperal breast abscesses are found in young women in the peripartum period. These are located in the peripheral breast tissue and are usually caused by *Staphylococcus aureus*. Blockage of lacrimal ducts and bacterial overgrowth are felt to be responsible.

These patients typically present with tenderness, fever, and tachycardia. Fluctuance is not always palpable. For small, localized abscesses without systemic effects and minimal cellulites, needle aspiration can be considered, although it must be repeated frequently. For larger abscesses or any patients with systemic findings, incision and drainage should be undertaken. Depending on the size of the abscess, this may require general anesthesia. All loculations should be broken down and a biopsy of the cavity wall should be obtained to evaluate for breast cancer, although it is uncommon in this population. Options for management of the cavity include open packing, cavity obliteration, and dependant drain placement with closure of the cavity. Packing is the most conservative option and patients usually heal quickly.

Lactation can be continued throughout treatment and decompression of the breast by nursing or pumping is encouraged as it assists with drainage of the ductal system. The baby is at no risk from the bacteria.[31]

Duct Ectasia Breast Abscess

Duct ectasia breast abscess occurs most commonly in women over the age of 40. It is generally periareolar and is associated with other nipple abnormalities such as discharge or inversion. Bacteriology is variable including *Staphylococci*, *Streptococci*, *Bacteroides,* and *Enterococci.* Anaerobic and aerobic mixed infections are common. The pathophysiology of these abscesses is believed to be ductal ectasia with periductal mastitis.

Therapy for these patients is incision and drainage and antibiotic treatment. Given the age group, breast cancer is relatively more likely and biopsy tissue should be taken, either at the time of initial drainage or at subsequent surgery. These abscesses commonly recur and usually will require subareolar dissection and ductal system excision for cure. This should be done after the initial infectious process has resolved. For small abscesses without systemic symptoms, needle aspiration may be considered, although this may require repeated aspirations.[31]

DIAPHRAGM

PARAESOPHAGEAL HERNIA
Epidemiology
Paraesophageal diaphragmatic hernias are common but rarely present with acute symptoms requiring emergency intervention. Paraesophageal hernias represent only 3-15% of hiatal hernias. They are commonly seen in patients in their 70s and 80s with multiple comorbidities.

Pathophysiology
Dilation of the diaphragmatic opening and laxity of the gastrosplenic and gastrocolic ligaments results in upward displacement of the gastroesophageal junction. This may occur with (type III combined) or without (type I sliding) herniation of the greater curvature. Fixation of the gastroesophageal junction and rotation of the greater curvature of the stomach up into the left hemithorax (type II paraesophageal) may also uncommonly result in gastric volvulus with ischemia. Mucosal trauma from sliding of the stomach is common and results in bleeding (Fig. 4-7).

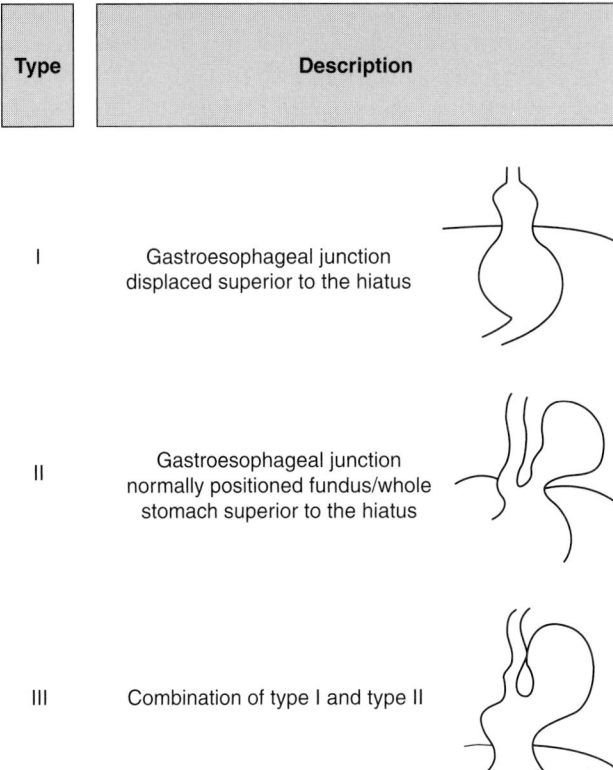

Type	Description
I	Gastroesophageal junction displaced superior to the hiatus
II	Gastroesophageal junction normally positioned fundus/whole stomach superior to the hiatus
III	Combination of type I and type II

Figure 4-7 *Types of hiatal hernia.*
Reproduced with permission from Stylopoulos N, Rattner DW. Paraesophageal hernia: when to operate? Adv Surg 2003;37:213-229.

The majority of patients report minor symptoms such as postprandial chest pain and reflux. Patients with known paraesophageal hernias who develop changes in symptoms, particularly constant chest pain, inability to vomit, or bleeding, require immediate evaluation. These patients should be assumed to have volvulus, incarceration, strangulation, or gastric outlet obstruction.

Operative Management
Chest radiographs are typically enough for diagnosis in patients with known hernia. Others may require either computed tomography or barium study to further delineate their hernia. Upper endoscopy can be helpful if the diagnosis is still in doubt. If a nasogastric tube can be passed, the stomach will usually decompress and the operative intervention can be done urgently rather than emergently.

In deteriorating patients or in those in whom the stomach cannot be decompressed, emergent operative therapy is needed. Further evaluation for reflux and manometry is usually not needed as correction of the mechanical problem (herniation) will resolve the symptoms. Failure to operate with gastric ischemia from either strangulation or volvulus results in gastric rupture into the chest and is frequently lethal.

Definitive Management
Surgical repair is the only certain method of correcting paraesophageal hernia. In extremely high-risk patients, percutaneous endoscopic gastrostomy has been used as a tacking method to keep the stomach intra-abdominal. Definitive operative repair may be performed via a transthoracic, transabdominal, or laparoscopic approach. Repair by laparotomy is most common. Regardless of the approach, several steps must be completed. The stomach is reduced into the abdomen, and the hernia sac is excised.

The diaphragmatic defect must then be closed. In some cases, direct suture of the diaphragmatic crura is possible. In the majority, however, these do not hold suture because of attenuation of the muscle. Additionally, the distance between them may result in unacceptable tension on the repair. In this case, mesh prosthesis, usually a polytetrafluoroethylene patch, is utilized to bridge the gap. Polypropylene may also be used; however, adhesions will form. Although these prevent recurrent herniation, they may also result in gastric or esophageal injury. Several series indicated lower recurrence rates with mesh than with direct closure. Another option is direct crural approximation with a relaxing incision in the diaphragm, which is then repaired with mesh. This prevents mesh placement adjacent to the esophagus and the associated potential of esophageal injury.

Lastly, the stomach must be secured to prevent reherniation. This may be accomplished by an antireflux procedure or gastrostomy tube placement. Generally, both are optimal. Because of the degree of dissection needed in these cases, patients usually require an antireflux procedure. An incomplete wrap is recommended in any patient who did not have preoperative manometry. The gastrostomy tube has low added morbidity and can be used for feeding as well. When patients have a shortened esophagus (less than 2.5 cm intra-abdominal length after mobilization), a lengthening procedure, such as a Collis gastroplasty, is necessary.

Postoperative Management

The mortality for emergency surgery of paraesophageal hernias is about 17% (0-40%), with complications occurring in 72% (life-threatening in 3.6%). In elective surgery, mortality is about 2% and morbidity is about 20%.[32]

Special Topics

Rare adult diaphragmatic hernias are uncommon but frequently present as emergencies. The majority of these are delayed presentations of posttraumatic diaphragmatic injuries. Extremely uncommonly, congenital lesions may not present until adulthood. Congenital diaphragmatic hernias (CDH) are found in about 1/2000-1/5000 births and two-thirds of these die before or at delivery. Up to 90% of the remainder are diagnosed and repaired in the first year of life. These rare entities account for less than 1% of diaphragmatic hernias treated in adulthood.[33,34]

Congenital hernias are caused by failure of fusion of the diaphragm during development. *Morgagni* hernias are located anteriorly parasternally and are typically right sided (90%). These are usually diagnosed incidentally on radiographs for other reasons and are often misdiagnosed. Symptoms are uncommon, and incarceration is rare. The majority of these will have a hernia sac. *Bochdaleck* hernias occur in the posterolateral diaphragm and are typically left sided (80%). Although occasionally found incidentally, most of these hernias are diagnosed as a result of symptoms from incarceration, particularly of the stomach, spleen, and colon. In addition to obstructive symptoms, respiratory compromise is common. Gastric and splenic volvulus also have been reported. A hernia sac is present in only 10-20%. Although these hernias may present at any time, the most common presentation is in the postpartum period, likely as a result of increased intra-abdominal pressures (Fig. 4-8).[33,34]

Traumatic diaphragmatic injuries may not be initially noted, particularly with small penetrating injuries without herniated viscera. These openings may later enlarge and present with radiographic findings or clinical symptoms. Up to 12% of all traumatic diaphragmatic hernias present in a delayed manner. They are more common on the left, likely as a result of the liver preventing herniation on the right.[34]

Symptomatic hernias must be repaired urgently. Asymptomatic, incidentally found hernias should be

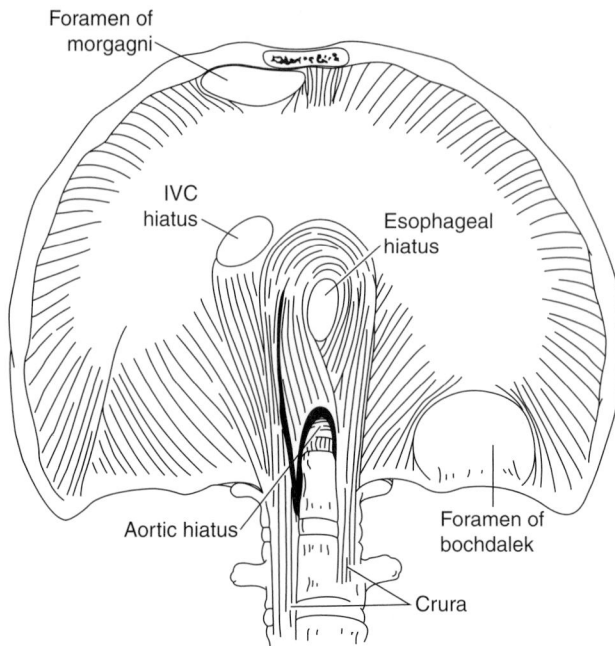

Figure 4-8 *Congenital diaphragmatic hernia. Reproduced with permission from Naunheim KS. Adult presentation of unusual diaphragmatic hernias.* Chest Surg Clin N Am *1998;8(2):359-369.*

repaired electively to prevent incarceration. Repair is undertaken via thoracotomy, laparotomy, thoracoscopy, or laparoscopy. Frequently direct suture closure is possible, otherwise mesh (usually polytetrafluoroethylene) closure is required. Morgagni hernias are more easily approached from the abdomen and via the laparoscope because of the anterior location, elective presentation, and presence of a hernia sac. Bochdalek hernias are more likely to require thoracotomy or combined thoraco/abdominal approach because of the posterior position and greater likelihood of adhesions. Delayed presentation of traumatic diaphragmatic hernias should be approached via thoracotomy as there is no hernia sac and adhesions to the lung are typically extensive. Elective repair of all these defects has good results. Emergency repair has higher mortality and morbidity, particularly if gastric or intestinal ischemia or perforation has occurred.[33,34]

SUMMARY

Although the majority of chest surgical procedures will be performed electively by surgical specialists, knowledge of the diverse pathology is necessary for the acute care surgeon as he or she may be called on to manage emergency interventions. These diseases are a challenge to care for; however, with rapid resuscitation and early surgical management, outcomes can be greatly improved.

REFERENCES

1. Dailey RH. Acute upper airway obstruction. *Emerg Med Clin North Am* 1983 Aug;1(2):261-277.
2. Aboussouan LS, Stoller JK. Diagnosis and management of upper airway obstruction. *Clin Chest Med* 1994 Mar;15(1):35-53.
3. Swanson KL, Edell ES. Tracheobronchial foreign bodies. *Chest Surg Clin N Am* 2001 Nov;11(4):861-872.
4. Rafanan AL, Mehta AC. Adult airway foreign body removal. What's new? *Clin Chest Med* 2001 Jun;22(2):319-330.
5. Smith SW, Biros M. Relief of imminent respiratory failure from upper airway obstruction by use of helium-oxygen: a case series and brief review. *Acad Emerg Med* 1999 Sep;6(9):953-956.
6. Beamis JF Jr. Interventional pulmonology techniques for treating malignant large airway obstruction: an update. *Curr Opin Pulm Med* 2005 Jul;11(4):292-295.
7. Sahn SA, Heffner JE. Spontaneous pneumothorax. *N Engl J Med* 2000 Mar 23;342(12):868-874.
8. Baumann MH. Management of spontaneous pneumothorax. *Clin Chest Med* 2006 Jun;27(2):369-381.
9. Van Schil PE, Hendriks JM, De Maeseneer MG, Lauwers PR. Current management of spontaneous pneumothorax. *Monaldi Arch Chest Dis* 2005 Dec;63(4):204-212.
10. Korom S, Canyurt H, Missbach A, et al. Catamenial pneumothorax revisited: clinical approach and systematic review of the literature. *J Thorac Cardiovasc Surg* 2004 Oct;128(4):502-508.
11. Sherman SC. Reexpansion pulmonary edema: a case report and review of the current literature. *J Emerg Med* 2003 Jan;24(1):23-27.
12. Jean-Baptiste E. Clinical assessment and management of massive hemoptysis. *Crit Care Med* 2001 May;29(5):1098.
13. Karmy-Jones R, Cuschieri J, Vallieres E. Role of bronchoscopy in massive hemoptysis. *Chest Surg Clin N Am* 2001 Nov;11(4):873-906.
14. Lenner R, Schilero GJ, Lesser M. Hemoptysis: diagnosis and management. *Compr Ther* 2002 Spring;28(1):7-14.
15. Sekkal S, Cornu E, Christides C, et al. Swan-Ganz catheter induced pulmonary artery perforation during cardiac surgery concerning two cases. *J Cardiovasc Surg (Torino)* 1996 Jun;37(3):313-317.
16. Feng WC, Singh AK, Drew T, Donat W. Swan-Ganz catheter-induced massive hemoptysis and pulmonary artery false aneurysm. *Ann Thorac Surg* 1990 Oct;50(4):644-6.
17. Mullerworth MH, Angelopoulos P, Couyant MA, et al. Recognition and management of catheter-induced pulmonary artery rupture. *Ann Thorac Surg* 1998 Oct;66(4):1242-1245.
18. Klafta JM, Olson JP. Emergent lung separation for management of pulmonary artery rupture. *Anesthesiology* 1997 Nov;87(5):1248-1250.
19. Wiedemann HP, Rice TW. Lung Abscess and Empyema. *Semin Thorac Cardiovasc Sur* 1995 Apr; 7(2): 119-128.
20. Cowen ME, Johnston MR. Thoracic empyema: causes, diagnosis, and treatment. *Compr Ther* 1990 Oct;16(10):40-45.
21. Wallenhaupt SL. Surgical management of thoracic empyema. *J Thorac Imaging* 1991 Jul;6(3):80-88.
22. Younes Z, Johnson DA. The spectrum of spontaneous and iatrogenic esophageal injury: perforations, Mallory-Weiss tears, and hematomas. *J Clin Gastroenterol* 1999 Dec;29(4):306-317.
23. Duncan M, Wong RK. Esophageal emergencies: things that will wake you from a sound sleep. *Gastroenterol Clin North Am* 2003 Dec;32(4):1035-1052.
24. Brinster CJ, Singhal S, Lee L, et al. Evolving options in the management of esophageal perforation. *Ann Thorac Surg* 2004 Apr;77(4):1475-1483.
25. Zwischenberger JB, Savage C, Bidani A. Surgical aspects of esophageal disease: perforation and caustic injury. *Am J Respir Crit Care Med* 2002 Apr 15;165(8):1037-1040.
26. Brady PG. Esophageal foreign bodies. *Gastroenterol Clin North Am* 1991 Dec;20(4):691-701.
27. Lum DF, McQuaid K, Lee JG. Endoscopic hemostasis of nonvariceal, non-peptic ulcer hemorrhage. *Gastrointest Endosc Clin N Am* 1997 Oct;7(4):657-670.
28. Steffes C, Fromm D. The current diagnosis and management of upper gastrointestinal bleeding. *Adv Surg* 1992;25:331-361.
29. Chong HH, Plotnick GD. Pericardial effusion and tamponade: evaluation, imaging modalities, and management. *Compr Ther* 1995 Jul;21(7):378-385.
30. Cobbe SM. Pericardial effusions. *Br J Hosp Med* 1980 Mar;23(3):250, 252-255.
31. Benson EA. Management of breast abscesses. *World J Surg* 1989 Nov-Dec;13(6):753-756.
32. Stylopoulos N, Rattner DW. Paraesophageal hernia: when to operate? *Adv Surg* 2003;37:213-229.
33. Swain JM, Klaus A, Achem SR, Hinder RA. Congenital diaphragmatic hernia in adults. *Semin Laparosc Surg* 2001 Dec;8(4):246-255.
34. Naunheim KS. Adult presentation of unusual diaphragmatic hernias. *Chest Surg Clin N Am* 1998 May;8(2):359-369.

Chapter 5

EMERGENCY SURGERY FOR STOMACH AND DUODENUM INJURIES

Ronald Jou, MD, David A. Spain, MD, and Susan I. Brundage, MD, MPH

INTRODUCTION

Injuries of the stomach and duodenum are uncommon, and a systematic approach to evaluation and management are required to prevent excess morbidity and mortality associated with delays in diagnosis and missed injuries.[1,2] In the setting of blunt trauma, hollow viscus injuries are much less common than solid organ injuries, and it has been found that the severity of solid organ injury predicts hollow viscus injury.[3-5] In a large multi-institution analysis from the Eastern Association for the Surgery of Trauma, the incidence of hollow viscus injury was approximately 3% in all patients admitted for blunt abdominal trauma, with injuries to the small bowel and colon being most common.[6] Hollow viscus injuries are more common in the setting of penetrating trauma, where the most commonly injured organ is the small bowel followed by the colon and stomach.[7]

OPERATIVE MANAGEMENT

GASTRIC INJURIES

Gastric injury following blunt trauma is rare, with reported incidence of 0.05% of all blunt trauma admissions and comprising 4% of all blunt hollow viscus injuries in a large series.[6] The stomach is a hollow, thick-walled, mobile organ that is relatively resistant to blunt injury. A distinction has been made in some reports between blunt gastric rupture and blunt gastric laceration.[8] Rupture was more commonly seen as a solitary lesion in the setting of having a full stomach and associated with left-sided and thoracic injuries, and laceration was more commonly associated with injuries of the spleen, liver, pancreas, and duodenum. Although anterior wall injuries are more common, the location of injury is variable and can occur in both anterior and posterior walls, as well as at both lesser and greater curvatures. The incidence of penetrating injury of the stomach is reported as 9% of all potentially penetrating abdominal trauma,[9] 17% of all penetrating traumas requiring laparotomy,[7] and 19% of abdominal gunshot wounds.[10] Most common associated injuries were injuries of the liver, diaphragm, and colon.[11]

In the setting of trauma, gastric injuries are diagnosed at the time of laparotomy, usually necessitated by hemodynamic instability or signs and symptoms of peritonitis. Positive (Diagnostic Peritoneal Lavage) DPL, positive (Focused Assessment with Sonography in Trauma) FAST, bloody nasogastric aspirate may also necessitate operation. Because gastric injuries are seldom immediately life threatening, management of hemorrhage from vascular injuries and injuries to solid organs usually take precedence. Operative management of gastric injuries should include adequate mobilization and inspection of anterior and posterior aspects of the stomach as well as the lesser and greater curvatures. The lesser sac should be opened for examination of the posterior wall of the stomach. Simple gastric injuries should be treated with primary closure without resection. Full-thickness injuries can be repaired in one or two layers. Partial thickness injuries should be repaired in a single layer. Superficial serosal injuries do not require repair. More extensive or multiple injuries may require emergency gastrectomy although there are no well-defined guidelines for injuries that require resection.[12,13] Pyloroplasty should be reserved for severe injuries of the pylorus or where there is a question of damage to the Vagus nerves.

Complications of gastric injury are related to infection, intra-abdominal abscess, and sepsis secondary to gross contamination.[11] Aggressive intraoperative lavage and broad-spectrum perioperative antibiotics are recommended.[14] Patients may require abscess drainage.[14]

Nasogastric decompression is also recommended. Intra-abdominal abscess formation is related to concomitant injury to the colon, age, and hemorrhage requiring blood transfusion.[15] Pulmonary complications are related to associated diaphragmatic injury.[11] Mortality because of gastric injury in recent series ranges from 0% to 27%. In blunt gastric injury, mortality is influenced by the severity of associated injuries.[14,16] Mortality from infection and sepsis is more common in the setting of penetrating injury.[11]

DUODENAL INJURIES

Compared to gastric injuries, duodenal injuries are also uncommon, but they do present more difficult diagnostic and therapeutic dilemmas. Its fixed location anterior to the lumbar spinal column makes the duodenum susceptible to blunt injury, and it also susceptible to deep penetrating trauma. Its close proximity to other viscera and major vascular structures means that isolated injury of the duodenum is uncommon. In a large series, incidence of blunt duodenal injury was 0.1-0.2% of all blunt trauma admissions comprising 4-19% of all blunt hollow viscus injuries, with perforating injuries accounting for less than one-third.[6,17] Motor vehicle crash is the most common mechanism of injury.[2] Blunt duodenal injury occurs more commonly in children, and whereas motor vehicle crash is still the most common mechanism, handlebar injuries also occur.[18-20] Blunt injuries to the liver, spleen, and pancreas are the most commonly associated lesions. Duodenal injuries are found in 11% of patients requiring operation for abdominal gunshot wounds and in 1.4% of patients requiring operation for abdominal stab wounds. Associated penetrating injuries of the colon, small bowel, liver, pancreas, and major blood vessels are most common.[21]

Suspicion of duodenal injury may be raised based on mechanism of injury or physical exam, but there is no diagnostic modality that can accurately make this diagnosis. Most duodenal injuries are identified on laparotomy,[21] and exploration remains the ultimate diagnostic test. When no clear indication for exploratory laparotomy exists, other diagnostic tests can be helpful, especially in the setting of blunt trauma. Neither DPL nor FAST evaluates retroperitoneal structures directly, although they may identify other associated injuries. Computed tomography (CT) is noninvasive and allows visualization of both intra- and retroperitoneal structures and has supplanted DPL as the diagnostic test of choice in evaluating hemodynamically stable trauma patients. In a small retrospective series of patients with blunt duodenal injury, CT findings were present in 87% of cases. There were delays in diagnosis, particularly in patients who did not undergo immediate exploration. In retrospect, delays in diagnosis were attributed to the subtlety of CT findings, and the authors concluded that CT findings suggestive of blunt duodenal injury

should be considered indications for operation.[17] Patients under high suspicion for duodenal injury with equivocal findings should undergo repeat CT scanning or laparotomy.

Duodenal hematomas usually occur in the setting of blunt abdominal injury in children and may be diagnosed by CT or at the time of laparotomy.[22] These intramural lesions are generally considered nonoperative, although they may cause a gastric outlet obstruction. Patients with isolated duodenal hematomas are managed expectantly with nasogastric decompression and parenteral nutrition,[23] this approach is successful in about 90% of cases.[19,20] Recommendations for the duration of nonoperative management vary from 5 days to 3 weeks,[23,24] but there is a consensus that obstructing duodenal hematomas that do not resolve after this period require further intervention.[22] Although there have been some case reports of using ultrasound guidance to perform percutaneous drainage of nonresolving hematomas,[25-27] this expertise is not widely available. An additional concern in the setting of persistent gastric outlet obstruction is the presence of occult duodenal or pancreatic injury. For this reason, authors have traditionally recommended exploratory laparotomy for nonresolving hematomas.[22] When a duodenal hematoma is seen on exploration, either initially during a laparotomy for a separate indication or after a period of nonoperative management, successful incision and drainage has been reported as a definitive procedure.[19,20]

A thorough operative evaluation of the duodenum requires extensive mobilization.[22] The Kocher maneuver exposes the second and third parts. Next, entry into the lesser sac provides exposure of the first and second parts of the duodenum. Mobilization of the ligament of Treitz provides additional exposure of the third and fourth parts. This may require mobilization of the colon and small bowel from their retroperitoneal attachments. The duodenum should be rigorously examined for any signs of bile staining or perforation.

Operative management of duodenal injuries should be directed at providing adequate repair while reducing the risk of duodenal fistula. In the critically ill patient with multiple injuries, an additional objective is to perform the safest and least extensive procedure, often favoring an abbreviated or damage control procedure over a definitive one. Minor injuries of the duodenum, involving less than 20% of the duodenal circumference, should be repaired by primary closure in one or two layers.[28] Longitudinal injuries should be closed in a transverse orientation if the length of the injury is less than 50% of the circumference. For larger defects, several techniques have been suggested, including mucosal pedicle graft using jejunum or gastric island and serosal patch. None of these techniques reliably prevents leaks; in some studies, they have been found to increase morbidity and mortality when compared to primary repair.

Complete transection of the duodenum should be repaired by mobilization, debridement, primary anastomosis, and drainage.[29] For injuries with a large amount of tissue loss or where mobilization of the duodenum is limited, approximation of the transected ends may not be possible without placing tension on the repair. In this situation, repair will require a more complex procedure, as discussed later in this chapter.

The most serious complication following the treatment of duodenal injury is the development of duodenal fistula from suture-line dehiscence. The incidence of duodenal fistula in patients repaired with primary closure ranges from 0% to 12% and is significantly higher in high-risk injuries.[21,30,31] Identified risk factors include combined pancreatic injury, shock, and delay in diagnosis.[21,30,32] The mortality rate associated with duodenal fistula is greater than 60%,[21] and various procedures have been developed to augment primary repair. More than 5 liters of fluid pass through the duodenum per day, and most strategies to protect duodenal repairs are aimed at controlling the amount of fluid that passes the suture line. Tube decompression was the earliest technique, consisting of various combinations of a gastrostomy tube for diverting gastric contents, a retrograde jejunostomy to decompress the duodenum, and an antegrade jejunostomy for enteral feeding.[33] This technique was found by some investigators to reduce the fistula rate in small series,[34] but these results could not be replicated in other series, and one report found that tube decompression was associated with excess morbidity and mortality.[35]

Duodenal diverticulization has been advocated in the setting of combined duodenal and pancreatic injury or severe duodenal injury. This procedure consists of a distal Billroth II gastrectomy, closure of the duodenal wound, placement of a decompressive tube duodenostomy, and placement of a drain around the repair, possibly with vagotomy and biliary drainage.[36] Disadvantages of this approach are the complexity and extent of the procedure, which may not be appropriate for a severely injured or hemodynamically unstable patient. Furthermore, the appropriateness of a gastrectomy in a patient with a normal stomach has been called into question.

Pyloric developed has a less extensive and reversible method to protect a duodenal repair. As initially described,[37] a gastrostomy is made in anterior wall of the antrum. The pyloric ring is grasped, elevated, and closed with staples or continuous suture. A loop gastrojejunostomy is then constructed to further divert enteric contents away from the repair. The pylorus reopens spontaneously after several weeks, restoring gastrointestinal continuity. In a series of patients examined with upper gastrointestinal studies, 94% of patients had patency of the pylorus when examined 3 weeks or more after the operation.[38] In an animal model, it was shown that pyloric reopening occurs regardless of whether absorbable suture, nonabsorbable suture, or staples are used.[38] A controlled reopen technique utilizing a continuous suture and slipknot has also been reported.[39] Several series have suggested a remarkable decrease in rate of duodenal fistula after the introduction of pyloric exclusion to augment primary repair.[37,38,40] Spontaneous reopening of the pylorus does not appear to influence the rate of fistula healing if a leak does develop.[37] The incidence of marginal ulceration at the site of the gastrojejunostomy has been reported to be from 8 to 33%.[38] Some authors have shown that vagotomy can be performed to reduce this risk,[41] whereas others have shown that pyloric exclusion can be performed without concomitant gastrojejunostomy (Ginzburg Procedure).[42] In this case, a gastrostomy tube and a jejunostomy feeding tube should be placed, and absorbable sutures should be used to promote spontaneous reopening of the pylorus.

In rare instances, more severe or complex injuries may require more extensive procedures such as pancreaticoduodenectomy. In the setting of severe periampullary injury or devascularizing injuries of the duodenum and pancreas, primary repair may not be feasible. Damage control, with control of bleeding, control of gross contamination, and ligation of common bile and pancreatic ducts, is the appropriate operation for the severely injured or hemodynamically unstable patient. Definitive pancreaticoduodenectomy and reconstruction can then be undertaken within the next 48 to 72 hours when the patient is stable.

IATROGENIC INJURIES OF THE STOMACH AND DUODENUM

Iatrogenic injuries of the stomach and duodenum are uncommon problems that ultimately may require an emergency operation. Unlike injuries due to trauma, iatrogenic injuries are often isolated. Most iatrogenic injuries are perforations due to endoscopy, many commonly associated with therapeutic instrumentation, rather than purely diagnostic procedures.

The incidence of gastric perforation due to flexible endoscopy has been estimated to be 0.1%. The diagnosis is suggested by postprocedural abdominal pain and distension progressing to peritonitis and eventually frank sepsis, and can be confirmed by the detection of free air on plain radiograph or extravasation of water-soluble oral contrast on a CT of the abdomen. In cases where gastric perforation is noted at the time of endoscopy, successful endoscopic repairs have been reported. Small contained gastric perforations with minimal symptoms and no signs of sepsis can be managed with nonoperative management including intensive care unit admission, bowel rest, intravenous fluids, intravenous proton-pump inhibitor, nasogastric decompression, and intravenous broad-spectrum antibiotics. The feasibility of endoscopic repair with metallic clips or omental patch have been reported,[43,44] but this expertise is not widely available. For patients who fail nonoperative or endoscopic therapy or for patients with uncontained perforation, peritonitis, or signs of sepsis, an emergency operation is indicated. Such perforations can be approached with laparoscopy and primary repair with omental patch or open laparotomy.

Iatrogenic duodenal perforation is marked by the same pitfalls as traumatic duodenal injuries, namely, the difficulty of diagnosing retroperitoneal injuries and the significant morbidity and mortality due to delays in diagnosis. Injuries may be seen directly or visualized at the time of ERCP if contrast dye is observed outside the bowel lumen or bile duct. Upright chest radiograph and abdominal radiographs may detect free air when an intraperitoneal perforation exists, but the most sensitive diagnostic test for duodenal perforation is contrast-enhanced CT of the abdomen. For small retroperitoneal perforations, if the diagnosis is made at the time of endoscopy, immediate endoscopic repair should be attempted with metallic clips. If the diagnosis of a small retroperitoneal perforation is made after the endoscopic procedure is completed, patients can initially be managed nonoperatively with bowel rest, nasogastric decompression, intravenous fluids, intravenous broad-spectrum antibiotics, intravenous proton pump inhibitor, and nutritional support. Patients failing to respond rapidly to nonoperative management or those with small intraperitoneal perforations and minimal symptoms should undergo primary laparoscopic repair. Patients with large perforations or peritonitis should undergo open repair, and pyloric exclusion should be considered.

HEMORRHAGE

Upper gastrointestinal bleeding is defined as bleeding from a source proximal to the ligament of Treitz and often involves the stomach or duodenum. Acute hemorrhage most often presents as hematemesis or melena, although hematochezia also can be due to massive upper gastrointestinal hemorrhage and often is associated with syncope or shock. History of previous gastrointestinal hemorrhage, peptic ulcer disease, portal hypertension, nonsteroidal anti-inflammatory drug (NSAID) use, anticoagulation, or toxic ingestion may help to elucidate the causative lesion.

Patients who are unable to protect their airway or who are hemodynamically unstable should be intubated. Two peripheral large-bore intravenous catheters should be inserted, and resuscitation should be initiated with administration of isotonic crystalloid. Blood should be drawn for laboratory testing, blood typing, and crossmatching. Ongoing or massive hemorrhage will require blood product transfusion to correct anemia and coagulation defects. Adequacy of resuscitation should be measured by monitoring urine output with a Foley catheter.

Management of acute upper gastrointestinal hemorrhage requires identification of the bleeding source. A large-caliber orogastric or nasogastric tube should be inserted and aspirated to examine the gastric contents, reduce the risk of aspiration, and improve visibility during subsequent examination. Intravenous H_2-receptor antagonist and proton-pump inhibitor therapy have been found to reduce the rates of rebleeding and need for surgical intervention and should be administered. Following these initial considerations, endoscopy is the essential modality for accurate diagnosis and effective management. In cases where expertise is available, endoscopy within 24 hours of admission is associated with reduced ICU stay, reduced hospital stay, reduced risk of recurrent bleeding, and reduced risk of operation so long as an accurate diagnosis and an appropriate intervention are made.[45] Source of upper gastrointestinal hemorrhage is identified at initial esophagogastroduodenoscopy (EGD) in about 90% of patients.[45,46] Validated endoscopic interventions include thermocoagulation, clipping, band ligation, epinephrine injection, and sclerosant injection. Rates of initial hemostasis for a variety of nonvariceal lesions including bleeding peptic ulcers, Dieulafoy lesions, and Mallory-Weiss tears are greater than 90% and greater than 95% when active bleeding or a nonbleeding visible vessel is seen. Accordingly, rates of diagnostic failure or initial failure to control nonvariceal hemorrhage are low. Variceal upper gastrointestinal hemorrhage, usually found in the setting of cirrhosis and portal hypertension, should be considered a distinct entity and will be discussed separately.

In the large majority of cases where initial endoscopy is successful, the greatest concern is recurrent bleeding. Rebleeding is the most important predictor of mortality, and it occurs in 10-30% of patients, with 97% of recurrent bleeding occurring within 96 hours of the initial endoscopy. Several risk assessment systems have been proposed to risk-stratify patients with upper GI hemorrhage to better predict risk of rebleeding and clinical outcomes.

Endoscopic variables, in particular the Forrest classification, predict a high risk of rebleeding for lesions with active bleeding (Forrest I) or signs of recent bleeding including a visible blood vessel or adherent clot (Forrest II).[47] Clinical factors such as advanced age, medical comorbidity, and amount of blood loss, and hematemesis have all been found to predict rebleeding and mortality.[48,49] The management of rebleeding has traditionally involved a surgical intervention, but recent studies suggest that repeat endoscopy may safely and effectively salvage up to half of rebleeding patients.[50] If retreatment fails, however, the morbidity and mortality associated with a surgical intervention is high.[50] Overall, 20% of patients fail endoscopic therapy because of initial failure to control hemorrhage or due to early recurrent hemorrhage.

For stable patients, endovascular intervention has been shown to be effective in controlling acute arterial hemorrhage.[51] Local vasoconstrictive therapy is reported to be successful in 50-90% of cases with an approximately 20% rate of rebleeding,[52-54] and embolization is initially successful in more than 70% of cases with about a 10% rate of rebleeding.[55] The major drawbacks of these interventions are tissue ischemia or infarction, although these complications are uncommon in the upper gastrointestinal tract where collateral blood supply is ample. Data comparing interventional radiology measures with more traditional endoscopic or surgical management is scarce, and this level of expertise is not widely available.

For nonvariceal upper gastrointestinal hemorrhage, traditional indications for operation are active hemorrhage refractory to endosopic measures, significant recurrent hemorrhage after endoscopic intervention, an ongoing transfusion requirement, or transfusion requirements exceeding six units of packed red blood cells in a 24-hour period. With current advances in endoscopic treatment, the decision to operate should be made on an individual basis, taking into consideration the patient characteristics, availability and expertise of endoscopic interventions, severity of hemorrhage, and availability of critical care support. There may be patients, such as those over the age of 60, in whom early surgical intervention provides better outcomes, but this subset of patients has not been well defined.[56]

OPERATIVE MANAGEMENT

Operative planning for nonvariceal upper gastrointestinal hemorrhage depends on the lesion encountered as well as the hemodynamic stability of the patient. The goals of operation are first to identify the lesion, second to control hemorrhage, third to prevent rebleeding, and third to rule out malignancy. If the location of the lesion is still unknown at the time of emergent operation, intraoperative endoscopy can be a useful technique to identify the source of bleeding.

For the bleeding gastric ulcer, the traditional recommendation of gastric resection with or without vagotomy is still considered the most effective operation for controlling hemorrhage and preventing rebleeding.[57] For unstable patients with bleeding from a gastric ulcer, controversy still exists regarding the role of a limited procedure compared to resection. Some investigators have shown that limited ulcer excision or oversewing may be useful, particularly for unstable or high-risk patients in whom gastric resection could be associated with excess morbidity.[58,59] Others have found that limited operation is not superior[60] and may even be associated with a higher mortality due to rebleeding. Although data exist supporting both hypotheses, no recent data exists that takes into account current experience with endoscopy, antiulcer medications, and *H. pylori* eradication. Gastric ulcers are associated with malignancy in approximately 15% of cases,[61-64] and biopsies should be obtained at the time of operation to evaluate for cancer. Unusually firm or suspicious tissue should be sampled and sent for frozen section if available, as the presence of malignancy necessitates a more extensive resection. Options for reconstruction include Billroth I or Billroth II procedures.

The decision to perform an antisecretory procedure during an emergency operation for gastric ulcers has traditionally been based on the location of the lesion. Pyloric or prepyloric lesions, type II and III gastric ulcers according to the modified Johnson criteria,[65] are thought to be due to acid hypersecretion, and the recommendation is to perform bilateral truncal vagotomy for such ulcers. A gastric-emptying procedure will be required if the pylorus is intact and not bypassed. Some authors advocate a parietal cell vagotomy to preserve gastric emptying in stable patients who are able to tolerate a longer antisecretory procedure.

Control of hemorrhage from bleeding duodenal ulcers requires direct exposure of the ulcer within the duodenum. An upper midline incision should be made, and the duodenum should be mobilized via the Kocher maneuver. Pressure through the anterior duodenal wall may temporarily control brisk hemorrhage from an ulcer in the posterior duodenal wall. The ulcer is exposed via either longitudinal duodenotomy or duodenopyloromyotomy. Bleeding vessels should be controlled with direct suture ligature with nonabsorbable suture. Occasionally, four-quadrant suture ligation around the perimeter of ulcer may be required. Rarely, ligation of the gastroduodenal artery may be necessary to control hemorrhage. Older reports advocate truncal vagotomy and antrectomy (TV&A) as a definite procedure with the lowest rate of recurrent hemorrhage.[57] In the era of *H. pylori* eradication and medical treatment, however, less invasive procedures have been advocated to avoid the morbidity associated with gastric resection. Truncal vagotomy with pyloroplasty and oversewing of the ulcer is considered an adequate procedure for the acutely bleeding duodenal ulcer,[66] especially when *H. pylori* eradication, antisecretory medications, or withdrawal of nonsteroidal anti-inflammatory agents are expected to make a significant impact on the disease process. By contrast, for chronic bleeding refractory to medical management and not associated with *H. pylori* infection, the procedure of choice is TV&A followed by Billroth I or Billroth II reconstruction.

Nonulcer causes of upper gastrointestinal hemorrhage are not as common, representing about 30% of nonvariceal bleeding.[67] Dieulafoy lesions due to an anomalous artery can be secured with suture ligature. Upper gastrointestinal angiodysplasia is an uncommon mucosal lesion associated with end-stage renal disease, congestive heart failure, cirrhosis, and a variety of systemic illnesses. Most hemorrhage due to angiodysplasia is occult, but acute bleeding has been reported. Endoscopy is the mainstay of diagnosis and management, and the need for an emergency antrectomy, partial gastrectomy, or total gastrectomy is rare.[68] Upper gastrointestinal hemorrhage is sometimes attributed to gastritis in the setting of ingestion, erosive gastritis, and stress gastritis in critically ill patients. Discrete lesions refractory to endoscopic management are exposed via a longitudinal gastrotomy and oversewn. Where no discrete lesion can be identified, gastric devascularization,[69,70] partial gastrectomy,[71] or total gastrectomy[72] may be required, depending on the extent of involvement. Gastric devascularization includes ligation of right and left gastric arteries and right and left gastroepiploic arteries, sparing the short gastric arteries, followed by bilateral truncal vagotomy.

Mechanical lesions due to gastric volvulus[73,74] or strangulated paraesophageal hernia[75] can sometimes present with hematemesis, although obstruction is a more common presentation.

Acute upper gastrointestinal hemorrhage can complicate both benign and malignant gastroduodenal tumors. Endoscopic therapy is usually successful in controlling hemorrhage in this situation. When an emergency operation is indicated, a curative resection and lymph node dissection should be done if the patient is stable. If the patient is unstable, a limited resection to control hemorrhage should be performed, and a definitive cancer operation can be performed in a staged manner.[76,77]

VARICEAL BLEEDING

In the setting of portal hypertension, acute upper gastrointestinal hemorrhage is due to bleeding from varices in the upper alimentary tract. Although esophageal varices are the most common lesions, gastric varices occur in approximately 20% of patients with portal hypertension, either in isolation or in combination with esophageal varices.[78] The most common gastric varices are located in the cardia. These cardial varices are considered extensions of esophageal varices and should be treated accordingly with endoscopic sclerotherapy.[79] Gastric varices that arise in the fundus are sometimes extensions of esophageal varices but are also sometimes found in isolation. Isolated varices can also be found in the antrum, corpus, or near the pylorus. Bleeding from these varices is difficult to control with endoscopic sclerotherapy,[80,81] and is associated with significant rebleeding rates. A recent advancement in endoscopic management involves injection of cyanoacrylate compounds or thrombin into the varix to solidify or induce thrombosis. These techniques have been shown to be useful in the management of acute bleeding

from fundal and isolated gastric varices.[82-84] If endoscopic therapy is unsuccessful, patients should be considered for further interventions. For patients in whom bleeding gastric varices are the consequence of splenic vein thrombosis and isolated left-sided portal hypertension, interruption of splenogastric venous drainage is effective. The traditional approach is splenectomy,[85] although successful management with splenic artery embolization has been reported.[86] For patients awaiting liver transplantation, Transcutaneous Intrahepatic Portocaval Shunt (TIPS) is effective for controlling bleeding from gastric varices with 96% initial hemostasis and 28% rebleeding rate in a small series.[87] In a series of 30 patients with preserved liver function, the distal splenorenal shunt procedure was shown to control bleeding in 87% of cases with a 10% rate of rebleeding.[88] Some authors have recommended underrunning of actively bleeding gastric varices with 2-0 absorbable suture via a high anterior gastrotomy,[81] with or without ligation of the left gastric vein.[89] In these small series, the mortality rate associated with emergency operation was as high as 50%.[89]

Duodenal varices are uncommon lesions that arise in the setting of portal hypertension. Although most duodenal varices are limited to the submucosa are of limited clinical significance, acute hemorrhage has been reported. Successful management with a variety of modalities has been reported including the use of endoscopic injection,[90,91] endoscopic banding,[92] endovascular obliteration,[93] TIPS,[94,95] suture ligation,[96] and resection.[97]

PERFORATION

Free perforation of the upper alimentary tract is usually heralded by severe abdominal pain. Patients will have signs of peritonitis, and fever and leukocytosis are common. An upright chest radiograph will demonstrate pneumoperitoneum. In older or debilitated patients, the presentation may be less dramatic, and even though perforation may not be initially suspected, abdominal computed tomography scan will reveal the presence of free air.

Most patients who present with free perforation will require an emergency operation, and the choice of procedure will depend on the patient factors such as history, comorbidities, stability, as well as the cause and location of the lesion.

For stable patients under the age of 70 with perforated gastric or duodenal ulcer, the validity of a trial of nonoperative management (fluid resuscitation, nasogastric decompression, broad-spectrum antibiotics, and acid suppression) has been demonstrated in a randomized trial.[98] Patients over the age of 70 had poorer outcomes when operation was delayed. Patients showing no clinical improvement in 12 hours require operative management.

The primary goal of the operation is to repair the perforation. Secondary goals are to investigate the possibility of malignancy and decrease the risk of recurrence. Perforated duodenal ulcers are not associated with malignancy and should be repaired with simple closure or omental patch closure. The decision whether or not to perform an antisecretory procedure is controversial. In patients infected with *H. pylori*, eradication after simple closure is sufficient to prevent recurrence.[99] Unfortunately, *H. pylori* status and NSAID history are not always known at the time of emergency operation. If unknown, *H. pylori* status should be established with mucosal biopsies at the time of operation. One reasonable approach is to perform simple repair for patients with unknown or untreated *H. pylori* status if they do not require the long-term use of ulcerogenic medications. Although perforations of so-called giant duodenal ulcers have been reported, omental patch closure is technically feasible for defects as large as 3 cm.[100] For extremely large duodenal defects, defunctionalization of the upper gastrointestinal tract has been suggested. One report suggested a tube decompression procedure similar to the one developed for duodenal injuries in the setting of trauma.[101] It is possible that other procedures developed for duodenal injuries may be useful in this exceedingly rare situation.

For perforated duodenal ulcers, an antisecretory procedure should be reserved for stable, low-risk patients who have previously failed *H. pylori* eradication, have demonstrated dependency on chronic NSAID therapy, or are known to be *H. pylori* negative.[102] Simple repair can be performed either by laparoscopic or open procedure,[103-110] although experience with laparoscopic antisecretory procedures is limited.

Perforated gastric ulcers are similar to perforated duodenal ulcers with the important difference that gastric ulcers are associated with malignancy in approximately 15% of cases.[61-64] Operative procedures include ulcer excision, omental plication, and gastrectomy. In recent studies, simple repair with ulcer excision or omental plication has been shown to be a safe and effective procedure for the majority of patients.[111-113] If a nonresectional procedure is performed, biopsies should be taken to evaluate *H. pylori* status and risk of malignancy. Although vagotomy and pyloroplasty were traditionally performed after nonresectional repair, the value of adding an antisecretory procedure in the era of *H. pylori* eradication has not been conclusively demonstrated. One reasonable approach is to reserve bilateral truncal vagotomy for hemodynamically stable patients with a long history of refractory peptic ulcer disease. Parietal cell vagotomy is a lengthy procedure, and is probably not appropriate for an emergency operation.

Resectional procedures for perforated gastric ulcers include antrectomy and distal gastrectomy. Resection

has been advocated for perforated gastric ulcer in a variety of scenarios including patients with prepyloric lesions, patients with so-called giant ulcers, patients with lesions near the incisura angularis, and patients with chronic ulcers refractory to treatment.[111,114,115] By contrast, simple repair with ulcer excision or omental plication has been shown been an equivalent emergency procedure that avoids excess mortality associated with gastric resection.[111-113,116-118] One reasonable approach is to routinely perform simple repair, either by open or laparoscopic procedure.[103] Gastric resection should be reserved for patients in whom simple repair is not technically feasible. If gastric resection is performed, an antisecretory procedure is not needed.[116] Peritoneal lavage should be performed in all cases of perforation.

Essential postoperative medical therapy for perforated gastric ulcers includes *H. pylori* eradication, discontinuing ulcerogenic medication, and acid suppression. For patient managed nonoperatively, interval endoscopy should be performed after 3 weeks to assess ulcer healing and to perform repeat biopsies if non-healing is encountered.[61]

Perforation is an uncommon presentation for gastric malignancy and usually occurs in elderly patients with advanced disease.[119,120] If malignancy is known or discovered at the time of operation for gastric perforation, the feasibility of performing a cancer operation should be considered. The diagnosis of gastric adenocarcinoma is diagnosed preoperatively or intraoperatively in approximately thirty percent of patients with perforated gastric cancer.[120] When this is the case, the choice of emergency procedure depends primarily on the status of the patient at the time of operation. Early evidence indicated that long-term survival was possible for the minority of patients with early stage who underwent immediate gastrectomy.[121-124] This long-term survival is only meaningful, however, if the morbidity of a radical emergency operation can be minimized. Furthermore, adequacy of resection is unlikely to have a significant impact for the majority of patients with advanced disease. If the patient is unstable or the extent of disease precludes immediate gastrectomy, omental patch closure is an adequate procedure for management of the perforation.[123] Otherwise, an immediate gastrectomy should be performed with the extent of resection depending on the location of the cancer. A formal lymphadenectomy significantly prolongs operative time and may contribute to excess morbidity, and several authors have advocated a two-stage approach to perforated gastric cancer.[119,120,125] The initial operation is directed at managing the perforation and peritonitis, and the second operation is directed at tumor staging with a formal lymphadenectomy.

Gastric lymphoma can sometimes lead to perforation,[126,127] but surgical resection has a limited role in management of lymphoma. In this situation, simple repair of perforation is an appropriate procedure. Other uncommon gastric neoplasms such as leiomyoma, carcinoid, gastrointestinal stromal tumor, and sarcoma all have the potential to cause perforation, though few cases have been published. Perforated duodenal cancers are also uncommon. In the setting of an emergency operation, unless the pathologic diagnosis is certain, the safest operation is to take adequate biopsies and perform simple repair with peritoneal lavage.

Perforation can be encountered in the advanced stages of gastric volvulus[73,74] or strangulated paraesophageal hernia,[75] although obstruction is a more common presentation. Emergency management of these lesions is discussed later in this chapter.

OBSTRUCTION

Upper gastrointestinal obstruction presents with nausea and vomiting. Patients may have chronic or progressive symptoms and are often significantly hypovolemic and malnourished. Initial measures include volume resuscitation, nasogastric decompression, and correction of electrolyte imbalances.

Initial diagnostic evaluation includes plain abdominal radiographs, upper gastrointestinal contrast studies, and upper gastrointestinal endoscopy.

In this situation, the need for a truly emergent operation is uncommon, and most patients will benefit from a delay in operative intervention to allow for decompression and optimization of volume and nutritional status. Nonemergent causes of gastric outlet obstruction include gastric peptic ulcer disease, gastric cancer, periampullary cancer, extrapulmonary tuberculosis, gallstone obstruction, and bezoar.

If acute abdominal pain, hematemesis, or signs of perforation are present, however, an emergent operation may be necessary. The triad of epigastric pain, inability to vomit, and inability to pass a nasogastric tube suggest impending strangulation and gastric necrosis. This acute presentation suggests the presence gastric volvulus or incarcerated paraesophageal hernia, and often both lesions are present.

Attempts to reduce the lesion by passing a nasogastric tube are rarely successful,[74] and urgent laparotomy is indicated. Goals of the operation are to reduce the lesion, resect any compromised tissue, and prevent recurrence.

Gentle traction may be all that is required to reduce the lesion, but in the situation of a severely distended stomach, a short gastrotomy may be helpful for decompression.[74] The stomach should be reduced and inspected for signs of gangrene or perforation. Tissue that appears nonviable after reduction should be resected, and, in rare cases, a subtotal or total gastrectomy may be required. If a diaphragmatic defect is encountered, it should be repaired with interrupted sutures. The decision to excise the hernia sac is controversial.[75] The stomach should be returned to an anatomic position and an anterior gastropexy should be performed by suturing the stomach to the posterior rectus sheath.[75] In unstable patients, no further intervention should be considered. In stable patients with significant history of reflux, an antireflux procedure such as a Nissen fundoplication can be considered.[75] Patients with mild reflux symptoms can be managed medically.

REFERENCES

1. Sung CK, Kim KH. Missed injuries in abdominal trauma. *J Trauma* 1996;41(2):276-282.
2. Allen GS, Moore FA, Cox CS, Jr., Wilson JT, Cohn JM, Duke JH. Hollow visceral injury and blunt trauma. *J Trauma* 1998;45(1):69-75; discussion 78.
3. Kemmeter PR, Hoedema RE, Foote JA, Scholten DJ. Concomitant blunt enteric injuries with injuries of the liver and spleen: a dilemma for trauma surgeons. *Am Surg* 2001;67(3):221-225; discussion 225-226.
4. Miller PR, Croce MA, Bee TK, Malhotra AK, Fabian TC. Associated injuries in blunt solid organ trauma: implications for missed injury in nonoperative management. *J Trauma* 2002;53(2):238-242; discussion 242-244.
5. Nance ML, Peden GW, Shapiro MB, Kauder DR, Rotondo MF, Schwab CW. Solid viscus injury predicts major hollow viscus injury in blunt abdominal trauma. *J Trauma* 1997;43(4):618-622; discussion 622-623.
6. Watts DD, Fakhry SM. Incidence of hollow viscus injury in blunt trauma: an analysis from 275,557 trauma admissions from the East multi-institutional trial. *J Trauma* 2003;54(2):289-294.
7. Nicholas JM, Rix EP, Easley KA, et al. Changing patterns in the management of penetrating abdominal trauma: the more things change, the more they stay the same. *J Trauma* 2003;55(6):1095-1108; discussion 1108-1110.
8. Shinkawa H, Yasuhara H, Naka S, et al. Characteristic features of abdominal organ injuries associated with gastric rupture in blunt abdominal trauma. *Am J Surg* 2004;187(3):394-397.
9. van Haarst EP, van Bezooijen BP, Coene PP, Luitse JS. The efficacy of serial physical examination in penetrating abdominal trauma. *Injury* 1999;30(9):599-604.
10. Adesanya AA, Afolabi IR, da Rocha-Afodu JT. Civilian abdominal gunshot wounds in Lagos. *J R Coll Surg Edinb* 1998;43(4):230-234.
11. Coimbra R, Pinto MC, Aguiar JR, Rasslan S. Factors related to the occurrence of postoperative complications following penetrating gastric injuries. *Injury* 1995;26(7):463-466.
12. Nanji SA, Mock C. Gastric rupture resulting from blunt abdominal trauma and requiring gastric resection. *J Trauma* 1999;47(2):410-412.
13. Hirsch EF, Gould EA. Emergency gastrectomy for spontaneous double gastric perforation: report of one case. *Am Surg* 1966;32(4):278-280.

14. Pikoulis E, Delis S, Tsatsoulis P, et al. Blunt injuries of the stomach. *Eur J Surg* 1999;165(10):937-939.

15. Croce MA, Fabian TC, Patton JH, Jr., et al. Impact of stomach and colon injuries on intra-abdominal abscess and the synergistic effect of hemorrhage and associated injury. *J Trauma* 1998;45(4):649-655.

16. Bruscagin V, Coimbra R, Rasslan S, et al. Blunt gastric injury. A multicentre experience. *Injury* 2001;32(10): 761-764.

17. Allen GS, Moore FA, Cox CS, Jr., Mehall JR, Duke JH. Delayed diagnosis of blunt duodenal injury: an avoidable complication. *J Am Coll Surg* 1998;187(4):393-399.

18. Ladd AP, West KW, Rouse TM, et al. Surgical management of duodenal injuries in children. *Surgery* 2002;132(4):748-752; discussion 751-753.

19. Desai KM, Dorward IG, Minkes RK, Dillon PA. Blunt duodenal injuries in children. *J Trauma* 2003;54(4): 640-645; discussion 645-646.

20. Clendenon JN, Meyers RL, Nance ML, Scaife ER. Management of duodenal injuries in children. *J Pediatr Surg* 2004;39(6):964-968.

21. Timaran CH, Martinez O, Ospina JA. Prognostic factors and management of civilian penetrating duodenal trauma. *J Trauma* 1999;47(2):330-335.

22. Degiannis E, Boffard K. Duodenal injuries. *Br J Surg* 2000;87(11):1473-1479.

23. Touloukian RJ. Protocol for the nonoperative treatment of obstructing intramural duodenal hematoma during childhood. *Am J Surg* 1983;145(3):330-334.

24. Thoms CA, Ricketts RR. Intramural duodenal hematoma in children: reappraisal of current management. *South Med J* 1988;81(8):985-988.

25. Lloyd GM, Sutton CD, Marshall LJ, Jameson JS. Case of duodenal haematoma treated with ultrasound guided drainage. *ANZ J Surg* 2004;74(6):500-501.

26. Jain R, Sawhney S, Ghose R, Berry M. Percutaneous management of duodenal and retroperitoneal hematoma. *AJR Am J Roentgenol* 1991;156(5): 1112-1113.

27. Aizawa K, Tokuyama H, Yonezawa T, et al. A case of traumatic intramural hematoma of the duodenum effectively treated with ultrasonically guided aspiration drainage and endoscopic balloon catheter dilation. *Gastroenterol Jpn* 1991;26(2):218-223.

28. Nassoura ZE, Ivatury RR, Simon RJ, Kihtir T, Stahl WM. A prospective reappraisal of primary repair of penetrating duodenal injuries. *Am Surg* 1994;60(1):35-39.

29. Ivatury RR, Nassoura ZE, Simon RJ, Rodriguez A. Complex duodenal injuries. *Surg Clin North Am* 1996;76(4):797-812.

30. McKenney MG, Nir I, Levi DM, Martin L. Evaluation of minor penetrating duodenal injuries. *Am Surg* 1996;62(11):952-955.

31. Jansen M, Du Toit DF, Warren BL. Duodenal injuries: surgical management adapted to circumstances. *Injury* 2002;33(7):611-615.

32. Cogbill TH, Moore EE, Feliciano DV, et al. Conservative management of duodenal trauma: a multicenter perspective. *J Trauma* 1990;30(12):1469-1475.

33. Stone HH, Fabian TC. Management of duodenal wounds. *J Trauma* 1979;19(5):334-339.

34. Hasson JE, Stern D, Moss GS. Penetrating duodenal trauma. *J Trauma* 1984;24(6):471-474.

35. Ivatury RR, Gaudino J, Ascer E, Nallathambi M, Ramirez-Schon G, Stahl WM. Treatment of penetrating duodenal injuries: primary repair vs. repair with decompressive enterostomy/serosal patch. *J Trauma* 1985;25(4):337-341.

36. Berne CJ, Donovan AJ, White EJ, Yellin AE. Duodenal "diverticulization" for duodenal and pancreatic injury. *Am J Surg* 1974;127(5):503-507.

37. Vaughan GD, 3rd, Frazier OH, Graham DY, Mattox KL, Petmecky FF, Jordan GL, Jr. The use of pyloric exclusion in the management of severe duodenal injuries. *Am J Surg* 1977;134(6):785-790.

38. Martin TD, Feliciano DV, Mattox KL, Jordan GL, Jr. Severe duodenal injuries. Treatment with pyloric exclusion and gastrojejunostomy. *Arch Surg* 1983;118(5): 631-635.

39. Fang JF, Chen RJ, Lin BC. Controlled reopen suture technique for pyloric exclusion. *J Trauma* 1998;45(3): 593-596.

40. Degiannis E, Krawczykowski D, Velmahos GC, Levy RD, Souter I, Saadia R. Pyloric exclusion in severe penetrating injuries of the duodenum. *World J Surg* 1993;17(6):751-754.

41. Buck JR, Sorensen VJ, Fath JJ, Horst HM, Obeid FN. Severe pancreatico-duodenal injuries: the effectiveness of pyloric exclusion with vagotomy. *Am Surg* 1992;58(9):557-560; discussion 561.

42. Ginzburg E, Carrillo EH, Sosa JL, Hertz J, Nir I, Martin LC. Pyloric exclusion in the management of duodenal trauma: is concomitant gastrojejunostomy necessary? *Am Surg* 1997;63(11):964-966.

43. Binmoeller KF, Grimm H, Soehendra N. Endoscopic closure of a perforation using metallic clips after snare excision of a gastric leiomyoma. *Gastrointest Endosc* 1993;39(2):172-174.

44. Hashiba K, Carvalho AM, Diniz G, Jr., et al. Experimental endoscopic repair of gastric perforations with an omental patch and clips. *Gastrointest Endosc* 2001;54(4):500-504.

45. Chak A, Cooper GS, Lloyd LE, Kolz CS, Barnhart BA, Wong RC. Effectiveness of endoscopy in patients admitted to the intensive care unit with upper GI hemorrhage. *Gastrointest Endosc* 2001;53(1):6-13.

46. Makela J, Haukipuro K, Laitinen S, Kairaluoma MI. Endoscopy for the diagnosis of acute upper gastrointestinal bleeding. *Scand J Gastroenterol* 1991;26(10):1082-1088.

47. Forrest JA, Finlayson ND, Shearman DJ. Endoscopy in gastrointestinal bleeding. *Lancet* 1974;2(7877): 394-397.

48. Guglielmi A, Ruzzenente A, Sandri M, et al. Risk assessment and prediction of rebleeding in bleeding gastroduodenal ulcer. *Endoscopy* 2002;34(10):778-786.

49. Vreeburg EM, Terwee CB, Snel P, et al. Validation of the Rockall risk scoring system in upper gastrointestinal bleeding. *Gut* 1999;44(3):331-335.

50. Lau JY, Sung JJ, Lam YH, et al. Endoscopic retreatment compared with surgery in patients with recurrent bleeding after initial endoscopic control of bleeding ulcers. *N Engl J Med* 1999;340(10):751-756.

51. Funaki B. Endovascular intervention for the treatment of acute arterial gastrointestinal hemorrhage. *Gastroenterol Clin North Am* 2002;31(3):701-713.

52. Clark RA, Colley DP, Eggers FM. Acute arterial gastrointestinal hemorrhage: efficacy of transcatheter control. *AJR Am J Roentgenol* 1981;136(6):1185-1189.

53. Eckstein MR, Kelemouridis V, Athanasoulis CA, Waltman AC, Feldman L, van Breda A. Gastric bleeding: therapy with intraarterial vasopressin and transcatheter embolization. *Radiology* 1984;152(3):643-646.

54. Rosch J, Dotter CT, Antonovic R. Selective vasoconstrictor infusion in the management of arterio-capillary gastrointestinal hemorrhage. *Am J Roentgenol Radium Ther Nucl Med* 1972;116(2):279-288.

55. Aina R, Oliva VL, Therasse E, et al. Arterial embolotherapy for upper gastrointestinal hemorrhage: outcome assessment. *J Vasc Interv Radiol* 2001;12(2):195-200.

56. Cochran TA. Bleeding peptic ulcer: surgical therapy. *Gastroenterol Clin North Am* 1993;22(4):751-778.

57. Herrington JL, Jr., Davidson J, 3rd. Bleeding gastroduodenal ulcers: choice of operations. *World J Surg* 1987;11(3):304-314.

58. Rogers PN, Murray WR, Shaw R, Brar S. Surgical management of bleeding gastric ulceration. *Br J Surg* 1988;75(1):16-17.

59. Schein M, Gecelter G. APACHE II score in massive upper gastrointestinal haemorrhage from peptic ulcer: prognostic value and potential clinical applications. *Br J Surg* 1989;76(7):733-736.

60. Doberneck RC. Limited operation for bleeding or perforated gastric ulcer in high risk patients. *Am Surg* 1993;59(7):472-474.

61. Mountford RA, Brown P, Salmon PR, Alvarenga C, Neumann CS, Read AE. Gastric cancer detection in gastric ulcer disease. *Gut* 1980;21(1):9-17.

62. Bustamante M, Devesa F, Borghol A, Ortuno J, Ferrando MJ. Accuracy of the initial endoscopic diagnosis in the discrimination of gastric ulcers: is endoscopic follow-up study always needed? *J Clin Gastroenterol* 2002;35(1):25-28.

63. Nelson RS, Urrea LH, Lanza FL. Evaluation of gastric ulcerations. *Am J Dig Dis* 1976;21(6):389-392.

64. Tragardh B, Haglund U. Endoscopic diagnosis of gastric ulcer. Evaluation of the benefits of endoscopic follow-up observation for malignancy. *Acta Chir Scand* 1985;151(1):37-41.

65. Johnson HD. Gastric ulcer: classification, blood group characteristics, secretion patterns and pathogenesis. *Ann Surg* 1965;162(6):996-1004.

66. Hunt PS, McIntyre RL. Choice of emergency operative procedure for bleeding duodenal ulcer. *Br J Surg* 1990;77(9):1004-1006.

67. Rockall TA, Logan RF, Devlin HB, Northfield TC. Risk assessment after acute upper gastrointestinal haemorrhage. *Gut* 1996;38(3):316-321.

68. Novitsky YW, Kercher KW, Czerniach DR, Litwin DE. Watermelon stomach: pathophysiology, diagnosis, and management. *J Gastrointest Surg* 2003;7(5):652-661.

69. Richardson JD, Aust JB. Gastric devascularization: a useful salvage procedure for massive hemorrhagic gastritis. *Ann Surg* 1977;185(6):649-655.

70. Udassin R, Nissan S, Lernau OZ, Vinograd I, Goldberg MD. Gastric devascularization—an emergency treatment for hemorrhagic gastritis in the neonate. *J Pediatr Surg* 1983;18(5):579-580.

71. Stremple JF, Elliott DW. Hemorrhage due to diffuse erosive gastritis. *Arch Surg* 1975;110(5):606-612.

72. Vinograd I, Granot E, Ron N, Klin B, Tauber T, Segal M. Chronic diffuse varioliform gastritis in a child. Total gastrectomy for acute massive bleeding. *J Clin Gastroenterol* 1993;16(1):40-44.

73. Godshall D, Mossallam U, Rosenbaum R. Gastric volvulus: case report and review of the literature. *J Emerg Med* 1999;17(5):837-840.

74. Haas O, Rat P, Christophe M, Friedman S, Favre JP. Surgical results of intrathoracic gastric volvulus complicating hiatal hernia. *Br J Surg* 1990;77(12):1379-1381.

75. Geha AS, Massad MG, Snow NJ, Baue AE. A 32-year experience in 100 patients with giant paraesophageal hernia: the case for abdominal approach and selective antireflux repair. *Surgery* 2000;128(4):623-630.

76. Lee HJ, Park DJ, Yang HK, Lee KU, Choe KJ. Outcome after emergency surgery in gastric cancer patients with free perforation or severe bleeding. *Dig Surg* 2006;23(4):217-223.

77. Kasakura Y, Ajani JA, Mochizuki F, Morishita Y, Fujii M, Takayama T. Outcomes after emergency surgery for gastric perforation or severe bleeding in patients with gastric cancer. *J Surg Oncol* 2002;80(4):181-185.

78. Sarin SK, Lahoti D, Saxena SP, Murthy NS, Makwana UK. Prevalence, classification and natural history of gastric varices: a long-term follow-up study in 568 portal hypertension patients. *Hepatology* 1992;16(6):1343-1349.

79. Sarin SK. Long-term follow-up of gastric variceal sclerotherapy: an eleven-year experience. *Gastrointest Endosc* 1997;46(1):8-14.

80. Korula J, Chin K, Ko Y, Yamada S. Demonstration of two distinct subsets of gastric varices. Observations during a seven-year study of endoscopic sclerotherapy. *Dig Dis Sci* 1991;36(3):303-309.

81. Millar AJ, Brown RA, Hill ID, Rode H, Cywes S. The fundal pile: bleeding gastric varices. *J Pediatr Surg* 1991;26(6):707-709.

82. Sarin SK, Jain AK, Jain M, Gupta R. A randomized controlled trial of cyanoacrylate versus alcohol injection in patients with isolated fundic varices. *Am J Gastroenterol* 2002;97(4):1010-1015.

83. Lo GH, Lai KH, Cheng JS, Chen MH, Chiang HT. A prospective, randomized trial of butyl cyanoacrylate injection versus band ligation in the management of bleeding gastric varices. *Hepatology* 2001;33(5):1060-1064.

84. Przemioslo RT, McNair A, Williams R. Thrombin is effective in arresting bleeding from gastric variceal hemorrhage. *Dig Dis Sci* 1999;44(4):778-781.

85. Hosking SW, Johnson AG. Gastric varices: a proposed classification leading to management. *Br J Surg* 1988;75(3):195-196.

86. McDermott VG, England RE, Newman GE. Case report: bleeding gastric varices secondary to splenic vein thrombosis successfully treated by splenic artery embolization. *Br J Radiol* 1995;68(812):928-930.

87. Chau TN, Patch D, Chan YW, Nagral A, Dick R, Burroughs AK. "Salvage" transjugular intrahepatic portosystemic shunts: gastric fundal compared with esophageal variceal bleeding. *Gastroenterology* 1998;114(5):981-987.

88. Thomas PG, D'Cruz AJ. Distal splenorenal shunting for bleeding gastric varices. *Br J Surg* 1994;81(2):241-244.

89. Greig JD, Garden OJ, Anderson JR, Carter DC. Management of gastric variceal haemorrhage. *Br J Surg* 1990;77(3):297-299.

90. Ota K, Shirai Z, Masuzaki T, et al. Endoscopic injection sclerotherapy with n-butyl-2-cyanoacrylate for ruptured duodenal varices. *J Gastroenterol* 1998;33(4): 550-555.

91. Bhasin DK, Sharma BC, Sriram PV, Makharia G, Singh K. Endoscopic management of bleeding ectopic varices with histoacryl. *HPB Surg* 1999;11(3):171-173.

92. Tan NC, Ibrahim S, Tay KH. Successful management of a bleeding duodenal varix by endoscopic banding. *Singapore Med J* 2005;46(12):723-725.

93. Zamora CA, Sugimoto K, Tsurusaki M, et al. Endovascular obliteration of bleeding duodenal varices in patients with liver cirrhosis. *Eur Radiol* 2006;16(1): 73-79.

94. Jonnalagadda SS, Quiason S, Smith OJ. Successful therapy of bleeding duodenal varices by TIPS after failure of sclerotherapy. *Am J Gastroenterol* 1998;93(2):272-274.

95. Sort P, Elizalde I, Llach I, et al. Duodenal variceal bleeding treated with a transjugular intrahepatic portosystemic shunt. *Endoscopy* 1995;27(8):626-627.

96. Cottam DR, Clark R, Hayn E, Shaftan G. Duodenal varices: a novel treatment and literature review. *Am Surg* 2002;68(5):407-409.

97. Qiao HQ, Liu B, Dai WJ, Jiang HC. Resection for ruptured duodenal varices secondary to portal hypertension. *Chin Med Sci J* 2004;19(4):301-302.

98. Crofts TJ, Park KG, Steele RJ, Chung SS, Li AK. A randomized trial of nonoperative treatment for perforated peptic ulcer. *N Engl J Med* 1989;320(15):970-973.

99. Ng EK, Lam YH, Sung JJ, et al. Eradication of Helicobacter pylori prevents recurrence of ulcer after simple closure of duodenal ulcer perforation: randomized controlled trial. *Ann Surg* 2000;231(2):153-158.

100. Gupta S, Kaushik R, Sharma R, Attri A. The management of large perforations of duodenal ulcers. *BMC Surg* 2005;5:15.

101. Cranford CA, Jr., Olson R, Bradley EL, 3rd. Gastric disconnection in the management of perforated giant duodenal ulcer. *Am J Surg* 1988;155(3):439-442.

102. Stabile BE. Redefining the role of surgery for perforated duodenal ulcer in the Helicobacter pylori era. *Ann Surg* 2000;231(2):159-160.

103. Sanabria AE, Morales CH, Villegas MI. Laparoscopic repair for perforated peptic ulcer disease. *Cochrane Database Syst Rev* 2005;(4):CD004778.

104. Kaiser AM, Katkhouda N. Laparoscopic management of the perforated viscus. *Semin Laparosc Surg* 2002;9(1): 46-53.

105. Katkhouda N, Mavor E, Mason RJ, Campos GM, Soroushyari A, Berne TV. Laparoscopic repair of perforated duodenal ulcers: outcome and efficacy in 30 consecutive patients. *Arch Surg* 1999;134(8):845-848; discussion 9-50.

106. Lunevicius R, Morkevicius M. Comparison of laparoscopic versus open repair for perforated duodenal ulcers. *Surg Endosc* 2005;19(12):1565-1571.

107. Naesgaard JM, Edwin B, Reiertsen O, Trondsen E, Faerden AE, Rosseland AR. Laparoscopic and open operation in patients with perforated peptic ulcer. *Eur J Surg* 1999;165(3):209-214.

108. Siu WT, Chau CH, Law BK, Tang CN, Ha PY, Li MK. Routine use of laparoscopic repair for perforated peptic ulcer. *Br J Surg* 2004;91(4):481-484.

109. Tsumura H, Ichikawa T, Hiyama E, Murakami Y. Laparoscopic and open approach in perforated peptic ulcer. *Hepatogastroenterology* 2004;51(59):1536-1539.

110. Vettoretto N, Poiatti R, Fisogni D, Diana DR, Balestra L, Giovanetti M. Comparison between laparoscopic and open repair for perforated peptic ulcer. A retrospective study. *Chir Ital* 2005;57(3):317-322.

111. Turner WW, Jr., Thompson WM, Jr., Thal ER. Perforated gastric ulcers. A plea for management by simple closures. *Arch Surg* 1988;123(8):960-964.

112. Hewitt PM, Krige J, Bornman PC. Perforated gastric ulcers: resection compared with simple closure. *Am Surg* 1993;59(10):669-673.

113. Madiba TE, Nair R, Mulaudzi TV, Thomson SR. Perforated gastric ulcer—reappraisal of surgical options. *S Afr J Surg* 2005;43(3):58-60.

114. Di Quinzio C, Phang PT. Surgical management of perforated benign gastric ulcer in high-risk patients. *Can J Surg* 1992;35(1):94-97.

115. Tsugawa K, Koyanagi N, Hashizume M, et al. The therapeutic strategies in performing emergency surgery for gastroduodenal ulcer perforation in 130 patients over 70 years of age. *Hepatogastroenterology* 2001;48(37): 156-162.

116. McDonald MP, Broughan TA, Hermann RE, Philip RS, Hoerr SO. Operations for gastric ulcer: a long-term study. *Am Surg* 1996;62(8):673-677.

117. Noguiera C, Silva AS, Santos JN, et al. Perforated peptic ulcer: main factors of morbidity and mortality. *World J Surg* 2003;27(7):782-787.

118. Wysocki A, Biesiada Z, Beben P, Budzynski A. Perforated gastric ulcer. *Dig Surg* 2000;17(2):132-137.

119. Roviello F, Rossi S, Marrelli D, et al. Perforated gastric carcinoma: a report of 10 cases and review of the literature. *World J Surg Oncol* 2006;4:19.

120. Kasakura Y, Ajani JA, Fujii M, Mochizuki F, Takayama T. Management of perforated gastric carcinoma: a report of 16 cases and review of world literature. *Am Surg* 2002;68(5):434-440.

121. Larmi TK. Perforation of gastric carcinoma. *Acta Chir Scand* 1962;123:222-227.

122. Siegert TA, Donegan WL. Acute perforation of gastric carcinoma. *Wis Med J* 1982;81(10):17-21.

123. Stechenberg L, Bunch RH, Anderson MC. The surgical therapy for perforated gastric cancer. *Am Surg* 1981;47(5):208-210.

124. Wilson TS. Free perforation in malignancies of the stomach. *Can J Surg* 1966;9(4):357-364.

125. Lehnert T, Buhl K, Dueck M, Hinz U, Herfarth C. Two-stage radical gastrectomy for perforated gastric cancer. *Eur J Surg Oncol* 2000;26(8):780-784.

126. Yabuki K, Tamasaki Y, Satoh K, Maekawa T, Matsumoto M. Primary gastric lymphoma with spontaneous perforation: report of a case. *Surg Today* 2000;30(11): 1030-1033.

127. Attard-Montalto S, Kingston JE, Eden OB. Gastric perforation in non-Hodgkin's lymphoma. *Pediatr Hematol Oncol* 1993;10(1):101-103.

Chapter 6

NONTRAUMATIC EMERGENCY SURGERY OF THE SMALL INTESTINE

David H. Livingston, MD, and Chirag Badami, MD

INTRODUCTION

As the longest organ in the gastrointestinal tract, the small intestine plays a critical role in numerous functions including digestion, absorption of nutrients, maintaining electrolyte balance, and the immunologic defense against environmental factors. Ensuring the optimal functioning of the small bowel requires a complex interaction of structural and endocrine processes. The small intestine ranges in size from 5 to 6 m in the adult, beginning just distal from the pyloric sphincter and extending all the way to the ileocecal valve. Even though it is a very large organ, and it has such important functions, there is a surprising lack of intrinsic pathology seen in the small bowel. In this chapter, we will focus on the most common disorders that require emergency surgical consultation and care. Trauma to the small bowel will be covered in a separate chapter.

ANATOMY

The small intestine is divided into three major segments: the duodenum, jejunum, and ileum. The duodenum is the shortest part of the small intestine, approximately 20-25 cm long, extends from the pylorus to the ligament of Treitz. The duodenum itself is divided into four parts, which include the bulb, descending, transverse, and ascending duodenum. The jejunum begins at the ligament of Treitz, which creates the duodenojejunal angle. At times adhesions and bands make it difficult to identify the actual location of the ligament of Treitz. In these cases, a useful landmark is to identify the inferior mesenteric vein in the retroperitoneum, which leads the surgeon to the exit of the duodenum from the retroperitoneum. There is no clear anatomic delineation between the jejunum and the ileum. During emergency surgery when a patient has recently eaten, lacteals can be better identified in the jejunum and there is a gradual change in the architecture of the arterial supply in the mesentery. In the jejunum, the vasa recta are longer and straighter, whereas in the ileum they are shorter and more branched. Classically, the jejunum is represented by the first 40% of the small bowel. The arterial supply of the small intestine is delivered by the celiac and superior mesenteric arteries from the aorta. The duodenum has the most complicated blood supply with multiple branches off the celiac trunk. The jejunum and ileum are supplied by branches of intestinal arteries from the superior mesenteric artery. The venous drainage parallels the artery supply for the small intestine.

SMALL BOWEL OBSTRUCTION

EPIDEMIOLOGY

Obstruction is the most common small bowel pathology that will require emergency surgical consultation and accounts for 20% of all acute surgical admissions.[1] Over 60,000 patients a year are admitted with bowel obstruction at a cost of more than $800 million annually. Although small bowel obstruction (SBO) can be caused by numerous pathologies, postoperative adhesions are far and away the most common cause accounting for two-thirds to three-quarters of all patients.[2] Malignancies (9%), hernias (8%), inflammatory bowel disease (5%), and other miscellaneous causes (4%) account for the rest.[3] Categorization by etiology is also useful as it has impact on the treatment and eventual need for emergent surgical intervention. Simply put, the presence of small bowel obstruction in the patient who has never had a prior abdominal operation or those patients with an incarcerated and irreducible hernia require urgent surgical intervention. In contrast, most of the time and effort of the acute care surgeon is related to determining the optimal care of those patients with obstruction due to postoperative adhesions.

The most common previous operations that lead to SBO include appendectomy (23%), colorectal resection

(21%), gynecological surgery (12%), upper gastrointestinal (gastric, biliary, or splenic) surgery (9%), small bowel surgery (8%), and more than one previous abdominal operation (24%).[2] Considering whether the patient had an open surgical procedure may also be important. Evidence has shown that laparoscopy produces fewer intra-abdominal adhesions when compared to open surgery.[4] This may be due to less manipulation and mobilization of intra-abdominal contents. Nonetheless, SBO has been reported following laparoscopic procedures and the location of the port sites may aid the surgeon in identifying what operation was performed previously. Many studies have also shown that SBO is more common after lower abdominal and pelvic operations.[2,5] The proposed explanation is that the bowel is normally tethered more cephalad at the root of the mesentery and therefore adhesions within the lower portion of the abdomen and pelvis are more likely to lead to an obstruction and torsion of the small bowel based solely on mechanical considerations.

Malignancies are the second most common cause of obstruction, and the diagnosis should be entertained if a patient presents with SBO that has not had any previous abdominal surgery. Although previously it was uncommon to make these diagnoses prior to emergent celiotomy, the liberal use of CT scanning in patients presenting with abdominal pain and signs of obstruction makes the preoperative identification of a mass likely. Primary malignant tumors of the small bowel are a heterogeneous group of tumors and are uncommon compared to tumors in other locations of the gastrointestinal tract. SBO is more likely due to a secondary malignant cause[6,7] with the obstruction caused by direct extension of other primary GI tumors or other metastatic lesions including lymph nodes in the abdominal cavity. Primary small bowel tumors are difficult to diagnose and the first sign of presentation maybe a surgical emergency, whether it is a perforation, bleeding, or obstruction. One study demonstrated a correlation between type of small bowel tumors and clinical emergency presentation of the patient: gastrointestinal stromal tumors (GIST) presented with GI bleeding, carcinoids with SBO, lymphomas with free perforations, and metastasis from melanoma resulting in intussusception.[8]

Although hernias comprise a small percentage of all patients presenting with SBO, this group is at high risk for intestinal strangulation and is of considerable importance to acute care surgeons.[9] External hernias include groin (inguinal and femoral) and all types of ventral/abnormal wall hernias. The diagnosis should be relatively straightforward, provided a good physical examining is carried out. It is unfortunately all too common to be called in consultation for a patient with suspected bowel obstruction only to find an incarcerated hernia after the patient is finally disrobed and appropriately examined. Making the diagnosis of an external hernia causing SBO on CT scanning is merely a sign of poor clinical skills. These should all be able to be identified with a good physical examination. Internal hernias may masquerade as adhesive obstruction, especially in those patients with prior abdominal procedures. When suspicion of a hernia exists, the patient should be observed closely, as earlier if not immediate surgical intervention may be needed.

Other uncommon causes of small bowel obstruction can include Crohn disease, gallstone ileus, pregnancy, intra-abdominal abscesses, bezoars, intussusceptions, and familial Mediterranean fever. In the pediatric population, possible causes include intussusception, pyloric stenosis, and congenital intestinal atresia.[5]

PREOPERATIVE

CLINICAL MANIFESTATIONS

The overall goal in the management of bowel obstruction is to determine which patients need acute operative intervention and which do not. Although distinction appears simple when written in black and white, when facing a postoperative patient with abdominal distension and pain, low grade fever, and tachycardia who may or may not be passing flatus, the issue becomes much more gray. Unfortunately, with the exception of better imaging using CT scanning, little has changed in the overall management of the patients with SBO in the past two decades.[1]

In a patient with prior abdominal surgery, a good history and physical will quickly rule out hernias and will lead the surgeon to a rapid diagnosis of adhesive obstruction. On questioning, abdominal pain, although nonspecific, is the most common complaint. Pain that is crampy and intermittent is more prevalent in simple obstruction, where the bowel is not ischemic.[10] Pain that occurs for a shorter duration and is colicky and associated with bilious vomiting may indicate a relative proximal obstruction, whereas pain that is longer lasting associated with more feculent vomitus may be more indicative of a distal obstruction.[11] Pain that starts out crampy but increases and becomes constant has been associated with strangulated or ischemic bowel. Nonetheless, putting too much emphasis on the duration and quality of pain will likely lead the examiner astray as there is great overlap in symptoms between those patients with compromised bowel and those who do not. Other symptoms will include nausea and vomiting with an inability to keep food or liquids down. Anorexia is also common. The lack of passing flatus has an association with complete obstruction; however, early on, patients may experience diarrhea or normal bowel movements as a colonic response to the more proximal obstruction. Again, there is great spectrum of symptoms and the most important issue is not to identify the precise anatomic location of the obstruction but to determine whether urgent operative intervention is required.

As outlined earlier, the physical symptoms are common in obstruction but are not very specific. Even with compromised bowel, the young healthy patient may have no change in their vital signs. Slight tachycardia is often present and may be merely secondary to pain or more importantly dehydration as a result of limited oral intake, vomiting, and the third spacing of fluid into the bowel lumen. Obstruction, whether partial or complete, leads to an accumulation of bowel contents, including gastrointestinal secretions and air, proximal to the obstruction resulting in dilatation of the bowel loops proximal to the obstruction. The dilatation of bowel leads into a cycle of increased intraluminal pressures, causing additional water and electrolytes to continuously be secreted into the lumen of the bowel causing fluid "third spacing" and worsening dehydration. Electrolyte disturbances are frequent and commonly result in a hypochloremic, hypokalemic contraction metabolic alkalosis. Of course, with more long-standing obstruction and bilious vomiting, a mixed electrolyte abnormalities may be observed. In contrast to early SBO where peristalsis is increased, small bowel edema and intraluminal fluid leads to fatigue and less muscle activity as the obstruction persists. Thus the patient's pain may actually be improved during this time period as their crampy pain is relieved. Further fluid sequestration may lead to increased intra-abdominal pressure, bowel wall ischemia, pulmonary dysfunction, and renal dysfunction. At this point, intravascular volume should be rapidly corrected and urgent surgical intervention is warranted.

Radiographic Studies

Even with these signs on history and physical suggestive of SBO, radiographic studies are invaluable to both confirm the diagnosis of bowel obstruction and also to aid in the managment.[12] The initial step should be abdominal radiographs. These can be usually performed quicker than abdominal computed tomography (CT) scan and may provide sufficient information to proceed with immediate surgical intervention without further radiographic studies. Although it may be difficult for the current generation of house offices and medical students to understand, an abdominal CT scan is not an absolute prerequisite to get into the operating room. Optimally, both supine and upright abdominal radiographs should be obtained. In patients that cannot stand, lateral decubitus films may be substituted. The characteristic findings seen on plain radiographs will be dilated loops of small bowel with air fluid interfaces at multiple levels (especially in more distal obstructions) without colonic distention (Fig. 6-1). Edema of the bowel may be observed by increased space between the bowel loops as well as a widening of the valvulae conniventes. The valvulae markings are usually closely spaced and should be within 1 to 4 mm of each other, but this distance

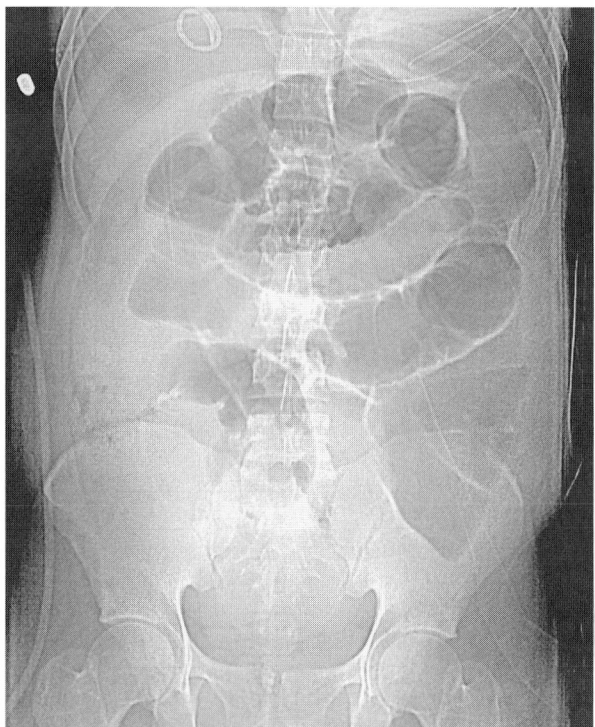

Figure 6-1 *Plain abdominal film demonstrating several features of small bowel obstruction. Small bowel loops are both dilated (midabdomen) and fluid-filled (right lower quadrant and pelvis). There does not appear to be a significant degree of edema in the small bowel. There is a paucity of gas in the left and right colon and only some air present in the transverse colon. An NG tube has been inserted, which may decrease the ability to see the degree of proximal dilatation. From this single film, it cannot be determined whether this patient has a complete or partial obstruction, although it appears that the point of obstruction is in the distal small bowel.*

increases with small-bowel distention and edema. A lack of small bowel distension may be present if the site of obstruction is in the proximal jejunum. In these cases, a distended air/fluid filled stomach or even duodenum may be observed if the patient has not vomited recently or a nasogastric tube has not been placed. If any signs of free air are seen on the film, that patient should be taken to the operating room immediately for exploratory laparotomy. Plain radiographs are reasonable as a first-line screening examination, but diagnostic failure rates of as much as 30% have been reported.[14] In two studies, the sensitivity of plain radiographs were reported as 75%, and specificity was reported to be 53%.[12-14]

Abdominal CT scanning has emerged as the radiologic study of choice for SBO. CT scanning is over 90% sensitive and specific in diagnosing SBO (Fig. 6-2).[13-14] In addition, CT scanning has proved useful in distinguishing extrinsic causes such as adhesions and hernia from intrinsic causes such as neoplasms or Crohn disease. It also differentiates the above from intraluminal

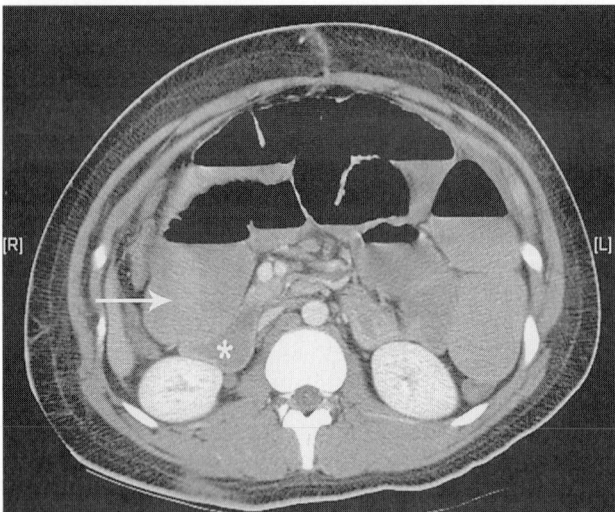

Figure 6-2a *Representative CT scans from the patient in Fig. 6-1 demonstrating the dilated loops of small bowel with obvious air-fluid levels (arrow) and the bowel just proximal to the transition zone (∗). There is no gas present in the left colon, which can be seen below the dilated fluid filled loop of small bowel.*

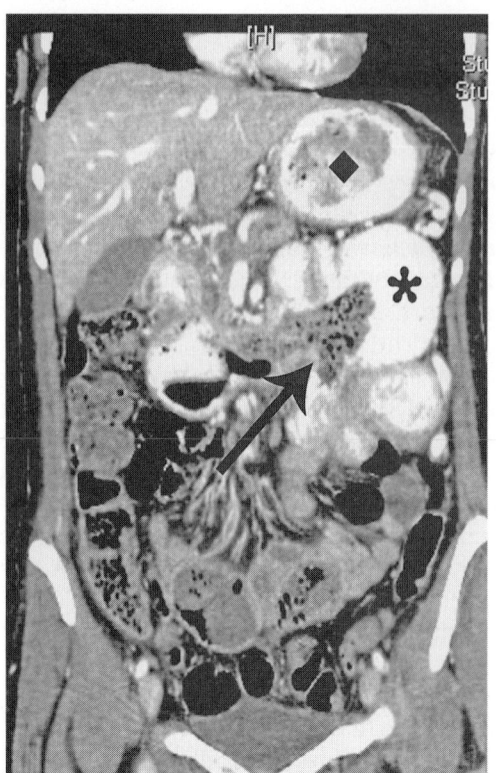

Figure 6-3 *The utility of CT scanning in managing SBO is demonstrated in this coronal reconstruction of a patient with bezoars at multiple levels. The patient had a significant amount of hair removed from her stomach endoscopically, but the follow-up CT here shows residual material in the stomach, which would probably pass (♦), but additional inspissated material (arrow) and dilated proximal small bowel (∗), which required exploration and evacuation of the material.*

causes such as bezoars (Fig. 6-3).[15] The level of obstruction may be determined by identifying the change in the lumen of the bowel from dilated to collapsed loops of bowel (the transition zone). The degree of collapse and the amount of residual content in the distal bowel beyond the obstruction are useful to note. The passage of contrast material into the distant collapsed segment indicates that the obstruction is partial or incomplete. CT scans rarely identify an adhesive band but, rather, the diagnosis of adhesions is based on the identifying the transition zone in the small bowel without another identifiable cause of the obstruction cause. It is also important in pinpointing the location of the obstruction and has the ability to detect early signs of bowel ischemia. Ischemia is manifested by bowel wall thickening, poor enhancement of the bowel wall, target sign, mesenteric stranding and congestion, ascites, and pneumatosis intestinalis. Thus, CT scanning may result in findings that have prognostic significance and lead to the identification of patients who may be observed compared to those who require urgent surgical intervention.

Other radiologic methods include enterolysis and ultrasound. Enterolysis involves the placement of barium or Gastrografin contrast usually via a postpyloric nasogastric tube to view the intestinal obstruction under direct fluoroscopy. This seems to be more useful in chronic obstructive patients. Ultrasound may also be used in pregnant patients in order to prevent radiation exposure. Recently capsule endoscopy, even without prior radiological examination, has been used to interrogate some patients with possible strictures and

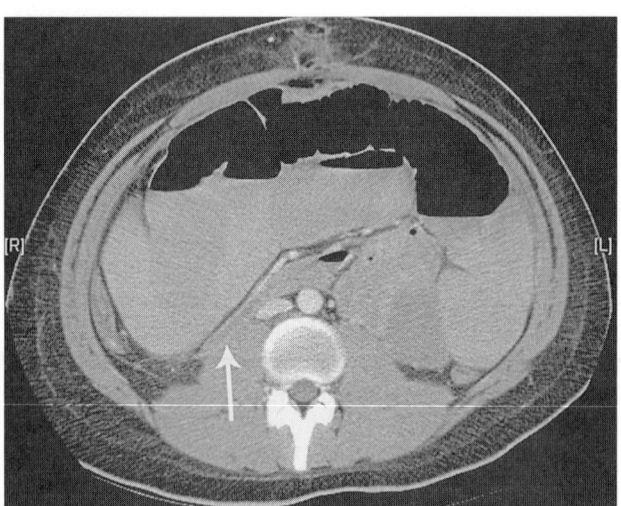

Figure 6-2b *CT scan just lower to that shown in Fig. 6-2a showing the collapsed loop of small bowel (arrow) just after the transition zone. This finding clearly demonstrates complete obstruction. At exploration, the patient had several thick adhesions, resulting in torsion of the small bowel in the distal ileum.*

chronic obstructive symptomatology. The utility of this modality remains under investigation and is not applicable to those patients with acute obstruction.

The optimal management of adhesive small bowel obstruction remains controversial. From a surgical standpoint, the goal is to operate on only those patients who will not resolve their obstruction and to do so before bowel ischemia or compromise necessitate bowel resection. Not surprisingly, delays in surgery and the need for bowel resection have been clearly associated with an increase in complications and mortality.[16-17] Therefore, those patients who manifest obvious signs and symptoms of peritonitis or possible strangulated obstruction require urgent operation on presentation. In this group, the decision making and care is relatively straightforward. Thankfully, most patients do not fall into this group and usually receive trial "conservative" treatment unless, as stated earlier, there is suspicion of bowel strangulation. Unfortunately, the optimal duration of this trial conservative treatment is not clear and there has been no definite answer as to when conservative treatment should be considered unsuccessful and the patient should undergo surgery.

Initial treatment in either scenario should begin with fluid resuscitation and nasogastric decompression. As discussed, these patients are often dehydrated secondary to intraluminal fluid sequestration vomiting and lack of oral intake. Careful attention to electrolyte abnormalities and acid-base balance, especially in those patients with long-standing obstruction, is required, and patients often will need electrolyte replacement. Adequate fluid resuscitation can usually be monitored by urine output but elderly patients or those with preexisting cardiopulmonary morbidities may require central venous or even pulmonary artery pressure monitoring. Antibiotics should be reserved for those patients with signs of perforation or peritonitis or those patients on the way to the operating room. Despite experimental evidence that intestinal obstruction causes an increase in bacterial translocation there is *no* role for routine antibiotic administration in patients with simple obstruction.[18]

The next step in the treatment of simple obstruction would involve intestinal decompression via a nasogastric tube. The tube is placed into the stomach and attached to wall suction device. Previously, much debate and many resident hours were utilized to pass long intestinal tubes. Thankfully prospective randomized trials have shown no significant difference.[19] Depending on the series, such treatment is reported to be successful in 73%-90% of cases involving patients who present with simple obstruction that will resolve without any surgical intervention.[20-22] However, surgical treatment may be required in one-third of patients because of significant complications, such as strangulation, which can develop when surgery is delayed for more than 48 hours.[23-24] In reality, these patients have noncomplete obstruction that will resolve over time or

that decompression of the proximal bowel will allow the remainder of the small bowel to "detort" and regain function. Patients who fail are those patients who have complete obstruction at the time of presentation. Only time will differentiate the two groups and, as stated earlier, the goal is to identify those patients who require surgical intervention prior to the development of bowel compromise. There are no hard and fast evidence-based guidelines for the length of time that should be allotted to tube decompression. If the patient shows signs of a worsening condition, early rather than late, intervention should be instituted. Several studies have shown a trial of 3 days of nonoperative management and, in some cases, up to 5 days in order to resolve the obstruction.[18] In patients with clear evidence of partial obstruction, several weeks of conservative therapy haven been utilized, although this delay clearly increases hospital length of stay. Ultimately, many of these patients eventually go on to operative intervention.

Thus, the real goal in the care of a patient who presents with adhesive obstruction would be to determine who has a complete obstruction and requires a lysis of adhesion, and who will resolve with nonoperative management. Administration of Gastrografin has emerged as a useful modality to determine which patients will resolve their obstruction versus those who are complete.[25-29] This technique involves the administration of a bolus of Gastrografin with radiologic follow-up studies. The contrast should appear in the colon within 24 hours. An early prospective randomized trial showed that the average time to pass stool decreased from 23 to 6 hours and the hospital stay went from 4 to 2 days in the group treated with contrast.[21] Subsequent randomized studies demonstrated that use of Gastrografin in adhesive small bowel obstruction is safe and reliable to determine which patients required surgery.[25-28] It was initially postulated that the mechanism of action was promoting the movement of fluid from the intestinal wall, reducing bowel wall edema, improving intestinal motility, and increasing the pressure gradient across the obstruction. As more data has come forward, it remains unclear if this technique truly reduces the need for surgical intervention or if it merely better identifies those patients. In a structured review and meta-analysis of the available literature, Abbas et al found strong evidence supporting the routine use of water-soluble contrast as a predictive test for nonoperative resolution of adhesive small bowel obstruction.[28] Although they could not find conclusive data supporting the finding that Gastrografin administration decreased the number of patients who required operative intervention, it clearly reduced hospital stay in those patients who did resolve their obstruction. Recently, Chen et al, in a small randomized prospective series of 128 patients, utilized an oral regimen of magnesium oxide, *Lactobacillus. acidophilus* and simethicone, and found that it was safe and effective in hastening the resolution of conservatively treated partial adhesive small-bowel obstruction and shortening the hospital stay (4 days versus 1 day).[29] As this therapy was compared to standard nasogastric decompression, it is unknown whether it is better than Gastrografin.

OPERATIVE MANAGEMENT

Surgical intervention remains an integral part of the care of patients with suspected strangulated obstruction or those in whom conservative treatment with emergent laparotomy being the mainstay of treatment for patients with peritonitis. However, as experience with advanced minimally invasive surgical techniques increases, its use in simple bowel obstruction (a previously relative contraindication) has also expanded.[30] Kirshtein in a small and undoubtedly selected series of 65 patient reported that about half were able to be successfully corrected using laparoscopy alone, 20% required a limited incision, and 30% required conversion to a formal laparotomy.[31] Because the obstruction in many cases is a result of a single or few adhesive bands, there is no doubt that laparoscopic techniques will play a definite role in the care of selected patients. When operating on a patient with bowel distention by any technique, great care must be taken when manipulating the bowel as it may be very friable or thinned out. Even the use of "nontraumatic clamps" may lead to perforation of compromised bowel. Manipulation of the mesentery or large segments of intestine preferred in order to accomplish the reduction and detorsion of the obstructed bowel. Precise sharp dissection of adhesive bands is preferred to prevent tearing long areas of the distended bowel. A useful technique to relieve the intraluminal distension is to pass the nasogastric tube into the duodenum or to "milk back" the intestinal contents into the stomach. Although it is time-consuming and labor-intensive, this technique also can aid in closing the laparotomy incision and decreasing the incidence of intra-abdominal hypertension in the postoperative period. Again, great care must be taken not to damage the bowel. At the conclusion of all cases and especially those cases where the obstruction has been long-standing, the bowel must be inspected for viability.

Any clinical suspicion of strangulated obstruction demands an immediate laparotomy. Obviously, nonviable or perforated intestine demands resection. The intraoperative decision making in these cases stems from what should be the limit of resection and whether the patient should undergo primary anastomosis during this setting. Although clearly black or pulseless bowel requires resection, the decision whether dilated, hemorrhagic, or congested bowel is viable, especially in the face of long-standing obstruction or a patient with marginal perfusion due to hemodynamic compromise can be challenging. Following relief of the obstruction, the bowel should be wrapped in warm saline soaked laparotomy pads and allowed to recover for 5-10 minutes to see if there is a return of color of the bowel serosa. It is important to have patience, as 5-10 minutes "doing nothing" in the operating room can feel like an eternity; however, overaggressive resection of potentially viable bowel does nothing to help a patient who may later require reoperation for the same condition. In addition, evaluation of the arterial supply in the mesentery by inspection or Doppler examination, looking for a biphasic arterial pulse, is useful. A fluorescein test also has been advocated by some, and one prospective randomized trial investigating ischemic injury to the intestines found that it was superior to clinical judgment alone.[32] Finally, adopting an approach for the trauma literature or those patients who undergo mesenteric vascular occlusion, the bowel can be left in discontinuity and returned the abdominal cavity with a planned reexploration within 24 hours. Care should be taken to make sure that the remaining bowel is well decompressed so as to not further compromise the intestinal microcirculation. The patients should be monitored carefully and returned to the operating room earlier than 24 hours if their condition deteriorates.

SMALL BOWEL PERFORATION

Primary small bowel perforations are uncommon and are often only diagnosed when a patient undergoes emergency laparotomy for free air or peritonitis. Prolonged obstruction is a very common cause, but other causes include ulcers, inflammatory bowel disease, ischemia, neoplasms, cytomegalovirus infection, trauma, iatrogenesis during endoscopy and surgery, and foreign bodies. Not surprisingly, there is a paucity of data on nontraumatic small bowel perforations.[33-34] If one includes the proximal duodenum, then ulcer disease is the major cause of nontraumatic small bowel perforations. Although significant advances in the diagnosis and treatment of *H. pylori* as a cause of ulcer disease, a significant number of patients will present first with perforation with duodenal perforations two to three times more than with gastric perforations.[35] Excluding ulcer disease, the three most common etiologies of nontraumatic small bowel perforations are Crohn disease, foreign body perforations, and strangulated obstructions.

PREOPERATIVE

CLINICAL MANIFESTATIONS

Patients most commonly will present as an emergency with peritonitis. A history of inflammatory bowel disease will identify those patients with a likely perforation secondary to Crohn. As a reasonable percentage of patients will present with a perforation as their first indication of ulcer disease, there may be no specific antecedent history. Foreign body perforation has been associated with edentulous patients as well as the use of toothpicks, but almost always the diagnosis made at the time of celiotomy. Information regarding medication usage, such as aspirin, nonsteroidal anti-inflammatory drugs (NSAIDs), or steroids should be obtained, but as these drugs are so commonly used, the information may only be relevant in retrospect. Almost all patients will complain of abdominal pain. Nausea and vomiting are unlikely to be symptoms of a perforation but may be present if the patient has obstruction. Also, the patient may complain of hiccups as a current or previous symptom, and that may be a sign of free air in the peritoneal cavity. Patients with peritonitis, especially those with tachycardia, fever, or a decrease in blood pressure, require urgent resuscitation prior to emergent surgical exploration. The goal is not to restore the patient to "normal physiology" but merely to begin a resuscitative process that will continue in the intra- and postoperative periods.

Classic radiographic imaging begins with an upright chest film looking for evidence of pneumoperitoneum (Fig. 6-4). The most common finding of intraperitoneal air should be subdiaphragmatic on an upright chest radiograph. However, radiographs will not show any free air in 30% of patients with intestinal perforations,[36] especially in perforations more distal in the GI tract. If a large amount of air is in the abdominal cavity, there may be a visible falciform ligament, extending from the right upper quadrant to the umbilicus. Another method of identifying a pneumoperitoneum is by ultrasonography. Ultrasound may be much better at detecting free air than a plain radiograph and

pneumoperitoneum appears as a linear area of increased echogenicity with distal ringdown or reverberation artifact.[28] CT scanning has emerged as the best of choice in evaluating patients with suspected intra-abdominal process. However, if the diagnosis of free air is made in plane radiographs CT is a waste of time and money. CT has the ability to detect loculated free air or an intra-abdominal abscess, which would suggest intestinal perforation. As stated previously, a majority of nontraumatic small bowel perforations will be diagnosed in the operating room. The optimal treatment of subgroup of patients with perforations secondary to ulcer disease is discussed in a separate chapter; however, almost all patients present with perforations smaller than 1 cm and can be treated by either simple closure with omental buttressing or a Graham patch using omentum or falciform ligament. Following closure, patients should be treated for *Helicobacter pylori*. Discontinuation of aspirin and NSAIDS is also appropriate.

OPERATIVE MANAGEMENT

The optimal treatment for primary small bowel perforations depends on the underlying pathology and the physiology of the patient. In general, the goal for patients with Crohn disease is to treat the perforation at the same time avoiding potentially unnecessary and extensive bowel resections as these patients are likely to require additional procedures in the future. Free perforations are uncommon, as the transmural inflammation often leads to significant adhesions between the inflamed bowel and surrounding viscera. Abscesses also often respond to medical therapy and when indicated percutaneous drainage. Thus, the indications for surgery in this group of patients are free perforations and those perforations unresponsive to medical management. Resection of gross disease along with a small margin of macroscopically disease-free bowel (about 5 cm) is optimal.

In patients with perforations secondary to foreign bodies, usually all that is needed is to resect the perforated segment back to the noninflamed bowel. Patients with perforations secondary to strangulated obstructions or ischemia may have a significant amount of dusky or compromised bowel. In these patients, simple resection of the perforated segment, followed by resuscitation and a second-look operation in 24 hours, may allow the surgeon to save intestinal length.

SMALL BOWEL BLEEDING

PREOPERATIVE

Gastrointestinal (GI) bleeding is a very common problem accounting for 1-2% of all acute hospital admissions

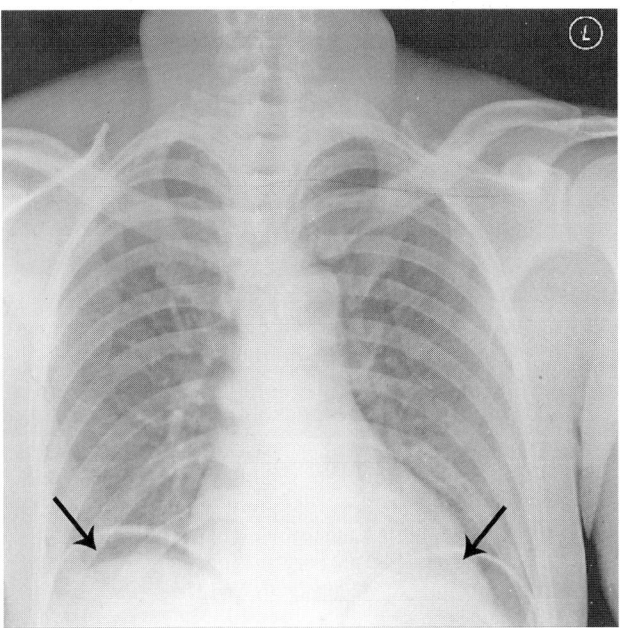

Figure 6-4 *Upright chest radiograph demonstrating free air under both diaphragms (see arrows).*

with a reported incidence of 170 per 100,000 adults per year.[37-38] Although bleeding can occur anywhere from the mouth to rectum, excluding bleeding ulcers, primary small bowel hemorrhage is uncommon, accounting for 1-5% of all cases of GI bleeding. GI bleeding from ulcer disease is usually easily detected and managed by esophagogastroduodenoscopy (EGD). Similarly, patients with colonic bleeding can usually be diagnosed via colonoscopy. In contrast, the diagnosis of GI bleeding from the small bowel distal to the second portion of the duodenum to ileocecal valve can be challenging as this area is much more difficult to access and isolate. Often a patient will present with one or more bouts of GI bleeding with "negative" upper and lower endoscopic evaluations. If a nasogastric tube has been inserted, it is most often free of blood. Unless the bleeding is rapid, the stool will be either guaiac-positive or show some signs of melena. Blood tests may show a microcytic anemia and low iron stores in patients with chronic ongoing bleeding. Unless the patient is exsanguinating, rarely is he or she immediately taken to the operating room because it is challenging even to find the source of bleeding under direct visualization. Other methods of treatment have been developed and are much more accurate in locating the bleed. Radiographic methods include enteroclysis, which involves a series of abdominal radiographs following ingestion of contrast to visual bowel wall irregularities. This method is a first-line evaluation for small bowel bleeding but does not provide a treatment and can easily miss AVMs.

Methods of visualization of the small intestine beyond the ligament of Treitz have used a pediatric colonoscope or a long videoenteroscope; however, it still remains a challenge.[39-40] Small bowel endoscopy can be broken down into three major methods. These involve a "push" endoscopy, an intraoperative endoscopy, and a wireless capsule endoscopy. "Push" endoscopy involves the use of a pediatric endoscopy, and extending past the ligament of Treitz. An intraoperative endoscopy consists of a laparotomy and directly placing the endoscope into the small bowel and may disclose arteriovenous malformations by transillumination. A wireless capsule endoscopy involves a capsule that is swallowed by the patient. This capsule, about the size of a large pill, is allowed to transit the entire small bowel while capturing images. Several studies have shown the benefit of capsule endoscopy, especially when comparing it to other endoscopic methods.[41-43] If endoscopy is unsuccessful or cannot be performed, or if the patient is rapidly hemorrhaging, selective mesenteric angiography is a good method to locate and possibly embolize the bleeding. Contrast is injected via the artery in order to visualize extravasation in the bleeding vessels. In order for this to occur, the bleeding must be occurring at a rate greater than 0.5 cc per minute. Finally, if all of these methods are deemed unsuccessful, a bleeding scan using ^{99m}technetium (Tc)-labeled red blood cells could be performed.[44] This is a good method for visualizing bleeding at lower rates, but the isotope does accumulate in the intestine and is pushed down via peristalsis, making it difficult to locate the exact site of bleeding. Bleeding located by angiography also may be embolized by coils to control or subdue the hemorrhaging.

OPERATIVE MANAGEMENT

Treatment for acute GI bleeds starts with resuscitation with fluid and blood and correction of any coagulopathy followed by identification of the source of the bleeding. Treatment of small bowel bleeding is managed based on the pathology and the rapidity of the bleeding. Bleeding from neoplastic disease requires operation and resection. Slow or intermittent bleeds from AVMs often can be managed conservatively. Rapid bleeding may be able to be treated at least initially with angiographic embolization. In the operating room, the blood will tend to suffuse through the entire small bowel. The one caveat for surgical management in these patients is to avoid blind resections as it is often "embarrassing" to resect what is throughout to be the offending segment of bowel, only to have the patients rebleed in the recovery room. Enterotomy with intraoperative endoscopy also has been employed, with some success.

REFERENCES

1. Bass KN, Jones B, Bulkley GB. Current management of small-bowel obstruction. *Adv Surg* 1997;31:1-34.
2. Cox MR, Gunn IF, Eastman MC, et al. The operative etiology and types of adhesions causing small bowel obstruction. *Aust N Z J Surg* 1993;63(11):848-852.
3. Bizer LS, Liebling RW, Delany HM, Gliedman ML. Small bowel obstruction: the role of nonoperative treatment in simple intestinal obstruction and predictive criteria for strangulation obstruction. *Surgery* 1981;89(4):407-413.
4. Garrard CL, Clements RH, Nanney L, et al. Adhesion formation is reduced after laparoscopic surgery. *Surg Endosc* 1999;13(1):10-13.
5. Hayanga AJ, Bass-Wilkins K, Bulkley GB. Current management of small-bowel obstruction. *Adv Surg* 2005;39:1-33.
6. Mucha P, Jr. Small intestinal obstruction. *Surg Clin North Am* 1987;67(3):597-620.
7. Barclay TH, Schapira DV. Malignant tumors of the small intestine. *Cancer* 1983;51(5):878-881.
8. Catena F, Ansaloni L, Gazzotti F, et al. Small bowel tumours in emergency surgery: specificity of clinical presentation. *ANZ J Surg* 2005;75(11):997-999.
9. Miller G, Boman J, Shrier I, Gordon PH. Etiology of small bowel obstruction. *Am J Surg* 2000;180(1):33-36.

10. Shatila AH, Chamberlain BE, Webb WR. Current status of diagnosis and management of strangulation obstruction of the small bowel. *Am J Surg* 1976;132(3): 299-303.

11. Holder WD, Jr. Intestinal obstruction. *Gastroenterol Clin North Am* 1988;17(2):317-340.

12. Daneshmand S, Hedley CG, Stain SC. The utility and reliability of computed tomography scan in the diagnosis of small bowel obstruction. *Am Surg* 1999;65(10):922-996.

13. Frager DH, Baer JW. Role of CT in evaluating patients with small-bowel obstruction. *Semin Ultrasound CT MR* 1995;16(2):127-140.

14. Frager D, Medwid SW, Baer JW, et al. CT of small-bowel obstruction: value in establishing the diagnosis and determining the degree and cause. *AJR Am J Roentgenol* 1994;162(1):37-41.

15. Balthazar EJ, George W. Holmes Lecture. CT of small-bowel obstruction. *AJR Am J Roentgenol* 1994;162(2): 255-261.

16. Bickell NA, Federman AD, Aufses AH, Jr. Influence of time on risk of bowel resection in complete small bowel obstruction. *J Am Coll Surg* 2005;201:847-854.

17. Fevang BT, Fevang J, Stangeland L, Soreide O, Svanes K, Viste A. Complications and death after surgical treatment of small bowel obstruction: a 35-year institutional experience. *Ann Surg* 2000 231:529-537.

18. Deitch EA. Simple intestinal obstruction causes bacterial translocation in man. *Arch Surg* 1989;124(6): 699-701.

19. Richards WO, Williams LF, Jr. Obstruction of the large and small intestine. *Surg Clin North Am* 1988;68(2): 355-376.

20. Seror D, Feigin E, Szold A, et al. How conservatively can postoperative small bowel obstruction be treated? *Am J Surg* 1993;165:121-125.

21. Assalia A, Schein M, Kopelman D, et al. Therapeutic effect of oral Gastrografin in adhesive, partial small-bowel obstruction: a prospective randomized trial. *Surgery* 1994;115:433-437.

22. Brolin RE. Partial small bowel obstruction. *Surgery* 1984;95:145-149.

23. Sosa J, Gardner B. Management of patients diagnosed as acute intestinal obstruction secondary to adhesions. *Am Surg* 1993;59:125-128.

24. Shih SC, Jeng KS, Lin SC, et al. Adhesive small bowel obstruction: How long can patients tolerate conservative treatment? *World J Gastroenterol* 2003;9:603-605.

25. Choi HK, Chu KW, Law WL. Therapeutic value of gastrografin in adhesive small bowel obstruction after unsuccessful conservative treatment: a prospective randomized trial. *Ann Surg* 2002;236:1-6.

26. Biondo S, Pares D, Mora L, Marti Rague J, Kreisler E, Jaurrieta E. Randomized clinical study of Gastrografin administration in patients with adhesive small bowel obstruction. *Br J Surg* 2003;90:542-546.

27. Kapoor S, Jain G, Sewkani A, Sharma S, Patel K, Varshney S. Prospective evaluation of oral gastrografin in postoperative small bowel obstruction. *J Surg Res* 2006;131:256-260.

28. Abbas S, Bissett IP, Parry BR. Oral water soluble contrast for the management of adhesive small bowel obstruction. *Cochrane Database Syst Rev* 2005;5:CD004651.

29. Chen SC, Lee CC, Yen ZS, et al. Specific oral medications decrease the need for surgery in adhesive partial small-bowel obstruction. *Surgery* 2006;139:312-316.

30. Franklin ME, Jr., Dorman JP, Pharand D. Laparoscopic surgery in acute small bowel obstruction. *Surg Laparosc Endosc* 1994;4:289-296.

31. Kirshtein B, Roy-Shapira A, Lantsberg L, Avinoach E, Mizrahi S. Laparoscopic management of acute small bowel obstruction. *Surg Endosc* 2005;19:464-47.

32. Bulkley GB, Zuidema GD, Hamilton SR, et al. Intraoperative determination of small intestinal viability following ischemic injury: a prospective, controlled trial of two adjuvant methods (Doppler and fluorescein) compared with standard clinical judgment. *Ann Surg* 1981;193(5):628-637.

33. Kimchi NA, Broide E, Shapiro M, Scapa E. Non-traumatic perforation of the small intestine. Report of 13 cases and review of the literature. *Hepatogastroenterology* 2002;49:1017-1022.

34. Leijonmarck CE, Fenyo G, Raf L. Nontraumatic perforation of the small intestine. *Acta Chir Scand* 1984;150: 405-411.

35. Lau WY, Leow CK. History of perforated duodenal and gastric ulcers. *World J Surg* 1997;21(8):890-896.

36. Baker SR. Plain films and cross-sectional imaging for acute abdominal pain: unresolved issues. *Semin Ultrasound CT MR* 1999;20:142-147.

37. Peura DA, Lanza FL, Gostout CJ, Foutch PG. The American College of Gastroenterology Bleeding Registry: preliminary findings. *Am J Gastroenterol* 1997;92(6):924-928.

38. Yavorski RT, Wong RK, Maydonovitch C, et al. Analysis of 3,294 cases of upper gastrointestinal bleeding in military medical facilities. *Am J Gastroenterol* 1995;90(4):568-573.

38. Leduc LJ, Mitchell A. Intestinal ischemia after laparoscopic cholecystectomy. JSLS 2006;10(2):236-238.

39. Kovacs TO, Jensen DM. Recent advances in the endoscopic diagnosis and therapy of upper gastrointestinal, small intestinal, and colonic bleeding. *Med Clin North Am* 2002;86(6):1319-1356.

40. Rossini FP, Pennazio M. Small-bowel endoscopy. *Endoscopy* 2002;34(1):13-20.

41. Adler DG, Knipschield M, Gostout C. A prospective comparison of capsule endoscopy and push enteroscopy in patients with GI bleeding of obscure origin. *Gastrointest Endosc* 2004;59(4):492-498.

42. Ell C, Remke S, May A, et al. The first prospective controlled trial comparing wireless capsule endoscopy with push enteroscopy in chronic gastrointestinal bleeding. *Endoscopy* 2002;34(9):685-689.

43. Fireman Z, Eliakim R, Adler S, Scapa E. Capsule endoscopy in real life: a four-centre experience of 160 consecutive patients in Israel. *Eur J Gastroenterol Hepatol* 2004;16(9):927-931.

44. Suzman MS, Talmor M, Jennis R, et al. Accurate localization and surgical management of active lower gastrointestinal hemorrhage with technetium-labeled erythrocyte scintigraphy. *Ann Surg* 1996;224(1):29-36.

Chapter **7**

THE COLON

Thomas J. Schroeppel, MD, and Timothy C. Fabian, MD

INTRODUCTION

This chapter will address the multiple acute pathologic conditions of the colon. These disease states demand knowledge of anatomy, physiology, and pathology for adequate diagnosis. Common problems such as appendicitis are generally straightforward, but the acute care surgeon must also be versed with more unusual colonic pathology. Colonic cancer is the third most commonly diagnosed malignancy with 104,950 new cases diagnosed in 2005.[1] Up to 25% of the time, it presents as an obstruction requiring prompt and decisive treatment. Other obstructive processes include benign strictures and volvulus. Common infectious processes include diverticulitis and appendicitis. Lower gastrointestinal bleeding refractory to medical management may also present emergently requiring prompt treatment. Inflammatory bowel disease may lead to fulminant colitis, toxic megacolon, fistulas, hemorrhage, and perforation requiring decisive action. The end result of many of these diseases is perforation requiring urgent surgical intervention. The acute care surgeon must be versed with these conditions, including workup and treatment options in order to provide optimal patient care.

APPENDICITIS

EPIDEMIOLOGY

In the United States, acute appendicitis is the most common surgical emergency in the abdomen, annually occurring in 250,000 patients.[2,3] The lifetime cumulative risk of acute appendicitis in industrialized nations is 7%. Appendicitis is slightly more common in males at 1.4 to 1 with a lifetime risk of 8.6% in men and 6.7% in women.[2-5] It is primarily a disease of young adults and adolescents with increased morbidity and mortality at the extremes of age.

ANATOMY

Anatomically, the appendix lies at the base of the cecum 2.5 cm inferior to the ileocecal valve where the three tenia coalesce. It varies in length from 5 to 10 cm and in width from 0.5 to 1.0 cm.[2] Its position in relation to the cecum can vary: paracolic, retrocecal, preileal, postileal, promonteric, pelvic, and subcecal.[2] The exact pathophysiology has not been completely elucidated, but it is hypothesized that luminal obstruction and continued mucus secretion lead to bacterial overgrowth and these processes produce increased intraluminal pressure. Obstruction may result from stasis, fecoliths, or lymphoid hyperplasia.[2,3] The increased pressure leads to venous stasis, ischemia, ulcerated mucosa, and eventually perforation. The responsible organisms are colonic flora with greater than 10 organisms cultured on average composed predominantly of aerobic and anaerobic gram-negative rods.[2]

PREOPERATIVE MANAGEMENT

The typical presentation of acute appendicitis is a vague abdominal pain that worsens over a 12- to 24-hour period. In 95% of patients, pain begins in the periumbilical region and migrates to the right lower quadrant (RLQ).[2,6] Other common symptoms include isolated RLQ pain, anorexia, and nausea (Table 7-1).[2,6] Physical examination findings include mild tachycardia, fever, decreased bowel sounds, and tenderness to palpation at McBurney point (one-third distance from anterior superior iliac spine to umbilicus).[7] Other variable physical findings include psoas sign, pain elicited with the patient in left lateral decubitus with extension of the thigh; Rovsing sign, referred pain to the right lower quadrant with palpation in the left lower quadrant; obturator sign, pain elicited on internal rotation in the adductors of the flexed thigh.[2] These signs are variable and depend on the location of the appendix and inflammatory reaction anatomically.[2,3] All patients with abdominal pain require a rectal examination and all females need a pelvic examination to evaluate for pelvic inflammatory processes or abscesses.

Laboratory findings reveal mild leukocytosis in most patients.[2-4,6,8,9] Urinalysis will be abnormal with pyuria, hematuria, or bacteria in 40% of patients with

Table 7-1 Symptoms of Appenditicis[3,7]	
Pain migrating to the RLQ	95%
RLQ Pain	90%
Anorexia	90%
Nausea	60-80%

acute appendicitis due to the inflammatory process of the appendicitis overlying the ureter.[8]

Diagnostic Studies

Radiographic studies can be useful adjuncts in patients in whom the diagnosis is unclear, but are not necessary in patients with classic history and physical examination as they delay treatment and add costs. The two most useful radiographic studies to assist in the diagnosis are ultrasonography (US) and computed tomography (CT).

US is a noninvasive study with reported sensitivity and specificity rates of 77%-88% and 87%-95% respectively.[3,10-12] Findings on US consistent with appendicitis include an aperistaltic, noncompressible appendix with size greater than 6 mm.[4] Pitfalls of US include the fact that it is operator and interpreter dependent. US produces more equivocal or inconclusive studies than CT and it may also be difficult to obtain good quality images in patients with a large body habitus.[11] US studies should generally be reserved for those patients in whom ionizing radiation is dangerous (pregnancy, young) and for those in whom the diagnosis is in doubt.

CT is a relatively noninvasive study with sensitivity and specificity rates of 87%-98% and 92%-98%, respectively.[3,6,10,11,13] Accuracy rates are 74.5% to 98%.[6,9,10,13,14] CT criteria for appendicitis include a visualized appendix with size greater than 6 mm and periappendiceal thickening or wall thickening (Fig. 7-1).[5,11,13,15] Advantages of CT over US include better image quality, absence of operator dependency, visualization of the entire abdomen for additional pathology, retrocecal visualization, and extent of disease.[10] However, controversy persists in the literature regarding the utility of preoperative CT for appendicitis. Some authors suggest that it assists in making the diagnosis and lowers the negative appendectomy rate.[5,6,15-17] Others have shown no significant difference in the rates with the assistance of CT.[9,14,18] CT's role is most prevalent in areas of diagnostic uncertainty, including atypical symptoms, women of childbearing age, and at extremes of age.[13,17,19]

OPERATIVE MANAGEMENT

Treatment of acute appendicitis is predominantly surgical unless perforated appendicitis with abscess is diagnosed.

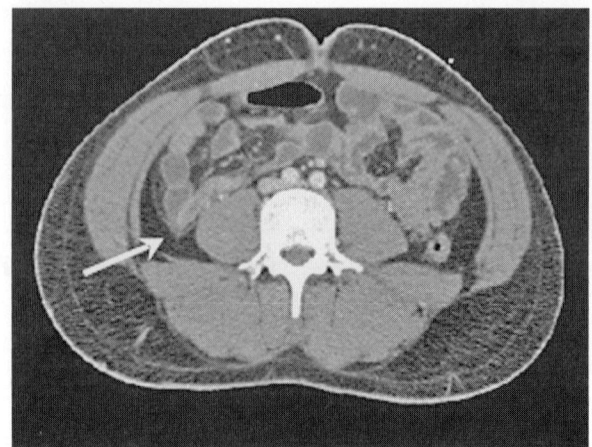

Figure 7-1   *CT image of acute appendicitis. The arrow points to the inflamed appendix.*

Perforated appendicitis at presentation accounts for 15% to 30% of all cases (Figs. 7-2, 7-3).[2,4,5,20,21] In cases of perforation with a well-localized abscess, treatment may consist of percutaneous drainage, antibiotics, and interval appendectomy in 6-12 weeks.[3] The first open appendectomy (OA) with a muscle splitting incision was described by McBurney in 1889.[7] This procedure with several modifications became the standard of care for acute appendicitis for nearly a century until Semm introduced laparoscopic appendectomy (LA) in 1983.[22] Controversy began at that point and continues today with advocates of both the OA and LA. Proposed benefits of LA include reduced wound infection rate, decreased pain, shorter length of stay, and earlier return to work. Many retrospective studies, randomized trials, and meta-analyses have looked at this issue in the last 15 years. Findings of decreased wound

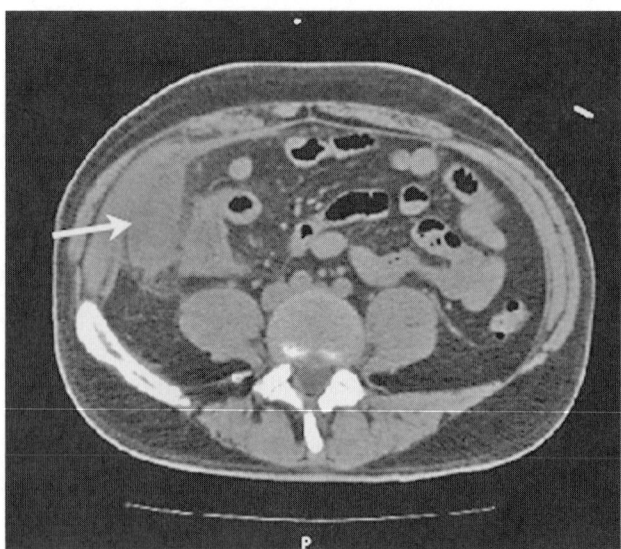

Figure 7-2   *CT image of perforated appendicitis. The arrow points to the abscess.*

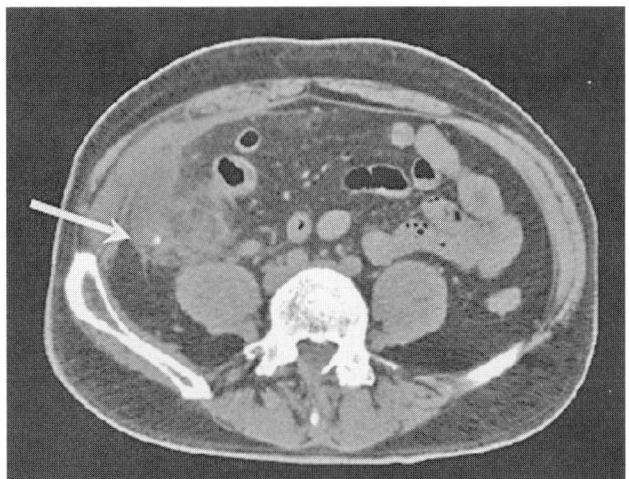

Figure 7-3 *CT image of perforated appendicitis. The arrow points to an appendicolith within an abscess.*

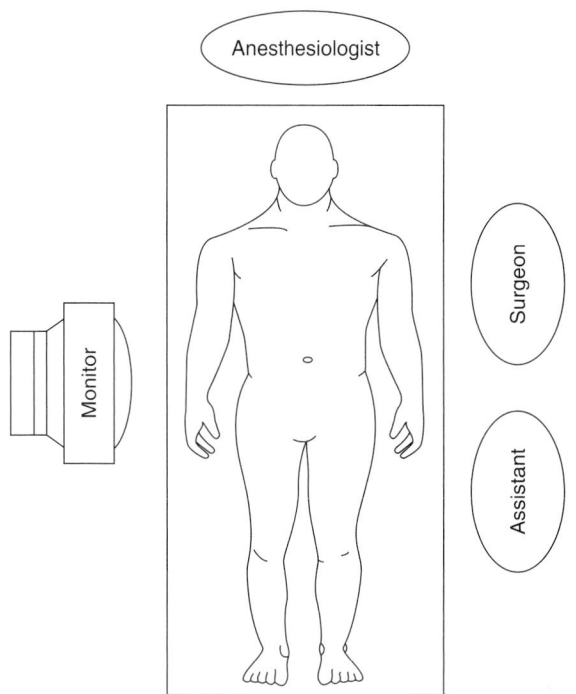

Figure 7-4 *Operating room setup for laparoscopic appendectomy.*

infections, LOS, and equivalent or decreased abscess rates have been reported for LA by some authors.[20,21,23-28] Other authors have noted no significant differences between the LA and OA.[29-33] Operative times and cost have also been consistently reported as longer and higher respectively in LA.[20,21,24,33] Although some of the differences found in studies may reach statistical significance, clinical significance must still be questioned given the low rates of complications and small differences in other variables. Ultimately, the decision should be based on surgeon and patient preferences.[20,21,33] Although not supported by the data, special consideration should be given to performing LA in patients in which there is a diagnostic dilemma or in obese patients as the wound morbidity is lower with LA.

LAPAROSCOPIC TECHNIQUE

LA is typically performed with three trocars placed in the abdomen with the patient supine and the left arm tucked. The monitor can initially be placed at the patient's feet and then rotated to the right side of the patient after the assistant and operating surgeon are both on the patient's left (Fig. 7-4). Initial trocar placement is in the midline infra- or supraumbilical position in an open manner initially described by Hasson.[34] Once access to the abdomen has been obtained, CO_2 pneumoperitoneum is obtained and diagnostic laparoscopy is performed. If the diagnosis is confirmed to be acute appendicitis, then additional trocars are placed. The placement of these trocars varies depending on patient habitus and location of the appendix. Typical positioning includes a 5-mm suprapubic trocar and one additional trocar. In a small patient with an easily accessible appendix, an additional trocar may be placed in the midline between the Hasson port and the suprapubic port. This requires the use of a 5-mm laparoscope to facilitate the passage of a

stapling device through the camera port. Standard trocar placement for more difficult cases includes a 12-mm trocar placed either in the right upper quadrant or left lower quadrant for passage of the stapler (Fig. 7-5). Patient positioning is very important as gravity may be used to retract the viscera to assist in exposure. Once

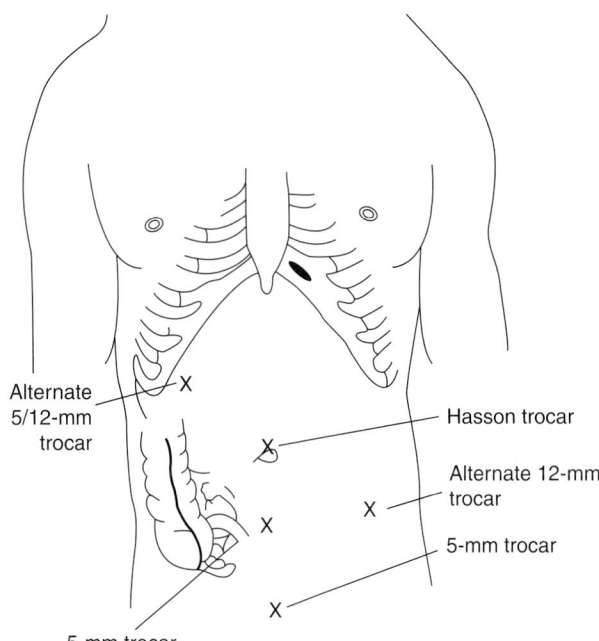

Figure 7-5 *Options for trocar placement for laparoscopic appendectomy.*

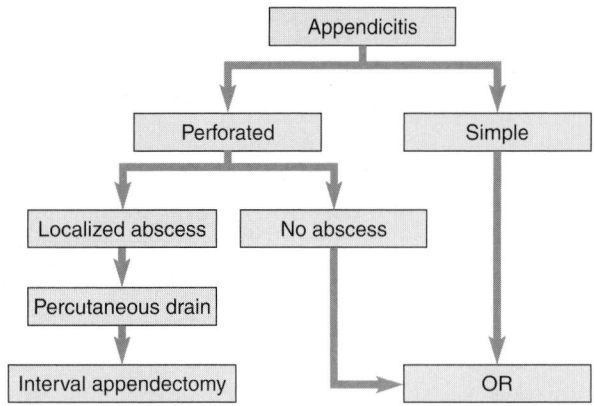

Figure 7-6 *Management algorithm for acute appendicitis.*

access is obtained the patient should be airplaned to the left and placed into Trendelenberg position for maximal exposure. The appendix may then be freed from surrounding adhesions and attachments in order to get to the base. Once the base of the appendix is identified, a window is created with blunt dissection between the mesoappendix and cecum. Endoscopic staplers or endoloop devices are then used to divide the appendix and mesoappendix. The appendix is then placed into an endoscopic retrieval bag and removed from the abdomen. The abdomen is then inspected for hemostasis. Suctioning and irrigation can then be done at the discretion of the surgeon. The trocars are removed under direct visualization to ensure no abdominal wall hemorrhage. The management algorithm for appendicitis is shown in Fig. 7-6.

DIVERTICULITIS

EPIDEMIOLOGY

Diverticular disease of the colon is a common colonic condition in the elderly of Western societies. Diverticulosis occurs in up to one-third of the population over the age of 45 and up to two-thirds of the population over the age of 85.[37] Most patients with diverticulosis are asymptomatic, approximately 20% develop diverticulitis and 3-5% develop severe hematochezia.[38]

Diverticulitis has been hypothesized to occur in a process similar to appendicitis. A diverticulum becomes obstructed with inspissated stool in the neck resulting in a fecalith. The fecalith then abrades the mucosa of the sac, causing inflammation and expansion of usual bacterial flora with diminished venous outflow and localized ischemia. This leads to bacterial overgrowth, translocation, perforation, and subsequent abscess.[39]

The main symptom of diverticulitis is left lower quadrant abdominal pain. The pain may be intermittent or constant in nature and is usually associated with a change in bowel habits. Anorexia, nausea, and emesis may also be symptoms. Atypical symptoms may include pelvic pain or pain in the right lower quadrant caused by redundant or floppy sigmoid colons.

PREOPERATIVE MANAGEMENT

Physical examination reveals left lower quadrant tenderness and occasionally a palpable abdominal mass. Fever is present in most cases and the white blood cell is usually elevated.

In individuals with this classic presentation, empiric treatment with antibiotics directed toward gram-negative bacteria and anaerobes is warranted without further workup. Diet may be restricted to clear liquids. In patients able to maintain oral intake and without severe pain, outpatient management may be employed with antibiotics for 7 to 10 days. If a response is not seen within 3 days, further investigation is warranted.[39]

In patients in whom a complication is suspected or response to empiric treatment is inadequate, further workup is mandatory.

Diagnostic Studies

Chest and abdominal radiographs are obtained to screen for pneumoperitoneum, ileus, and dilated large or small intestine. Computed Tomography (CT) scanning of the abdomen and pelvis is the procedure of choice for diagnosing diverticulitis. CT is helpful by demonstrating colonic wall thickening, pericolic fatty infiltration, and abscess (Fig. 7-7). Sensitivity and specificity of 93%-98% and 75%-100%, respectively, have consistently been reported in CT obtained for diverticulitis.[39] Flexible endoscopy is avoided in the acute setting to avoid the risk of perforation.

Complicated Diverticulitis

If outpatient antibiotic therapy fails or pain is too severe for oral medications, admission is warranted. Initial treatment includes intravenous antibiotics,

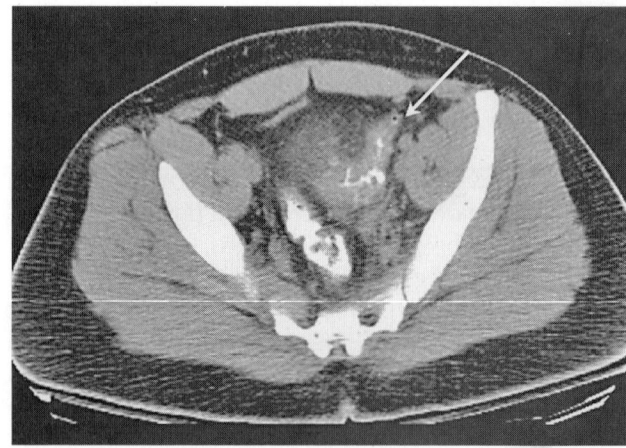

Figure 7-7 *CT image of diverticulitis. The arrow points to inflamed, thickened sigmoid colon.*

fluids, narcotics, and observation. Improvement should be seen within 2 to 4 days. If improvement does not occur in this time frame, a diligent search should be made for complications of diverticulitis. If a response is seen, discharge may take place when oral intake is tolerated and treatment with antibiotics should be continued for 7 to 10 days.[39]

OPERATIVE MANAGEMENT

Complications of diverticulitis include perforation, abscess, fistulas, and obstruction. Perforation of a diverticulum can lead to a localized inflammatory process (phlegmon), formation of pericolic or intraabdominal abscess, and purulent or feculent peritonitis.[37] Hinchey et al described a grading system for the degree of perforation: stage I, diverticulitis associated with pericolic abscess; stage II, diverticulitis associated with a distant abscess; stage III, diverticulitis associated with purulent peritonitis; and stage IV, diverticulitis associated with feculent peritonitis (Table 7-2).[40] Treatment options depend on the stability of the patient, presence or absence of peritonitis, location, accessibility, and size of any abscess. Small pericolic abscesses will likely resolve with conservative management. Larger abscesses or the presence of peritonitis necessitates further therapy.

Large abscesses require drainage in addition to antibiotics. Accessible abscesses can undergo CT or US guided percutaneous drainage in the absence of peritonitis in the stable patient. Seventy to ninety percent of abscesses that are accessible for percutaneous drainage can be managed in this way.[37] Advantages of this approach include avoiding of a two-stage procedure and stoma, allowing the inflammation to subside, and the possibility of a laparoscopic approach for sigmoid colon resection. If the abscess is drained percutaneously and clinical symptoms persist or worsen, then surgical intervention is mandated.

The procedure of choice acutely is resection with primary anastomosis (RPA). If there is significant contamination (feculent peritonitis), inflammation, or obstruction, the procedure of choice becomes a Hartmann procedure (resection with colostomy, HP).[37] A three-stage procedure should be avoided unless significant concern exists about the safety of proceeding due to unclear anatomy or patient instability. If this concern exists, diversion and drainage will allow the inflammation to subside, allowing a safe definitive resection.

Diverticulitis associated with free perforation, Hinchey stage III or IV, is a surgical emergency that requires prompt operative intervention. The procedure of choice is the HP with removal of the involved segment. Mortality for this stage is reported as 6%-35% and depends on the degree of fecal contamination, the general physiologic status of the patient, and the timeliness of surgical intervention.[37]

Fistulas can also develop as a result of diverticular disease. The organs most commonly involved include the urinary bladder, vagina, integument, intestine, and uterus. Colovesical fistulas are the most common and make up 65% of diverticular fistulas.[37] Although diverticular disease is the most common cause of these fistulas, other etiologies need to be excluded including malignancy, inflammatory bowel disease, and radiation.[37] Colovesical fistula symptoms include pneumaturia, fecaluria, and recurrent urinary tract infections in a male. Cystography, cystoscopy, and contrast enemas may show the fistula tract.[39] Colovaginal fistulas are the next most common representing about 25% of fistulas.[38] Passage of stool or flatus via the vagina is pathognomic. Frequent vagina infections or copious discharge should prompt thorough investigation.[39] Treatment of these conditions includes resection of the involved colon and repair of the affected contiguous organ.

ELECTIVE COLON RESECTION

Elective resection following multiple episodes of simple diverticulitis or a single episode of complicated diverticulitis remains an area of controversy. The current recommendations by the American Society of Colon and Rectal Surgeons is elective resection following one complicated attack of diverticulitis or two uncomplicated attacks.[37,41] Multiple authors have disputed these recommendations stating the risk of recurrent attacks and recurrent complicated attacks are much lower than previously thought.[42-44] Elective resections of the sigmoid colon are also being more commonly done laparoscopically or with a hand-assisted laparoscopic (HALS) approach, greatly reducing the morbidity of resection. This remains an area of debate, which will likely not be resolved until a prospective study is performed. The management algorithm for diverticulitis is shown in Fig. 7-8.

BOWEL PREPARATION

The standard of care for elective colon surgery from the 1970s until recently has included mechanical bowel preparation (MBP). The proposed advantages of preparing the bowel include removing solid feces, decreasing the bacterial load, and improving the handling characteristics of the colon. Choices for bowel preparation include large volume polyethylene glycol

Table 7-2	Hinchey et al. Grading System for Degree of Perforation[39]
Stage I	Diverticulitis with a pericolic abscess
Stage II	Diverticulitis with a distant abscess
Stage III	Diverticulitis with purulent peritonitis
Stage IV	Diverticulitis with feculent peritonitis

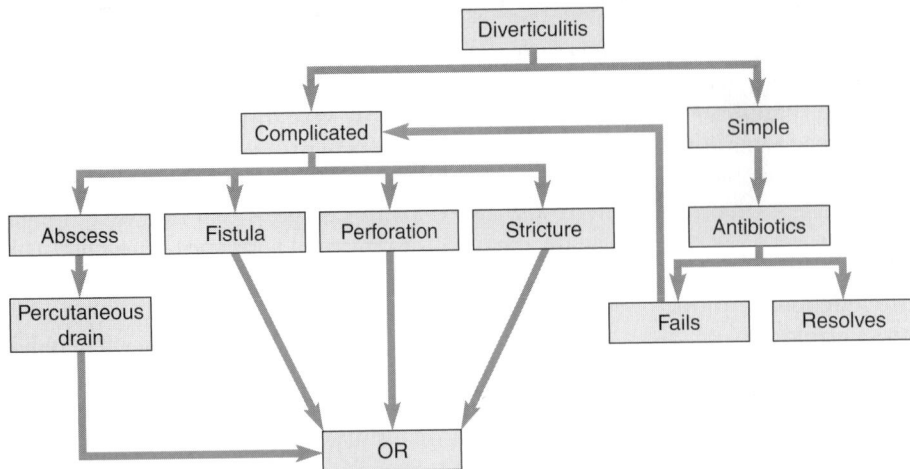

Figure 7-8 *Management algorithm for diverticulitis.*

solutions, sodium phosphate solutions, and antibiotics. Recently, the utility of MBP has been questioned. The practice of MBP is based mainly on historical, noncontrolled, small sample studies published before the routine introduction of antibiotic prophylaxis and on a small number of animal studies.[35] Several recent studies and a meta-analysis have called this practice into question finding equivalent or lower leak and infection rates in the patients who did not undergo a MBP.[35,36] The burden of MBP, especially polyethylene glycol solutions, to complete with the resulting physiologic consequences including electrolyte abnormalities and dehydration must also be considered. Although methods of on-table colonic lavage have been described, the data supporting no MBP calls these burdensome approaches into question.

LOWER GASTROINTESTINAL BLEEDING

EPIDEMIOLOGY

Lower gastrointestinal (GI) bleeding is defined as intestinal blood loss that occurs distal to the ligament of Treitz. The annual incidence in the general population is 0.03%, but rises dramatically with a 200-fold increase from the second to eighth decade of life.[38] The mean age of patients with lower GI bleeding is 63 to 77 years with a mortality rate of 2%-4%.[38] Ten to fifteen percent of upper GI bleeds can present with severe hematochezia and the appearance of a lower GI bleed. The other most common causes are diverticulosis, hemorrhoids, ischemic colitis, and angiodysplasias or arteriovenous malformations.[38]

PREOPERATIVE MANAGEMENT

As with any patient evaluated acutely, the starting point should be the history and physical examination. Stability should be assessed and resuscitation begun by starting two large bore intravenous catheters, placing a Foley catheter, drawing labs for electrolytes, type and crossmatch, coagulation parameters, and complete blood count. The duration of the bleeding, medication history (especially Nonsteroidal Anti-inflammatory Drugs [NSAIDs]), symptoms of orthostasis, prior episodes, and family history of cancer should all be included in the focused history. Symptoms of pallor, fatigue, chest pain, palpitations, dyspnea, tachypnea, tachycardia, postural changes, or syncope are suggestive of hemodynamic compromise.[38] Orthostatic hypotension with a decrease of the systolic blood pressure of greater than 10 mm Hg or an increase in the heart rate of more than 10 beats per minute indicates an acute blood loss of at least 15% of the blood volume.[45] The American College of Surgeons Advanced Trauma Life Support course offers a nice description to the degree of hemorrhage and estimated fluid and blood loss based on patient presentation (Table 7-3).[46] Using this classification scheme can give an objective estimate on the severity of hemorrhage, amount of blood loss, and a starting point for resuscitation and volume replacement. If any of these symptoms are present, immediate resuscitation must ensue with correction of intravascular volume and coagulation parameters.

Physical examination follows with emphasis placed on cardiac, pulmonary, abdominal, and rectal examinations. Stigmata of cirrhosis should also be evaluated including caput medusa at the umbilicus, ascites, and palpable liver edge. The patient should likewise be examined for signs of malignancy and masses in the abdomen and nodal basins. Any positives on examination will direct the workup appropriately.

The majority of patients admitted with a lower GI bleed will resolve spontaneously. Those who continue to bleed with persistent hematochezia, falling hematocrit, or hemodynamic compromise require further workup.

Diagnostic Studies

All patients should have a nasogastric tube inserted as the first step in the workup. If gross blood is returned, an esophagogastroduodenoscopy (EGD) is warranted as the first intervention. Return of bilious fluid suggests the bleeding source is distal to the ligament of Treitz.

Table 7-3 ACS ATLS Estimated Fluid and Blood Losses Based on Patient's Initial Presentation[46]

	Class 1	Class 2	Class 3	Class 4
Blood loss (mL)	Up to 750	750-500	1500-2000	> 2000
Blood loss (% blood volume)	Up to 15%	15%-30%	30%-40%	> 40%
Pulse rate	< 100	>100	>120	>140
Blood pressure	Normal	Normal	Decreased	Decreased
Pulse pressure	Normal or increased	Decreased	Decreased	Decreased
Respiratory rate	14-20	20-30	30-40	> 35
Urine output (mL/hr)	> 30	20-30	5-15	Negligible
CNS/Mental Status	Slightly anxious	Mildly anxious	Anxious, confused	Confused, lethargic
Fluid replacement (3:1 rule)	Crystalloid	Crystalloid	Crystalloid and blood	Crystalloid and blood

Colonoscopy should be the initial diagnostic study once the diagnosis of lower GI bleed is confirmed. Diagnostic accuracy of colonoscopy ranges from 72% to 86%.[38] Urgent colonoscopy should be performed within the first 8 to 24 hours in an attempt to localize and potentially treat the bleeding source.[45] Endoscopic diagnosis and treatment rates are 88% and 12%, respectively.[45] A careful examination of the anorectal region with anoscopy should always be performed to exclude bleeding hemorrhoids as a source of hemorrhage.

If the bleeding source cannot be localized by flexible endoscopy, radiographic options are available to attempt to localize the bleeding source. Study selection depends on the rate of hemorrhage. If hemorrhage rates are 0.5 to 1.0 ml per minute, angiography of the mesenteric vasculature will localize the bleeding source 40%-78% of the time.[45] If the bleeding source is localized, selective angioembolization may be considered for control of the site of hemorrhage.[45] Rebleeding rates of 15%-40% are reported after embolization.[45] Experience has been reported with selective vasopressin infusion of the bleeding vessel with control rates of 91%, but a major complication rate of 10% to 20% including arrhythmias, pulmonary edema, hypertension, and ischemia limit its utility.[45] Adverse effects of vasopressin are due to its profound vasoconstrictive properties, including reduction of coronary blood flow and decreased oxygen delivery leading to cardiac ischemia, intestinal ischemia, and persistent acidosis.

If the bleeding rate is slower or unable to be localized on angiography, radionuclide imaging may be able to identify the site. Bleeding rates of 0.1 to 0.5 mL/min can be detected with accuracy of 24% to 91%.[45] Two techniques exist for localizing including technetium sulfur colloid and ^{99m}Tc pertechnetate labeled red blood cells (RBCs). Technetium sulfur colloid can localize bleeding rates as low as 0.1 ml/min,

but is limited by its short half life to bleeding ongoing during the injection.[45] [99m]Tc pertechnetate tagged RBCs have a much longer half life and may be accurately imaged for up to 24 hours expanding the utility of this study.[45] Controversy persists over the utility of these studies due to the intermittent nature of lower GI bleeding and the fact that bleeding must be occurring for the scan to be positive. The diagnostic yield for bleeding scans varies from as low as 15% to 70% but is below 50% in most studies.[47,48] Results for our center have also been poor. Its use should be reserved for those patients who continue to bleed when all other tests are negative.

Ten to 20% of patients will continue to hemorrhage without a localized site.[48] The majority of these patients will resolve spontaneously, but for those that rebleed diagnostic options include small bowel capsule endoscopy, enteroscopy, small bowel follow through, enteroclysis, and exploratory laparotomy. If all other options have been exhausted and exploratory laparotomy is performed, adjuncts in the operating room to assist with localization include intraoperative endoscopy and catheter directed injection of methylene blue via a super selective catheter placement at the time of a diagnostic arteriogram.[49] Fortunately, these scenarios are rare, less than 5%, as the localization techniques previously described will localize the site in the majority of cases.[48]

OPERATIVE MANAGEMENT

Indications for surgical intervention in lower GI bleeding occur in two settings: massive lower hemorrhage and recurrent bleeding.[45] Some authors have put a transfusion total on indications for surgical intervention with greater than 4 units in a 24-hour period or 10 units total during the admission.[45] Recent data on transfusion triggers have been called into question

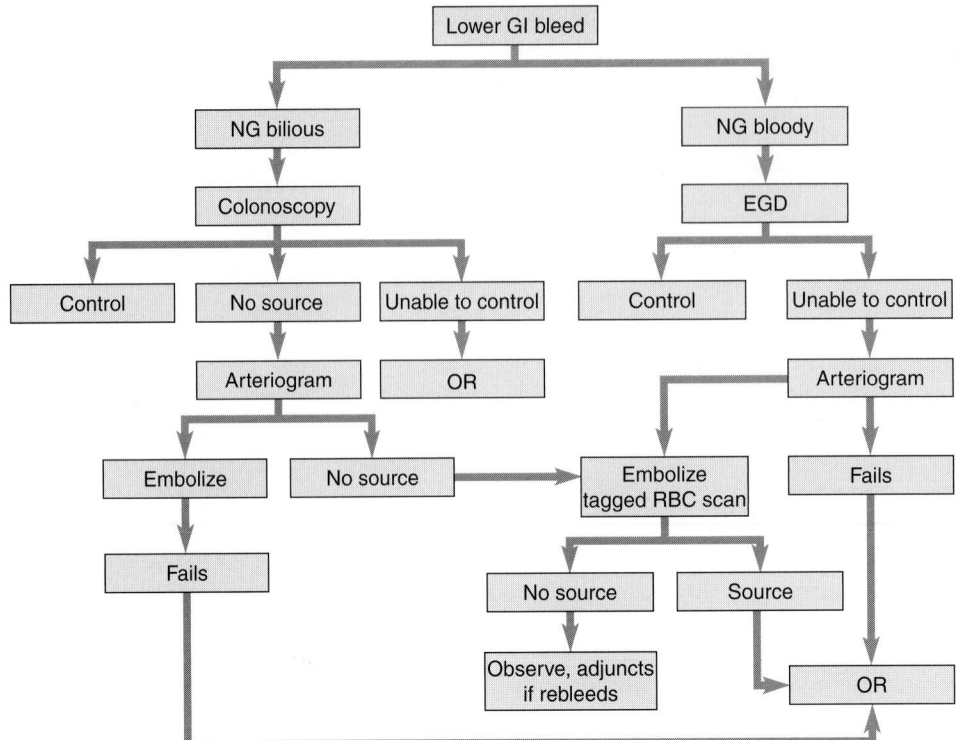

Figure 7-9 *Management algorithm for lower GI bleeding.*

with many authors showing the safety of lower hemoglobin values of 7 to 9 mg/dL in the hemodynamically stable patient.[50-52] Surgical intervention may be avoided by using these more restrictive transfusion triggers as the majority of lower GI bleeding will resolve spontaneously. All efforts should be made to localize the site of hemorrhage prior to surgical intervention. Blind segmental colectomy is contraindicated with a prohibitively high rebleed rate of 42%.[38] If the site of hemorrhage can be localized, then a segmental colectomy can be performed safely with a mortality of 10%.[45] If the site of bleeding is unable to be localized, total abdominal colectomy should be performed with mortality ranging from 5% to 33%.[47]

Overall mortality rates for lower GI bleeding are in the range of < 5%, historically less than for upper GI bleeds.[47] The management algorithm for lower GI bleeding is shown in Fig. 7-9.

COLONIC OBSTRUCTION

EPIDEMIOLOGY

Despite widespread screening for colorectal cancer, approximately one fourth of all cancer patients present with obstruction. Furthermore, 85% of all colonic emergencies present as malignant obstruction.[54] Colonic cancer with obstruction generally presents at an advanced stage, with 27% having hepatic metastasis at the time of diagnosis.[54] Other causes of obstruction are listed in Table 7-4. Malignant obstruction will be covered in this section with volvulus and diverticular disease covered prior or subsequently.

PREOPERATIVE MANAGEMENT

Specific findings for metastatic disease should be sought on the physical examination including adenopathy and palpable masses. Laboratory values should be obtained and corrected in a timely fashion prior to surgical intervention. Plain radiographs should be obtained to evaluate the bowel gas pattern and assess for free air. Important differences on radiographs between small and large bowel obstruction are seen in Table 7-5. Additional information may be obtained from computed tomography of the abdomen and pelvis, or appropriate enema studies depending on the location of the obstruction.

OPERATIVE MANAGEMENT

Obstructing colon cancers can occur anywhere in the colon. However, in a recent study, the obstructing

Table 7-4	Colonic Obstruction Etiology
Malignancy	
Inflammatory stricture (Diverticulitis, IBD)	
Ischemic stricture	
Extrinsic compression	
Volvulus	
Colonic pseudoobstruction	

Table 7-5	Comparison SBO versus LBO			
	SB	Colon	Air/Fluid Levels	Rectum
SBO	Dilated	Normal	Present	Gas Present
LBO	Dilated	Dilated	Present	Gas Absent

lesion was at or proximal to the splenic flexure 44% of the time and distal to the splenic flexure 56% of the time.[55] This differentiation is important as the surgical options vary depending on the location. Lesions located at or proximal to the splenic flexure are managed with right hemicolectomy or extended right hemicolectomy with primary anastomosis. The reported leak rates for these procedures vary from 2.5% to 13.8%.[55-57] Management options with lesions distal to the splenic flexure are more controversial. The classic three-stage procedure has largely been abandoned secondary to the high morbidity and mortality reported. Current options include HP, RPA, RPA with on table lavage, and subtotal colectomy. Many authors are now advocating RPA with or without on table colonic lavage (described later in this chapter). Authors that advocate resection with HP report a lower mortality of 9%, but a higher morbidity as two procedures are required. Forty percent to 50% of patients that undergo HP will not undergo colostomy closure, resulting in a permanent stoma.[54,58] Appropriate circumstances for this operation may include an unstable patient or if diffuse feculent peritonitis precludes performing a safe anastomosis.

RPA with on-table lavage of the colon reduces the amount of fecal load that passes the anastomosis but also adds length to the operative time and can potentially increase the amount of fecal contamination of the abdomen if not carefully done. The reported mortality for this operation ranges from 3% to 10%.[54] The technique for intraoperative lavage involves cannulating the appendix with a Foley catheter (terminal ileum if appendix is absent) and complete mobilization of the left colon and splenic flexure. The left colon is then placed into a plastic bag and normal saline lavage is performed until effluent is clear.[59] A colocolic anastomosis is then performed with reported leak rates of 4% to 6.6%.[54,55,58,59]

A different decompression technique, described by Hsu, includes complete mobilization of the sigmoid colon, descending colon, and splenic flexure. The distal end of the colon is then placed into a basin. A colotomy is then made proximal to the tumor and the feces are then decompressed into the basin without either antegrade or retrograde irrigation. He reports a leak rate of 2.3% for colocolic anastomoses performed in this fashion.[57]

Subtotal colectomy with either ileosigmoid or ileorectal anastomosis are advocated by some authors for obstructing left-sided lesions. The advantages are removal of all dilated colon, ileocolic anastomosis, and removal of potential synchronous lesions which occur in 3.3% to 6.8% of patients with an obstructed colon.[58,60] Disadvantages include a longer operation, more frequent bowel movements, and removal of healthy colon unnecessarily. The reported mortality for this operation ranges from 3% to 10% with leak rates 4% to 7.6%.[54,55,58] Mean stool frequency ranges from two to eight bowel movements per day with most not requiring antimotility medications.[54,60] Although this operation can be performed safely with a low morbidity, it should be reserved for those individuals with identified synchronous tumors or impending or frank perforation of the cecum.

A final option for those patients who are unresectable or unstable at the time operation is simple diversion with a loop colostomy. This procedure should be reserved for those without options for resection as acceptable results can be obtained with resection and diversion (HP) or RPA. The management algorithm for obstruction is shown in Fig. 7-10.

VOLVULUS

EPIDEMIOLOGY

Volvulus is defined as the axial twisting of an organ on its vascular pedicle. It occurs when a large, mobile segment of colon has a narrow, fixed mesenteric attachment, which readily allows axial rotation to occur.[61] Once twisted, gas and fluid accumulates in the closed loop, leading to distension, ischemia, gangrene, and perforation.[61] Volvulus of the colon primarily occurs in the cecum and sigmoid colon with reported frequencies of 22% to 52% and 43% to 74%, respectively.[62-66] Volvulus also occurs at the splenic flexure and at the transverse colon, but these locations are less common. Presenting symptoms are those of a bowel obstruction including abdominal pain, distension, nausea and

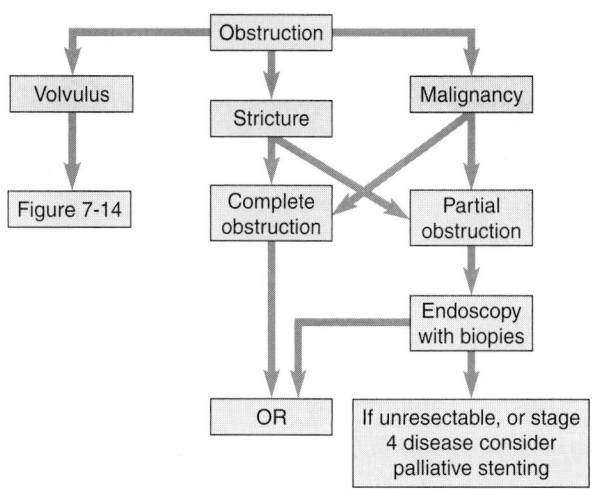

Figure 7-10 *Management algorithm for obstruction.*

emesis, and constipation or obstipation. The typical patient is a chronically ill, bedridden resident of a long-term care facility.

PREOPERATIVE MANAGEMENT

Physical examination reveals a tender distended abdomen consistent with an obstruction.

Diagnostic Studies

Plain abdominal radiographs reveal the diagnosis in 37% to 85% of patients.[62,64-68] The typical radiograph shows the "bent inner tube" sign arising from the left lower quadrant (Fig. 7-11).[67] Contrast enemas can be very accurate showing a "bird's beak" or "ace of spades" sign but should not be obtained if the diagnosis is clear following plain radiographs, as this will not provide any additional information and will delay definitive treatment.

OPERATIVE MANAGEMENT

The management of sigmoid volvulus begins with sigmoidoscopic decompression and placement of a rectal tube (Fig. 7-12). Reduction can be accomplished with the rigid sigmoidoscope, flexible sigmoidoscope, or the colonoscope. An explosive rush of gas and stool will accompany reduction of the volvulus. Following evacuation of the contents in the segment of reduced colon, careful inspection for necrosis should ensue followed by placement of the rectal tube.[68] Reduction rates can be as high as 95%, which allows time for

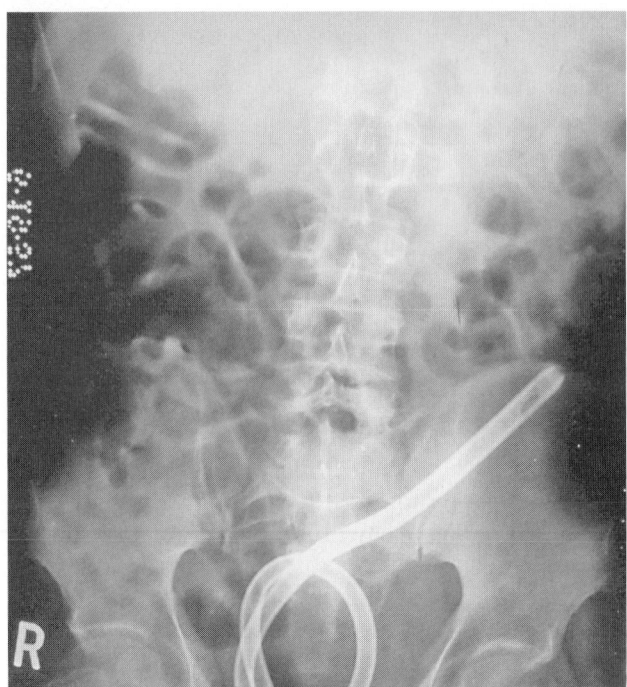

Figure 7-12 *Abdominal x-ray of reduced sigmoid volvulus with placement of rectal tube.*

decompression and urgent resection.[69] If reduction is successful, resection should be performed unless the patient is unable to tolerate surgery as the recurrence ranges from 29% to 90%.[63-67,69-71] If the volvulus is unable to be reduced endoscopically, emergency surgery is the only option. Emergency resection with HP is associated with mortality ranging from 17% to 80%.[65,66] Procedural options include simple detorsion if the colon is viable, detorsion with sigmoidopexy, RPA, and resection with HP. Simple detorsion with or without sigmoidopexy have largely been abandoned secondary to recurrence rates as high as 38%.[68] RPA is the procedure of choice for those patients able to be reduced. In those patients with gangrenous bowel and or undergoing an emergency procedure, resection with HP is a safer procedure. Mortality rates for resection differ for emergency resection, gangrenous colon, and urgent resection. Mortality rates for emergency resection range from 17% to 80%.[62,66,67,71] Mortality rates for gangrenous colon vary from 25% to 47%.[63,69] The lowest mortality rates reported are for urgent resection after reduction ranging from 5% to 22%.[62,63,65,67,69-72] The treatment of choice is thus reduction with urgent resection and primary anastomosis. Excellent results with low mortality and morbidity can be achieved with this algorithm.

CECAL VOLVULUS
Epidemiology

Cecal volvulus occurs in two forms: a full proximal volvulus and a cecal bascule. Cecal bascule or a proximal anterior folding of the cecum on itself accounts

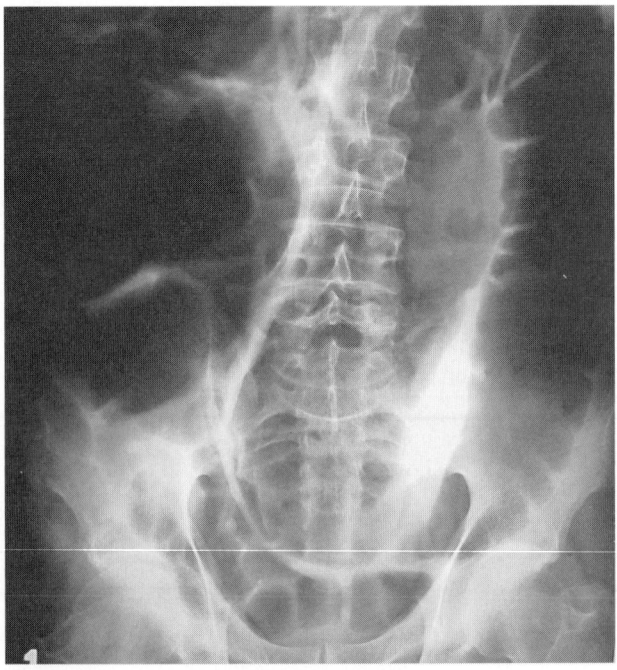

Figure 7-11 *Abdominal x-ray of sigmoid volvulus. Massive colonic distension with "bent inner tube" sign arising from the left lower quadrant.*

for 10% of cecal volvulus.[64] The age range for cecal volvulus is 53 to 64 years.[61,65,66,72] The diagnosis is rarely made on clinical grounds and adjunctive studies are needed.

PREOPERATIVE MANAGEMENT
Plain abdominal radiographs establish the diagnosis from 25%-90% of the time.[61,64-66,68,72] Typical findings on a plain radiograph include the "coffee bean" colon with the point directed toward the left upper quadrant (Fig. 7-13).[68] Barium enema or KUB will show a "birds beak" sign at the point of obstruction.[68] Caution must be used when considering performance of a contrast enema secondary to the risk of perforation.

OPERATIVE MANAGEMENT
Cecal volvulus is a surgical emergency. Endoscopic decompression has been reported, but secondary to concerns about perforation and high recurrence rate is not recommended.[61] Treatment options depend on the viability of the colon at the time of operative intervention. A gangrenous colon requires resection with either a mucous fistula and ileostomy or a primary anastomosis with reported mortality rates of 9% to 33%.[64,65] In the scenario of a viable cecum after detorsion, the treatment options are somewhat controversial. Detorsion alone is associated with a high recurrence rate of 25% to 75% and is not recommended.[61] Operative cecopexy following detorsion involves suturing the tenia of the cecum to the peritoneal reflection to prevent torsion. The recurrence following this treatment ranges from 0% to 40% in recent

literature.[61] In a patient with a high surgical risk, this may be a viable option. The other nonresectional option is that of cecostomy. This treatment anchors the cecum by fixation from the placement of the cecostomy tube. Morbidity and mortality are higher for cecostomy with rates of 52% and 32%, respectively.[72] This treatment has largely fallen out of favor with the exception of the poorest surgical candidates. Resection is the procedure of choice for the majority of cases. The reported mortality rates for resection with viable colon are 0% to 12%.[61,64,65]

TRANSVERSE COLON AND SPLENIC FLEXURE VOLVULUS
Volvulus of the transverse colon and splenic flexure can also occur, accounting for 4% and 1%, respectively.[66] The signs and symptoms of volvulus at these locations are similar to the other sites. Diagnosis is often made on contrast enema or at operation. Volvulus of the transverse colon is most often treated with resection. An extended right hemicolectomy can be performed with an ileocolic anastomosis. Splenic flexure volvulus can be treated with resection and HP. The management algorithm for volvulus is shown in Fig. 7-14.

INFLAMMATORY BOWEL DISEASE

EPIDEMIOLOGY
Chronic inflammatory conditions of the intestinal tract are typically associated with symptoms of diarrhea, crampy abdominal pain, and variable amounts of bleeding.[73] Systemic manifestations of the inflammatory process may also be present including fever, weight loss, and fatigue.[73] Surgical intervention for inflammatory bowel disease (IBD) may be necessary in 25% to 30% of patients with ulcerative colitis (UC) and up to 75% of patients with Crohn disease (CD).[74] Specific indications for surgical intervention include failure of medical management, toxic megacolon, massive hemorrhage, free perforation, an acute abscess with sepsis,

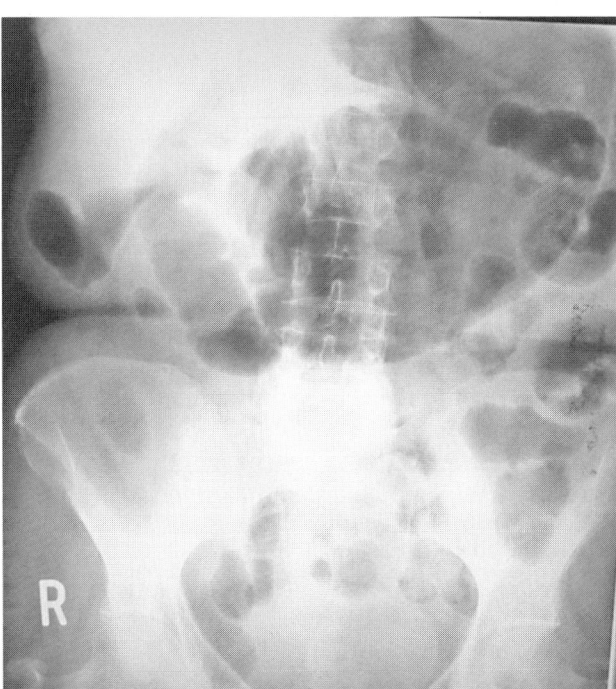

Figure 7-13 *Abdominal x-ray of cecal volvulus. Massively dilated cecum pointed to the left upper quadrant.*

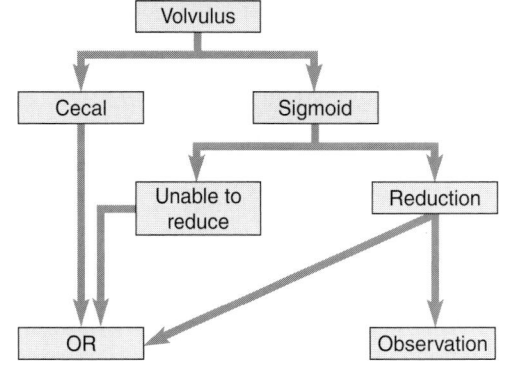

Figure 7-14 *Management algorithm for volvulus.*

fistulas, and complete obstruction.[74,75] Emergency interventions are often required for these problems and swift surgical management can limit the morbidity and mortality associated with these complications of IBD.

FULMINANT COLITIS

Fulminant colitis with or without megacolon can be a life-threatening complication of IBD and occurs in up to 10% of patients with UC and 6% of patients with CD.[75] The presentation includes an abrupt onset of bloody diarrhea, abdominal tenderness, colicky pain, and anorexia.[75] A patient is considered to be toxic if, in addition to severe colitis two of the following are present: fever greater than 38.6°C, tachycardia, leukocytosis greater than $10.5 \times 10^3/L$, and hypoalbuminemia (less than 3.0 g/100 mL).[75] Toxic megacolon is present if, in addition to fulminant colitis, either total or segmental dilation of the colon occurs greater than 6 cm.[75,76] Fulminant colitis may be the initial presentation of IBD in up to 33% of patients.[73]

PREOPERATIVE MANAGEMENT

Initial management includes obtaining large bore intravenous access and resuscitation. Initial laboratory values will likely show anemia, leukocytosis, and hypokalemia.[76,77] Aggressive resuscitation and medical management are the first line therapies unless the physical examination reveals peritonitis, which mandates an exploratory laparotomy.

Diagnostic Studies

Plain abdominal radiographs should be obtained to evaluate the size of the colon and to exclude the presence of free air. Abdominal CT may also be of value in localizing the presence of free air, abscess, or inflammatory changes in the colon including wall thickening and size.[76]

OPERATIVE MANAGEMENT

Medical management includes broad spectrum antibiotics, bowel rest, total parenteral nutrition, and high dose corticosteroids.[73,75-77] Daily radiographs of the abdomen should be obtained to evaluate colonic size. Medical treatment should continue for at least 7 days if signs of clinical deterioration are absent.[75] If no response to medical treatment is seen within 48 to 72 hours or deterioration is noted at any time, prompt surgical intervention is warranted.[73,75-78] If corticosteroid therapy fails, but clinical deterioration is absent cyclosporin may be added after 7 days with an initial response of 67%.[75] Medical management may obviate the need for surgery in 50% to 75% of patients.[73,78]

TOXIC MEGACOLON
Epidemiology

Toxic megacolon is fulminant colitis with a transverse colon diameter of at least 6 cm.[73,75,76,78] Toxic megacolon occurs in the setting of fulminant colitis with an incidence from 10% to 18% of patients with UC and from 6% to 7.8% of patients with CD.[73,75] Risk factors include barium enemas, drugs that slow colonic motility (narcotics, anticholinergics, and antidiarrheals), hypokalemia, and endoscopy.[73,75,76,79,80]

PREOPERATIVE MANAGEMENT

Initial management in the absence of perforation, peritonitis, or uncontrolled hemorrhage may be medical, as described for fulminant colitis, for 48 to 72 hours with response rates up to 50%.[73,75,78,80] Adjuncts to the previously described medical management include the use of position changes (prone) and upper gastrointestinal decompression (NG or long tubes).[76] If deterioration is noted at anytime, prompt surgical intervention is the rule.

OPERATIVE MANAGEMENT

The optimal surgical approach continues to stir controversy. Operative approaches vary from subtotal colectomy with ileostomy and mucous fistula or HP to total proctocolectomy. If perforation has already occurred, some advocate the decompressive procedure described by Turnbull to limit the amount of fecal contamination followed by elective colectomy.[76,81,82] The most common procedure recommended currently is either a subtotal colectomy or total colectomy with ileostomy and HP depending on the extent of the disease.[75-79,82,84] This will limit the amount of time in the operating room allowing more time to treat the patient medically in the intensive care unit once the offending organ is out. This disease continues to carry a significant mortality with reported rates from 2.4% to 27% and increasing to 40% if perforation has occurred prior to surgery.[75-83,85]

PERFORATION
Epidemiology

Colonic perforation in the absence of toxic megacolon is rare in UC and an unusual occurrence occurring in 1%-3% of patients with CD.[72,75,86-88] The etiology for free perforation in Crohn disease remains a mystery; however, corticosteroids and distal obstruction have been implicated.[86] Presentations of patients are very similar to that of fulminant colitis, with the exception of peritonitis on examination.

Pneumoperitoneum may only be present in up to 20% of patients on radiographs.[75] Most patients are also on corticosteroids, so the condition may be masked by the blunted inflammatory response.

OPERATIVE MANAGEMENT

Surgical treatment of the perforation must never be limited to simple suture plication due to the substantial morbidity and mortality of 25% to 44% and 33% to 45%, respectively.[86] In the setting of fulminant colitis or toxic megacolon, a subtotal colectomy or total colectomy with ileostomy and HP should be the procedure of choice.[75] Segmental colitis with perforation in the right colon in the absence of distal obstruction may undergo RPA through grossly normal bowel. All other locations should undergo resection with diversion and HP.

HEMORRHAGE
Epidemiology
Chronic blood loss in IBD is common occurring in 45% of patients.[89] Severe hemorrhage from IBD is a rare complication occurring with a frequency of 0.9% to 6% in those with UC and CD.[75,89,90] Severe hemorrhage is defined variably, but usually represents transfusion requirements of 4 to 6 units of packed red blood cells.[75,89,90] Although its occurrence is unusual in IBD, it accounts for up to 10% of urgent colectomies for UC.[75]

PREOPERATIVE MANAGEMENT
The management of severe hemorrhage for UC is straightforward. Initial efforts include examination, large bore IV access, laboratories, type and cross, and placement of a Foley catheter. If the diagnosis of ulcerative colitis is known, indications for surgery include transfusion requirements of four to six units, recurrent hemorrhage, or other indications for bowel resection.[75] Severe hemorrhage occurs in the setting of pancolitis in UC.[75] If a patient meets these requirements, then laparotomy and subtotal colectomy with ileostomy and HP should be performed.[75]

Severe hemorrhage associated with CD is more difficult to manage. Hemorrhage secondary to CD can occur anywhere in the gastrointestinal tract, therefore localization becomes more paramount. Diagnosis and management should proceed as described above in the lower GI bleed section. Spontaneous cessation will occur in up to 48% of patients, but 30% of these patients will have recurrent bleeding.[89]

OPERATIVE MANAGEMENT
Once the site of bleeding has been localized, resection should proceed. Recurrence can be decreased to 3.5% with a low operative mortality of 3%.[90] If the site of hemorrhage cannot be localized and the patient has recurrent episodes of hemorrhage, exploratory laparotomy should be performed with resection of all diseased bowel up to and including subtotal colectomy.

OBSTRUCTION
Epidemiology
Colonic obstruction due to strictures can occur with either CD or UC, but is more common with CD occurring in 5% to 17% of patients.[75,91] The risk of malignancy in patients with CD is 4 to 20 times that of the general population, and malignancy can occur in 6.8% of strictures.[75,91] Therefore, it is paramount to exclude malignancy in these patients prior to definitive management.

PREOPERATIVE MANAGEMENT
Initial workup of these patients includes complete history and physical examination, laboratories, and radiographs. Computed tomography may be helpful in defining the location of the obstructive process and evaluate for any associated infectious process or abscess. Radio-contrast enemas may also be helpful in determining the exact location and ruling out any additional masses or strictures. In the absence of a complete obstruction, endoscopy with multiple biopsies of the stricture to exclude malignancy should follow. Benign strictures due to exacerbations of the disease or with associated abscess may be treated medically with drainage of the abscess, antibiotics, and corticosteroids with resolution of the obstruction in the majority of cases.[75]

OPERATIVE MANAGEMENT
Surgical indications include failure of medical management or progressing disease. Surgical options depend on the disease process (UC vs CD) and location. UC should be managed with subtotal colectomy with ileostomy and HP. This allows removal of most disease and allows options for reconstruction with ileal pouch anal anastomosis (IPAA) at a later date.[75] Total proctocolectomy with IPAA may be considered at the first surgery if the patient is optimized medically and not acutely ill. CD strictures should be managed by RPA or resection and HP depending on the location, extent of disease, and illness of the patient. On rare occasions, the inflammatory response and location of disease precludes safe resection and should be managed with diverting ostomy and resection at a later date.

Malignant strictures must be managed with the appropriate oncologic operation. UC malignant strictures should be managed with total colectomy, ileostomy, and HP. CD malignant strictures should be managed with appropriate operations depending on the location of the tumor and completeness of obstruction. Please see the section on colonic obstruction for more information.

FISTULAS
Epidemiology
Fistulas are common complications of CD occurring in 17% to 43% of patients, with up to 33% of patients having perianal disease.[92,93] Other locations of fistulas include coloenteric, colovesical, colovaginal, and colocutaneous.

PREOPERATIVE TREATMENT
Following control of infection, medical management of CD is attempted. Initial medications for the control of CD and fistulas should be corticosteroids and metronidazole. Corticosteroids induce remission in 48% of patients and improve symptoms in an additional 32% within 30 days from initiation.[94] Twenty percent of patients are resistant from initiation, and at 1 year 45% are dependent on corticosteroids.[94] Direct

effects of corticosteroids on fistula disease have not been reported. Metronidazole has initial fistula closure rate of 56% at higher doses and improvement in 28%, but relapse occurs in 72% after discontinuation.[92] Chronic immunosuppression has also been evaluated with azathioprine (AZA) and 6-mercaptopurine (6MP) for closure of fistulas and suppression of active disease. Closure rates up to 54% have been reported with therapy, but relapse is common.[92] Cyclosporin with a parenteral loading dose followed by enteral therapy has closure or improvement rates of up to 80% but is limited by toxicity and frequent relapse after discontinuation of therapy.[92] Infliximab is a parenteral chimeric monoclonal immunoglobulin antibody to tumor necrosis factor composed of human constant and murine variable regions.[94] Induction infusions for refractory fistulas at 0, 2, and 6 weeks result in closure rates of 46% and improvement of 16%, but relapse is common after cessation of therapy.[92] Maintenence therapy can induce a sustained response for those with initial closure.[93]

OPERATIVE MANAGEMENT

Surgical management of fistulas associated with CD initially is limited to local control of infection and drainage of any associated abscesses.[75] Percutaneous techniques may also be used initially if the location is amenable to drainage.[75] Surgery should be the treatment of last resort following control of localized abscesses and sinus tracts. Fecal stream diversion via either a colostomy or ileostomy can result in sustained healing, but necessitates a stoma with the associated complications. Proctectomy should be reserved for those with hemorrhage or disease refractory to all other management options. The management algorithms for IBD are shown in Figs. 7-15 and 7-16.

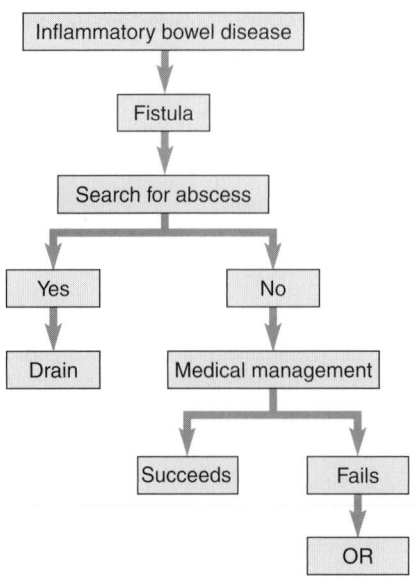

Figure 7-16 *Management algorithm for fistulas arising from inflammatory bowel disease.*

PERFORATION

EPIDEMIOLOGY

The end result of many of the pathologic processes of the colon discussed previously is perforation. Appendicitis, diverticulitis, volvulus, obstruction due to malignancy, interventions for lower GI bleeding, and inflammatory bowel disease can all lead to perforation of the colon. As perforation for each of these entities was discussed earlier, this section will focus on iatrogenic perforation from endoscopy.

Colonoscopy is a commonly performed procedure for many indications including cancer screening,

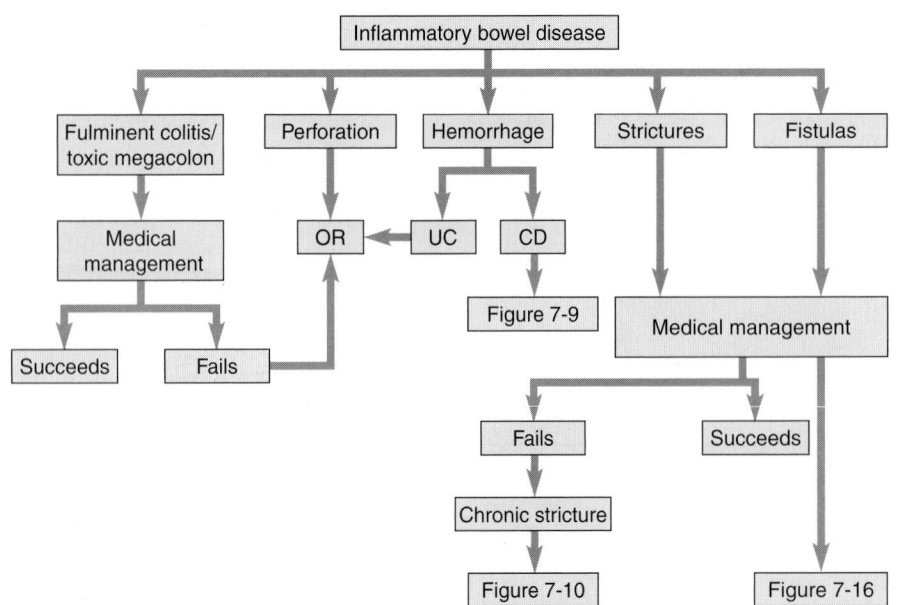

Figure 7-15 *Management algorithm for inflammatory bowel disease.*

diarrhea, guaiac positive stools, and almost any symptom referable to the colon. Complications occur with any procedure, and colonoscopy is no exception. The perforation rates for colonoscopy vary from 0.03% to 0.65%.[95-104] Some authors suggest that the perforation rates for therapeutic colonoscopy may be slightly higher from 0.073% to 2.14%.[99,100] Risk factors for perforation include the need for large amounts of sedation, force applied by the endoscopist during the procedure, and a "difficult exam."[95,104] Rapid recognition of the perforation and definitive management plans are important to keep morbidity low.

PREOPERATIVE MANAGEMENT

Following the procedure, most endoscopists will have a suspicion of perforation secondary to the difficulty of the exam, loss of ability to insufflate, or the presence of pain and need for heavy sedation. Almost all patients with perforation will have pain that does not resolve in a timely fashion.[98,100,103,105] Exam findings can range from diffuse peritonitis to subtle localized tenderness over the area of perforation.[101,102] Fever and tachycardia are also occasionally present.[100,104,105] Leukocytosis may be present depending on the duration of time from the perforation.[100,105] Plain abdominal x-rays will show free air in up to 87% of patients.[104] Retroperitoneal air may also be present on plain x-ray.[103] Other findings that may be present on x-ray include pneumomediastinum, pneumopericardium, pneumothorax, and pneumatosis intestinalis.[100] CT of the abdomen and pelvis is more sensitive for visualizing the area of injury and pneumoperitoneum than plain x-ray.[100] A water-soluble contrast enema study may be helpful to evaluate for a gross perforation in a patient without peritonitis who may be managed nonoperatively.[100,106]

OPERATIVE MANAGEMENT

The management algorithm for colonoscopic perforation depends on the extent of the perforation and duration of time from perforation to diagnosis. Treatment options vary from nonoperative to resection and colostomy. Those patients with obvious perforation, peritonitis on exam, and free air on abdominal x-ray should be taken to the operating room for laparotomy. Options in the operating room range from simple repair to HP if there is significant contamination or soilage and the patient is hemodynamically unstable. Simple colorrhaphy without diversion may be considered if the laceration is small, contamination is minimal, bowel prep is adequate, laparotomy is performed within 8 hours of perforation, and there is no underlying colonic pathology.[95,100,101] If these same criteria are met, but there is underlying colonic pathology, then RPA should be performed.[95,100,101]

If findings in the operating room are of large contamination or the patient is hemodynamically unstable, then HP should be performed. The majority of patients should be able to be managed with either colorrhaphy or RPA.

A small subgroup of patients exists in this population who may have signs and symptoms of perforation without diffuse peritonitis. These patients have localized tenderness and may have free air on abdominal x-ray. These select patients may be managed nonoperatively with bowel rest, antibiotics, intravenous fluids, and serial exams.[102] Other criteria for nonoperative management include late diagnosis, absence of peritonitis, a healthy patient, stable pneumoperitoneum, absence of a distal obstruction, and improving condition.[96] If any of these criteria are not met or change, a prompt trip to the operating room is warranted. Other authors recommend a water-soluble contrast enema in these patients to evaluate for frank extravasation.[100,106] In the presence of frank contrast extravasation, an urgent trip to the operating room is required with definitive intervention.[100,106] In the absence of extravasation, these patients may be managed conservatively with bowel rest, intravenous fluids, antibiotics, and serial exams. The algorithm is then followed for conservative management of the perforation. Even with prompt recognition and management mortality rates of 10% to 16% have been reported increasing to 33% with delays of greater than 24 hours.[98] As indications for colonoscopies increase and the number of exams performed increase, the acute care surgeon must be astute and prompt with recognition and definitive management of colonoscopic perforation to keep morbidity and mortality rates low. The management algorithm for perforation is shown in Fig. 7-17.

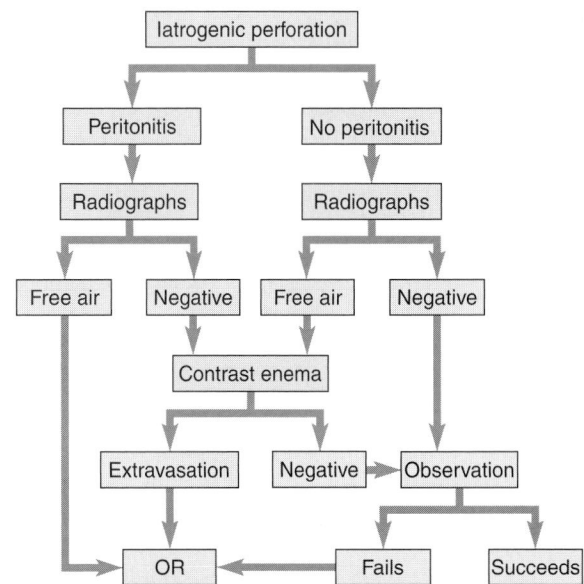

Figure 7-17 *Management algorithm for iatrogenic perforation.*

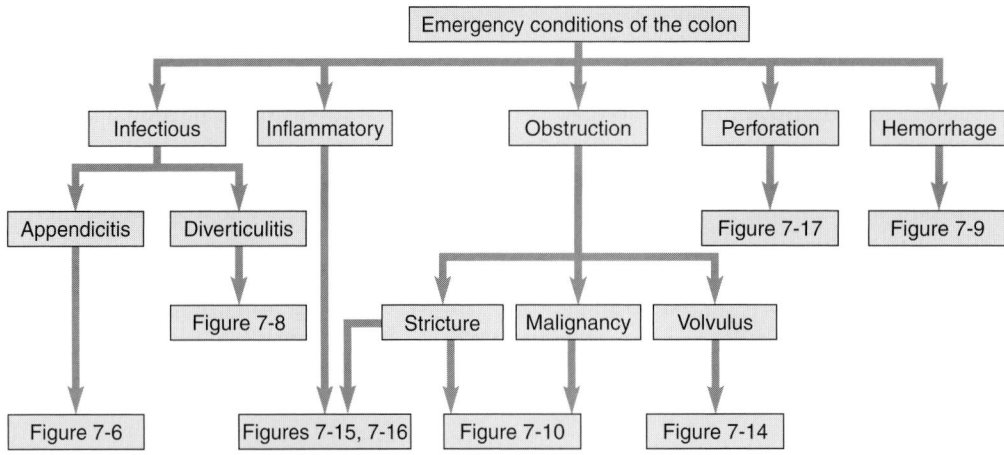

Figure 7-18   *Definitive management algorithm for acute colonic pathology.*

CONCLUSIONS

The acute care surgeon must be familiar with all aspects of the workup and treatment options for pathology of the colon, which is the most common organ affected by emergency pathology. Rapid diagnosis, resuscitation, and surgical intervention can limit the morbidity and mortality of emergency colonic pathology. An organized approach with algorithms as demonstrated in this chapter can expedite and facilitate this process and improve care (Fig. 7-18).

REFERENCES

1. http://www.nccn.org
2. Prystowsky JB, Pugh CM, Nagle AP. Appendicitis. *Curr Prob Surg* 2005;42:694.
3. Shelton T, McKinlay R, Schwartz RW. Acute appendicitis: current diagnosis and treatment. *Curr Surg* 2003;60:502.
4. Humes DJ, Simpson J. Acute appendicitis. *BMJ* 2006;333:530.
5. Jones K, Pena AA, Dunn EL, et al. Are negative appendectomies still acceptable? *Am J Surg* 2004; 188:748.
6. Rao PM, Rhea JT, Novelline RA, et al. Effect of computed tomography of the appendix on treatment of patients and use of hospital resources. *N Eng J Med* 1998;338:141.
7. McBurney C. Experience with early operative interference in cases of disease of the vermiform appendix. *NY Med J* 1889;50:676.
8. Paulson EK, Kalady MF, Pappas TN. Suspected appendicitis. *N Eng J Med* 2003;348:236.
9. Lee SL, Walsh AJ, Hung SH. Computed tomography and ultrasonography do not improve and may delay the diagnosis and treatment of acute appendicitis. *Arch Surg* 2001;136:556.
10. Doria AS, Moineddin R, Kellenberger CJ, et al. US or CT for diagnosis of appendicitis in children and adults? a meta-analysis. *Radiology* 2006;241:83.
11. Keyzer C, Zalcman M, De Maertelaer V, et al. Comparison of US and unenhanced multi-detector row CT in patients suspected of having acute appendicitis. *Radiology* 2005;236:527.

12. Wilcox RT, Traverso LW. Abdominal emergencies: has anything changed? Have the evaluation and treatment of acute appendicitis changed with new technology? *Surg Clin North Am* 1997;77:1356.
13. Morris KT, Kavanagh M, Hansen P, et al. The rational use of computed tomography scans in the diagnosis of appendicitis. *Am J Surg* 2002;183:547.
14. Perez J, Barone JE, Wilbanks TO, et al. Liberal use of computed tomography scanning does not improve dignositic accuracy in appendicitis. *Am J Surg* 2003;185:194.
15. Neumayer L, Kennedy A. Imaging in appendicitis: a review with special emphasis on the treatment of women. *Obstet Gynecol* 2003;102:1404.
16. McGory ML, Zingmond DS, Nanayakkara D, et al. Negative appendectomy rate: influence of CT scans. *Am Surg* 2005;71:803.
17. Bendeck SE, Nino-Murcia M, Berry GJ, Jeffrey RB. Imaging for suspected appendicitis: negative appendectomy and perforation rates. *Radiology* 2002;225:131.
18. Martin AE, Vollman D, Adler B, Caniano DA. CT scans may not reduce the negative appendectomy rate in children. *J Ped Surg* 2004;39:886.
19. Naoum JJ, Mileski WJ, Daller JA, et al. The use of abdominal computed tomography scan decreases the frequency of misdiagnosis in cases of suspected appendicitis. *Am J Surg* 2002;184:587.
20. Golub R, Siddiqui F, Pohl D. Laparoscopic versus open appendectomy: a metaanalysis. *J Am Coll Surg* 1998;186:545.

21. Chung RS, Rowland DY, Li P, Diaz J. A meta-analysis of randomized controlled trials of laparoscopic versus conventional appendectomy. *Am J Surg* 1999;177:250.
22. Semm K. Endoscopic appendectomy. *Endoscopy* 1983;15:59.
23. Yagmurlu A, Vernon A, Barnhart DC, et al. Laparoscopic appendectomy for perforated appendicitis: a comparison with open appendectomy. *Surg Endosc* 2006;20:1051.
24. Harrell AG, Lincourt AE, Novitsky YW, et al. Advantages of laparoscopic appendectomy in the elderly. *Am Surg* 2006;72:474.
25. Guller U, Hervey S, Purves H, et al. Lapaorscopic versus open appendectomy. Outcomes comparison based on a large administrative database. *Ann Surg* 2004;239:43.
26. Mancini GJ, Mancini ML, Nelson HS. Efficacy of laparoscopic appendectomy in appendicitis with peritonitis. *Am Surg* 2005;71:1.
27. Guller U, Nitin J, Peterson ED, et al. Laparoscopic appendectomy in the elderly. *Surgery* 2004;135:479.
28. Aziz O, Athanasiou T, Tekkis PP, et al. Laparoscopic versus open appendectomy in children: a meta-analysis. *Ann Surg* 2006;243:17.
29. Moberg AC, Berndsen F, Palmquist I, et al. Randomized clinical trial of laparoscopic versus open appendicectomy for confirmed appendicitis. *Br J Surg* 2005;92:298.
30. Cothren CC, Moore EE, Johnson JL, et al. Can we afford to do laparoscopic appendectomy in an academic hospital? *Am J Surg* 2005;190:973.
31. Hoehne F, Ozaeta M, Sherman B, et al. Laparoscopic versus open appendectomy: is the postoperative infectious complication rate different? *Am Surg* 2005;71:813.
32. Wang YC, Yang HR, Chung PK, et al. Laparoscopic appendectomy in the eldery. *Surg Endosc* 2006;20:887.
33. Katkhouda N, Mason RJ, Towfigh S, et al. Laparoscopic versus open appendectomy. A prospective randomized double-blind study. *Ann Surg* 2005;242:439.
34. Hasson HM, Rotman C, Rana N, Kumari NA. Open laparoscopy: 29 year experience. *Obstet Gynecol* 2000;96:763.
35. Bucher P, Mermillod B, Gervaz P, Morel P. Mechanical bowel preparation for elective colorectal surgery: a meta-analysis. *Arch Surg* 2004;139:1359.
36. Fa-Si-Oen P, Roumen R, Buitenweg J, et al. Mechanical bowel preparation or not? outcome of a multicenter, randomized trial in elective open colon surgery. *Dis Colon Rectum* 2005;48:1509.
37. Roberts P, Abel M, Rosen L, et al. Practice parameters for sigmoid diverticulitis-supporting documentation. *Dis Colon Rectum* 1995;38:126.
38. Bounds BC, Friedman LS. Lower gastrointestinal bleeding. *Gastroenterol Clin N Am* 2003;32:1107.
39. Stollman N, Raskin JB. Diverticular disease of the colon. *Lancet* 2004;363:631.
40. Hinchey EF, Schaal PG, Richards GK. Treatment of perforated diverticular disease of the colon. *Adv Surg* 1978;12:85.
41. Wong WD, Wexner SD, Lowry A, et al. Practice parameters for the treatment of sigmoid diverticulitis—supporting documentation. *Dis Colon Rectum* 2000;43:290.
42. Janes S, Meagher A, Frizelle FA. Elective surgery after acute diverticulitis. *Br J Surg* 2005;92:133.
43. Broderick-villa G, Burchette RJ, Collins JC, et al. Hospitalization for acute diverticulitis does not mandate routine elective colectomy. *Arch Surg* 2005;140:576.
44. Guzzo J, Hyman N. Diverticulitis in young patients: is resection after a single attack always warranted? *Dis Colon Rectum* 2004;47:1187.
45. Green BT, Rockey DC. Lower gastrointestinal bleeding—management. *Gastroenterol Clin N Am* 2005;34:665.
46. Acker JE, Ali J, Aprahamian C, et al. *ATLS Student Course Manual.* 7th ed. Chicago: American College of Surgeons; 2004:74.
47. Olds GD, Cooper GS, Chak A, et al. The yield of bleeding scans in acute lower gastrointestinal hemorrhage. *J Clin Gastroenterol* 2005;39:273.
48. Lin S, Rockey DC. Obscure gastrointestinal bleeding. *Gastroentero Clin N Am* 2005;34:679.
49. McDonald ML, Farnell MB, Stanson AW, et al. Preoperative highly selective catheter localization of occult small-intestinal hemorrhage with methylene blue dye. *Arch Surg* 1995;130:106.
50. Hebert PC, Wells G, Blajchman MA, et al. A multicenter, randomized, controlled clinical trial of transfusion requirements in critical care. *N Engl J Med* 2006;340:409.
51. Vincent JL, Baron JF, Reinhart K, et al. Anemia and blood transfusion in critically ill patients. *JAMA* 2002;288:1499.
52. Corwin HL, Gettinger A, Pearl RG, et al. The crit study: anemia and blood transfusion in the critically ill-current clinical practice in the United States. *Crit Care Med* 2004;32:39.
53. Zuckerman GR, Prakash C. Acute lower intestinal bleeding, part II: etiology, therapy, and outcomes. *Gastrointest Endosc* 1999;49:228.
54. Deans GT, Krukowski ZH, Irwin ST. Malignant obstruction of the left colon. *Br J Surg* 1994;81:1270.
55. Lee YM, Law WL, Chu KW, Poon RT. Emergency surgery for obstructing colorectal cancers: a comparison between right-sided and left-sided lesions. *J Am Coll Surg* 2001;192:719.
56. Biondo S, Pares D, Frago R, et al. Large bowel obstruction: predictive factors for postoperative mortality. *Dis Colon Rectum* 2004;47:1889.
57. Hsu TC. Comparison of one-stage resection and anastomosis of acute complete obstruction of the left and right colon. *Am J Surg* 2005;189:384.
58. MacKenzie S, Thomson SR, Baker LW. Management options in malignant obstruction of the left colon. *Surg Gynecol Ostet* 1992;174:337.
59. Biondo S, Pares D, Kreisler E, et al. Anastomotic dehiscence after resection and primary anastomosis in left-sided colonic emergencies. *Dis Colon Rectum* 2005;48:2272.
60. Arnaud JP, Bergamaschi R. Emergency subtotal/total colectomy with anastomosis for acutely obstructed carcinoma of the left colon. *Dis Colon Rectum* 1994;37:685.
61. Madiba TE, Thomson SR. The management of cecal volvulus. *Dis Colon Rectum* 2002;45:264.
62. Grossman EM, Longo WE, Stratton MD, et al. Sigmoid volvulus in department of Veterans' Affairs medical centers. *Dis Colon Rectum* 2000;43:414.

63. Brothers TE, Strodel WE, Eckhauser FE. Endoscopy in colonic volvulus. *Ann Surg* 1987;206:1.

64. Ballantyne GH, Brandner MD, Beart RW, Ilstrup DM. Volvulus of the colon: incidence and mortality. *Ann Surg* 1985;202:83.

65. Hiltunen KM, Hannu S, Matikainen M. Colonic volvulus: diagnosis and results of treatment in 82 patients. *Eur J Surg* 1992;158:607.

66. Theuer C, Cheadle WG. Volvulus of the colon. *Am Surg* 1991;57:145.

67. Friedman JD, Odland MD, Bubrick MP. Experience with colonic volvulus. *Dis Colon Rectum* 1989;32:409.

68. Frizelle FA, Wolff BG. Colonic Volvulus. *Adv Surg* 1996;29:131.

69. Mangiante EC, Croce MA, Fabian TC, et al. Sigmoid volvulus: a four decade experience. *Am Surg* 1989;55:41.

70. Geer DA, Arnaud G, Beitler A, et al. Colonic volvulus: the army medical center experience 1983-1987. *Am Surg* 1991;57:295.

71. Bak MP, Boley SJ. Sigmoid volvulus in elderly patients. *Am J Surg* 1986;151:71.

72. Rabinovici R, Simansky DA, Kaplan O, et al. Cecal volvulus. *Dis Colon Rectum* 1990;33:765.

73. Roy MA. Abdominal emergencies: has anything changed? *Surg Clin North Am* 1997;77:1419.

74. Oberhelman HA. Inflammatory disease of the bowel: indications for surgery. *Dis Colon Rectum* 1976;19:582.

75. Berg DF, Bahadursingh AM, Kaminski DL, Longo WE. Acute surgical emergencies in inflammatory bowel disease. *Am J Surg* 2002;184:45.

76. Gan SI, Beck PL. A new look at toxic megacolon: an update and review of incidence, etiology, pathogenesis, and management. *Am J Gastroenterol* 2003;98:2363.

77. Cunsolo A, Bragaglia RB, Arena N, et al. Toxic megacolon complicating ulcerative colitis and crohn's disease. *Int Surg* 1985;70:339.

78. D'Amico C, Vitale A, Angriman I, et al. Early surgery for the treatment of toxic megacolon. *Digestion* 2005;72:146.

79. Heppell J, Farkouh E, Dube S, et al. Toxic megacolon: an analysis of 70 cases. *Dis Colon Rectum* 1986;29:789.

80. Soyer MT, Aldrete JS. Surgical treatment of toxic megacolon and proposal for a program of therapy. *Am J Surg* 1980;140:421.

81. Fry PD, Atkinson KG. Current surgical approach to toxic megacolon. *Surg Gyn Obstet* 1976;143:26.

82. Turnbull RB, Hawk WA, Weakley FL. Surgical treatment of toxic megacolon: ileostomy and colostomy to prepare patients for colectomy. *Am J Surg* 1971;122:325.

83. Marshak RH, Korelitz BI, Klein SH, et al. Toxic dilation in the course of ulcerative colitis. *Gastroenterology* 1960;38:165.

84. Defriend D, Hill J. A review of emergency colonic surgery. *Br J Hosp Med* 1996;56:326.

85. Sirinek KR, Tetirick CE, Thomford NR, Pace WG. Total proctocolectomy and ileostomy: procedure of choice for acute toxic megacolon. *Arch Surg* 1977;112:518.

86. Katz S, Schulman N, Levin L. Free perforation in Crohn's disease: a report of 33 cases and review of the literature. *Am J Gastroenterol* 1986;81:38.

87. Bundred NJ, Dixon JM, Lumsden AB, et al. Free perforation in Crohn's colitis: a ten year review. *Dis Colon Rectum* 1985;28:35.

88. Greenstein AJ, Mann D, Heimann T, et al. Spontaneous perforation and perforated abscess in 30 patients with Crohn's disease. *Ann Surg* 1987;205:72.

89. Robert JR, Sachar DB, Greenstein AJ. Severe gastrointestinal hemorrhage in Crohn's disease. *Ann Surg* 1991;213:207.

90. Cirocco WC, Reilly JC, Rusin LC. Life-threatening hemorrhage and exsanguinations from Crohn's disease. *Dis Colon Rectum* 1995;38:85.

91. Yamazaki Y, Ribeiro MB, Sachar DB, et al. Malignant colorectal strictures in Crohn's disease. *Am J Gastroenterol* 1991;86:882.

92. Pare P. Management of fistulas in patients with Crohn's disease: antibiotic to antibody. *Can J Gastroentero* 2001;15:751.

93. Sands BE, Anderson FH, Bernstein CN, et al. Infliximab maintenance therapy for fistulizing Crohn's disease. *N Eng J Med* 2004;350:876.

94. Rutgeerts P, Assche GV, Vermeire S. Optimizing anti-TNF treatment in inflammatory bowel disease. *Gastroenterology* 2004;126:1593.

95. Vincent M, Smith LE. Management of perforation due to colonoscopy. *Dis Colon Rectum* 1983;26:61.

96. Carpio G, Albu E, Gumbs MA, Gerst PH. Management of colonic perforation after colonoscopy: report of three cases. *Dis Colon Rectum* 1989;32:624.

97. Hall C, Dorricott NJ, Donovan IA, Neoptolemos JP. Colon perforation during colonoscopy: surgical versus conservative management. *Br J Surg* 1991;78:524.

98. Gedebou TM, Wong RA, Rappaport WD, et al. Clinical presentation and management of iatrogenic colon perforations. *Am J Surg* 1996;172:454.

99. Anderson ML, Pasha TM, Leighton JA. Endoscopic perforation of the colon: lessons from a 10-year study. *Am J Gastroenterol* 2000;95:3418.

100. Damore LJ, Rantis PC, Vernava AM, Longo WE. Colonoscopic perforations: etiology, diagnosis, and management. *Dis Colon Rectum* 1996;39:1308.

101. Araghizadeh FY, Timmcke AE, Opelka FG, et al. Colonoscopic perforations. *Dis Colon Rectum* 2001;44:713.

102. Christie JP, Marrazzo J. Mini-perforation of the colon—not all postpolypectomy perforations require laparotomy. *Dis Colon Rectum* 1991;34:132.

103. Tulchinsky H, Madhala-Givon O, Wasserberg N, et al. Incidence and management of colonoscopic perforations: 8 years experience. *World J Gastroenterol* 2006;12:4211.

104. Farley DR, Bannon MP, Zietlow SP, et al. Management of colonoscopic perforations. *Mayo Clin Proc* 1997;72:729.

105. Kavin H, Sinicrope F, Esker AH. Management of perforation of the colon at colonoscopy. *Am J Gastroenterol* 1992;87:161.

106. Clements RH, Jordan LM, Webb WA. Critical decisions in the management of endoscopic perforations of the colon. *Am Surg* 2000;66:91.

Chapter 8

THE RECTUM AND ANUS

Craig A. Reickert, MD, Sadaf Khan, MBBS, and Scott A. Dulchavsky, MD, PhD

INTRODUCTION

The management of surgical diseases of the rectum and perianal region is a critical skill for acute care surgeons.

PERIANAL ABSCESS AND FISTULOUS DISEASE

Perianal infections are usually caused by suppuration in one of the anal gland crypts.[1] Other infectious processes can occur in the skin and soft tissues near the anal canal (hidradenitis suppurativa, sebaceous cyst infection, Bartholin gland infection, etc); however, due to the composition of the perianal skin (absence of hair follicles and sweat glands), it is more common to have infection in the skin and soft tissues that is associated with the anal canal crypts.

Perianal infections are usually caused by obstruction of an anal canal gland which results in an infection in the gland. There are usually 9-15 of these glands at the level of the dentate line, arranged around the anal canal and clustered toward the midline anteriorly and posteriorly. Because the glands have a variable depth (internal sphincter, extending into the intersphincteric groove, and into the external sphincter), there are several potential spaces into which the infectious process can extend. The "cryptoglandular" etiology has been supported by anatomic, microscopic, and operative findings.[12] Over 90% of perianal abscesses and fistulas are cryptoglandular in origin.[2] Table 8-1 lists noncryptoglandular causes.

Patients commonly present with complaints of localized pain (~90%), swelling (~50%), and fever.[2] Exquisitely severe pain and associated difficulty with urination may suggest either an intersphincteric or supralevator abscess.

Physical examination is frequently a source of great anxiety for the patient. In general, reassurance and gentle retraction of the gluteal cheeks will expose the perianal area with little or no additional discomfort. Careful communication with the patient and discussion of the process prior to performance of an exam is imperative. An area of erythema and swelling and possible fluctuance is usually identified. A subset of patients may present with an opening from the area of swelling that is draining pus, or express pus from the anal canal with perianal pressure over the fluctuant area.

Some abscesses (intersphincteric, and supralevator abscesses) may not have significant external findings on exam. Similarly, patients with immunocompromise may also have a lack of significant external findings. Rectal exam is often too uncomfortable to tolerate for the patient but will confirm the area of tenderness and swelling. A vaginal examination can be useful to confirm the findings in patients without a clear perirectal abscess.

Radiologic imaging is generally not required for the diagnosis and management of perianal infections. Computed tomography is occasionally useful in patients with complex, supralevator infections; however, when no specific external findings are present, or there is suspicion of an intersphincteric or supralevator abscess. Generally, the patient is best examined and treated in the operating room. Lighted anal retractors or a headlight can provide additional visualization to facilitate examination deep in the anal canal.

A fistula-in-ano is a persistent epithelialized connection between an anal gland and the skin which can occur following a perianal infection. The external opening is a small dimpled area of granulation tissue or scar with drainage of pus or blood on manual compression. Frequently, a thin cordlike structure may be palpated representing the fistula tracking into the anal canal.[3] Patients with relapsing abscess with recurrence in the same location should raise the possibility of an undiagnosed fistula. Anoscopy and proctoscopy are important components of the rectal examination to evaluate perianal fistulas; however, this is not required during an episode of acute perianal abscess.

The guiding principle for treatment of perianal abscess is adequate incision and drainage. Nonoperative or antibiotic therapy is usually unsuccessful, prolongs the discomfort for the patient, and can lead to progression of

Table 8-1   Non-cryptoglandular causes of perianal infections

Inflammatory Bowel Disease
Crohn disease
Ulcerative colitis (much less common)

Infections
    Tuberculosis
    Actinomycosis
    Lymphogranuloma Venereum (Chlamydia Trachomatis)

Traumatic
    Impalement
    Foreign Body
    Open Pelvis Fracture

Postsurgical

Malignancy
    Carcinoma
    Leukemia
    Lymphoma

Radiotherapy

the disease with an increased risk of sphincter involvement. Rarely, perianal abscess is associated with the development of perineal necrotizing soft tissue infection and death.[4]

The majority of drainage procedures for perianal infections can be performed outside an operating room setting. Complex perianal infections, suspicion of supralevator involvement, and very large (> 5 cm) infections should be drained in an operating room setting. Patient cooperation can also be an important consideration regarding where drainage is performed. Preprocedure antibiotics are not required unless the patient is diabetic, immunocompromised, or has a prosthetic device in place.

The patient is placed in left lateral position or the prone jackknife position. The buttocks are gently retracted by an assistant; wide cloth tape can also be used to provide retraction. The perianal area is prepped with an antiseptic solution and anesthetized with 1% xylocaine without epinephrine using a 22-Gauge or 24-Gauge needle and slow injection technique in a field block fashion to minimize discomfort. Topical agents do not provide adequate anesthesia for optimal incision and drainage. A calm voice and reassurance during the procedure will help allay any anxiety from the patient.

A cruciate incision is made over the point of maximal fluctuancy. Localization with an 18-Gauge needle can be used in patients without obvious fluctuancy to guide the skin incision. Gentle exploration with a hemostat should be performed to break up any loculations. Successful resolution of the infection is dependent on adequate drainage. Removal of the skin edges or insertion of a 12-16 French mushroom–tipped

catheter)[5] will facilitate decompression and prevent sealing of the cavity prior to healing. Deep packing of the abscess cavity is not routinely required and adds to patient discomfort. Care must be taken to minimize additional injury to the sphincter muscle. If the patient is too uncomfortable to tolerate adequate drainage, the patient should be taken to the operating room for definitive examination and treatment under anesthesia.

Postprocedure pain and anticonstipation medications are an essential component to satisfactory treatment of perianal infections. The drainage catheter is removed during follow-up in 1-2 weeks. Immunocompromised and diabetic patients should be given an antibiotic with broad coverage; extensive cellulitis, necrotizing soft tissue infection, or signs of sepsis mandate hospital admission for intravenous antibiotics. Diligent monitoring of response is essential in patients with sepsis or large soft tissue infections; repeated examination under anesthesia may be required to allow careful evaluation while maintaining patient comfort.

There is limited benefit in attempting to identify an internal opening at the time of treatment for perianal abscess. Less than 50% of patients with a perirectal abscess will develop a fistula making the addition of a fistulotomy often unnecessary and potentially dangerous.[6] The risk of false passage of a probe, or iatrogenic damage to the sphincter complex, is heightened in inflamed tissues; therefore, routine fistulotomy at the time of treatment for abscess is not advised.

INTERSPHINCTERIC ABSCESS

Intersphincteric abscesses require special care to avoid incontinence during surgical drainage procedures. The abscess is drained by incising the internal sphincter over the point of maximal swelling, from the lower end to the dentate line, extensive dissection proximally is unnecessary and increases the risk of incontinence.

SUPRALEVATOR ABSCESS

Supralevator abscess may present with minimal external physical findings. Rectal examination may reveal perirectal fullness with tenderness; if there is associated intra-abdominal pathology, lower abdominal tenderness, rebound, or a mass may be noted.

The etiology of the supralevator abscess influences surgical therapy. Supralevator abscesses, which occur secondary to upward extension of an intersphincteric abscess should be drained directly into the rectum. Supra-levator abscesses which are the result of extension of ischioanal infections, are best drained via the ischioanal fossa. Supralevator abscesses may be caused by extrapelvic disease including Crohn disease, diverticulitis, or appendicitis. These patients usually present with abdominal complaints and systemic illness. Radiologic imaging can be useful in determining the etiology in these challenging patients. The supralevator abscess can be drained via the rectum or the ischioanal fossa; however, the primary abdominal pathology must be addressed.[1]

HORSESHOE ABSCESS

Perianal infections that extend bilaterally in the ischioanal tissue planes form a horseshoe abscess. The majority of these infections begin in the posterior midline. General or regional anesthesia is required to allow adequate examination and drainage in patients with a horseshoe abscess. Midline drainage in proximity to the sphincter with counterincisions in each ischial fossa provides excellent drainage while minimizing tissue disruption. Large drains, extensive packing, and repeated debridement are not usually required. Local wound care, sitz baths, and adequate pain control will usually result in an excellent outcome in patients with this type of infection.

MASSIVE LOWER GI BLEEDING

Massive lower gastrointestinal bleeding secondary to anorectal pathology is fortunately rare. A proctoscopic examination should be considered in any patient presenting with rapid nonmelanic bleeding to exclude an anorectal source of bleeding.[7] Gastrointestinal bleeding secondary to internal hemorrhoidal disease can be managed by rubber band ligation.[8] Suture ligation or electrocautery are very effective adjuncts for bleeding from hemorrhoids, rectal fissure, trauma, or stercoral ulcers.[9] Rectal varices may be initially managed with ligation; however, the bleeding recurrence rate is very high unless definitive treatment of portal hypertension is undertaken.[10,11,12] Significant bleeding secondary to radiation proctitis is discussed later in this chapter.

RADIATION PROCTITIS

Radiation proctitis is a common and occasionally significant problem in patients treated for pelvic malignancies. Early signs and symptoms of radiation proctitis are tenesmus and hematochezia. These symptoms usually resolve within 3 months with supportive management.[13] Chronic radiation proctitis develops as a result of progressive submucosal fibrosis and endarteritis obliterans. This results in formation of neovasculature that is fragile and prone to bleeding. The associated mucosal ischemia is also predisposed to ulcer formation. Symptoms vary in intensity from mild hematochezia associated with bowel movements, to brisk bleeding requiring emergency evaluation and intervention. Medical treatment with topical steroid, topical or oral sulfasalazine and sucralfate enemas are usually unsuccessful in the control of severe bleeding. Endoscopic intervention such as argon plasma coagulation, bipolar cautery, and heater probes are effective

and should be considered as primary treatment methods in patients with significant GI bleeding secondary to radiation proctitis. Topical formalin has been reported to be an effective adjunct with response rates ranging from 70% to 100%.[13]

Hyperbaric oxygen therapy has been used with limited success in patients with refractory radiation proctitis; the efficacy and cost-effectiveness has not yet been defined. In rare and severe cases, diverting colostomy or proctectomy with colostomy may be necessary.

ACUTE HEMORRHOIDAL DISEASE

Hemorrhoids are cushions of vascular tissue located in the anal canal. Hemorrhoidal tissue is present at birth and may undergo time-dependent changes resulting in pathology. There are three well-defined hemorrhoidal bundles—right anterior, right posterior and left lateral; there can be additional secondary cushions between these bundles which can result in symptoms. Hemorrhoidal tissue extends from the anal canal to the anal margin. Internal hemorrhoids are covered by mucosa and occur above the dentate line. External hemorrhoids are located below the dentate line. They are covered by squamous epithelium of the anoderm. Patients seek emergent or urgent therapy for hemorrhoidal disease due to bleeding, swelling, prolapse, or thrombosis of external hemorrhoids that may progress to ischemia, thrombosis, and gangrene.[8]

THROMBOSED EXTERNAL HEMORRHOID

Thrombosis of an external hemorrhoid results in significant pain. The pathogenesis is unclear; however, it is often preceded by straining or constipation. Thrombosed hemorrhoids can result in bleeding if ulceration of the overlying skin and clot extrusion occurs. The management of thrombosed hemorrhoids is dependent on the duration and severity of symptoms. Discomfort is most severe for the first 3-4 days with gradual improvement over the next week.[8] Mild discomfort and a small thrombus may be managed conservatively with sitz baths, topical astringents, anti-inflammatory agents, and oral analgesics. Larger thrombi are generally associated with significant pain or ulceration. Large thrombosed external hemorrhoids are best managed by early excision in the office or emergency room.[14]

HEMORRHOIDAL BLEEDING

Acute hemorrhoidal bleeding requiring emergency intervention is rare. Additional sources of bleeding should be excluded prior to rubber band ligation for internal hemorrhoids or suture ligation under anesthesia.[14]

HEMORRHOIDAL PROLAPSE

Patients with intermittent hemorrhoidal prolapse can progress to nonreducible (grade 4) hemorrhoidal prolapse. Patients with grade 4 prolapse may present with significant pain, local edema, and inflammation which can progress to thrombosis and local tissue ischemia; therefore, careful clinical evaluation is necessary. Signs of significant tissue necrosis warrant emergency surgical excision.[15] Patients with prolapsed external hemorrhoids who do not have thrombosis can be conservatively managed with sitz baths, topical analgesics, astringents, and anti-inflammatory agents with good success.

HEMORRHOIDAL SWELLING

Acute swelling of internal and external hemorrhoids can generally be managed nonsurgically in the acute phase. Patients with frequent episodes benefit from elective surgical hemorrhoidectomy. Patients who do not respond to medical management, who have severe pain or thrombosis, or show signs of infection, benefit from emergent surgical hemorrhoidectomy.

Acute hemorrhoidal crisis, consisting of severe pain, engorgement of hemorrhoids, and possibly thrombosis can occur during pregnancy. The principles of management do not differ in pregnant patients; surgical intervention can be undertaken with acceptable risk for mother and fetus.[16,17]

POSTHEMORRHOID TREATMENT COMPLICATIONS

Postsurgical complications following treatment for hemorrhoidal disease most commonly consist of bleeding, infection, and recurrence. Bleeding after surgical hemorrhoidectomy is the most common single complication occurring in approximately 1% of cases. Patients with significant bleeding require examination under anesthesia with ligation of the bleeding vessel. Submucosal injection of the bleeding area with 1/10,000 epinephrine solution has been described also.[18]

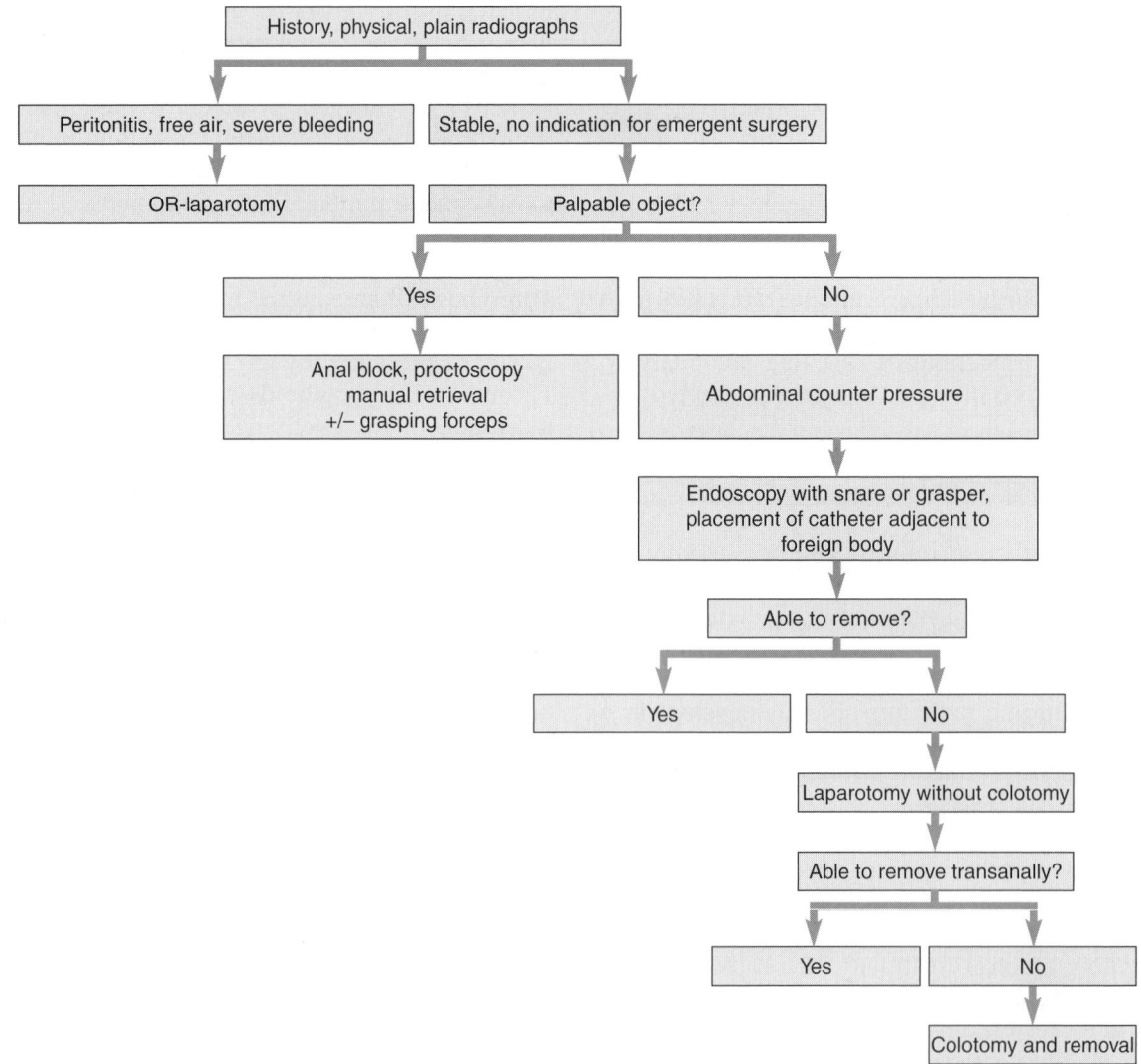

Figure 8-1 *Algorithm for the management of rectal foreign bodies.*

Patients may also have post-hemorrhoidectomy surgical urinary retention, which is usually managed with catheter decompression of the bladder and pain control.

A rapidly progressive infection has been rarely associated with hemorrhoid treatment (surgical or even office-based), which presents as pelvic pressure, pain, and inability to void. Careful examination and monitoring of the perineum is crucial in patients presenting with these symptoms to avoid progression of this potentially devastating infection. A low threshold for inpatient management of these patients should be maintained unless the patient has improving symptoms, resolving pain, and does not have signs of sepsis.[19,20,21]

RECTAL FOREIGN BODY

Anorectal foreign body is an infrequent presenting complaint. It is important to have a calm and private area for history and examination. Many patients will present with a history of consenting activity with rectal foreign body insertion during sexual activity. However, any implication of nonconsensual treatment mandates that the physician take a thorough history and evaluate for other trauma or rape findings. In such a case, any retrieved foreign body must be treated as evidence should a criminal case be initiated.

The varieties of foreign bodies that have been found and retrieved are myriad. Techniques for retrieval for many kinds of objects have been described in the literature.[22,23] An algorithm for the management of rectal foreign bodies is presented in Fig. 8-1. Key themes in the management of foreign body are to start with a careful evaluation of the abdomen. Any evidence of peritonitis, free-air, or other suspicion of perforation mandates laparotomy and removal of the foreign body under anesthesia. Many patients may present late due to obvious reluctance at seeking medical attention; therefore, specific questioning about the duration of presence of the foreign body, evidence of bowel obstruction, and a history of incontinence symptoms occurring prior to evaluation. Plain AP and lateral radiographs can help identify the foreign body and evaluate for free-air.

In stable patients without evidence of peritonitis, most foreign bodies of the rectum can be managed in the clinic or emergency room. For narrow, thin foreign bodies, a gentle rectal exam, using 2% xylocaine jelly as lubricant, relaxes the sphincter and allows manual retrieval of the object, especially when combined with a Valsalva maneuver by the patients. For larger diameter (> 2-3 cm) foreign bodies, the addition of a local anesthesia anal block can allow further relaxation of the sphincter and better tolerance for the insertion of an anoscope and a grasping instrument to retrieve the object.

In many situations, the foreign body is difficult to remove because of a vacuum effect in the bowel above the foreign body. The insertion of a small Foley catheter above the object and instilling air into the lumen of the bowel, followed by inflation of the balloon with saline has been effective in assisting with removal of foreign bodies.[22] Other removal aids, including grasping tenaculum, snare, or forceps via an anoscope can be useful. Extreme care must be taken with fragile glass objects (lightbulbs in particular)[23] due to the risk of laceration if the object is damaged during withdrawal. Several series have reported frequent success with foreign body removal transanally.[24] It is of primary importance to slowly dilate the sphincter to allow large objects to be retrieved without significant sphincter injury.

After removal of a foreign body, it is essential to evaluate for damage to the bowel.[25] Endoscopy and water-soluble contrast studies are effective in ruling out perforations. Observation in the hospital can be used in equivocal cases.

If extraction with local anesthesia is unsuccessful, a combination of a general anesthetic and abdominal counter pressure with transanal grasping and retrieval can be utilized. These steps should be attempted before performing laparotomy. Laparotomy and laparoscopic assisted retrieval are rarely required. When needed, an abdominal approach will allow the object to be advanced toward the rectum, allowing retrieval by a surgeon operating at the perineum. In very rare instances, a colotomy can be used to retrieve the object, followed by primary repair and evaluation for other bowel injuries from the foreign body.[26]

REFERENCES

1. Parks, AG. Pathogenesis and treatment of fistula-in-ano. *Br Med J* 1961;1:463-469.
2. Chrabot CM, Prasad ML, Abcarian H. Recurrent anorectal abscesses. *Dis Colon Rectum* 1984;27:126-30.
3. Scoma JA, Salvati EP, Rubin RJ. Incidence of fistulas subsequent to anal abscesses. *Dis Colon Rectum* 1974;17:357-9.
4. Bubrick MP, Hitchcock CR. Necrotizing anorectal and perineal infections. *Surgery* 86:655-62, 1979.
5. Beck DE, Fazio VW, Lavery IC, et al. Catheter Drainage of ischiorectal abscesses. *South Med J* 1988; 81:444-6.
6. Vasilevsky CA, Gordon PH. The incidence of recurrent abscess or fistula-in-ano following anorectal suppuration. *Dis Colon Rectum* 1984;27:126-130.
7. Kluiber RM, Wolff BG. Evaluation of anemia caused by hemorrhoidal bleeding. *Dis Colon Rectum* 1994; 37:1006-1007.
8. Thomsom WHF. The nature of hemorrhoids. *Br J Surg* 1975;62:542-552.
9. Hosking SW, Johnson AG, Smart HL, et al. Anorectal varies, haemorrhoids and portal hypertension. *Lancet* 1989;1(8634):349-52.

10. Johnson K, Bardin J, Orloff MJ. Massive bleeding from hemorrhoidal varices in portal hypertension. *JAMA* 1980;244:2084-5.

11. Chawla Y, Dilawari JB. Anorectal varices—their frequency in cirrhotic and non-cirrhotic portal hypertension. *Gut* 1991;32:309-311.

12. Wilson SE, Stone RT, Christie JP, et al. Massive lower gastrointestinal bleeding from intestinal varices. *Arch Surg* 1979;114:1158-61.

13. Parikh S, Hughes C, Salvati EP, et al. Treatment of hemorrhagic radiation proctitis with 4 percent formalin. *Dis Colon Rectum* 2003;46:596.

14. Barron J. Office ligation treatment of hemorrhoids. *Dis Colon Rectum* 1963;6:109-113.

15. Armstrong DN. Multiple hemorrhoidal ligation. *Dis Colon Rectum* 2003;46(2):179-186.

16. Medich DS, Fazio VW. Hemorrhoids, anal fissure, and carcinoma of the colon, rectum, and anus during pregnancy. *Surg Clin North Am* 1995;75(1):77-78.

17. Saleeby RG Jr, Rosen L, Stasik JJ, et al. Hemorrhoidectomy during pregnancy: risk or relief? *Dis Colon Rectum* 1991;34(3):260-1.

18. Bleday R, Pena JP, Rothenberger DA, et al. Symptomatic hemorrhoids: current incidence and complications of operative therapy. *Dis Colon Rectum* 1992;35:477.

19. Russell TR, Donohue JH. Hemorrhoidal banding. A warning. *Dis Colon Rectum* 1985;28:291-293.

20. Scarpa FJ, Hillis W, Sabetta JR. Pelvic cellulitis: a life-threatening complication of hemorrhoidal banding. *Surgery* 1988;103:383-385.

21. Bat L, Melze E, Koler M, et al. Complications of rubber band ligation of symptomatic internal hemorrhoids. *Dis Colon Rectum* 1993;36(3):287-90.

22. Barone JE, Yee J, Nealon TF, Jr. Management of foreign bodies and trauma of the rectum. *Surg Gyn and Obstet* 1983;156:453.

23. Garber HI, Rubin RJ, Eisenstat TE. Removal of glass foreign body from the rectum. *Dis Colon Rectum* 1981;24:323.

24. Nehme-Kingsley A, Abcarian H. Colorectal foreign bodies. Management update. *Dis Colon Rectum* 1985;28:941-4.

25. Rocklin MS, Apelgren KN. Colonoscopic extraction of foreign bodies from above the rectum. *Am Surg* 1989;55:119.

26. Fry RD. Anorectal trauma and foreign bodies. *Surg Clin North Am* 1994;74(6):1491-1505.

Chapter **9**

THE LIVER

Elliott R. Haut, MD, David T. Efron, MD, and Edward E. Cornwell, III, MD

INTRODUCTION

Acute care surgical management of patients with liver pathology encompasses a wide range of possible diagnostic and therapeutic dilemmas. Not all liver-related diagnoses require surgical intervention, but many liver-related issues are managed by acute care surgeons. Nontraumatic acute surgical emergencies of the liver (ie, liver infection and liver tumor complications) are relatively uncommon entities. However, when they do occur, wide-ranging approaches to both the nonsurgical and operative approaches are often necessary.

Managing common surgical diseases in patients with acute or chronic liver disease is the more likely scenario. Patients with preexisting liver disease, ascites, or cirrhosis present extremely difficult management decisions for what are otherwise straightforward general surgical issues. Appropriate preoperative surgical decision making depends on the specific risk of surgery and appropriate patient risk stratification based on the severity of their liver disease. Special intraoperative techniques are often necessary to render care to these severely ill individuals. Postoperative management of problems unique to cirrhotic patients must also be considered.

MANAGEMENT OF THE CIRRHOTIC PATIENT

RISK STRATIFICATION OF NONTRANSPLANT SURGERY IN PATIENTS WITH HEPATIC DYSFUNCTION SURGICAL RISK

Assessing the risk of nontransplant operative intervention in patients with cirrhosis or end-stage liver disease is of paramount importance for those being considered for elective procedures. However, understanding the risk in such patients is also vital to the care of the same population of patients who present with acute care surgical disease. A number of different descriptive scoring systems have been employed to predict such operative mortality including evolving versions of the Acute Physiology and Chronic Health Evaluation (APACHE), the Child-Turcotte-Pugh (CTP) classification, and, more recently, the Model for End-Stage Liver Disease (MELD).

The Child-Turcotte-Pugh classification is a liver-specific assessment of hepatic function.[1,2] It was originally derived empirically to stratify risks for patients undergoing portal decompressive shunt surgery. It is based on laboratory values (albumin, bilirubin, INR), the symptoms and degree of encephalopathy, and the presence and degree of ascites. Table 9-1 describes the CTP classification system.[3-5] It has been demonstrated in several studies to correlate well with mortality following nontransplant surgery. For patients undergoing abdominal operations, the operative morality for patients with Childs A, B, and C have been reported as 10, 30, and 60-80%, respectively. Emergent surgery carries a greater risk than elective surgery for all three classes of liver dysfunction.

One of the major criticisms of the CTP classification system is that subjective evaluation exerts a significant influence on prognostic class. This was recently replaced with an alternative scoring system, the Model for End-Stage Liver Disease (MELD).[6] MELD scoring is derived purely from objective data including serum total bilirubin, INR, and creatinine. A numeric rank is assigned according to the following equation:

$$\text{MELD score} = 3.8[\text{Log (e) (serum total bilirubin(mg/dL))}] + 11.2[\text{Log (e) (INR)}] + 9.6[\text{Log (e) (serum creatinine(mg/dL))}] + 6.4$$

The MELD was originally derived to predict the postprocedural survival of patients undergoing transjugular intrahepatic portosystemic shunt (TIPS). However, because it is based on objective criteria and on its applicability across hepatic disease of multiple etiologies, MELD has become the standard by which resource allocation is determined for liver transplantation.[7] Although there are several other considerations for such resource utilization that affect the MELD

Table 9-1	Child-Turcotte-Pugh Classification		
Assigned Points	1	2	3
Lab/Symptoms/Signs			
Serum albumin	> 3.5	2.8-3.5	< 2.8
Serum total bilirubin	< 2.0	2.0-3.0	> 3.0
INR	< 1.7	1.7-2.3	> 2.3
Prothrombin time (seconds prolonged)	< 4	4-6	> 6
Encephalopathy	None	Minimal	Severe
Ascites	None	Small	Moderate
Total sum points: Class A: 5-6; Class B: 7-9; Class C: 10-15			

scoring for priority, the MELD score itself has also been validated as a predictor of outcomes of nontransplant surgery in patients with liver disease. A MELD score of 14 or greater has been shown to be a potentially better predictor of outcome than the CTP C score,[8] whereas a MELD score of 25-30 caries a 50% mortality following nontransplant abdominal surgery.[9]

SURGICAL DISCRETION
Patients with advanced liver disease, cirrhosis, and portal hypertension carry the burden of several additive risks to emergent surgical conditions. These include coagulopathy, thrombocytopenia and platelet dysfunction, abdominal venous hypertension and varices, ascites, poor nutrition, encephalopathy, and marginal renal status. When truly emergent, the operation proceeds without delay and these factors are taken into account in a simultaneous manner. However, many acute care surgical issues are urgent and allow (if not mandate) correction of these abnormalities and/or adjustment of therapeutic options for successful outcome.

BLEEDING RISK
Patients with elevated INR benefit from Vitamin K administration and correction of coagulopathy with transfusion of fresh frozen plasma or cryopreciptate.[10] Although complete correction to normalization of laboratory values might not be an option (depending on the urgency of the problem), plasma products may also be used as a resuscitative fluid in the intra- and postoperative periods. More recently, the introduction of Factor VIIa has provided another potential option in severely coagulopathic patients,[11-13] but has yet to be proven to be advantageous in this setting and remains very expensive. Thrombocytopenia, although potentially multifactorial, should be corrected with platelet transfusion in the setting of ongoing bleeding with a goal of 50,000-100,000 platelets/μL, although little data exists regarding a specific target platelet count. Arginine vasopressin (desmopressin, DDVAP)

therapy is also an option for patients with platelet dysfunction reflected by elevated bleeding times.[14-15] Judicious choice of venous access and preoperative availability of blood products are essential.

VARICES AND VENOUS HYPERTENSION
Esophageal varices are an infrequent problem in the perioperative period for cirrhotic patients undergoing operations for other abdominal pathology; however, the presence of intra- and extra-abdominal varices is particularly hazardous. Varices in the anterior abdominal wall make entry into the abdominal cavity a treacherous task that may be accompanied by massive blood loss. These vessels are often enormous in diameter, are rarely amenable to control by cautery alone, and require ligation. In some patients for whom rapid access to the abdominal cavity is needed (trauma or other causes of hemorrhage), rapid entry may be facilitated by overlapping serial clamping of the abdominal wall at the fascia. Once initial packing is in place, the vessels may be oversewn, either individually or with a running (and potentially locking) suture. Dissection within the peritoneal cavity must also proceed with great care, as variceal dilatation may be present throughout.

When venous hypertension is reflected across the scarred and fragile parenchyma of a cirrhotic liver, injury to the liver itself can cause catastrophic blood loss. The bleeding from this liver bed is poorly controlled with cautery alone and is also difficult to stop as the friable liver tissue does not hold suture well. Careful and precise dissection of adhesions is the safest course, though not without risk. For the patient with cholecystitis (acute or chronic), the plane between the gallbladder and the liver bed is often indistinct; entry into the gallbladder during dissection is balanced against injury to the liver parenchyma along the gallbladder fossa. In order to avoid potential massive hemorrhage it is often advantageous to perform a subtotal cholecystectomy, in which the dissection is carried out from within the gallbladder.[16,17] The anterior aspect of the gallbladder can be removed, leaving the back wall adherent to the liver bed. The cystic duct orifice is identified and oversewn. The remaining gallbladder tissue is cauterized in its entirety (*in situ*) to obliterate residual mucosal tissue. A drain should be left in place.

ASCITES
Patients with severe liver disease and ascites pose a significant problem in the management of abdominal surgery. Ascites formation in the cirrhotic patient with portal hypertension is the result of sodium (and subsequently water) retention. To combat this patients are instructed to abide by a low sodium diet (less than 2000 mg/day). Most patients subsequently require a diuretic regimen consisting of spironolactone (starting at 100 mg/day and ranging up to 400 mg/day) and furosemide (starting at 40 mg/day and ranging up to 160 mg/day).[18] This diuretic regimen places the

patient at risk for electrolyte imbalance as well as hypovolemia in the setting of acute surgical disease and added third space fluid losses.

The postoperative management of ascites is among the most challenging features of emergent abdominal surgery in cirrhotic patients. Adequate decompression of the intra-abdominal cavity is vital to allow abdominal wall wound sealing, healing, and retention of domain.[19] Gastrointestinal anastomoses are best protected from bathing in ascites to facilitate sealing and healing of these tissues. A number of strategies have been proposed to reduce the potential for hazardous postoperative ascites accumulation and leak. Options include open portosystemic shunting, transcutaneous intrahepatic portosystemic shunting (TIPS), the use of transverse incisions (allowing multilayered closure) as well as delay of operative management to optimize ascites in the preoperative stage.

For those patients for whom the operation is truly emergent and ascites is not adequately controllable in the preoperative setting, the operative placement of intraperitoneal drains for their use in the immediate postoperative period achieves this goal. Diuretic therapy during the immediate postoperative period is not indicated for continued control of ascites as third spacing in addition to constant ascites formation results in severe intravascular volume depletion. Some surgeons favor large, soft, closed suction drains placed over the liver and in the pelvis to capture dependent fluid on both the recumbent and upright positions. The successful use of a peritoneal dialysis catheter as a large bore decompression drain has also been described.[20] The degree of drainage required depends on the volume of ascites production. Most patients with significant ascites production require frequent drain emptying to prevent the accumulation of tense ascites, which in turn necessitates intensive nursing care.

Care must be taken in the postoperative setting to replenish the fluid losses to prevent severe hypovolemia. Fluid may be replenished with crystalloid or very occasionally with some degree of albumin for patients with massive fluid output. Over the period of several days, the ascites is allowed to gently reequilibrate while diuretic therapy is reintroduced. Ordinary transabdominal drains are removed and a cutaneous purse-string suture functions to control the drain site. Removal of a peritoneal dialysis catheter requires a return to the operating room, but this may be performed under local anesthetic.

Uncompensated, poorly controlled (often due to noncompliance), and refractory ascites results in intra-abdominal hypertension and elevated risk of umbilical hernia complications. Patients with leaking ascites from umbilical erosion require surgical intervention, although, in the absence of incarcerated abdominal contents, these patients potentially may be optimized for surgery. The placement of a sterile occlusive dressing with control of ascitic leakage allows for better management of ascites, coagulopathy, and malnutrition with subsequent operative repair of the erosion in the ensuing days.[21,22] Given the high morbidity of surgical intervention in patients with advanced cirrhosis, perhaps elective repair of such hernias may be best deferred until the time of liver transplantation.

ENCEPHALOPATHY AND NUTRITION

Encephalopathic patients are at increased risk in the postoperative period for complications from their delirium and inability to participate in care.[10] Restriction of dietary protein and elimination of other sources of ammonia such as hypokalemia (which increases renal ammonia production), upper gastrointestinal bleeding, or intestinal bacterial overgrowth helps limit the production of ammonia.[23] Enhanced elimination of ammonia by the gastrointestinal route (via the use of lactulose) may be somewhat hindered by ileus or the need for bowel rest.

Often, cirrhotic patients are malnourished demonstrating low albumin and evidence of other compromised nutritional parameters.[24] Total protein intake should be limited to less than 70 g/day to prevent exacerbation of encephalopathy; however, a positive protein balance is sought for those in a malnourished state. Nutrition support is key to optimal healing and individual titration of protein load is often necessary to avoid exacerbation of encephalopathy in these patients.

RENAL STATUS

Patients with cirrhosis and liver failure are at particular risk for renal failure. Hepatorenal syndrome is progressive renal failure in the setting of end-stage liver disease or cirrhosis.[25] It is felt to be the combined result of splanchnic vasodilatation with concomitant profound compensatory renal vasoconstriction resulting in significant reduction in glomerular filtration. Although hepatorenal syndrome is a prerenal disease, it must be distinguished from true prerenal hypovolemia and intrarenal toxicities as the prognosis for hepatorenal syndrome is markedly worse. Cirrhotic patients with acute surgical issues are also at risk for hypovolemia (prerenal state), sepsis or nephrotoxicity (contrast, aminoglycosides); however, these are frequently reversible insults. Early in the evolution of hepatorenal syndrome, intravenous clonidine improves splanchnic flow and GFR. Improvement in liver function or liver transplant has the best success in recovering renal function.

POTENTIAL OPTIONS FOR LIVER REPLACEMENT

Supportive care for patients with severe hepatic failure is the mainstay of therapy. Patients with acute fulminant hepatic failure or end-stage chronic liver disease can have excellent outcomes with liver transplantation. However, not every patient is a candidate for transplantation and suitable livers are not available in a timely fashion for all patients in need. Modern medicine has mechanical or artificial replacements for many organ systems such as hemodialysis, mechanical ventilation, and mechanical cardiac support devices that can be used as temporary or permanent organ replacement. However, artificial liver support systems are still in the research, development, and clinical trial stages. A recent systematic review of the literature reports that there may be some mortality benefit compared to standard medical therapy when these systems are used for acute-on-chronic liver failure. However, no benefit was found in patients with acute liver failure.[26]

The current models fall into two main categories: bioartificial (cell-based) and non-cell-based systems. Bioartificial liver support systems function using living hepatocytes (porcine or immortalized human). These cells are incorporated into some extracorporeal device which is in direct contact with the patient's bloodstream to remove both water-soluble and protein-bound toxins. The systems that have shown the most promise include the HepatAssist, Amsterdam Medical Centre Bioartificial Liver (AMC-BAL), Extracorporeal Liver Assist Device (ELAD), and Modular Extracorporeal Liver Support (MELS) systems. The non-cell-based methods that have been tested have used techniques for detoxification such as hemofiltration, hemodialysis, hemopurification, or hemoabsorption (using charcoal or albumin). The two currently used systems are the Molecular Adsorbents Recalculating System (MARS) and the Fractionated Plasma Separation, Adsorption and Dialysis (FPAD—Promethium) systems.[27]

ACUTE LIVER TUMOR COMPLICATIONS

Acute complications of hepatic malignancies are often the first presentation of primary liver tumors. Three main acute presentations are possible. The most common malignancy-related presentation is a patient with biliary obstruction and jaundice (as discussed in the biliary chapter). The most severe and immediately life-threatening is free intra-abdominal tumor rupture. Other patients with known malignancy can have abscess formation in the center of large, necrotic tumors, especially after chemoembolization.

SPONTANEOUS HEPATOCELLULAR CARCINOMA (HCC) RUPTURE

Spontaneous rupture of hepatocellular carcinoma (HCC) with ensuing hemorrhage is a rare, but potentially life-threatening, occurrence. The patient will likely present with severe onset of sudden abdominal pain, which is most often associated with shock in 33-90% of patients. In the hemodynamically stable patient, conservative management with close monitoring and correction of coagulopathy is undertaken until the bleeding stops and the patient can be further evaluated for definitive HCC therapy. The unstable patient needs immediate resuscitation and a procedure

for hemostasis. Open surgical therapy for hemorrhage control via liver packing, suture placation, ethanol injection, hepatic artery ligation, or liver resection has been the historical treatment of choice. However, the advent of transarterial embolization (TAE), which is commonly performed in the elective setting for liver tumors and in the emergency setting after liver trauma, has changed the current management algorithm for patients with spontaneous hepatocellular carcinoma rupture. Patients treated with TAE have a lower 30-day mortality rate (0-37%) than patients treated with conventional open surgical hemostasis (28-75%).[28]

After hemostasis is achieved, assessment and staging of the HCC will direct the decision for staged liver resection (the only potential cure) or palliative treatment. Patients undergoing delayed liver resection after initial hemostasis and staging have higher resection rates (21%-56% vs. 13%-31%) and lower in-hospital mortality rates (0%-9% vs 17%-100%) than patients treated by single stage emergency liver resection. In appropriately chosen candidates, staged liver resection after TAE also can have acceptable long-term survival rates (1-year survival, 54.2%-100%; 3-year survival, 21.2%-48%; 5-year survival, 15%-21.2%).[28]

LIVER INFECTIONS

PYOGENIC LIVER ABSCESS

Patients with liver abscess may present with a wide variety of symptoms. Early symptoms may simply include low-grade fever and malaise, whereas later symptoms may include severe abdominal pain, tachycardia, sepsis, or shock. Laboratory studies may demonstrate an elevated white blood count and possibly an elevated total bilirubin level if biliary obstruction is the underlying cause. Early broad-spectrum intravenous antibiotics must be given as soon as liver abscess is suspected. Antibiotics should be initially directed at the common bacteria that are encountered in patients with pyogenic liver abscess including gram-negative bacilli (ie, *E. coli, Klebsiella*), gram-positive cocci (ie, Streptococci, Staphylococci), and anaerobes (ie, *Bacteroides,* Clostridia).[29] Fungal liver abscess was a rare entity in the past, but this phenomenon has increased significantly in recent years. This rise may be due to the identification of liver abscess in patients at higher risk for fungal infection (immunocompromised, malignancy) or the increased use of broad-spectrum antibiotics. Amphotericin B treatment should be initiated early in all patients with hematologic malignancies. Otherwise, antimycotic treatment is reserved for patients with mixed fungal/pyogenic hepatic abscesses who do not improve with drainage and broad-spectrum antibiotics.[30]

Pyogenic liver abscesses are most frequently caused by another underlying intra-abdominal infection. In the past, the most common primary cause was appendicitis leading to pylephlebitis (air in the portal venous system) with ensuing bacterial infection of the liver and pyogenic liver abscess. Currently, these abscesses are more commonly from a biliary source (most commonly malignant biliary obstruction) or from hematogenous spread via the hepatic artery. Other potential causes include posttraumatic, direct extension, or cyptogenic.[29,31]

Historically, before the era of abdominal imaging, surgery was the mainstay for diagnosis (and treatment) for pyogenic liver abscess. However, in the era of modern imaging, other less invasive means are commonly used for diagnosis and treatment. CT scanning and ultrasonography can obtain excellent imaging of liver abscess. Ultrasound demonstrates fluid-filled (and often septate) cavities within the liver. CT scanning will show similar findings and may give more precise anatomic detail, especially when IV contrast is used to help localize the anatomic relationships of the abscess to the underlying normal vascular anatomy (see Fig. 9-1).

As with most other abscesses, liver abscesses must be physically drained in addition to treating with antibiotics. Percutaneous interventional radiologic procedures to drain these lesions are most often performed under real-time ultrasound or CT guidance. Aspiration of abscess contents for Gram stain and culture is imperative to tailor antibiotic therapy based on bacteria identified and their sensitivities. Percutaneous placement of large bore drains (often because of viscous material) is the current mainstay of therapy. However, open surgical approaches to drainage must be in the armamentarium of all acute care surgeons. Surgical drainage is used in patients whose abscess cannot be drained percutaneously, have abscess rupture, or who undergo abdominal exploration for associated pathology.[32] Pyogenic liver abscesses should be simply

incised and drained with closed suction drains. Formal liver resection is discouraged at the initial operation but may be considered for refractory cases. Other authors have suggested that primary surgical intervention for large liver abscess leads to higher success rates, fewer secondary procedures, and shorter hospitalizations, with equivalent mortality.[33]

Liver abscess due to tumor necrosis requires additional consideration and potentially may be managed differently from an abscess in a patient without tumor. Percutaneous drainage should be avoided if possible due to the potential risk of tumor seeding along the tract. If these patients have minimal clinical signs of infection, antibiotic treatment to sterilize the bloodstream followed by liver resection may be a viable option. However, in those with more clinically apparent infection, percutaneous drainage still may be necessary as a patient with sepsis is not an ideal candidate for a major liver resection.

PARASITIC LIVER DISEASES
Amebic Liver Abscess

Amebic liver abscess is a common entity, as 10% of the population worldwide is chronically infected with *Entamoeba histolytica*. These abscesses are usually solitary and in the right lobe. The abscess is filled with sterile pus and has the pathognomonic "anchovy paste" texture of liquefied necrotic liver. Patients with amebic liver abscess present with pain and appear acutely ill with symptoms including fever, night sweats, diarrhea, weight loss, nausea, or vomiting. The definitive diagnosis is based on the clinical presentation and associated serologic and radiographic findings. The erythrocyte sedimentation rate and white blood count will be elevated, but should not contain eosinophils. Serologic testing with amebic titers will also help determine the diagnosis, except in endemic areas due to prior infection.[34] Ultrasound is the radiographic test of choice, showing a thick-walled hypoechoic fluid collection. The treatment of amebic liver abscess is nonsurgical with a majority of cases responding to treatment with metronidazole treatment alone. Ultrasound guided aspiration should be used in patients who do not respond to initial medical therapy[35,36] or patients who have large lesions (> 10 cm) with impending peritoneal, pleural, or pericardial rupture.[34] Open surgical therapy is only indicated in case of free rupture or nonresponse to other less invasive measures.[34]

HYDATID CYSTS (ECHINOCOCCUS)

Hydatid disease of the liver is caused by *Echinococcus*, an intestinal tapeworm (cestode). The primary hosts are dogs (or other canine) and sheep are the most common intermediate hosts. Humans are accidental hosts, becoming infected with the eggs through the fecal-oral route. Endemic areas include the Mediterranean region, Middle East, Far East, and South America.[34] Patients may present clinically with

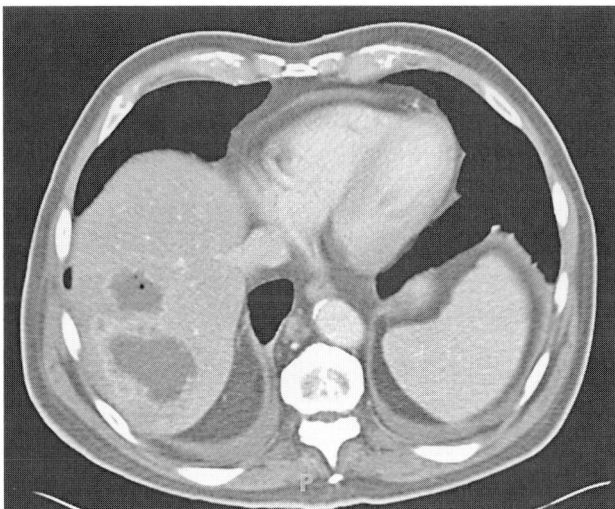

Figure 9-1 *CT scan showing liver abscess with rim enhancement and multiple loculated areas containing air.*

abdominal pain and/or a palpable abdominal mass. Other patients may be asymptomatic and have the cyst identified on imaging studies. Serologic testing can be of some benefit, but noninvasive imaging with ultrasound or CT scanning will be most likely to confirm the diagnosis. Anatomic findings include a unilocular or complex thick-walled cyst, often with calcification. Cysts often contain smaller "daughter cysts" or hydatid "sand," a white sediment which is formed by scolices within the cyst, which causes echogenicity on ultrasound.[37] Management of most hepatic hydatid disease is surgical to prevent increase in cyst size and eventual rupture. Only small completely calcified lesions (signifying complete death of all parasites) may be treated nonoperatively. Mabendazole or albendazole medical therapy is often used in conjunction with surgical treatment or in patients who are unfit surgical candidates.

Many different options exist for surgical treatment of hepatic *Echinococcus*. Options range from simple drainage to radical liver resection. No matter what method is selected, the surgeon should make every effort to prevent spilling the cyst contents (including live scolices) into the abdominal cavity to avoid formation of intraperitoneal cysts. Scolicidal agents including hypertonic saline, ethanol, or povidone-iodine have been used to kill any living parasites. Early studies of the treatment options have shown that any type of more definitive surgical management is better than external drainage.[38] More current data shows that more aggressive procedures such as partial cystectomy with omentoplasty, cyst excision, pericystectomy, laparoscopic drainage, and radiofrequency ablation have lower complication rates than external drainage, primary closure, and marsupialization. These authors suggest that more conservative approaches such as cystectomy with omentoplasty should be the surgery of choice if possible.[39]

GASTROINTESTINAL BLEEDING IN THE CIRRHOTIC PATIENT

The gastrointestinal hemorrhagic sequelae of portal hypertension are one of the most challenging clinical problems that might be faced by an acute care surgical specialist. Therapeutic advances have led to an evolution in the clinical strategies for managing bleeding such that the surgeon is now a member of the multidisciplinary team approaching these patients. Gastroenterologists, interventional radiologists, critical care intensivists, and transplant surgeons are frequently other essential parts of the team that assists in the management of the cirrhotic patient with variceal bleeding.

Variceal hemorrhage is the most immediately life-threatening complication the acute care surgeon will face in the cirrhotic patient. The mortality ranges from 40 to 70% for cirrhotic patients (compared with 5 to 10% mortality with the first episode of variceal hemorrhage in a noncirrhotic). Variceal hemorrhage typically presents as hematemesis, and the tendency to lose massive amounts of blood over a short period of time mandates that a management algorithm be promptly applied.

A rapid ABC approach to the patient with acute variceal bleeding serves the clinician well as it does in other scenarios of acute surgical bleeding. The airway must be protected because of the high risk of aspiration and the potential for further respiratory deterioration in encephalopathic patients and those who will soon be undergoing endoscopy. A low threshold for endotracheal intubation should be promptly followed by aggressive resuscitation with crystalloids and blood products via adequate intravenous access. Early platelet and fresh frozen plasma (FFP) use is often indicated in this patient population due to baseline thrombocytopenia and coagulopathy. Patients with known esophageal varices are at risk for other sources of upper gastrointestinal bleeding (ie, peptic ulcer disease, gastritis, Mallory-Weiss tear) and therefore early diagnostic flexible endoscopy (EGD—esophagogastroduodenoscopy) is essential to rule out these sources. Endoscopy is important in cases of varices for direct visualization as well as affording the opportunity for injection sclerotherapy. The skilled endoscopist must use extreme caution as mechanical stress on the walls of the esophagus can exacerbate variceal hemorrhage.

Once the diagnosis of variceal hemorrhage is confirmed, the first line of therapy is *pharmacologic*, and that is aimed at decreasing splanchnic blood flow and portal venous pressure.[40] Octreotide, a long acting somatostatin analogue, is administered in a 250-μg bolus followed by 25 to 50 μg/hour for 2 to 4 days. Vasopressin is a splanchnic vasoconstrictor and may also utilized as a 20 units intravenous bolus (over 20 minutes), followed by an infusion of 0.2 to 0.4 units per minute. Nitroglycerin is often added as a vasodilator to decrease potential cardiac ischemia in patients receiving vasopressin. Octreotide and vasopressin appear to have similar efficacy, although vasopressin may carry a higher risk of cardiovascular side effects and should be considered a second line drug.[41] In addition, administration of octreotide has been shown to improve the success rate of hemorrhage control in combination with sclerotherapy when compared to sclerotherapy alone.[42]

Endoscopic sclerotherapy involves the injection of a sclerosant (usually 5% sodium morrhuate) either into or around the esophageal varix. This produces obliteration of the varix via submucosal fibrosis to prevent rupture. Endoscopic therapy has replaced balloon tamponade as the mechanical treatment of choice in patients who do not respond to pharmacologic therapy. Prospective randomized analyses suggest that endoscopic sclerotherapy produces better hemorrhage control, less rebleeding, and in a subset of patients, improved long-term survival when compared with patients undergoing balloon tamponade with the Sengstaken-Blakemore tube.[43-45] Furthermore, Sengstaken-Blakemore tube does not add any additional benefit to patients whose active hemorrhage stops with endoscopic sclerotherapy.[43] Both a meta-analysis and a randomized controlled clinical trial suggest that there is similar efficacy with regard to hemorrhage control when endoscopic therapy is compared to medical pharmacotherapy, but the complications appear to be higher with sclerotherapy (esophageal strictures, pneumonias, and other infections).[46,47] A randomized trial comparing endoscopic variceal band ligation with sclerotherapy has suggested that it is at least as effective, and associated with fewer complications.[48] In practice, pharmacotherapy and endoscopic sclerotherapy are commonly used concurrently.

Although the specific devices have evolved since its introduction in 1950, the basic therapeutic principle of *balloon tamponade* remains to apply upward pressure against varices at the esophagogastric junction.[49] The Sengstaken-Blakemore tube is inserted in the stomach and the gastric balloon is initially inflated to 40 to 50 cc of air. Once an abdominal x-ray ensures appropriate position of the gastric balloon below the diaphragm, it is further inflated to about 300 cc and pulled upward with external traction. If hemorrhage persists, the esophageal balloon is inflated to a pressure of approximately 35 mm Hg and individual suction is applied to both a gastric and esophageal ports to reduce the risk of aspiration[50] (see Fig. 9-2). These patients should be intubated for airway protection. Although balloon tamponade therapy is effective in controlling acute hemorrhage in over 90% of cases, its use has become limited because of the high incidence of recurrent

bleed after the therapy ceases. Its associated significant complication rate of gastric or esophageal perforations, aspiration, and potential airway obstruction have led to it being used predominantly in variceal hemorrhage refractory to pharmacologic or endoscopic therapy, or as a bridge to transjugular intrahepatic portosystemic shunt (TIPS) or surgical portal systemic shunting.

Now that a quarter of a century of clinical experience has accrued, *transjugular intrahepatic portosystemic shunting (TIPS)* has earned a place in the therapeutic armamentarium against acute variceal hemorrhage.[51] The procedure is performed typically via internal jugular vein cannulation with a catheter placed into a hepatic vein. At this point, a needle is advanced from the hepatic vein through the liver parenchyma into a branch of the portal vein. A guide wire passed through the needle allows the tract to be dilated with a balloon, and finally, an expandable stent (see Fig. 9-3). The stent effectively produces a nonselective portosystemic shunt.[52] Meta-analyses have been done comparing TIPS to endoscopic therapy (with or without pharmacotherapy) in acute variceal hemorrhage.[53] Although TIPS generally demonstrates a favorable incidence of hemorrhage

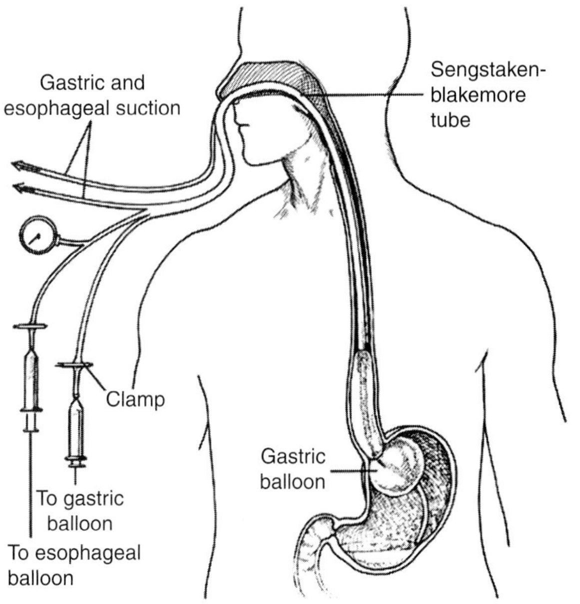

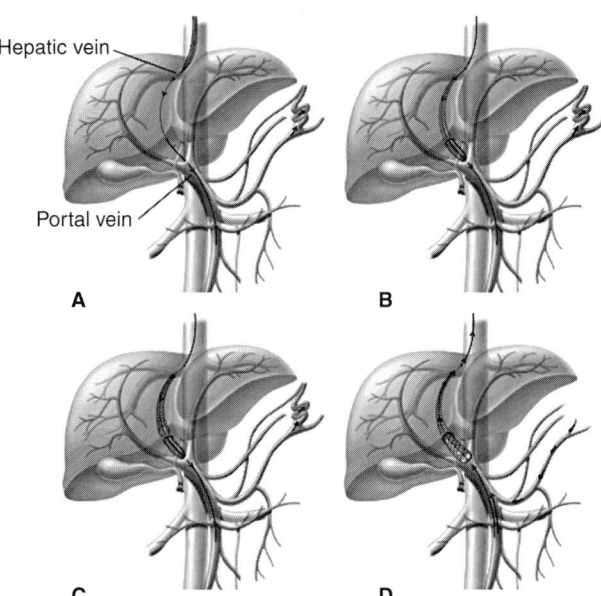

Figure 9-3 *Technique for performing transjugular intrahepatic portosystemic shunting (TIPS). (A) A needle is passed under radiologic guidance from a hepatic vein into a major portal venous branch, and a guide wire is advanced through this needle. (B) A balloon is passed over the guide wire, creating a tract in the hepatic parenchyma. (C) An expandable stent is placed though this tract. (D) The effective result is a nonselective portosystemic shunt. Reproduced, with permission, from Cho CS, Rikkers LF: Portal hypertension: Gastrointestinal tract and abdomen. In: Souba WW, Fink MJ, Jurkovich GJ, et al, eds. ACS Surgery: Principles and Practice. New York, NY: WebMD Inc, 2004. http://www.acssurgery.com/acs/figures/ch0510-f3.htm.*

Figure 9-2 *Sengstaken-Blakemore tube placement. Reproduced, with permission, from Cho CS, Rikkers LF: Portal hypertension: Gastrointestinal tract and abdomen. In: Souba WW, Fink MJ, Jurkovich GJ, et al, eds. ACS Surgery: Principles and Practice. New York, NY: WebMD Inc, 2004. http://www.acssurgery.com/acs/figures/ch0510-f2.htm.*

control, these patients have an increased incidence of hepatic encephalopathy. Contraindications to TIPS include right heart failure, polycystic liver disease, and portal vein thrombosis as a relative contraindication.

In view of the aforementioned clinical studies, a treatment algorithm in the approach to the patient with acute variceal bleeding can be generated (see Fig. 9-4—algorithm). Rapid attention to airway protection and resuscitation with blood and blood products progresses, and goes hand in hand with the first line of pharmacotherapy with octreotide +/– vasopressin. This pharmacotherapy is continued periprocedurally in patients who do not have rapid cessation of bleeding as they move on to endoscopic therapy with either sclerosis or band ligation. Balloon tamponade is then used as a bridge for those patients who are refractory to pharmacotherapy and sclerotherapy with the recognition that it only provides acute hemorrhage control, but with the known caveat of significant rates of rebleeding and complications. If TIPS is readily available to patients who are refractory to pharmacotherapy and endoscopic treatment, then this should be utilized as the salvage therapy of choice, and progression to balloon tamponade can be skipped. The combined efficacies of the aforementioned therapies explain the substantial decrease in surgical management for acute variceal bleeding. Surgery is now applied only to those patients who have proven to be

Algorithm for Evaluation and Management of Patient with Potential Variceal Bleed

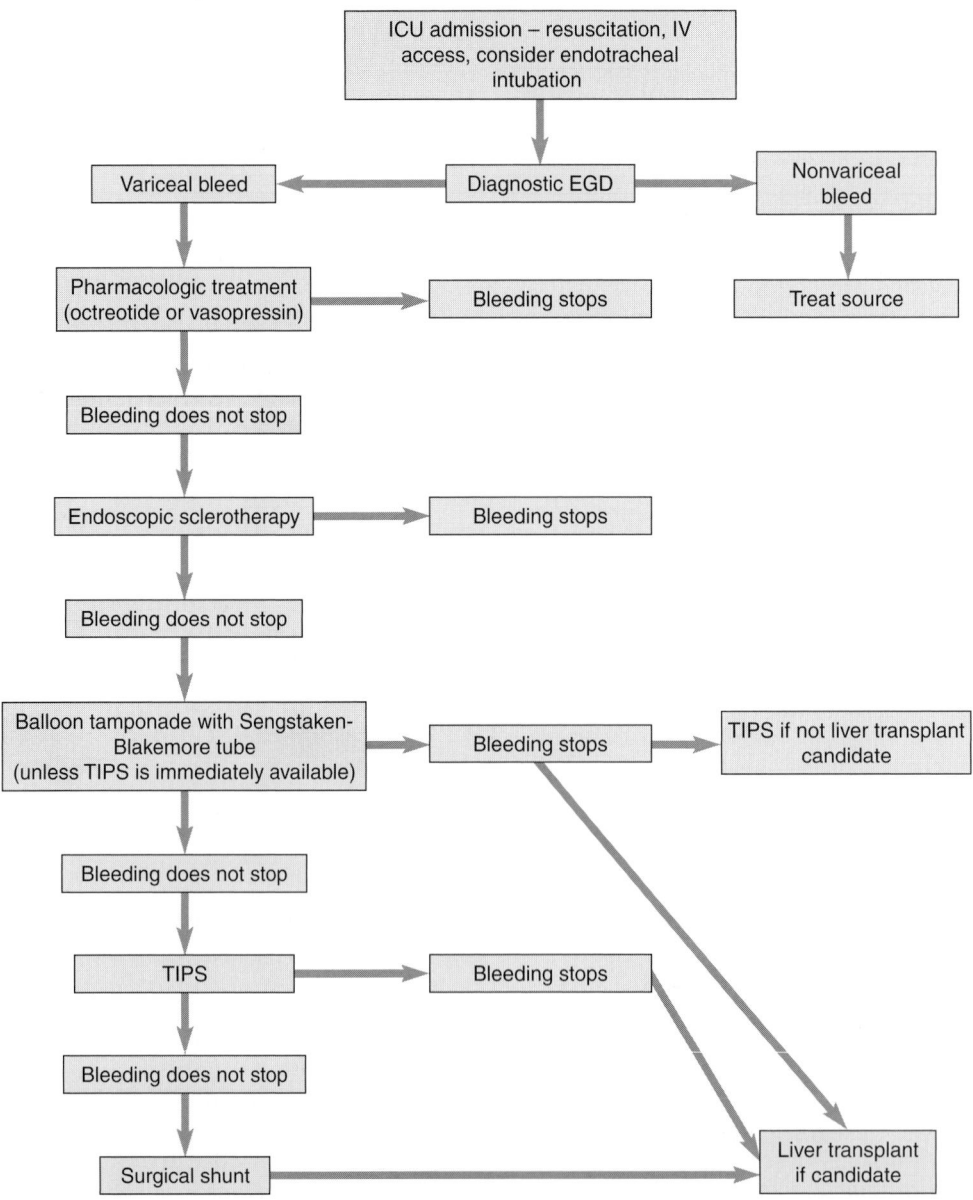

Figure 9-4 *Algorithm for evaluation and management of patient with potential variceal bleed. TIPS, transjugular intrahepatic portosystemic shunting.*

refractory to pharmacotherapy, endoscopic treatments, balloon tamponade, and TIPS. At the same time, these patients are assessed for their adequacy as a candidate for liver transplantation. Surgical therapy in the acute phase for esophageal bleeding includes esophageal transection with an end-to-end anastomosis or a variety of portosystemic shunting operations.

REFERENCES

1. Child CG, Turcotte JG. Surgery and portal hypertension. *Major Probl Clin Surg.* 1964;1:1-85.
2. Pugh RN, Murray-Lyon IM, Dawson JL, Pietroni MC, Williams R. Transection of the oesophagus for bleeding oesophageal varices. *Br J Surg.* 1973;60:646-649.
3. Ziser, A, Plevak, DJ, Wiesner, RH, et al. Morbidity and mortality in cirrhotic patients undergoing anesthesia and surgery. *Anesthesiology* 1999;90:42.
4. Garrison RN, Cryer HM, Howard DA, et al. Clarification of risk factors for abdominal operations in patients with hepatic cirrhosis. *Ann Surg* 1984;199:648.
5. Mansour A, Watson W, Shayani V, Pickleman J. Abdominal operations in patients with cirrhosis: Still a major surgical challenge. *Surgery* 1997;122:730.
6. Malinchoc M, Kamath PS, Gordon FD, et al. A model to predict survival in patients undergoing transjugular intrahepatic portosystemic shunts. *Hepatology* 2000; 31:864.
7. Kamath PS, Kim WR. The model for end-stage liver disease (MELD). *Hepatology.* 2007;45:797-805.
8. Befeler AS, Palmer DE, Hoffman M, et al. The safety of intra-abdominal surgery in patients with cirrhosis: model for end-stage liver disease score is superior to Child-Turcotte-Pugh classification in predicting outcome. *Arch Surg* 2005;140:650.
9. Northup PG, Wanamaker RC, Lee VD, Adams RB, Berg CL. Model for End-Stage Liver Disease (MELD) predicts nontransplant surgical mortality in patients with cirrhosis. *Ann Surg.* 2005;242:244-251.
10. Wiklund RA. Preoperative preparation of patients with advanced liver disease. *Crit Care Med.* 2004;32: S106-S115.
11. Vincent JL, Rossaint R, Riou B, Ozier Y, Zideman D, Spahn DR. Recommendations on the use of recombinant activated factor VII as an adjunctive treatment for massive bleeding—a European perspective. *Crit Care.* 2006;10:R120.
12. Levy JH, Fingerhut A, Brott T, Langbakke IH, Erhardtsen E, Porte RJ. Recombinant factor VIIa in patients with coagulopathy secondary to anticoagulant therapy, cirrhosis, or severe traumatic injury: review of safety profile. *Transfusion.* 2006;46:919-933.
13. Bosch J, Thabut D, Bendtsen F, et al. Recombinant factor VIIa for upper gastrointestinal bleeding in patients with cirrhosis: a randomized, double-blind trial. *Gastroenterology.* 2004; 127:1123-1130.
14. Cattaneo M, Tenconi PM, Alberca I, Garcia VV, Mannucci PM. Subcutaneous desmopressin (DDAVP) shortens the prolonged bleeding time in patients with liver cirrhosis. *Thromb Haemost.* 1990;64:358-360.
15. Agnelli G, Parise P, Levi M, Cosmi B, Nenci GG. Effects of desmopressin on hemostasis in patients with liver cirrhosis. *Haemostasis.* 1995;25:241-247.

16. Bornman P, Terblanche J. Subtotal cholecystectomy: for the difficult gallbladder in portal hypertension and cholecystitis. *Surgery* 1985;98: 1-6.
17. Palanivelu C. Rajan PS, and Jani K, et al. Laparoscopic cholecystectomy in cirrhotic patients: the role of subtotal cholecystectomy and its variants. *J Am Coll Surg* 2006;203:145-151.
18. Sandhu BS, Sanyal AJ. Management of ascites in cirrhosis. *Clin Liver Dis.* 2005;9:715-732.
19. Fuster J, Llovet JM, Garcia-Valdecasas JC, et al. Abdominal drainage after liver resection for hepatocellular carcinoma in cirrhotic patients: a randomized controlled study. *Hepatogastroenterology.* 2004;51: 536-540.
20. Slakey DP, Benz CC, Joshi S, Regenstein FG, Florman SS. Umbilical hernia repair in cirrhotic patients: utility of temporary peritoneal dialysis catheter. *Am Surg.* 2005;71:58-61.
21. Lemmer JH, Strodel WE, Knol JA, Eckhauser FE. Management of spontaneous umbilical hernia disruption in the cirrhotic patient. *Ann Surg.* 1983;198:30-34.
22. Fagan SP, Awad SS, Berger DH. Management of complicated umbilical hernias in patients with end-stage liver disease and refractory ascites. *Surgery.* 2004;135: 679-682.
23. Cordoba J, Blei AT. Treatment of hepatic encephalopathy. *Am J Gastroenterol.* 1997;92:1429-1439.
24. O'Keefe SJD, El-Zayadi AR, Carraher T, et al. Malnutrition and immuno-incompetence in patients with liver disease. *Lancet* 1980;2:615-617.
25. Cardenas A, Gines P. Hepatorenal syndrome. *Clin Liver Dis.* 2006;10:371-385.
26. Kjaergard LL, Liu J, Als-Nielsen B, Gluud C. Artificial and bioartificial support systems for acute and acute-on-chronic liver failure: a systematic review. *JAMA* 2003;289(2):217-222.
27. Stadlbauer V, Jalan R. Acute liver failure: liver support therapies. Curr Opin Crit Care. 2007;13(2):215-221.
28. Lai EC, Lau WY. Spontaneous rupture of hepatocellular carcinoma: a systematic review. *Arch Surg.* 2006;141(2):191-198.
29. Huang CJ, Pitt HA, Lipsett PA, et al. Pyogenic hepatic abscess. Changing trends over 42 years. *Ann Surg* 1996;223(5):600-607;discussion 607-609.
30. Lipsett PA, Huang CJ, Lillemoe KD, Cameron JL, Pitt HA. Fungal hepatic abscesses: Characterization and management. *J Gastrointest Surg* 1997;1(1):78-84.
31. Chu KM, Fan ST, Lai EC, Lo CM, Wong J. Pyogenic liver abscess. An audit of experience over the past decade. *Arch Surg* 1996;131(2):148-152.
32. Barakate MS, Stephen MS, Waugh RC, et al. Pyogenic liver abscess: a review of 10 years' experience in management. *Aust N Z J Surg* 1999;69(3):205-209.

33. Tan YM, Chung AY, Chow PK, et al. An appraisal of surgical and percutaneous drainage for pyogenic liver abscesses larger than 5 cm. *Ann Surg* 2005;241(3): 485-490.

34. Krige JE, Beckingham IJ. ABC of diseases of liver, pancreas, and biliary system. *BMJ* 2001;322(7285): 537-540.

35. McGarr PL, Madiba TE, Thomson SR, Corr P. Amoebic liver abscess—results of a conservative management policy. *S Afr Med J* 2003;93(2):132-136.

36. Akgun Y, Tacyildiz IH, Celik Y. Amebic liver abscess: changing trends over 20 years. *World J Surg* 1999;23(1): 102-106.

37. Pedrosa I, Saiz A, Arrazola J, Ferreiros J, Pedrosa CS. Hydatid disease: radiologic and pathologic features and complications. *Radiographics* 2000;20(3):795-817.

38. Balik AA, Basoglu M, Celebi F, Oren D, Polat KY, Atamanalp SS, Akcay MN. Surgical treatment of hydatid disease of the liver: review of 304 cases. *Arch Surg* 1999;134(2):166-169.

39. Safioleas MC, Misiakos EP, Kouvaraki M, Stamatakos MK, Manti CP, Felekouras ES. Hydatid disease of the liver: a continuing surgical problem. *Arch Surg* 2006;141(11):1101-1108.

40. D'Amico G, Pagliaro L, Bosch J. The treatment of portal hypertension: a meta-analytic review. *Hepatology* 22:332, 1995.

41. Avgerinos A, Klonis C, Rekoumis G, et al. A prospective randomized trial comparing somatostatin, balloon tamponade and the combination of both methods in the management of acute variceal hemorrhage. *J Hepatol* 1991;13(1):78-83.

42. Banares R, Albillos A, Rincon D, et al. Endoscopic treatment versus endoscopic plus pharmacologic treatment for acute variceal bleeding: a meta-analysis. *Hepatology* 2002;35:609.

43. Barsoum MS, Bolous FI, El-Rooby AA, et al. Tamponade and injection sclerotherapy in the management of bleeding esophageal varices. *Br J Surg* 1982;69(2):76-78.

44. Paquet KJ, Feussner H. Endoscopic sclerosis and esophageal balloon tamponade in acute hemorrhage from esophagogastric varices: a prospective controlled randomized trial. *Hepatology* 1985;5(4):580-583.

45. D'Amico G, Pietrosi G, Tarantino I, et al. Emergency sclerotherapy versus vasoactive drugs for variceal bleeding in cirrhosis: a Cochrane meta-analysis. *Gastroenterology* 2003;124:1277.

46. Larson AW, Cohen H, Zweiban B, et al. Acute esophageal variceal sclerotherapy. Results of a prospective randomized controlled trial. *JAMA* 1986;255(4): 497-500.

47. Escorsell A, Ruiz del Arbol L, Planas R, et al. Multicenter randomized controlled trial of terlipressin versus sclerotherapy in the treatment of acute variceal bleeding: the TEST study. *Hepatology* 2000;32:471.

48. Stiegmann GV, Goff JS, Michaletz-Onody PA, et al. Endoscopic sclerotherapy as compared with endoscopic ligation for bleeding esophageal varices. *N Engl J Med* 1992;326(23):1527-1532.

49. Sengstaken RW, Blakemore AH. Balloon Tamponage for the Control of Hemorrhage from Esophageal Varices. *Ann Surg* 1950;131(5):781-789.

50. McCormick PA, Burroughs AK, McIntyre N. How to insert a Sengstaken-Blakemore tube. *Br J Hosp Med* 1990;43(4):274-277.

51. Boyer TD. Transjugular intrahepatic portosystemic shunt: current status. *Gastroenterology* 2003;124(6): 1700-1710.

52. McCormick PA, Dick R, Chin J, et al. Transjugular intrahepatic portosystemic stent-shunt. *Br J Hosp Med* 1993;49(11): 791-73, 796-797.

53. Luca A, D'Amico G, La Galla R, et al. TIPS for prevention of recurrent bleeding in patients with cirrhosis: meta-analysis of randomized clinical trials. *Radiology* 1999;212(2):411-421.

Chapter **10**

BILIARY SURGERY

Benjamin Braslow, MD, Ernest L. Rosato, MD, and Karen A. Chojnacki, MD

INTRODUCTION

Biliary colic is typically defined by severe episodic pain in the epigastrium or the right hypochondrium, eventually radiating to the back. This pain usually presents suddenly and persists for intervals of 1 to 5 hours, often waking the patient during the night. The pain then gradually eases. Episodes of biliary colic typically occur postprandially and are often associated with diaphoresis, nausea, and emesis. The pain is not exacerbated by movement and not relieved by squatting maneuvers, bowel movements, or flatus. Although ingestion of fatty meals is theoretically linked to the inception of this pain, in reality, most foods can trigger the event.[1] The etiology of biliary colic is most commonly linked to the gallbladder contracting in response to hormonal or neural stimulation, forcing a stone (or possibly sludge or microlithiasis) against the gallbladder outlet or cystic duct opening, producing increased intraluminal pressure and pain. The stones then fall back into the lumen of the gallbladder when the gallbladder relaxes and the pain subsides. In most cases, the pain is not very severe and most patients undergo several bouts prior to seeking medical attention. The frequency of recurrent attacks is variable ranging from years to hours.[2] Prolonged or frequently recurrent cystic duct blockage can progress to total obstruction causing acute cholecystitis (see section later in this chapter). An episode of prolonged right upper quadrant pain (> 6 hours), especially if associated with fever or an elevated white blood cell count, should spur suspicion for acute cholecystitis as opposed to an attack of simple biliary colic. Other acute upper abdominal pain diagnoses such as peptic ulcer disease, acute or chronic pancreatitis, gastroesophageal reflux disease, hepatitis, renal colic, and irritable bowel syndromes must also be considered in such patients. Also, it is important to remember that many of these conditions are common in the general population and may coexist but be unrelated to gallstones.

PREOPERATIVE MANAGEMENT

DIAGNOSIS

Patients presenting with biliary colic symptoms should undergo evaluation to diagnose the presence of gallbladder stones or sludge. A thorough physical exam is paramount. Patients with simple biliary colic are not usually ill appearing and do not have fever or persistent tachycardia. Peritoneal signs should be absent and the pain poorly localized since the pain is purely visceral in the absence of gallbladder wall inflammation. This is in direct contrast to cholecystitis in which transmural gallbladder inflammation leads to localized right upper quadrant peritonitis. Here, the patient will experience a positive Murphy sign. This is elicited by palpating the area of the gallbladder fossa just beneath the liver edge while the patient is asked to inspire deeply, causing the gallbladder to descend toward the examining fingers. An inspiratory arrest is noted and cholecystitis is suspected.

Laboratory studies should be normal in patients with uncomplicated biliary colic both during asymptomatic periods and during acute attacks. However, several laboratory studies can help to rule out other diagnoses. The following are reasonable screening tests: liver function studies (serum AST, ALT, total bilirubin, and alkaline phosphatase), serum amylase and lipase (to evaluate for pancreatitis), complete blood count, and urinanalysis to rule out a renal or ureteral source of pain. A high leukocytosis (especially with a left shift) may be a warning sign of possible acute cholecystitis or cholangitis. The development of an obstructive pattern in liver function tests (elevated bilirubin and alkaline phosphatase) may suggest choledocholithiasis with possible extrahepatic duct obstruction.

Secondary Testing

Imaging studies are usually employed to confirm the presence of gallstones or sludge in a patient with a history suggestive of biliary colic. They may also be helpful in ruling out complications of cholelithiasis (ie, choledocholithiasis, cholecystitis, cholangitis, or gallstone pancreatitis). Transabdominal ultrasonography is generally considered to be the most useful test to evaluate the patient with biliary colic and detect the presence of gallstones. It is noninvasive, readily available, relatively inexpensive, and does not expose the patient to ionizing radiation. Biliary sludge appears as multiple, slightly echogenic signals, without acoustic shadowing, that occupy the dependent portion of the gallbladder.[3] Gallstones appear as hyperechoic foci with acoustic shadowing. It is more difficult to visualize gallstones in a contracted gallbladder. For this reason, the sensitivity of the study increases when patients have been NPO for 6 to 8 hours prior.[4] Gallstones are usually mobile, ie, they change position intraluminally when the patient's position is altered during the study. Mobility helps distinguish gallstones from gallbladder polyps (and masses) and from local calcifications of the gallbladder wall (porcelain gallbladder). Overall, the sensitivity (84-95%) and specificity (95-99%) is excellent and highest when the gallbladder stones are larger than 2 mm in diameter.[5]

Plain abdominal x-rays are generally not useful in looking for gallstones in symptomatic patients. The vast majority of gallstones lack sufficient quantities of calcium in their composition and are radiolucent. Likewise, the sensitivity of computed tomography (CT) for identification of gallstones is poor because most stones are isodense with bile and thus are not visible by this modality.[6] CT can be useful for screening patients for possible dissolution therapy because the presence of calcifications within gallstones (readily apparent on CT) greatly reduces the success rate of such therapy. To date, there is a limited role for magnetic resonance imaging (MRI) in the diagnosis of uncomplicated cholelithiasis. As with CT, MRI has limited sensitivity and specificity for detection of gallstones (68% and 23%, respectively, in recent studies).[7]

Oral cholecystography (OCG), once used commonly to diagnose gallstones and evaluate gallbladder function, has been all but replaced by the more sensitive and specific ultrasonography.[5] This modality is based on an orally administered contrast agent (iopanoic acid, sodium tyropanoate, or calcium ipodate) that is absorbed through the intestine, concentrated by the hepatocytes, and secreted into the bile. Gallstones appear as filling defects within the contrast. It is still occasionally used in patients who are being considered for medical dissolution therapy with ursodeoxycholic acid. False negative results can occur due to poor absorption from the intestines (malabsorption syndromes), diminished liver function (hepatitis, cirrhosis), or extrahepatic biliary obstruction. A gallbladder ejection fraction can be assessed by measuring the gallbladder diameter on sequential x-rays following administration of cholecystokinin. This can be helpful in the workup of biliary dyskinesia but again has a limited role for the acute care surgeon.

TREATMENT

For the acute care surgeon, the management of biliary colic involves two general principles: pain control and prophylactic treatment against recurrent attacks and/or the development of gallstone related complications. According to the natural history of biliary colic, approximately 70% of patients who have an initial episode of classic biliary colic will experience additional incidents over the next 21 months. Fortunately, the probability that a severe complication requiring urgent surgical intervention will develop in these patients is only ~1% per year.[8]

Pain control can usually be achieved with the intravenous administration of meperidine, which is preferred to morphine because it has less of an effect on sphincter of Oddi motility.[9] NSAIDs have also been shown to be effective against biliary colic pain and may have a theoretical benefit in the prevention of acute cholecystitis via inhibition of prostaglandin synthesis.[10] In fact, intravenous administration of ketorolac has been shown to provide equivalent analgesia as meperidine with fewer adverse effects like nausea and dizziness.[11]

To date, the most efficacious management option of symptomatic cholelithiasis is cholecystectomy, using the laparoscopic approach if feasible. It is generally accepted that symptomatic gallstone carriers have a high risk of recurrent biliary colic.[12-15] Additionally, patients who have had severe biliary colic or gallstone related complications (such as cholangitis, pancreatitis, cholecystitis, choledocholithiasis, or gallstone ileus) were shown to have approximately a 70% risk of recurrent symptoms or complications within 2 years after initial presentation.[16] For these reasons, it is felt that a patient presenting with biliary colic and confirmed to have cholelithiasis should be offered surgery in a timely manner. If the patient is to be admitted to the hospital for persistent pain control and intravenous hydration secondary to nausea and vomiting, it is appropriate to perform cholecystectomy during that admission. Otherwise, patients slated for discharge from the emergency department following a brief bout of less severe biliary colic should be instructed to follow-up expediently for surgical scheduling as an outpatient. For patients with significant comorbidities, a preoperative surgical risk assessment must be obtained prior to committing to surgical intervention. Nonsurgical options for the treatment of symptomatic cholelithiasis do exist such as dissolution therapy (with chenodeoxycholic acid and ursodeoxycholic acid) and extracorporeal shockwave lithotripsy, but their low efficacy and high recurrence rates make them far less attractive options compared to cholecystectomy.

ACUTE CHOLECYSTITIS

Acute cholecystits refers to a syndrome of right upper quadrant pain, fever, and leukocytosis associated with an acute inflammation of the gallbladder. Nearly 90 to

95% of cases of cholecystitis are calculous in origin and result from a persistent obstruction of the gallbladder outlet by a stone impacted in the neck of the gallbladder, Hartmann pouch, or the cystic duct. This obstruction results in gallbladder distention, subserosal edema, mucosal sloughing, venous and lymphatic congestion, and localized ischemia. The natural history of acute cholecystitis varies, depending on whether the obstruction becomes relieved, the development and extent of secondary bacterial invasion, the age of the patient and the scale of aggravating comorbidities. Most attacks resolve spontaneously without surgery or other specific therapy; however, some progress to free perforation with local abscess formation or generalized peritonitis. Other complications include sepsis, empyema (suppurative cholecystitis), gallstone ileus, and cholecystic enteric fistula. Repeated episodes of acute inflammation may lead to chronic cholecystitis in which the gallbladder wall becomes thick, infiltrated with inflammatory cells. The subsequent development of fibrosis leads to a loss of contractility and concentration function of the gallbladder.

The cause of acute cholecystitis is still partially speculative. It was once thought to be exclusively the result of stagnation of bile secondary to stone impaction and subsequent infection. However, recent data has shown that only 46% of patients with confirmed cholecystitis were found to have positive bile cultures.[17] Another recent study showed that only 15-30% of patients who received a cholecystectomy for cholecystitis had positive bile cultures.[18] Thus, inflammation of the gallbladder is not simply an infectious process but rather a multifactorial cascade of events initiated by gallstone obstruction of the gallbladder outflow tract. It is postulated that gallbladder wall trauma associated with stone impaction causes the release of phospholipase from the adjacent mucosal cells. This is followed by conversion of lecithin in bile to lysolecithin, which is a toxic compound that incites more inflammation. Local prostaglandin synthesis increases and further amplifies the inflammatory response. The edema and inflammation can often play a role in elevating the gallbladder wall away from the impacted stone, thus resulting in disimpaction and spontaneous drainage through the cystic duct.[19] Failure of spontaneous disimpaction results in continued cystic duct obstruction, biliary stasis, wall distention, venous congestion, gallbladder ischemia, and a subsequent systemic inflammatory response that necessitates operative intervention.

CLINICAL PRESENTATION
The main complaint of patients with acute cholecystitis is severe pain below the right costal margin. The pain frequently radiates to the back, the right scapula, or the right clavicular area. The vast majority of patients will recount a previous attack of biliary colic at first indistinguishable from the present illness. This new pain, however, does not mitigate and in fact worsens with time and is often associated with nausea, emesis, anorexia, and low-grade fever (38°C to 38.5°C). Mild icterus is present in about 10% of cases. Note that very high fevers with chills are uncommon and suggest the possibility of complications like cholangitis. Likewise, severe jaundice suggests the presence of common bile duct stones, cholangitis, or obstruction of the common hepatic duct by severe pericholecystic inflammation associated with an impacted large stone in Hartmann pouch, which mechanically obstructs the bile duct (*Mirizzi syndrome*). On physical examination, right upper quadrant (RUQ) tenderness to palpation is present. A palpable RUQ mass is present in about a third of all patients. This is often the result of not only gallbladder distention and swelling but also omentum that has migrated to the pericholecystic area in response to local inflammation. If instructed to breath deeply during palpation in the right subcostal region, the patient experiences accentuated tenderness and sudden inspiratory arrest (*Murphy sign*).

The white blood cell count (WBC) is usually elevated to 12,000-15,000/μL but normal counts are not uncommon. A very high WBC (> 20,000) should suggest further complications of cholecystitis like gangrene, perforation, or cholangitis. A mild elevation of the serum bilirubin (2-4 mg/dL) is common, presumably a result of secondary inflammation of the common bile duct. Values higher than this usually indicate the presence of common bile duct stones. Mild elevations in alkaline phosphatase, transaminases, amylase, and lipase may also be present. But again, dramatic elevations in any one or all of these laboratory values should clue one into the presence of complications.

IMAGING STUDIES
As in the evaluation of biliary colic, ultrasound is the first-line diagnostic modality of choice to identify cholecystitis with ~95% specificity and sensitivity for making the diagnosis. Ultrasound findings most suggestive of acute cholecystitis include gallbladder distention, gallbladder wall thickening (> 4 mm), pericholecystic fluid, an impacted stone, biliary sludge, and a positive sonographic Murphy sign. Comorbid factors like the presence of ascites decrease the specificity of this test.[20]

When ultrasound is equivocal, technically not possible, or negative in a patient with very high clinical suspicion for cholecystitis, the patency of the cystic duct can be assessed by performing cholescintigraphy. The test consists of intravenous administration of gamma-emitting ^{99}Tc-labled Hydroxyl iminodiacetic acid (HIDA) or diisopropyl iminodiacetic acid (DISIDA), which is rapidly taken up by hepatocytes and secreted into the bile. The scan is considered normal when radionucleotide is detected in the gallbladder, CBD, and small bowel within 30-60 minutes after injecting isotope. An abnormal or "positive scan" is defined as the nonvisualization of the gallbladder with preserved excretion into the CBD or small bowel. HIDA scanning has a high sensitivity and specificity (100% and 95%, respectively, and a diagnostic accuracy rate approaching 98% in patients with clinical evidence of acute calculous cholecystitis. A false positive scan, defined as the absence of isotope in the gallbladder in patients who do not have acute cholecystitis, is seen in patients who have fasted for more than 5 days, ie, critically ill patients who are receiving total parenteral nutrition. In this population of patients, false positive rates as high as 40 to 60% are common.[8] To reduce the frequency of false-positive scans, augmentation with morphine is often performed if the gallbladder has not visualized after 60 minutes. Morphine increases the pressure within the sphincter of Oddi, thereby directing bile into the gallbladder unless the cystic duct is obstructed.

Computed tomography (CT) with oral and intravenous contrast is usually utilized to assess late complications of previously undiagnosed or misdiagnosed cases of acute cholecystitis, such as perforation, abscess, or cholecystenteric fistula. Its role in an uncomplicated case of acute cholecystitis is limited unless other pathologic abdominal processes need to be ruled out first.

Magnetic resonance imaging (MRI) although fairly accurate in detecting acute cholecystitis (95% sensitivity, 70% specificity),[7] also has a limited role in uncomplicated cases. However magnetic resonance cholangiopancreatography (MRCP) is an excellent modality for detection of CBD stones that may complicate acute cholecystitis (see later in this chapter).

OPERATIVE MANAGEMENT

MANAGEMENT

Patients diagnosed with acute cholecystitis should be admitted to the hospital. As many of these patients have been ill for days prior to seeking medical attention, initial therapy should include intravenous hydration and correction of any associated electrolyte disorders.

The role of antibiotic prophylaxis in uncomplicated acute cholecystitis remains largely unproven.[21] Despite the limited number of positive bile cultures assayed from patients with acute cholecystitis in the literature, when identified, the most common pathogens include *E. coli*, enterococcus, klebsiella, and enterobacter. Even without clear evidence of benefit to support their use, broad spectrum intravenous antibiotics are given to most patients who are hospitalized for an episode of cholecystitis. When used, suggested regimens of antibiotics include (1) Metronidazole plus a third-generation cephalosporin or a fluoroquinolone or aztreonam, (2) piperacillin/tazobactam, (3) Ampicillin/sulbactam, (4) Ticarcillin-clavulanate, or (5) Imipenem.

Patients with elevated liver function test results (specifically serum total bilirubin and/or alkaline phosphatase) or dilated bile ducts (> 6 mm) on ultrasound should be further evaluated for the presence of CBD stones (see section on definitive workup and treatment options of CBD stones).

The definitive therapy for acute cholecystitis is cholecystectomy in all patients unless there are specific contraindications to operation (eg, serious concomitant disease). Overall, cholecystectomy, whether performed in an open or laparoscopic fashion, has been associated with very low complication rates: < 0.2% mortality, < 5% major morbidity, and a bile duct injury rate of ~0.4%.[22] More recently, the laparoscopic cholecystectomy has become the preferred operation and arguably the current standard of care. Four recent randomized controlled trials found that laparoscopic cholecystectomy reduced the duration of hospital stay, without an increase in the duration of surgery or intraoperative/postoperative complications compared with open cholecystectomy.[23-26] Extensive inflammation, adhesions, and increased oozing can make laparoscopic dissection of Calot triangle and recognition of the biliary anatomy hazardous and difficult. Therefore, conversion to open cholecystectomy remains an important treatment option to ensure patient safety in such difficult cases.

The timing of cholecystectomy for acute cholecystitis has been studied and debated for several decades. Ten to twenty percent of patients require immediate operative intervention (usually open laparotomy) as a result hemodynamic instability and or generalized peritonitis on presentation. These findings are suggestive of gangrene or perforation of the gallbladder and delays in operative intervention usually result in major morbidity or death. It is for the remaining 80-90% of patients with cholecystitis that the controversy regarding the timing of operation exists. Traditionally, delayed cholecystectomy was preferred in the setting of acute cholecystitis. Patients initially were managed nonoperatively (NPO, intravenous fluids, IV antibiotics) and discharged home after their symptoms resolved. Elective cholecystectomy (open or laparoscopic) was then performed 6 to 12 weeks later after the acute inflammation had resolved. More recent data showed that early cholecystectomy (within 72 hours of presentation) whether performed laparoscopically or open, reduced the duration of hospital stay compared with delayed open or laparoscopic cholecystectomy, with no significant difference in operative or perioperative complications and postoperative mortality. Also, 23% of people scheduled to undergo delayed cholecystectomy required urgent operation because of recurrent or worsening symptoms.[27,28] In head-to-head comparisons of early versus late laparoscopic cholecystectomy for cholecystitis, multiple trials (both prospective and retrospective) and meta-analyses have shown that early laparoscopic cholecystectomy (within 3 days of symptom onset) can be accomplished with a similar morbidity and mortality rate as delayed laparoscopic cholecystectomy. No significant differences were observed in the conversion rate to open cholecystectomy, overall morbidity, or mortality among patients undergoing early cholecystectomy versus those managed with delayed surgery. Hospital stay and overall costs, however, were significantly reduced in the early laparoscopic cholecystectomy groups.[29-35]

In high-risk surgical patients with acute cholecystitis, such as those in the ICU or with extensive cardiopulmonary disease, the mortality rates for emergent cholecystectomy can approach 50%. Gallbladder drainage by percutaneous cholecystostomy in conjunction with antibiotic therapy is currently considered to be the treatment of choice.[36-38] This procedure is now routinely performed by interventional radiologists using fluoroscopic or ultrasound guidance at most hospitals. The preferred route for tube insertion is transhepatic which serves to better stabilize the gallbladder during insertion and also promotes less leakage upon tube removal if this occurs prior to cholecystectomy. The transhepatic route is also preferred over the transperitoneal route in the setting of ascites because tract maturation occurs faster.[39] A < 5% major morbidity rate is quoted for this procedure (ie, catheter dislodgement, bleeding, liver hematoma, bile leakage, bowel perforation). If the percutaneous method is not readily available, a small right subcostal incision permitting visualization of the fundus is made under local anesthesia. The gallbladder is then needle decompressed as much as possible and a Malecot-type or similar catheter is inserted into the gallbladder and secured with a pursestring suture and exteriorized.

The optimal timing of cholecystostomy tube removal is a question of debate. Hatjidakis et al demonstrated that in the majority of patients with a transhepatic cholecystostomy, a 2-week period was sufficient for the tract to mature, whereas 3 weeks may be needed for those drained by the transperitoneal route.[40] Cholecystography should be performed via the tube after resolution of the cholecystitis. If contrast flows freely into the duodenum through a patent cystic and common duct, and no stones are present, the cholecystostomy tube can be removed and cholecystectomy is not necessarily needed. Patients with gallstones who recover from their acute illness and become improved surgical candidates should then undergo an elective laparoscopic cholecystectomy as ~80% of these patients will have recurrence of symptoms or further complications.[41,42] The laparoscopic approach to interval cholecystectomy is successful in the majority of critically ill patients who recover following percutaneous cholecystostomy. In a report by Spira et al, 31 of 52 (60%) patients who recovered following tube cholecystostomy underwent an interval cholecystectomy that was accomplished safely laparoscopically in 24 patients with a conversion rate of 14%.[43]

COMPLICATIONS

Several complications of acute cholecystitis are common and often mandate prompt surgical intervention. These include empyema, emphysematous cholecystitis,

perforation, and cholecystenteric fistula. All are the consequence of gallbladder wall ischemia and can be associated with significant morbidity and mortality. All require immediate surgical intervention.

In *empyema* (suppurative cholecystitis), the gallbladder contains frank pus, and the patient becomes more toxic, with high spiking fevers (39°-40°C), chills and a markedly elevated WBC (15,000/μL or greater). Severe sepsis may accompany with hemodynamic instability and multisystem organ failure. Treatment consists of broad-spectrum antibiotics (including anaerobic coverage and possible antifungal coverage), and emergent cholecystectomy or cholecystostomy. Not surprisingly, cholecystostomy is sometimes inadequate to relieve the entire source of sepsis.

Emphysematous cholecystitis is characterized by bubbles of gas from anaerobic infection appearing in the gallbladder lumen, its wall, the pericholecystic space, and, on occasion, the bile ducts. Clostridia species are the most commonly implicated organism, but other gas forming anaerobes may be identified. Three times as many men as women are affected, and 20% of patients are diabetic. In contrast to the usual form of acute cholecystitis, this disease is a bacterial infection from the start and often not associated with the presence of gallstones.[44] Patients present with severe pain and are toxic appearing with high fevers and a significant leukocytosis. Abdominal x-rays or CT scans usually demonstrate air within the gallbladder lumen or wall. Broad-spectrum antibiotics including an anticlostridial agent need to be initiated immediately. Emergent cholecystectomy is indicated. If the patient is too unstable for surgery, cholecystostomy is often effective.

Perforation can occur when an ischemic gallbladder wall progresses to gangrene. Perforation may occur as early as 3 days after the onset of acute cholecystitis or not until late in the second week and beyond. Luckily, this occurs in < 10% of cases. Gallbladder perforation can be categorized as either being localized or free. Localized perforation generally results in the formation of a pericholecystic abscesses the omentum walls off the contamination limiting it to the right upper quadrant. Here, cholecystectomy (open or laparoscopic) with abscess drainage can be performed safely in many of these patients, but again if the patient is too unstable for surgery, cholecystostomy and percutaneous abscess drainage can temporize the situation.

Free perforation occurs much less frequently (~1%) and results when gangrene develops before adhesions wall off the inflamed gallbladder. Bile spills freely into the peritoneal cavity, causing a generalized peritonitis and often septic shock ensues. These patients need aggressive intravenous volume resuscitation and broad antibiotic coverage. Emergent exploratory laparotomy is indicated with generous abdominal cavity lavage and cholecystectomy.

Cholecystenteric fistula occurs in 1%-2% of patients with acute cholecystitis. Here, the inflamed gallbladder becomes adherent to a neighboring hollow viscus organ and necrosis develops at the site of this adhesion eventually leading to perforation into the adjacent lumen. The duodenum (~20%) and the hepatic flexure of the colon (~80%) are the most common sites but fistulas to the stomach are also reported. Generally, after the fistula forms, the episode of acute cholecystitis resolves as the gallbladder spontaneously decompresses. Rarely, patients vomit gallstones or steatorrhea, but in most cases the acute attack subsides and the cholecystenteric fistula remains clinically undetected. If a large gallstone passes from the gallbladder into the small intestine, a mechanical bowel obstruction may result, which is termed *gallstone ileus*. This occurs in 10 to 15% of patients with a cholecystenteric fistula. Patients present with signs and symptoms of small bowel obstruction including nausea, vomiting and generalized abdominal pain and distention. The pain may be episodic as the stone temporarily impacts at one site in the intestinal lumen, then dislodges and is peristalsed forward where it obstructs again. The terminal ileum is the usual final site of stone impaction at or near the ileocecal valve. Often, abdominal plain films will show dilated small bowel loops with air-fluid levels and pneumobilia and a calcified gallstone in the right lower quadrant.

The initial management of gallstone ileus includes removal of the obstructing stone usually via a proximal enterotomy in a segment of nonedematous small bowel. The stone should be milked back to this zone and extracted. The enterotomy is then closed in two layers.

Although there is no debate regarding the need to emergently relieve the obstruction, there still exists debate over when and if the cholecystenteric fistula should be addressed. Classic teaching favored treating the obstruction only at the initial setting especially in a sick patient with acute or chronic comorbid conditions. If symptomatic, the gallbladder may be removed on a semielective basis at a later time. This teaching was founded on the evidence that the vast majority of cholecystenteric fistula will close spontaneously with a < 5% recurrence rate of gallstone ileus.[45,46] Recently, several authors have revisited the issue citing that with improved preoperative and postoperative care as well as intraoperative technique, a one-stage procedure consisting of enterolithotomy, cholecystectomy, and fistula excision may be performed safely.[47] Some even advocate that the entire procedure can be performed safely and expediently via a laparoscopic approach.[48,49]

ACUTE ACALCULOUS CHOLECYSTITIS

INTRODUCTION

Acute acalculous cholecystitis accounts for 5%-10% of all patients with acute cholecystitis. The disease often has a more fulminant course than acute calculous cholecystitis and often progresses to empyema, or gangrene with perforation. There is a strong association with a variety of clinical conditions including recent nonbiliary surgery, major trauma, severe burns, sepsis/shock, immunosuppression, receiving total parenteral nutrition (TPN), diabetes mellitus, severe infections, prolonged mechanical ventilation, narcotic administration, coronary artery disease, cholesterol emboli, multiple transfusions, childbirth, and multiple connective tissue/rheumatologic disorders. Patients are usually critically ill, being cared for in an ICU, and the diagnosis usually follows a workup for unexplained fever, leukocytosis, sepsis, or vague abdominal discomfort. The conditions associated with acalculous cholecystitis lead to gallbladder stasis and ischemia, which result in a local inflammatory response in the gallbladder wall. Once a calculous cholecystitis is established, secondary infection with enteric pathogens, *E. coli*, *Enterococcus faecalis*, klebsiella, pseudomonas, proteus species, and bacteroides is common and antibiotic therapy should be directed against these organisms initially.[50] Signs and symptoms are generally identical to those of calculous cholecystitis with right upper quadrant tenderness, fever, elevated WBC count, and elevated liver enzymes. Up to 20% of patients are jaundiced secondary to partial biliary obstruction induced by inflammation extending into the common bile duct. This finding is in sharp contrast to calculous cholecystitis in which jaundice is quite uncommon. Often, the diagnosis of acalculous cholecystitis is delayed, as symptoms are difficult to detect in noncommunicative critically ill patients in the ICU. This, in part, accounts for the increased morbidity and mortality (up to 40% in some series) associated with this diagnosis compared to acute cholecystitis.[51] As in acute calculous cholecystitis, ultrasonography is the investigation of first choice.[52] Ultrasonographic features suggestive of acalculous cholecystitis include absence of gallstones or sludge, thickening of the gallbladder wall (> 5 mm) with pericholecystic fluid, a positive Murphy sign induced by the ultrasound probe in a conscious patient, emphysematous cholecystitis with gas bubbles present in the fundus of the gallbladder (Champagne sign), and, occasionally, failure to visualize the gallbladder secondary to too much surrounding inflammation. The reported accuracy of HIDA scans in these patients is variable, with a sensitivity of 70-80% and a specificity of 90-100%. Again, failure to opacify the gallbladder is the most sensitive and specific finding. Leakage of tracer into the pericholecystic space suggests perforation. The fact that a majority of patients who develop acute acalculous cholecystitis are not being fed enterally and are receiving TPN greatly reduces the accuracy of this test.[47]

Emergency cholecystectomy is the ultimate treatment once the diagnosis is established or the suspicion is high. Both open and laparoscopic techniques have been utilized successfully.[53] The gallbladder is often encased in an inflammatory mass, which makes the laparoscopic approach more complicated because of a higher risk of bile duct and vascular injuries. The incidence of gangrene, perforation, and empyema exceeds 50%; and, therefore, cholecystectomy rather than cholecystostomy is usually required in this setting, however, in the patient too critically ill to undergo a general anesthetic or unable to travel from the ICU percutaneous cholecystostomy is a viable temporizing modality. Occasionally, percutaneous cholecystectomy is more than a temporizing measure if the patient recovers and the underlying problem causing the cholecystitis resolves. Here, subsequent cholecystectomy is often unnecessary.[42,54] McLoughlin et al demonstrated in a series of 50 patients that only 24% with acalculous cholecystitis required cholecystectomy at a mean follow-up period of 12 months. Isolated cases of successful transpapillary endoscopic drainage of the gallbladder have also been reported.[55,56]

OPERATIVE MANAGEMENT

SURGICAL TIPS AND PITFALLS

Open cholecystectomy is usually performed via a right subcostal or vertical high midline incision. A 5 cm to 8 cm incision (a so-called minicholecystectomy, first described by Dubois and Barthelot in 1982) is usually adequate to provide ample exposure and visualization of the necessary anatomy. The old conventional 8-cm to 14-cm incision has been shown to be excessive in most instances, causing more muscle damage and postoperative discomfort than is necessary. In a prospective randomized controlled trial comparing minicholecystectomy to the conventional open incision for the management of acute cholecystitis, patients receiving the smaller incision (5.5 cm vs 13.5 cm) required less postoperative analgesia, had decreased hospital lengths of stay, and had an earlier return to normal daily activities. No significant differences were found between the two groups in length of operative time, operative morbidity, or mortality.[57] A "dome-down" technique (dissection from the fundus toward the cystic duct) is recommended. This method is preferred when there is significant inflammation and adhesions that prevent safe, adequate visualization of the delicate structures that exist in or near the triangle of Calot (cystic duct, common hepatic duct, common bile duct, cystic artery, and right hepatic artery). A distended gallbladder should be aspirated to facilitate manipulation with care taken not to spill bile in the operative field. Bile should be sent for Gram stain and culture to better direct antibiotic therapy. Clamps placed at the gallbladder fundus and laterally at the infundibulum (Hartmann pouch) allow for controlled mobilization of the gallbladder as dissection heads toward the cystic duct. Note that excessive traction during this dissection may angulate the common duct and can result in clamping and, even worse, transection, of the hepatic or common duct.

If identification of the ductal anatomy is difficult, an intraoperative cholangiogram (IOC) must be performed to clarify the relationship of the ducts. In addition to uncertain anatomy, other indications for IOC include known choledocholithiasis, history of pancreatitis or jaundice, suspected CBD injury, abnormal preoperative liver function test results, or dilated bile ducts on preoperative imaging. Injury to the right hepatic artery can result from mistaking this structure for the cystic artery. This injury can lead to future biliary strictures and long-term morbidity. The anatomic variations of the cystic, hepatic, and common ducts and arteries are common enough, especially in the setting of local inflammation causing distortion, to warrant no clamping, transaction, or ligation until all critical structures have been properly identified. The incidence of bile duct injury in open cholecystectomy is between 0.1% and 0.2%.[58] If an injury has occurred, repair is best if it can be done safely at the time of the original operation. Primary repair can be performed over a T-tube if the defect is small (< 1cm) and there is no crush or electrocautery burn injury. A Roux-en-Y hepatico- or choledochojejunostomy can be performed for larger defects or complete transactions with significant gap between viable duct ends.

Although drain placement at the conclusion of the cholecystectomy is not supported by any indisputable data, the presence of a drain allows for detection and expedient treatment of a persistent bile leak following cholecystectomy. Bile leaks occur in ~1% of open cholecystectomy cases and most commonly emanate from the cystic duct stump, an unidentified accessory duct, or intrahepatic bile ducts. Most leaks are self-limited, but if drainage persists for greater than 1-2 weeks, an endoscopic retrograde cholangiopancreatography (ERCP) is indicated. This study is both diagnostic (able to identify the source of the leak) and therapeutic if a transpapillary stenting or sphincterotomy are performed. These procedures serve to reduce the back pressures in the common bile duct that have been promoting ongoing patency of the leak and allow for sealing.[59]

In rare instances, completion of a planned cholecystectomy needs to be aborted secondary to an acute change in a patient's hemodynamic stability, severe anatomic abnormalities caused by inflammatory changes, or untoward bleeding in the setting of portal hypertension or cirrhosis. In this situation, a partial cholecystectomy may be performed although this is a less than ideal procedure.[60] The fundus of the gallbladder is opened and the contents evacuated. The surgeon then places a finger in the lumen and uses it as a guide while the entire anterior wall of the gallbladder above the cystic duct is removed using the bovie cautery. Impacted stones visualized or palpated in the cystic duct should be removed and the cystic duct ligated only if it is clearly identified. Alternatively, the cystic duct is left without further intervention and should seal, provided there is no common bile duct obstruction. The posterior wall of the gallbladder still attached to the liver is left in place and its mucosa is removed with a curette or fulgurated with electrocautery. The operative field is widely drained via closed suction drains. Drainage of bile usually stops spontaneously. The procedure avoids dissection in Calot triangle and reduces the risk of bile duct injury. In addition, it potentially makes the control of bleeding easier and avoids the need for a second look operation in very high-risk patients.[61]

Laparoscopic dissection is more difficult in acute cholecystitis as compared to uncomplicated cholelithiasis because of inflammatory changes in the gallbladder wall itself as well as the extensive pericholecystic inflammation and adhesions. Edematous, friable, vascular tissues obscure the anatomy around the triangle of Calot and are easily torn during retraction, resulting in bleeding or inadvertent injury. If the gallbladder is too tense and distended it should be aspirated through the fundus early in the procedure. This is done under direct vision utilizing a percutaneous angiocatheter or even a Verres needle.[62] Dense adhesions that may be present between the gallbladder and the omentum, duodenum, or colon should be dissected bluntly using a cotton swab ("peanut") dissector or with the suction-irrigator tip. Liberal use of suction and irrigation help keep the field free of blood and preserve clear visualization. Electrocautery should be used sparingly until the vital structures around Calot triangle are identified. When dissecting out the structures in the triangle of Calot, dissection should proceed close to the gallbladder wall. Dissection of the lower part of the gallbladder from the liver bed early in the operation may aid in identification of the gallbladder neck-cystic duct junction (similar to the retrograde dissection performed during open cholecystectomy). Retraction of the gallbladder neck laterally optimizes exposure of the triangle of Calot. Dislodgment or extraction of an impacted stone in Hartmann pouch will allow for better traction on this area with graspers. If the ductal anatomy remains obscure and dissection is tenuous, preliminary cholangiography via the decompressed gallbladder may indicate the position of the cystic duct in relationship to the common duct. If the obstructing stone responsible for the acute attack is found to lie in the cystic duct, it must be milked back into the gallbladder before the duct is clipped or ligated. A thickened, edematous cystic duct is often better controlled by ligation (either extracorporeal or via a ligating loop) than by clipping. Closed suction drains can be placed if cystic duct closure is deemed tenuous. Before complete transection of the cystic duct, an IOC should be performed if any of the indications listed here exist.

Conversion from laparoscopic to open cholecystectomy is indicated when laparoscopic cholecystectomy cannot be completed safely based on anatomic complications or on patient intraoperative physiology.

Conversion is also advocated for persistent uncontrollable bleeding or intraoperative injury to a duct other than the cystic duct or to bowel. Conversion should not be considered a complication of laparoscopic surgery, but a judicious surgical decision in a complicated case to avoid further morbidity and mortality. A wide variation in conversion rates for cholecystitis exists in the literature (0%[63,64] to 35%[65-68]), which may reflect not only the experience of the individual surgeons performing the procedures but also on the patient populations described and the timing of the surgery. Predictors of conversion have varied among reports and have included male gender, a history of biliary disease, a delay in surgery of more than 48 hours, marked leukocytosis (> 18,000/µL), and obesity.[69] Conversions, however, were invariably related to adhesions and inability to demonstrate the biliary anatomy.

Acute Cholecystitis in Pregnancy

Acute cholecystitis is the second most common nonobstetrical cause of acute abdomen during pregnancy, behind appendicitis. Cholelithiasis is the cause of cholecystitis in over 90% of cases.[70] The incidence of cholelithiasis in pregnant woman undergoing routine obstetric ultrasound examinations is 3.5-10%.[71] The progesterone-induced smooth muscle relaxation of the gallbladder promotes stasis of bile and increases the risk of cholelithiasis and subsequently of acute cholecystitis.[72] Additionally, elevated levels of estrogen during pregnancy increase the lithogenicity of bile, which further increases the risk of cholelithiasis and acute cholecystitis.

The symptomatology of acute cholecystitis is almost identical in pregnant and nonpregnant women but the differential diagnosis list must include HELLP syndrome and preeclampsia. LFTs (specifically alkaline phosphatase) and serum amylase values may be elevated as a result of the pregnancy rather than related to a specific pathological condition. Ultrasound remains the diagnostic procedure of choice with similar accuracy as in nonpregnant patients.

Because of the high incidence of fetal loss, early studies recommended medical management and delay in operation until after parturition.[73] Recently, surgery as a primary treatment has been used widely because of (1) reduced use of medications, (2) recurrence rate during pregnancy of 44-92%, depending on the trimester of presentation, (3) shorter hospital length of stay, and (4) minimizing the development of potentially life-threatening complications such as perforation, sepsis, and peritonitis, which are all indications for surgical treatment.[74] In addition, nonoperative management of symptomatic cholelithiasis increases the risk of gallstone pancreatitis up to 13%, which causes fetal loss in 10-20% of cases.[75,76] Nonoperative management has also been associated with higher incidences of spontaneous abortions, preterm labor, and preterm delivery than among those undergoing cholecystectomy.[77] The current recommendation is to perform laparoscopic cholecystectomy in the first, second, and early in the third trimester, if indicated, because the procedure is safe for both the mother and the fetus. The open technique (Hasson technique) for initial trocar insertion is essential to minimize organ injuries. This should be performed at a supraumbilical site. Transvaginal ultrasound for fetal assessment is ideal during laparoscopy. Other unique aspects of laparoscopic cholecystectomy in pregnant patients include reverse Trendelenburg positioning with left side down to preserve return blood flow in the vena cava, low-pressure pneumoperitoneum, and, if possible, laparoscopic ultrasound to rule out common bile duct stones.

There is disagreement on the use of operative cholangiography in the pregnant patient. Some authors feel that IOC is probably safe in the second and third trimester because only small amounts of radiation are used in a period when organogenesis is already complete. Shielding the uterus further reduces the risk of radiation exposure.[78] Liberman et al advocate routine IOC in all pregnant patients undergoing LC because of the increased incidence of common bile duct stones. In addition, a negative IOC can avoid unnecessary postoperative endoscopic retrograde cholangiography if jaundice develops later in pregnancy.[79] Others feel that IOC should be used only when there is a question of choledocholithiasis on the basis of clinical, biochemical, or ultrasonic evidence.[80] Alternative methods of investigating the common bile duct during surgery without x-ray exposure have been suggested. These include intraoperative ultrasonography, transcystic duct choledochoscopy, and endoscopic papillotomy performed under ultrasonographic guidance.

COMMON BILE DUCT STONES

INTRODUCTION

The acute care surgeon will encounter choledocholithiasis with a wide spectrum of presentations ranging from asymptomatic, incidentally found common bile duct (CBD) stones to acute cholangitis/biliary sepsis. Primary CBD stones are calculi that originate in the bile duct. These stones often result from impaired drainage of the common bile duct secondary to stricture or mass effect on the CBD or ampulla of Vater. These stones are caused by stasis within the CBD and consist of calcium bilirubinate. They are soft, brown, and form a "cast" of the bile duct. Operative intervention must include clearance of the duct as well as a drainage procedure. More commonly, CBD stones are secondary stones. These stones are formed within the gallbladder and migrate to the common bile duct. Secondary stones are predominately cholesterol stones formed by an imbalance of the three main components

of bile: bile salts, lecithin, and cholesterol. Cholesterol stones are often yellow, multiple, and faceted. The management of CBD stones is varied and dependent on the timing of diagnosis and the patient's presenting symptoms.

PREOPERATIVE MANAGEMENT

Patients with CBD stones have a diverse array of presenting symptoms. Most commonly patients will present with symptoms of cholecystitis, biliary colic, pancreatitis, jaundice, or cholangitis. Seven percent of patients with cholecystits, 16% with biliary colic, 20% with pancreatitis, and 45% with jaundice will have CBD stones.[81] The classic presentation of cholangitis is abdominal pain, fever, and jaundice—Charcot triad. Few patients may progress to sepsis with shock and altered mental status—Reynold pentad. Preoperative blood work may reveal elevations of alkaline phosphatase, glutamic oxaloacetic transaminase, lactate dehydrogenase, or bilirubin. If one of these values is elevated, CBD stones are present 20% of the time. If two of these values are elevated, choledocholithiasis will be present 40% of the time. However, normal serum liver enzymes do not ensure a clear common duct.[82] Five to twelve percent of patients with normal enzymes and minimal to no symptoms will have common bile duct stones.[83,84]

Once common bile duct stones are suspected, initial management of the patient depends on presenting symptoms. Most patients admitted will be dehydrated from inanition and/or vomiting therefore intravenous fluids should be administered. Placement of a nasogastric tube may be necessary for nausea and vomiting. If symptoms of infection such as fever and leukocytosis are present, antibiotics should be administered.[82]

Patients with cholangitis require close monitoring and aggressive support. Hypotension and tachycardia should be corrected with volume replacement. One measure of response to resuscitation is indicated by urinary output of 30 ml per hour; therefore, a Foley catheter should be placed. Patients failing to respond to volume resuscitation or patients with cardiovascular disease may require central venous pressure monitoring or determination of cardiac output and pulmonary artery pressures. Antibiotic therapy should be promptly initiated in all patients with cholangitis. The most commonly found pathogens in patients with cholangitis are *E. coli*, *Klebsiella* spp., *Enterobacter* spp., and *Enterococcus* spp.[85] Anaerobes are found in 3% of bile cultures.[86] Broad spectrum antibiotic therapy should be tailored to cover these gram-negative rods and gram-positive cocci. Penicillin derivatives such as piperacillin-tazobactam, ampicillin-sulbactam, and ticarcillin-clavulanic acid offer excellent coverage. Second- and third-generation cephalosporins with metronidazole also provide adequate therapy to treat the most common pathogens and anaerobes. If a patient has a history of vancomycin resistant enterococcus (VRE), combination therapy with linezolid should be instituted. Once the patient has been stabilized, imaging studies and therapeutic interventions can proceed.[82]

DIAGNOSIS
Ultrasound
Transabdominal ultrasonography is often the first imaging modality used to evaluate patients with biliary symptoms. Ultrasonography is excellent at detecting gallstones and common bile duct dilation. The sensitivity of ultrasound for detecting intra- and extrahepatic duct dilation compared to endoscopic retrograde cholangiopancreatography (ERCP) is 96%.[87] The sensitivity of ultrasonography at detecting common bile duct stones is much lower compared to endoscopic ultrasound (EUS) and ERCP, ranging between 25% and 63%.[88,89] However, if choledocholithiasis is detected by ultrasound, the specificity of this finding is 95%.[88]

COMPUTED TOMOGRAPHY (CT)
The sensitivity of conventional CT for choledocholithiasis is between 70 and 90%.[90,91] Oral contrast increases CT cholangiography sensitivity to 92%.[92]

MAGNETIC RESONANCE CHOLANGIOPANCREATOGRAPHY (MRCP)
MRCP is very reliable for the detection of common bile duct stones. The sensitivity, specificity, and accuracy of MRCP are 90%, 95%, and 95%, respectively. There is also excellent intraobserver agreement in the diagnosis of CBD stones.[93-95] In one study, all CBD stones greater than 5 mm were detected by MRCP. Sixty percent of stones less than 5 mm were detected.[96] An NIH consensus statement found that MRCP, ERCP, and EUS were comparable in their sensitivities, specificities, and accuracy rates for the detection of CBD stones.[97] MRCP has fewer potential complications than ERCP. The 30-day morbidity of ERCP has been reported as high as 15.9%. Procedure related mortality rates of 1% are also reported.[98] In addition to its lower side-effect profile, MRCP is 30% to 50% less costly than ERCP.[99]

ENDOSCOPIC RETROGRADE CHOLANGIOPANCREATOGRAPHY (ERCP)
ERCP is highly specific for detecting CBD stones. Its sensitivity is between 90 and 95%.[100,101] The advantage of ERCP is the ability to perform therapeutic removal of stones at the time of diagnosis. The disadvantage is the associated morbidity and mortality of the procedure, discussed above. Also, for up to 61% of patients undergoing ERCP, no CBD stones will be found. These patients will have been exposed to the risks of ERCP unnecessarily.[102,103] ERCP is best reserved for those patients for whom there is a high probability of CBD stones or for whom CBD stones have been documented by other studies.

ENDOSCOPIC ULTRASOUND (EUS)
This is also an accurate test for the diagnosis of CBD stones. The reported sensitivity of EUS is between 94 and 98%.[104,105] The specificity is 99%.[104] In some centers, EUS has been used in conjunction with ERCP to avoid unnecessary exposure to the risks of ERCP. EUS is performed first in patients with moderate suspicion of CBD stones. ERCP is performed only if the EUS demonstrates the presence of CBD stones.[26]

OPERATIVE MANAGEMENT

INTRAOPERATIVE EVALUATION FOR CBD STONES
Intraoperative Cholangiography (IOC)
IOC should be performed during laparoscopic cholecystectomy if CBD stones are suspected, there is a history of pancreatitis, jaundice, or abnormal liver function tests, the common bile duct is dilated, or there is difficulty in defining anatomy. Some centers perform routine IOC. With this approach, the incidence of CBD stones is between 10 and 14%.[106,107] The sensitivity and specificity of IOC are 98% and 94%, respectively.[108]

Laparoscopic Ultrasound (LUS)
LUS in an attractive alternative to IOC; however, most surgeons have little to no experience with this technique. Studies have shown that LUS is more sensitive than IOC and as accurate and specific as IOC. These studies have also shown it can be performed more quickly.[109,110]

OPERATIVE MANAGEMENT OF COMMON BILE DUCT STONES
If common bile duct stones are identified preoperatively, the surgeon has several options for management depending upon resources available and the surgeon's comfort with advanced laparoscopic techniques.

ERCP/ES followed by Laparoscopic Cholecystectomy
For centers without experience in laparoscopic common bile duct exploration, patients should undergo ERCP with endoscopic sphincterotomy (ES). ERCP with ES will be successful in clearing the CBD in 70 to more than 90% of cases.[111,112] Laparoscopic cholecystectomy should follow successful endoscopic clearance of the CBD. If ERCP with ES is unsuccessful, the common bile duct must be surgically cleared. Laparoscopic common bile duct exploration (LCBDE) or open common bile duct exploration should be performed depending on surgeon preference. In experienced hands, LCBDE has been shown to have a 100% success rate in salvaging failed preoperative ERCP/ES.[113] If the treating surgeon is not experienced with LCBDE, open cholecystectomy with common bile duct exploration should be performed. Contraindications for open or laparoscopic CBD exploration include portal hypertension, severe periportal inflammation, and a CBD

smaller than 5 mm. Choledochotomy should be avoided on a small CBD because of the high incidence of postsurgical stricture.[114] Other indications for open CBD exploration include the presence of primary duct stones and impacted stone at the ampulla of Vater. The presence of primary duct stones requires a drainage procedure such as choledochoduodenostomy or choledochojejunostomy. These biliary-enteric anastomoses can be done laparoscopically, but this requires advanced laparoscopic suturing capabilities. Stones impacted at the ampulla of Vater require sphincterotomy or sphincteroplasty. Elderly or debilitated patients with common bile duct stones can be treated by ERCP/ES without cholecystectomy. Studies have shown that 75 to 84% of patients remain symptom free with up to 70 months of follow-up.[115,116]

LAPAROSCOPIC COMMON BILE DUCT EXPLORATION (LCBDE)

For centers with experience in LCBDE, patients identified preoperatively with CBD stones may be taken directly to surgery without ERCP/ES. LCBDE is feasible for 85% of patients with CBD stones and is successful in 85% to 95% of cases.[117-119] This single stage approach is attractive for several reasons. The risks of ERCP/ES are avoided. LCBDE and ERCP/ES followed by LC have equivalent success rates but hospital stay is significantly reduced for LCBDE.[120] LCBDE has also been shown to be the most cost-effective approach.[121]

IRRIGATION TECHNIQUES

Common bile duct stones found/confirmed by IOC can be managed by a variety of techniques. Stones smaller than or equal to 3 mm often can be flushed through the CBD with saline or contrast material. Glucagon, 1 to 2 mg IV, should be administered to relax the sphincter of Oddi and relieve sphincter pressure. Passage of stones should be followed fluoroscopically.[122] Stones greater than 4 mm often will not pass with this irrigation technique.[124] Fifty percent of CBD stones that are clinically silent/incidentally found will pass spontaneously within 6 weeks regardless of number of stones or CBD size. These stones can be followed expectantly in the short term.[123] Symptomatic by irrigation techniques should be removed by other means.

TRANSCYSTIC TECHNIQUES CBD STONES THAT CANNOT BE FLUSHED FROM THE CBD

Successful LCBD through the cystic duct or by choledochotomy requires special equipment. A listing of recommended equipment is listed in Table 10-1. Many factors go into determining whether a transcystic approach or choledochotomy is most appropriate. A listing of these factors is included in Table 10-2.

BALLOON TECHNIQUES

Transcystic exploration of the CBD is highly effective and precludes the need for choledochotomy. During

Table 10-1	Laparoscopic Common Bile Duct Equipment
14 gauge IV catheter	
Fluoroscope (C-arm type)	
Glucagon, 1 to 2 mg (IV, given by anesthetist)	
Balloon tipped catheters (4 French)	
Segura type baskets	
0.035 inch diameter long guide wire (>90 cm)	
Mechanical over the wire dilators (7 to 12 Fr, found in most urology departments)	
High pressure "over the wire" pneumatic dilator	
IV tubing (for saline irrigation through the choledochoscope)	
Atraumatic grasping forceps (for choledochoscope manipulation)	
Flexible choledochoscope with light source	
Second camera	
Second monitor	
Video switcher (for simultaneous display of the choledochoscopic fluoroscopic, and/or laparoscopic images)	
Absorbable suture	
T-tube	

Adapted from: Petelin, JB, Pruett, CS (2004): Common Bile Duct Stones. In Cameron, JL editor: *Current Surgical Therapy*, ed 8, pg 393, Philadelphia, Elsevier Mosby.

port placement the midclavicular port should be placed within 2 cm of the rib cage. This facilitates access to the cystic duct.[82] A 4 Fr embolectomy balloon catheter is introduced, through the cystic duct, into the duodenum via the CBD. The balloon is inflated and the catheter withdrawn until it meets resistance at the sphincter. The balloon is then let down to withdraw the catheter 1 cm into the CBD. The balloon is gently reinflated and the catheter slowly withdrawn with the stone/s into the cystic duct.[124]

BASKET TECHNIQUES

A 5 Fr basket with four to six wires is introduced into the CBD under fluoroscopic guidance. The basket should be advanced past the stone and then opened. Advancing an open basket proximal to the stone may result in the basket with stone to enter the duodenum. The stone and basket can then become trapped in the duodenum requiring open extraction. Once the basket is closed around the stone, the stone and basket are withdrawn to the cystic duct for stone extraction.[82]

TRANSCYSTIC CHOLEDOCHOSCOPY

A flexible, bidirectional choledochoscope can be introduced into the CBD through the cystic duct for direct visualization of the common bile duct. The cystic duct

Table 10-2   Factors Influencing Approach

Factor	Transcystic Approach	Choledochotomy Approach
One stone	+	+
Multiple stones	+	+
Stones ≤ 6 mm diameter	+	+
Stones > 6 mm diameter	–	+
Intra-hepatic stones	–	+
Diameter of cystic duct < 4 mm	–	+
Diameter of cystic duct > 4 mm	+	+
Diameter of common duct < 6 mm	+	–
Diameter of common duct > 6 mm	+	+
Cystic duct entrance—lateral	+	+
Cystic duct entrance—posterior	–	+
Cystic duct entrance—distal	–	+
Inflammation—mild	+	+
Inflammation—marked	+	–
Suturing ability—poor	+	–
Suturing ability—good	+	+

+, Positive or neutral effect; –, negative effect.
Petelin, JB, Pruett, CS: Common Bile Duct Stones. In Cameron, JL editor: *Current Surgical Therapy*, ed 8, pg 394, Philadelphia, 2004, Elsevier Mosby.

may need to be dilated to accommodate the scope. This can be accomplished by the introduction of a guide wire into the cystic duct. Graduated dilators (7 to 12 Fr) can then be passed over the guide wire to dilate the cystic duct. The cystic duct can also be dilated by a balloon dilating catheter. The balloon is positioned, by fluoroscopy, with its proximal end in the cystic duct and the distal end in the CBD. The balloon is dilated to several atmospheres pressure (dependent on balloon size and manufacturers' recommendations) for several minutes. The balloon is deflated and then removed. The choledochoscope can then be passed into the cystic duct with or without the use of the guide wire. A stone basket is introduced through the scope's working channel to ensnare the stone under direct visualization. The stone, basket, and scope are withdrawn as one unit. Multiple passes are made until the duct is clear. Alternatively, a balloon catheter may be introduced next to the scope. The catheter is passed beyond the stone and then inflated. The catheter is then withdrawn trapping the stone between the balloon and the scope. The catheter, stone, and scope are all withdrawn together.[124]

At completion of transcystic LCBDE, a cholangiogram should be performed to ensure clearance of the common bile duct. Because of the aggressive manipulation of the duct, the cystic duct will often develop edema postoperatively. Therefore, the duct should be ligated rather than clipped to protect against cystic duct leak.[82] The duct should also be ligated if postoperative ERCP/ES may be required.

LAPAROSCOPIC CHOLEDOCHOTOMY

For stones greater than 6 mm or within the hepatic duct, choledochotomy must be performed. The CBD must be dilated to 6 mm or more for this approach. The anterior surface of the CBD is cleared. A 5- to 10- mm longitudinal choledochotomy, distal to the cystic duct junction, is made. A choledochoscope is then used to examine and clear the CBD as described earlier. The choledochotomy may be closed primarily or over a 12- or 14- Fr T-tube. Recent studies have shown comparable results.[124] Others have shown decreased complications with primary closure.[125,126] T-tubes should always be placed in cases of residual distal obstruction or retained stones after exploration. The common bile duct should be closed with fine absorbable suture using intracorporeal suturing techniques because of the fragility of the duct. Completion cholangiography should be performed.

Once laparoscopic CBDE is completed, cholecystectomy is performed in the usual manner. If a T tube has been placed it is brought out by the most direct route through one of the port sites. T-tube cholangiogram is performed prior to tube removal at 10 to 14 days. If retained stones are identified, the tube remains for percutaneous stone extraction. If the study is normal the tube is removed.

LCBDE is safe and has excellent results. Success rates in most series are between 88% and 100%. Most LCBDEs, 80% to 98%, can be performed by a transcystic approach.[120,127,128] A procedure related morbidity between 6% and 12% has been reported.[49] These complications included cystic duct avulsion, cystic duct leak, bile leak, entrapped basket and stone, intimal disruption/tear, bile duct puncture, and retained stone. The mortality rate has been reported between 0%-2%.[120,127-128] In expert hands, LCBDE adds 1 hour of operating time to the procedure. Length of stay for transcystic approaches are 1 to 2 days. Length of stay for laparoscopic choledochotomy is generally longer, between 2 and 7 days.

Other methods of stone clearance such as electrohydraulic or laser lithotripsy, pulsatile saline, and antegrade sphincterotomy have been described.[129] However, limited experience with these techniques has been reported. They also require equipment not readily available to the acute care surgeon and can cause severe injury to the common duct if not used properly.

POSTOPERATIVE MANAGEMENT
Postoperative ERCP/ES
Postoperative ERCP/ES must be considered if the CBD cannot be cleared at the time of cholecystectomy or if CBD stones are found postoperatively. Despite the advances in laparoscopic technique, LCBDE is sometimes unsuccessful. Some surgeons may not be comfortable with LCBDE. As LCBDE does lengthen the operation, some patients may be too ill to prolong the surgery. In these situations postoperative ERCP/ES may be required. This does require the patient undergo a second invasive procedure, but if successful, maintains the goals of minimally invasive surgery. In one study, 80 patients with CBD stones found at the time of laparoscopic cholecystectomy were randomized to LCBDE or postoperative ERCP/ES. Stone clearance was achieved in 100% of the LCBDE patients and 93% of the ERCP/ES patients. Hospital stay was decreased for the LCBDE group.[130] Even in experienced hands, ERCP/ES has a failure rate for CBD clearance of 4% to 18%.[131] Because of the uncertainty of postoperative ERCP/ES, a catheter can be left in the cystic duct. Through this, a guide wire can be advanced into the duodenum to assist with ERCP/ES cannulation of the common bile duct.[132] Certainly, conversion to open common bile duct exploration should be considered when laparoscopic duct clearance is not possible or fails. Figure 10-1 summarizes the approach to common bile duct stone management.

TREATMENT OF ACUTE CHOLANGITIS
Once the patient with acute cholangitis is stabilized, emergent or urgent decompression of the biliary tree is indicated. Endoscopic management is associated with less morbidity and mortality than surgical decompression.[133] A randomized prospective study has compared the safety and efficacy of endoscopic and surgical management of patients with severe cholangitis secondary to stones. In this study, patients treated with open common bile duct exploration had significantly higher morbidity (64% vs 34%) and mortality (32% vs 10%) than patients treated with ERCP/ES.[134] Endoscopic sphincterotomy can be performed and is successful in 97% of cases.[135] ES can drain the duct and can clear it of stones. If stones cannot be removed, a stent can be placed across the obstruction. Stents can also relieve obstruction caused by malignant and benign strictures.

Percutaneous transhepatic cholangiography (PTC) and placement of a percutaneous transhepatic biliary drain by intervention radiologists can also decompress an infected, obstructed biliary tree. PTC is performed if endoscopy is unavailable, unsuccessful, or not feasible because of patient anatomy (prior surgery, such as Billroth II or Roux-en-Y anatomy).

Rarely, surgical decompression is required. This can be done by laparoscopic or open techniques depending on surgeon preference and patient condition. Patient status also determines if simple drainage by choledochotomy and T-tube is performed or full exploration with duct clearance.

GALLSTONE PANCREATITIS

INTRODUCTION
Most cases of *acute* pancreatitis in North America are the result of gallstones migrating into the common bile duct and passing through the ampulla of Vater. The resultant pancreatic duct obstruction causes pancreatic and peripancreatic inflammation which can progress to a severe systemic illness in a small proportion of patients. Although initial management focuses on supportive care and severity staging, there can be a great deal of variation in the surgical and endoscopic management of patients who have experienced gallstone pancreatitis. The optimal management schema has yet to be devised. The following section reviews current trends in the evaluation and treatment of acute gallstone pancreatitis.

INCIDENCE
Worldwide, there has been an increased incidence of gallstone pancreatitis over the past four decades. Current European studies report an incidence of first attack gallstone pancreatitis in approximately 12 out of every 100000 population.[136] In the United States, studies have shown a 3.4% risk of developing pancreatitis in those patients followed for asymptomatic gallstones.[137] Although the incidence of alcoholic pancreatitis is two times greater in men than women, the incidence of gallstone pancreatitis is approximately

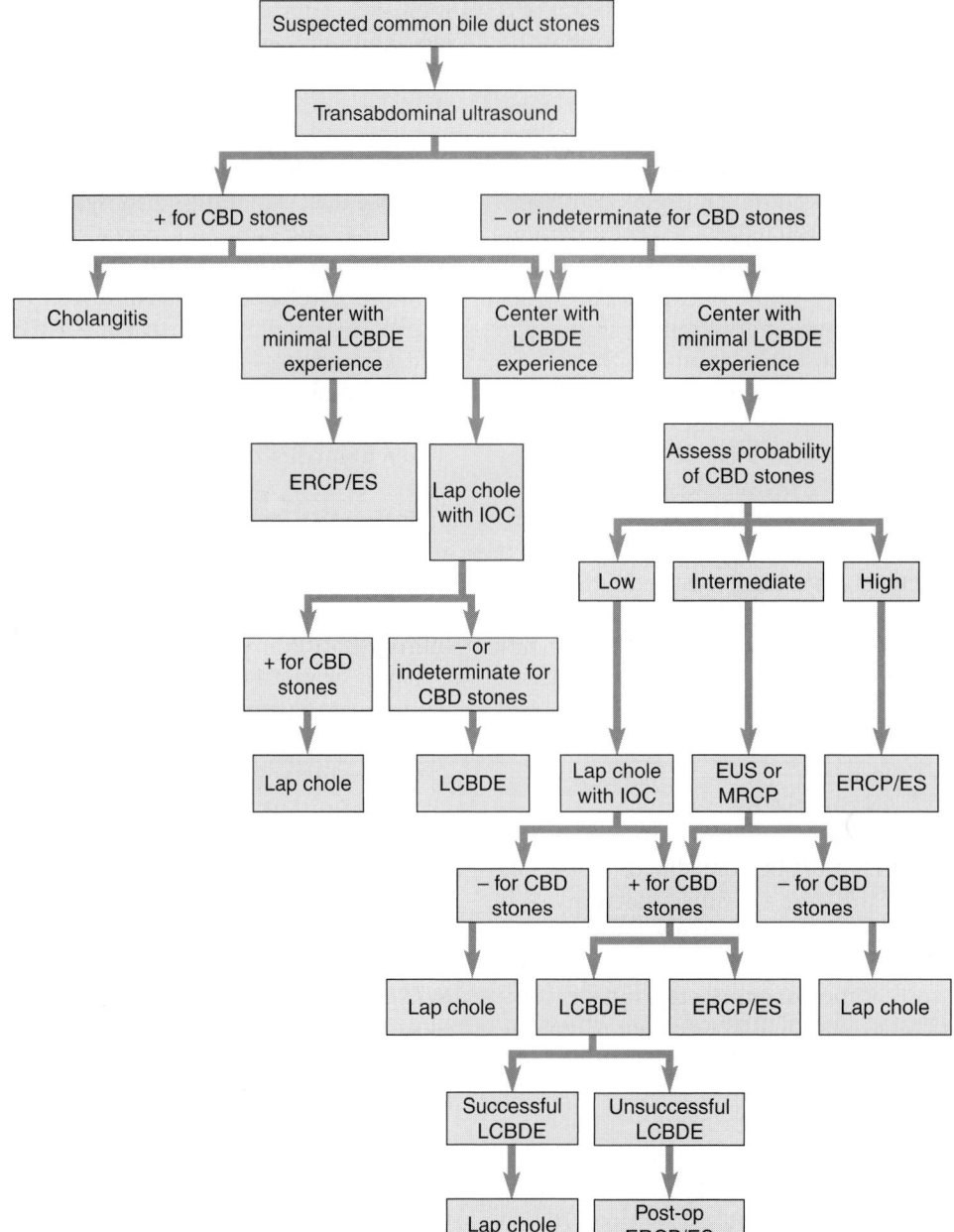

Figure 10-1 *Algorithm for management of common bile duct stones. CBD, common bile duct; ERCP, endoscopic retrograde cholangiopancreatography; ES, endoscopic sphincterotomy; EUS, endoscopic ultrasound; IOC, intraoperative cholangiography; lap chole, laparoscopic cholecystectomy; LCBDE, laparoscopic common bile duct exploration; MRCP, magnetic resonance cholangiopancreatography; postop, postoperative; +, positive; –, negative.*

equal in the two sexes. The incidence of all types of pancreatitis increases with age with a peak incidence in the sixth decade of life. As expected, cholecystectomy dramatically reduces the incidence of gallstone pancreatitis. Morrow et al calculated a decrease from approximately 14 cases of gallstone pancreatitis per 1000 patient years to 1.9 cases per 1000 patient years in those patients who completed cholecystectomy.[138] Gallstone size has also been implicated as a risk factor for the development of gallstone pancreatitis. Diehl et al investigated clinical factors associated with the risk of acute biliary pancreatitis. Multivariant analysis

showed that acute pancreatitis was associated with a stone diameter of less than 5.0 mm and with "mulberry" shaped gallstones.[138]

ETIOLOGY
Although gallstones remain the most common etiology for acute pancreatitis in North America, the exact cause of an acute episode of pancreatitis may not always be obvious on initial presentation. The absence of stones in the gallbladder in a patient with acute pancreatitis does not necessarily rule out a biliary etiology. Approximately 10-20% of gallstone pancreatitis

cases are the result of passage of a single gallstone. Gallbladder imaging will reveal no evidence of stones; however, acute bile duct dilation and elevated liver function testing usually help to make the proper diagnosis. Bile crystals and biliary sludge, which may be too small to be appreciated on standard transabdominal ultrasound, can also lead to acute pancreatitis. These microliths may be the etiology of many cases of previously reported "idiopathic" pancreatitis.[139] It is important to appreciate the other causes of acute pancreatitis when evaluating the patient in extremis. These other etiologies include alcohol, endoscopic retrograde cholangiopancreatography, hyperlipidemia, human immunodeficiency syndrome (HIV) infection, drugs (Table 10-3), viral infections including mumps, coxsackie-b, hepatitis B, CMV, herpes simplex II, and varicella zoster. Certain collagen vascular diseases including systemic lupus erythematosus, rheumatoid arthritis, and Sjogren syndrome may be causative of acute pancreatitis. Hypercalcemia associated with hyperparathyroidism and end-stage renal failure is a known cause, as is blunt or penetrating trauma to the pancreas (including penetrating posterior gastric and duodenal ulcers), and ischemia especially during coronary bypass procedures.

PATHOPHYSIOLOGY

In 1901, the "common channel" theory of gallstone pancreatitis was reported by Opie based on anatomic observations made during autopsy for a patient who suffered from acute pancreatitis requiring operative drainage at the Johns Hopkins University.[140] During the autopsy, a 7-mm-diameter stone was found lodged in the ampulla of Vater at a point that was 7 mm distal to the juncture of the pancreatic duct and common bile ducts. It was theorized that the reflux of bile into

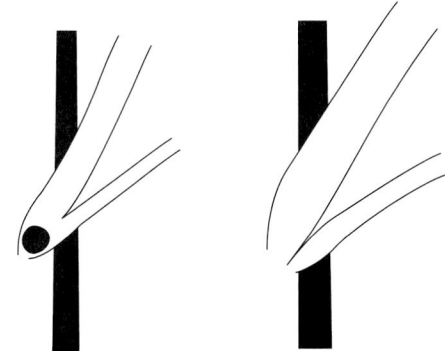

Figure 10-2 *Anatomy of the common channel theory.*

the pancreatic duct via this common channel incited an acute inflammatory process which resulted in the lethal pancreatitis (Fig. 10-2). This was subsequently confirmed in a dog model in which bile was injected directly into the pancreatic duct. More recently, studies have suggested that transient pancreatic duct hypertension without the influence of bile salt contamination may be the major inciting event in acute pancreatitis.[141] This pancreatic duct hypertension is more likely to occur in patients with a common biliopancreatic channel; however; the pancreatic and peripancreatic autodigestion appears to result from the activated secreted pancreatic enzymes: amylase, lipase, and ribonuclease. This can be associated with a local and systemic inflammatory response, which may be further damaging to the pancreas and surrounding organs.

PREOPERATIVE MANAGEMENT

Most patients with acute pancreatitis present with severe epigastric pain, which may radiate to the back. There is often associated nausea, vomiting, and significant abdominal distention. Fever usually develops within the first 48-72 hours. The pain of acute pancreatitis is sudden in onset and may mimic biliary colic or other causes of acute peritonitis (Table 10-4). Approximately 85-95% of patients will experience a mild form of pancreatitis with resolution of symptoms in 3-5 days.

Table 10-3   Drugs Implicated in the Development of Acute Pancreatitis
L-Asparaginase
Azaathioprine
Didanosine (anti-HIV)
Estrogen
Furosemide
Pentamidine
6-Mercaptopurine
Salicylates
Sulfonamide
Sulindac
Vincristine
Vinblastine

Table 10-4   Presentations That May Mimic Acute Pancreatitis
Perforated gastric ulcer
Perforated duodenal ulcer
Acute bowel obstruction with ischemia
Mesenteric ischemia
Acute bacterial peritonitis

A small percentage of patients admitted with acute pancreatitis will evolve into the severe, necrotizing form of the disease. This is usually manifested as persistent tachycardia, tachypnea, and hypotension. Pulmonary complications, including sympathetic effusions, atelectasis, and, in the most severe cases, adult respiratory distress syndrome (ARDS) may accompany patients with severe acute pancreatitis. Inflammatory changes in the lesser sac and retroperitoneum result in a profound ileus as well as third-space fluid accumulation. This results in significant abdominal distention, which in rare cases can produce an abdominal compartment syndrome. Flank edema and scrotal edema signify severe retroperitoneal inflammation. Flank ecchymoses (Grey Turner sign) or periumbilical ecchymoses (Cullen sign) are indicators of retroperitoneal hemorrhage from acute hemorrhagic pancreatitis. Jaundice indicates bile duct obstruction from pancreatic edema or persistent stone obstruction of the biliary tree. The presence of jaundice, fever, and abdominal pain (Charcot triad) is indicative of cholangitis. Early bile duct decompression may benefit patients with this presentation.

LABORATORY FINDINGS

Although most patients will have a marked elevation of amylase and lipase following the acute onset of pancreatitis, the absolute level of amylase elevation does not correlate well with the expected severity of the pancreatitis. In most patients, amylase elevations will resolve within 3 to 5 days following the initial attack. Persistent elevations beyond this time frame are suspicious for more severe ongoing pancreatitis, pancreatic ductal obstruction secondary to ampullary edema or stone impaction, or pseudocyst development. Serum lipase is always elevated with amylase in patients with acute pancreatitis. Isolated amylase elevations without lipase elevations are present in a number of disease states (Table 10-5), which are not associated with acute pancreatitis.

The systemic inflammatory response associated with severe pancreatitis results in serum electrolyte values that are consistent with severe dehydration. Hemoglobin and hematocrit are initially elevated. Blood urea nitrogen (BUN) and creatinine are increased, as well as their ratio. Serum glucose, likewise, can be elevated and is a good indicator of severe pancreatic parenchymal injury and systemic stress.[142]

Mild gallstone pancreatitis is associated with transient elevations of the liver function testing including bilirubin (direct and indirect) as well as the transaminases. These values usually normalize shortly after resolution of the abdominal pain. Persistent elevation of bilirubin, especially within the first 24-48 hours, is usually indicative of an impacted stone in the biliary tree. Mild elevations of the bilirubin are often seen in patients with pancreatic edema causing partial ductal obstruction and usually do not require any decompression unless associated with signs of biliary sepsis.

Severe pancreatitis can be associated with hypertriglyceridemia as well as hypocalcemia and hypoalbuminemia. Hemorrhagic pancreatitis is usually associated with a drop in hemoglobin in spite of significant dehydration. Severe pancreatitis may be associated with a disseminated intravascular coagulation (DIC) syndrome manifested as thrombocytopenia, elevated levels of fibrin split products, and decreased fibrinogen levels.

Measurement of serum C-reactive protein (CRP) has been proposed as a sensitive predictor of pancreatitis severity. CRP values are most useful more than 48 hours following onset of symptoms. The absolute value predictive of severe pancreatitis has varied between numerous studies; however, the Santorini Consensus Conference in 1999 recommended a "cut-off" value of greater than 15 mg/dL as a strong indicator of progression to severe necrotizing pancreatitis.[143]

Serum phospholipase A_2 (PLA_2) is a serum isoenzyme associated with acute pancreatitis. Marked increases in the PLA_2 level are considered to be evidence of systemic inflammation associated with multiple organ failure.[144]

DIAGNOSTIC IMAGING

In acute pancreatitis, the etiology and severity of the pancreatitis is determined by imaging studies performed early in the clinical course. The first imaging study should be an ultrasound of the abdomen to assess for the presence of gallstones and bile duct dilation. Ultrasound offers limited assessment of the pancreatic parenchyma due to surrounding edema and overlying bowel gas in most instances. Two-dimensional imaging with CT scan and MRI allows identification and assessment of the extent of pancreatic necrosis and peripancreatic inflammatory change which is important in determining prognosis.[145,146] Intravenous contrast administration is required to assess the degree of enhancement and estimate the area of necrosis from CT scan evaluation. A small unenhanced area seen during arterial enhancement phase is consistent with edematous pancreatitis, whereas a large unenhanced area is consistent with pancreatic necrosis (Fig. 10-3). Pancreatic necrosis is

Table 10-5   Causes of Isolated Hyperamylasemia
Parotid gland disorders
Perforated peptic ulcer
Esophagopleural fistula
Renal failure
Macroamylasemia
Drugs

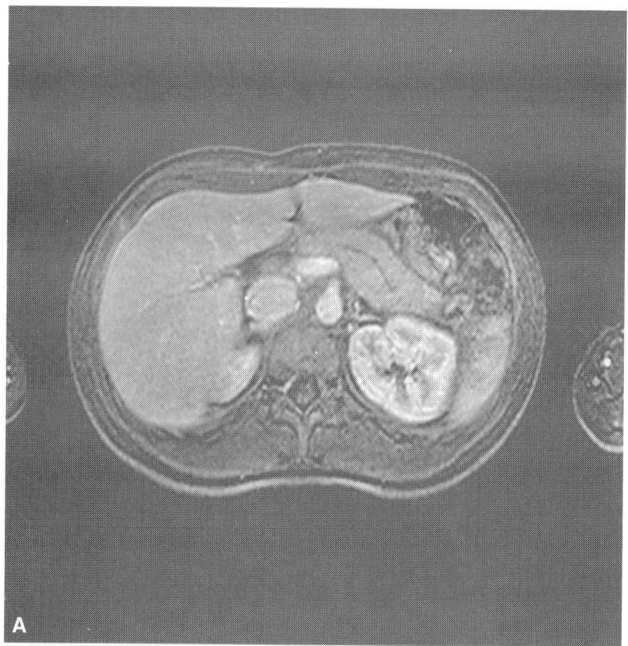

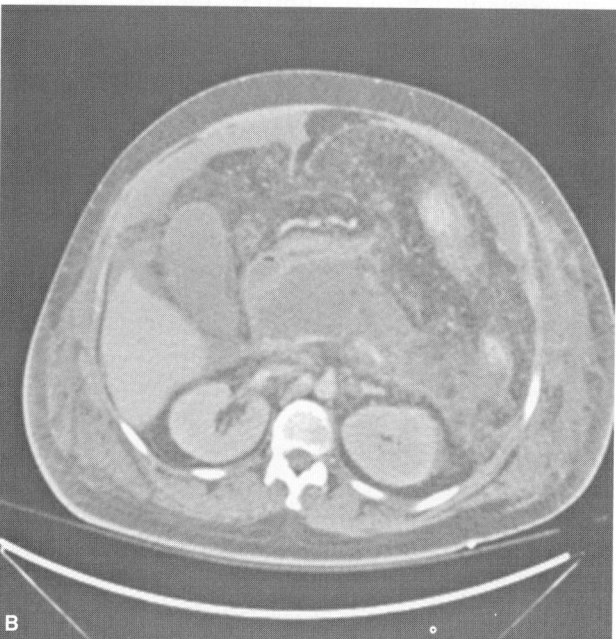

Figure 10-3 *A. Acute edematous pancreatitis. B. Acute necrotizing pancreatitis.*

requires some time to evolve before it is mature enough to be visualized on the most sensitive of imaging studies.

Not all patients are candidates for iodinated contrast dye on admission to the hospital. Severe dehydration and multisystem organ failure make the use of iodinated dyes dangerous in patients who have not been adequately resuscitated or who are progressing rapidly to severe pancreatitis. Recent reports have suggested that the use of intravenous contrast medium may actually exacerbate the underlying pancreatitis. Others have shown that contrast administration has no impact on clinical severity in patients with severe acute pancreatitis.[149,150] Most institutions utilize contrast enhanced CT scan as the initial evaluation for those patients who are felt to be adequately resuscitated and at low risk for renal complication from the administered dye.

Magnetic resonance imaging (MRI) is another useful study to evaluate the severity of acute pancreatitis.[151,152] Gadolinium, which is the contrast agent administered during MRI, has less nephrotoxicity than iodinated CT scan dyes, which makes its use more attractive in patients with contrast dye allergy or renal insufficiency. MRI also allows for assessment of the biliary and pancreatic ductal systems as well as surrounding vasculature. Magnetic resonance cholangiopancreatography (MRCP) has greater than 90% sensitivity in detecting common bile duct stones. This can be particularly helpful in patients with mild acute gallstone pancreatitis in whom assessment of the common bile duct may influence the course of treatment. Historically, patients with mild gallstone pancreatitis in whom liver function testing remained elevated during their hospital course, would be subjected to an endoscopic retrograde cholangiopancreatography (ERCP). This allowed for excellent visualization of the biliary tree as well as extraction of any impacted common bile duct stones. ERCP, however, is associated with significant morbidity (10%) and mortality (0.5-1.0%) and this newer modality of MRCP allows for selection of patients who will truly benefit from the therapeutic advantage of ERCP.[153]

SEVERITY ASSESSMENT OF GALLSTONE PANCREATITIS

Acute pancreatitis of any etiology is determined by two main factors: associated organ failure and the extent of pancreatic necrosis. The severity of the disease as marked by these two indicators allows for the proper selection of medical and surgical care to maximize the chance for recovery. Contrast-enhanced CT scans assesses the degree of pancreatic edema, necrosis, and peripancreatic inflammation. The CT severity index scores pancreatitis severity based on the presence and extent of pancreatic necrosis, and the extent of peripancreatic inflammatory change.[154] Table 10-6 reviews the CT findings associated with each grade of CT-assessed severity.

currently defined as a poorly perfused area with an increase in density after intravenous contrast enhancement of less than 30 Hounsfield units, covering more than 30% of the pancreas or measuring 3.0 cm or more in diameter.[147]

Most centers obtain contrast enhanced CT scan on admission in patients who are deemed adequate candidates to receive an intravenous iodine dye load. Studies have suggested, however, that the greatest sensitivity and specificity for pancreatic necrosis occurs between the 3rd and 10th days of hospital admission for acute pancreatitis.[148] This recommendation is based on the observation that pancreatic necrosis

Table 10-6   Balthazar Computed Tomography (CT) Grading System for Pancreatitis

Grade	CT Findings
A	Normal pancreas
B	Focal or diffuse enlargement of pancreas
C	Inflammation of pancreatic parenchyma and peripancreatic fat
D	One fluid collection
E	Two or more fluid collections

A number of assessment criteria have been put forth over the past 30 years in an attempt to stratify patients according to the severity of their pancreatitis. Ranson identified eleven prognostic indicators which were measured within the first 48 hours of acute pancreatitis. These were further modified to better characterize gallstone pancreatitis (Table 10-7)[155] Another system, the Glasgow score, is based on nine severity assessment criteria and was developed in the United Kingdom in 1978 and subsequently revised to its current form. Both the Ranson and Glasgow scoring systems have a sensitivity of between 70% and 80% for predicting the outcome from acute pancreatitis. One critical drawback is that both require at least 48 hours of disease evolution before their assessment can be complete.[156] The Apache II scoring system is based on 12 findings in the medical examination as well as the presence of chronic complications and age. It has the advantage of assessment of severity within the first 24 hours of pancreatitis. From a practical standpoint, the Apache II system is more complex and less frequently utilized than the Ranson criteria in the United States.

Table 10-7   Ranson Criteria

	Nonbiliary Pancreatitis	Billary Pancreatitis
Admission		
Age	> 55	> 70
WBC (mm^3)	> 16,000	> 18,000
Glucose (mg/dl)	> 200	> 220
LDH (iu/l)	> 350	> 400
AST (fu/l)	> 250	> 250
Within 48 hours		
BUN rise (mg/dl)	> 5	> 2
PaO$_2$ (mm Hg)	< 60	< 60
Serum calcium (mg/dl)	< 8	< 8
Hematocrit decrease (points)	> 10	> 10
Base default (meq/l)	> 4	> 5
Fluid sequestration (liter)	> 6	> 4

AST, Aspirate aminotransferase; *BUN*, blood urea nitrogen; *LDH*, lactate dehydrogenase; *WAC*, white blood cells.

Obesity is related to outcome. Body mass index greater than 30 kg/m squared or more has been associated with higher mortality. This is thought to be the result of respiratory complications from obesity.[157] Gastric intramucosal Ph, which is lowered during rapid reduction of circulating plasma volume, and is therefore an indicator of acute volume loss and circulatory failure, has been shown to be associated with significantly higher mortality when measured within the first 48 hours after admission.[158] Last, the serum concentration of certain molecular markers of inflammation may play a role in early severity assessment in acute pancreatitis. Interleukin VI, interleukin VIII, tumor necrosis factor receptor, ribonuclease, and endothelin-1 are molecular markers, which are being studied to hopefully enable better early severity assessment in all forms of pancreatitis.

OPERATIVE AND NONOPERATIVE MANAGEMENT

The initial treatment for gallstone pancreatitis includes admission to the hospital for fluid resuscitation and pain control. Close monitoring of vital signs and respiratory and cardiovascular support are critical in the early hospital course. Nasogastric tube decompression is only utilized in those patients with severe ileus or recurrent episodes of vomiting. H$_2$ blocker prophylaxis has not been found to be beneficial unless gastric ulceration develops.

Routine laboratory and imaging studies are performed to determine both the etiology and severity of the pancreatitis. Management is then based on the clinical course and severity assessment.

Those patients with mild gallstone pancreatitis (Ranson < 3) usually resolve their acute symptoms within 3-5 hospital days. Once, the acute abdominal pain has resolved, they can be restarted on a low fat diet. This is not predicated on the normalization of pancreatic enzymes, which may take several days longer to reach a normal status.

It is recommended that the gallstone bearing gallbladder be removed on the index admission to prevent any future attacks of pancreatitis. Approximately 25% of patients will experience a recurrent bout of gallstone pancreatitis within 3 months of the initial attack if the stone-bearing gallbladder is not removed. The surgical goal is removal of the gallbladder and evaluation and clearance of the biliary tree. This can be achieved in a number of ways based on availability of expertise in endoscopy and ERCP, surgeon expertise, and hospital resources. We prefer laparoscopic cholecystectomy with intraoperative cholangiogram and, if a stone is suspected, laparoscopic common bile duct exploration usually performed through a transcystic duct approach in patients with a small common bile duct. Larger bile ducts can be addressed by laparoscopic choledochotomy or in those surgeons who are more comfortable with the open approach: open cholecystectomy and common bile duct exploration.

If common bile duct stones are suspected preoperatively due to persistent elevation of liver function testing, or preoperative imaging studies showing stones (ultrasound, CT scan, or MRI), then we prefer preoperative ERCP and stone extraction to clear the duct prior to laparoscopic cholecystectomy.

In cases of severe gallstone pancreatitis (Ranson > 3), early ERCP and stone extraction has been debated. Several randomized controlled prospective studies have failed to conclusively show benefit for early stone extraction in severe pancreatitis.[159-161] The current consensus recommendation is that emergency endoscopic procedures should be performed in those patients who are categorized as moderate to severe pancreatitis with evidence of persistent bile duct obstruction and in cases complicated by cholangitis. In those patients in whom ERCP and duct clearance is unsuccessful, transhepatic cholangio catheter insertion for decompression or, in rare cases, open cholecystectomy and T-tube placement will enable duct decompression.

Patients who progress to severe necrotizing pancreatitis often require an extensive ICU and hospital course. Although mortality is based on the number of affected organ systems, degree of pancreatic necrosis, and infectious complications; the average mortality in this group ranges between 15% and 20%. Cholecystectomy is therefore delayed until clinical resolution of their pancreatitis and associated complications.

Certain patient populations present unique challenges. The elderly or severely debilitated patient may be considered too high-risk for general anesthesia or the stress of cholecystectomy. ERCP and sphincterotomy is protective against pancreatitis and cholangitis from most small stones and may serve as definitive therapy in this high-risk group. The pregnant patient who presents with gallstone pancreatitis will benefit from elective laparoscopic cholecystectomy and intraoperative cholangiography during the second trimester of pregnancy. This can be performed safely utilizing close fetal monitoring, proper patient positioning to avoid vena cava compression by the uterus, and adequate lead shielding of the fetus. Patients who present after the second trimester are usually managed expectantly until cholecystectomy can be performed following delivery of the fetus.

OUTCOMES

Approximately 85-95% of patients with acute gallstone pancreatitis develop only mild, self-limited pancreatitis and are ultimately offered cholecystectomy as definitive treatment. Mortality in this low-risk group ranges between 1% and 3%.[162] In the 10-20% of patients who develop severe acute pancreatitis, mortality remains high. The presence of infection within the necroses raises the mortality to approximately 34% as opposed to 7% mortality in those patients with sterile pancreatic necrosis.[163,164]

Those patients who survive severe pancreatitis will face long recoveries and may be subjected to long-term alterations in glucose control as well as malabsorption issues leading to nutritional challenges. Their initial and long-term management presents a great challenge to physicians and the health care system. Improvements in severity assessment and critical care techniques hopefully will allow us to improve outcomes in the most severe cases of gallstone pancreatitis.

REFERENCES

1. Rigas B, Torosis J, Mcdougall CJ, et al. The circadian rhythm of biliary colic. *J Clin Gastroenterol* 1990;12:409.

2. Festi D, Sottili S, Colecchia A, et al. Clinical manifestations of gallstone disease: evidence from the multicenter Italian study on cholelithiasis (MICOL). *Hepatology* 1999;30:839.

3. Ko CW, Sekijima JH, Lee SP. Biliary sludge. *Ann Intern Med* 1999;130:301-311.

4. Conrad MR, Janes JO, Dietchy J. Significance of low level echoes within gallbladder. *AJR AM J Roentgenol* 1979;132:967

5. Shea JA, Berlin JA, Escarce JJ, et al. Revised estimates of diagnostic test sensitivity and specificity in suspected biliary tract disease. *Arch Inten Med* 1994;154:2573

6. Barakos JA, Ralls PW, Lapin SA, et al. Cholelithiasis: evaluation with CT. *Radiology* 1987;162:415

7. Altun E, Semelka RC, Elias J, et al. Acute cholecystitis: MR findings and differentiation from chronic cholecystitis. *Radiology* 2007;244:174-183.

8. Browning J, Horton J. Gallstone disease and its complications. *Seminars in Gastrointest* Dis. 2003; 14:165-177.

9. Thompson, DR. Narcotic analgesic effects on the sphincter of Oddi: a review of the data and therapeutic implications in treating pancreatitis. *Am J Gastroenterol* 2001;96:1266.

10. Goldman G, Kahn PJ, Alon R, et al. Biliary colic treatment and acute cholecystitis prevention by prostaglandin inhibitor. *Dig Dis Sci* 1989;34:809-811.

11. Bernard, HR, Hartman TW.Complications after laparoscopic cholecystectomy. *AM J Surg* 1993;165:533.

12. Salman B, Yuksel O, Irkorucu O, et al. Urgent laparoscopic cholecystectomy is the best management for biliary colic. A prospective randomized study of 75 cases. *Dig Surg* 2005;22: 95-99.

13. Lawrentschuk N, Hewitt PM, Pritchard MG. Elective laparoscopic cholecystectomy: Implications of prolonged waiting times for surgery. *ANZ J Surg* 2003;73:890-893.

14. Rutledge D, Jones D, Rege R. Consequences of delay in surgical treatment of biliary disease. *Am J Surg* 2000;180: 466-469.

15. Venneman NG, van Erpecum KJ. Gallstone disease: primary and secondary prevention. *Best Practice & Research Clin Gastroenterol* 2006;20:1063-1073.

16. Thistle JL, Cleary PA, Lachin JM, et al. The natural history of cholelithiasis: the National Cooperative Gallstone Study. *Ann Inter Med* 1984;101:171.

17. Csendes A, Burdiles P, Maluenda F, et al. Simultaneous bacteriologic assessment of bile from gallbladder and common bile duct in control subjects and patients with gallstones and common duct stones. *Arch Surg* 1996;131:389.

18. Den-Hoed PT, Boelhouwer RU, Veen HF, et al. Infectious and bacteriologic data after laparoscopic and open gallbladder surgery. *J Hosp Infection* 1999;39: 27-37.

19. Sheth KR, Pappas TN. Operative management of cholecystitis and cholelithiasis. In Yeo CJ (ed) *Shackelford's Surgery of the Alimentary Tract* (6th ed), Vol 2. Philadelphia, PA: Saunders; 2007:1473-1481.

20. Ralls PW, Colletti PM, Lapin SA. Real-time sonography in suspected acute cholecystitis. *Radiology* 1985;155:767-771

21. Kanafani ZA, Khalife N, Kanj SS, et al. Antibiotic use in acute cholecystitis: practice patterns in the absence of evidence-based guidelines. *J of Infec* 2005;51:128-134.

22. Posther KE, Pappas TN. Acute Cholecystitis. In Cameron JL (ed) *Current Surgical Therapy* (8th ed). Philadelphia, PA: Mosby;2004:385-391.

23. Johansson M, Thune A, Nelvin L,et al. Randomized clinical trial of open versus laparoscopic cholecystectomy in the treatment of acute cholecystitis. *Br J Surg* 2005;92(1):44-49.

24. Eldar S, Sabo E, Nash E, et al. Laparoscopic versus open cholecystectomy in acute cholecystitis. *Surg Laparosc Endosc* 1997;7:407-414.

25. Kiviluoto T, Siren J, Luukkonen P, et al. Randomised trial of laparoscopic versus open cholecystectomy for acute and gangrenous cholecystitis. *Lancet* 1998;351: 321-325.

26. Schledeck THK, Schulte T, Gunarsson R, et al. Laparoscopic cholecystectomy in acute cholecystitis. *Minim Invasive Chirurg* 1997;6:48-51.

27. Papi C, Catarci M, D'Ambrosio, et al. Timing of cholecystectomy for acute calculous cholecystitis;a meta-analysis. *Am J Gastroenterol* 2004;99:147-155.

28. Shikata S, Noguchi Y, Fukui T. Early versus delayed cholecystectomy for acute cholecystitis: a meta-analysis of randomized controlled trials. *Surgery Today* 2005;35(7): 553-560.

29. Lo CM, Liu CL, Fan ST, et al. Prospective randomized study of early versus delayed laparoscopic cholecystectomy for acute cholecystitis. *Ann Surg* 1998;227:461.

30. Lai P, Kwong K, Leung K, et al. Randomized trial of early versus delayed laparoscopic cholecystectomy for acute cholecystitis. *Br J Surg.* 1998;85:764.

31. Tzovaras G, Zacharoulis D, Paraskevi L, et al. Timing of laparoscopic cholecystectomy for acute cholecystitis: A prospective non randomized study. *World J Gastroenterol* 2006;12(34):5528-5531.

32. Stevens KA, Chi A, Lucas LC, et al. Immediate laparoscopic cholecystectomy for acute cholecystitis: No need to wait. *Am J Surg* 2006;192:756-761.

33. Lau H, Lo CY, Patil NG, et al. Early versus delayed-interval laparoscopic cholecystectomy for acute cholecystitis. *Surg Endos* 2006;20:82-87

34. Soffer D, Blackbourne LH, Schulman CI, et al. Is there an optimal time for laparoscopic cholecystectomy in acute cholecystitis? *Surg Endosc* 2007;21:805-809.

35. Gurusamy KS, Samraj K. Early versus delayed laparoscopic cholecystectomy for acute cholecystitis. *Cochrane Database of Systematic Reviews* 2006; 4: Art No. CD005440.

36. Byrne MF, Suhocki P, Mitchell RM, et al. Percutaneous cholecystectomy in patients with acute cholecystitis: Experience of 45 patients at a U.S. referral center. *J Am Coll Surg* 2003;197:206-211.

37. Patel M, Miedema BW, James MA, et al. Percutaneous cholecystectomy is an effective treatment for high-risk patients with acute cholecystitis. *Am Surg* 2000: 66:33-37.

38. Davis CA, Landercasper j, Gundersen LH, et al. Effective use of percutaneous cholecystostomy in high-risk surgical patients: techniques, tube management, and results. *Arch Surg* 1999;134:727.

39. Teoh WM, Cade RJ, Banting SW, et al. Percutaneous Cholecystostomy in the management of acute cholecystitis. *ANZ J Surg* 2005: 75:396-398.

40. Hatjidakis AA, Karampekios S, Prassopoulos P, et al. Maturation of the tract after percutaneous cholecystostomy with regard to the access route. *Cardiovasc Intervent Radiol* 1998;21:36-40.

41. Berber et al. Selective use of tube cholecystectomy withinterval laparoscopic cholecystectomy in acute cholecystitis. *Arch Surg* 2000;135: 341

42. McLoughlin RF, Patterson EJ, Mathieson JR, et al. Radiologically guided percutaneous cholecystostomy for acute cholecystitis: long term outcome in 50 patients. *Can Assoc Radiol J* 1984;45:455-459.

43. Spira RM, Nissan A, Zamir O, et al. Percutaneous transhepatic cholecystostomy and delayed laparoscopic cholecystectomy in critically ill patients with acute calculus cholecystitis. *Am J Surg* 2002;183:62-66.

44. Garcia-sancho TL, et al. Acute emphysematous cholecystitis: report of twenty cases. *Hepatogastroenterology* 1999;46:2144.

45. Helou H, Gadacz TR. Gallstone Ileus. In: Cameron JL (ed) *Current Surgical Therapy* (8th ed). Philadelphia, PA: Mosby;2004:426-428.

46. Reisner RM, Cohen JR. Gallstone ileus: a review of 1001 reported cases. *Am Surg* 1994;60:441.

47. Rodriguez-Sanjuan JC, et al. Cholecystectomy and fistula closure versus enterolithotomy alone in gallstone ileus. *Br J Surg* 1997;82(supp 1): 634.

48. Allen JW. Totally laparoscopic management of gallstone ileus. *Surg Endosc* 2003;17:352.

49. Soto DJ. Laparoscopic management of gallstone ileus. *JSLS* 2001;5:279.

50. Wang AJ, Wang TE, Lin CC, et al. Clinical predictors of severe gallbladder complications in acute acalculous cholecystitis. *World J Gastroenterol* 2003;9:2821.

51. Ryu JK, Ryu KH, Kim KH. Clinical features of acute acalculous cholecystitis. *J Clin Gastroenterology* 2003;36:166.

52. Molenat F, Boussuges A, Valantin V, et al. Gallbladder abnormalities in the medical ICU patients: An ultrasonographic study. *Intensive Care Med* 1996;22:356.

53. Yang HK, Hodgson WJ. Laparoscopic cholecystectomy for acute acalculous cholecystitis. *Surg Endosc* 1996;10:673.

54. Sugiyama M, Tokuhara M, Atomi Y. Is percutaneous cholecystostomy the optimal treatment for acute cholecystitis in the very elderly? *World J Surg* 1998;22:459.

55. Huibregtse, K, van Amerongen, R, van Deventer, SJ. Drainage of the gallbladder in patients with acute acalculous cholecystitis by transpapillary endoscopic cholecystoxeransis. *Gastrointest Endosc* 1994;40:523.

56. Kjaer DW, Kruse A, Frunch-Jensen P. Endoscopic gallbladder drainage of patients with acute cholecystitis. *Endoscopy* 2007;39:304-308.

57. Assalia A, Kopelman D, Hashmonai M. Emergency minilaparotomy cholecystectomy for acute cholecystitis: prospective randomized trial—implications for the laparoscopic era. *World J Surg* 1997;21(5):534-539.

58. Roslyn JJ, Binns GS, Hughes EX, et al. Open cholecystectomy: A contemporary analysis of 42,474 patients. *Ann Surg* 1993;218: 219-229.

59. Sandha GS, Bourke MJ, Haber GB, et al. Endoscopic therapy for bile leak based on new classification: Results in 207 patients. *Gastrointest Endosc* 2004; 60: 567-574.

60. Douglas PR, Ham JM. Partial cholecystectomy. *ANZ J Surg* 1990;60:595-597.

61. Soleimani M, Mehrabi A, Mood ZA, et al. Partial cholecystectomy as a safe and viable option in the emergency treatment of complex acute cholecystitis: A case series and review of the literature. *Am Surg* 2007;73: 498-507.

62. Lee KT, Shan YS, Wang ST, et al. Verres needle decompression of distended gallbladder to facilitate laparoscopic cholecystectomy in acute cholecystitis: a prospective study. *Hepato-Gastroenterology* 2005;52(65): 1388-1392.

63. Madan A, Aliabadi-Wahle S, Tesi D, et al. How early is early in laparoscopic treatment of acute cholecystitis? *Am J Surg* 2002;183:232-236.

64. Bhattacharya D, Senapati PSP, Hurle R, et al. Urgent versus interval laparoscopic cholecystectomy for acute cholecystitis: a comparativestudy. *J Hepatobiliary Pancreat Surg* 2002;9:538-542.

65. Kolla SB, Aggrawal S, Kumar A, et al. Early vs delayed laparoscopic cholecystectomy for acute cholecystitis. *Surg Endosc* 2004;18:1323-1327.

66. Eldar S, Eitan A, Bickel A, et al. The impact of patient delay and physician delay on the outcome of laparoscopic cholecystectomy for acute cholecystitis. *Am J Surg* 1999;178:303-307.

67. Kum CK, Goh PM, Isaac JR, et al. Laparoscopic cholecystectomy for acute cholecystitis. *Br J Surg* 1994;81:1651-1654.

68. Rattner DW, Ferguson C, Warshaw AL. Factors associated with successful laparoscopic cholecystectomy for acute cholecystitis. *Ann Surg* 1993;217:233-236.

69. Rosen M, Brody F, Ponsky J. Predictive factors for conversion of laparoscopic cholecystectomy. *Am J Surg* 2002;184:254-258.

70. Lu EJ, Curet MJ, El-Sayed YY, et al. Medical versus surgical management of biliary tract disease in pregnancy. *Am J Surg* 2004;188:755-759.

71. Basso L, McCollum P, Darling M, et al. A study of cholelithiasis during pregnancy and its relationship with age, parity, menarche, breastfeeding, dysmenorrhea, oral contraception and a maternal history of cholelithiasis. *Gynecol Obstet* 1992;175:41-46.

72. Behar J. Clinical aspects of gallbladder motor function and dysfunction. *Curr Gastroenterol Rep* 1999;1:91-94.

73. Hiatt JR, Hiatt JC, Williams RA, et al. Biliary disease in pregnancy: strategy for surgical management. *Am J Surg* 1986;151:263-5.

74. Swisher S, Schmidt P, Hunt K, et al. Biliary disease during pregnancy. *Am J Surg* 1994;168:576-579.

75. Cosenza CA, Saffari B, Jabbour N, et al. Surgical management of biliary gallstone disease during pregnancy. *Am J Surg* 1999;178:545-548.

76. Scott LD. Gallstone disease and pancreatitis in pregnancy. *Gastroenterol Clin North Am* 1992;21: 803-815.

77. Curet MJ. Special problems in laparoscopic surgery: previous abdominal surgery, obesity, and pregnancy. *Surg Clin North Am* 2000;80: 1093-1110.

78. Eichenberg BJ, Vanderlinden J, Miguel C et al. Laparoscopic cholecystectomy in the third trimester of pregnancy. Am Surg 1996;62:874-877.

79. Liberman MA, Phillips EH, Carroll B et al. Management of choledocholithiasis during pregnancy: A new protocol in the laparoscopic era. *J Laparoendosc Surg* 1995;5:399-403.

80. Wilson RB, McKenzie RJ, Fisher JW. Laparoscopic cholecystectomy in pregnancy: Two case reports. *Aust NZ J Surg* 1994;64:647-649.

81. Hungness, ES, Soper, NJ. Management of common bile duct stones. In: Yeo CJ, Dempsey DT, Klein AS, Pemberton JH, Peters JH (eds) *Shackelford's Surgery of the Alimentary Tract*. Philadelphia, PA: Saunders; 2007: 1590-1596.

82. Halpin VJ, Soper NJ. The Management of Common Bile Duct Stones. In: Cameron JL (ed) *Current Surgical Therapy*. Philadelphia, PA: Mosby, pp 435-440, 2001.

83. Murison MS, Gartell PC, McGinn FP. Does selective preoperative cholangiography result in missed common bile duct stones? *J R Coll Surg Edinb* 38:220-224, 1993.

84. Rosseland AR, Glomsaker TB. Asymptomatic common bile duct stones. *Eur J Gastroenterol Hepatol* 12: 1171-1173,2000.

85. Lipsett PA, Pitt HA. Acute cholangitis. *Surg Clin North Am* 1990;70:1297.

86. Sawyer RG, Jones RS. Acute Cholangitis. In: Cameron JL (ed): *Current Surgical Therapy*. Philadelphia, PA: Mosby; 2004:407-410.

87. Scott MA, Farrands PA, Guyer PB et al. Ultrasound of the common bile duct in patients undergoing cholecystectomy. *J Clin Ultrasound* 1991;19(2):73-76.

88. Suiyama M, Atomi Y. Endoscopic ultrasonography for diagnosing choledocholithiasis: a prospective comparative study with ultrasonography and computed tomography. *Gastrointest Endosc* 1997;45(2): 143-146.

89. Amouyal P, Amouyal G, Levy P et al. Diagnosis of choledocholithiasis by endoscopic ultrasonography. *Gastroenterology* 1994;106:1062-1067.

90. Jeffrey RB, Federle MP, Laing FC et al. Computed tomography of choledochlithiasis. *Am J Roentgenol* 1983;140:1179-1183.

91. Baron RL, Stanley RJ, Lee JK et al. Computed tomographic features of biliary obstruction. *Am J Roentgenol* 1983;140:1173-1178.

92. Soto JA, Alvarez O, Munera F et al. Diagnosing bile duct stones: comparison of unenhanced helical CT, oral contrast enhanced CT cholangiograpjy, and MR cholangiography. *Am J Roentgenol* 2000;175: 1127-1134.

93. Reinhold C, Taourel P, Bret PM, et al. Choledocholithiasis: evaluation of MR cholangiography for diagnosis. *Radiology* 1998;209:435-432.

94. Chan YL, Chan AC, Lam WW, et al. Choledocholithiasis: comparison of MR cholangiography and endoscopic retrograde cholangiography. *Radiology* 1996;200:85-89.

95. Varghese JC, Liddell RP, Farrell MA, et al. Diagnostic accuracy of magnetic resonance cholangiopancreatography and ultrasound compared with direct cholangiography in the detection of choledocholithiasis. *Clin Radiol* 2000;55:25-35.

96. Boraschi P, Neri E, Braccini G, et al. Choledocholithiasis: diagnostic accuracy of MR cholangiopancreatography, three year experience. *Magn Reson Imaging* 1999;17:1245-1253.

97. NIH state of the science statement on endoscopic retrograde cholangiopancreatography (ERCP) for diagnosis an therapy. *NIH Consens State Sci Statements* 2002;19(1):1-26.

98. Christensen M, Matzen P, Schulze S, Rosenberg J. Complications of ERCP: A prospective study. *Gastrointest Endosc* 2004;60:721.

99. Prasad SR, Sahani D, Saini S. Clinical applications of magnetic resonance cholangiopancreatography. *J Clin Gastroenterol* 2001;33(5):362-366.

100. Laokpessi A, Bouillet P, Sauteereau D, et al. Value of magnetic resonance cholagiography in the preoperative diagnosis of common bile duct stones. *Am J Gastroenterol* 2001;96(8):2354-2359.

101. Frey CF, Burbige EJ, Meinke WB et al. Endoscopic retrograde cholangiopancreatography. *Am J Surg* 1982;144(1):109-114.

102. Nataly Y, Merrie AE, Stewart ID. Selective use of preoperative endoscopic retrograde cholangiopancreatography in the era of laparoscopic cholecystectomy. *ANZ J Surg* 2002;72:186.

103. Lakatos L, Mester G, Reti G, et al. Selection creiteria for preoperative endoscopic retrograde cholangiopancreatography before laparoscopic cholecystectomy and endoscopic treatment of bile duct stones: Results of a retrospective, single-center study between 1996-2002. *World J Gastroenterol* 2004;10:3495.

104. Buscarini E, Tansini P, Vallisa D, et al. EUS for suspected choledocholithiasis: do benefits outweigh costs? A prospective, controlled study. *Gastrointest Endosc* 1998;57(4):439-448.

105. Canto MI, Chak A, Stellato T et al. Endoscopic retrograde cholangiopancreatography and laparoscopic cholecystectomy. *Am J Surg* 1993;165(4): 474-478.

106. Fried GM, Feldman LS, Klassen DR. Cholecystectomy and common bile duct sexploration. In ACS Surgery: Principles and Practice, New York, NY: WebMD Professional Publishing; 2005: 1-22.

107. Fan S, Lai EC, Mok FP, et al. Early treatment of acute biliary pancreatitis by endoscopic papillotomy. *N Engl J Med* 1993;328:228.

108. Griniatsos J, Darvounis E, Isla AM. Limitations of fluoroscopic intraoperative cholangiography in cases suggestive of choledocholithiasis. *J Laparoendo and Adv Surg Tech* 2005;15(3): 312-317.

109. Tranter SE, Thompson MH. A prospective single-blinded controlled study comparing laparoscopic ultrasound of the common bile duct with operative cholangiogram. *Surg Endosc* 2003;17:216.

110. Stiegmann GV, McIntyre RC, Pearlman NW, et al. Laparoscopic intracorporeal ultrasound: An alternative to cholagiography? *Surg Endosc* 1994;8:167.

111. Caddy GR, Tham TCK. Symptoms, diagnosis, and endoscopic management of common bile duct stones. *Best Practice and Research Clin Gastro* 2006;20(6): 1085-1101.

112. Petelin JB, Pruett CS: Common bile duct stones. In Cameron JL (ed): *Current Surgical Therapy*. Philadelphia: Mosby; 2004: 392-399.

113. Tai CK, Tang CN, Ha JP, et al. Laparoscopic exploration of common bile duct in difficult choledocholithiasis. *Surg Endosc* 2004;18:910.

114. Hutter MM, Rattner DW. Open common bile duct exploration: when is it indicated? In Cameron JL (ed): *Current Surgical Therapy*. 2004, 8th edition. Philadelphia: Mosby:403-407.

115. Vazquez-Inglesias JL, Gonzalez-Conde B, Lopez-Roses L, et al. Endoscopic spincterotomy for prevention of the recurrence of acute biliary pancreatitis in patents with gallbladder in situ. *Surg Endosc* 2004;18:1442.

116. Schreurs WH, Vles WJ, Stuifbergen WH, et al. Endoscopic management of common bile duct stones leaving the gallbladder in situ: a cohort study with long term follow up. *Dig Surg* 2004;21:60.

117. Phillips EH, Carroll BJ, Pearlstein AR, et al. Laparoscopic choledochoscopy and extraction of common bile duct stones. *World J Surg* 1993; 17:22-28.

118. De Paula AL, Shashiba K, Bafutto M. Laparoscopic management of chledocholithiasis. *Surg Endosc* 1994;8:1399-1403.

119. Petelin J: Laparoscopic approach to common bile duct pathology. *Surg Laparosc Endosc* 1991;1:33-41.

120. Cuschieri A, Lezoche E, Morino M, et al. E.A.E.S. multicenter prospective randomized trial comparing two-stage versus single stage management of patients with gallstone disease and ductal calculi. *Surg Endosc* 1999;13:952.

121. Schroeppel TJ, Lambert PJ, Mathiason MA, et al. An economic analysis of hospital charges for choledocholithiasis by different treatment strategies. *Amer Surg* 2007;73:472-477.

122. Appel S, Krebs H, Fern D: Techniques for laparoscopic cholangiography and removal of common duct stones. *Surg Endosc* 1992;6:134-137.

123. Collins C, Maquire D, Ireland A, et al. A prospective study of common bile duct calculi in patients undergoing laparoscopic cholecystectomy: Natural history of choledocholithiasis. *Ann Surg* 2004;239:28.

124. Petelin JB: Laparoscopic common bile duct exploration. *Surg Endosc* 2003;17,1705-1715.

125. Isla AM, Griniatsos J, Karvounis E, et al. Advantages of laparoscopic stented choledochorrhaphy over T-tube placement. *Br J Surg* 2004;91:862.

126. Ha JP, Tang CN, Siu WT, et al. Primary closure versus T-tube drainage after laparoscopic choledochotomy for common bile duct stones. *Hepatogastroenterology* 2004;51:1605.

127. Rojas-Ortega S, Arizpe-Bravo D, Marin Lopez ER, et al. Transcystic common bile duct exploration in the management of patients with choledocholithiasis. *J Gastrointest Surg* 2003;7:492.

128. Thompson MH, Tranter SE. All-comers policy for laparoscopic exploration of the common bile duct. *Br J Surg* 2002;89:1608.

129. DePaula AL, Hashiba K, Bafutto M, et al. Laparoscopic antegrade sphincterotomy. *Surg Laparosc Endosc* 1993;3:157-160.

130. Rhodes M, Sussman L, Cohen L, et al. Randomized trial of laparoscopic exploration of common bile duct versus postoperative endoscopic retrograde cholangiography for common bile duct stones. *Lancet* 1998;351:159.

131. Tranter SE, Thompson MH. Comparison of endoscopic sphincterotomy and laparoscopic exploration of the common bile duct. *Br J Surg* 2002;89:1495.

132. Deslandres E, Gagner M, Pomp A. Intraoperative endoscopic sphincterotomy for common bile duct stones during laparoscopic cholecystectomy. *Gastrointest Endosc* 1993;39:54.

133. Foster PE, Traverso LW. Acute cholangitis. The management of common bile duct stones. In: Cameron JL (ed). *Current Surgical Therapy.* Philadelphia, PA: 2001;450-454.

134. Lai ECS, Mok FPT, Tan ESY, et al. Endoscopic biliary drainage for severe acute cholangitis. *N Eng J Med* 1992;326:1582.

135. Leung JWC, Chung SCS, Sung JJY et al. Urgent endoscopic drainage for acute suppurative cholangitis. *Lancet* 1989;1:1307.

136. Yadav D and Lowenfels AB. Trends in the epidemilogy of the first attack of acute pancreatitis: A systematic review. *Pancreas* 2006;33:323-330.

137. Morrow JA, Zinsmeister AR, Melton L III, DiMagno EP. Gallstone pancreatitis and the effect of cholecystectomy: A population based cohort study. *Mayo Clinic Proceedings* 1988;63: 466-473.

138. Diehl AK, Holleman DJ, Chapman JB, Schwesinger WH, Kurtin WE. Gallstone size and risk of pancreatitis. *Arch Intern Med* 1997;157:1674-1678.

139. Lee SP, Nicholls JF, Park HZ. Biliary sludge as a cause of acute pancreatitis. *NEJM* 1992;326:589.

140. Opie EL. The etiology of acute hemorrhagic pancreatitis. *Bull Johns Hopkins Hospital* 1901;12:182-192.

141. Lerch MM, Saluja AK, Runzi M, et al. Pancreatic duct obstruction triggers acute necrotizing pancreatitis in the opossum. *Gastroenterology* 1993;104:853-861.

142. Rajaratnam SG and Martin IG. Admission serum glucose level: an accurate predictor of outcome in gallstone pancreatitis. *Pancreas* 2006;33:27-30.

143. Dervenis C, Johnson CD, Bassi C, et al. Diagnosis, objective assessment of severity, and management of acute pancreatitis. Santorini Consensus Conference. *International J of Pancreatology* 1999;25:195-210.

144. Hietaranta A, Kemppainen E, Puolakkainen P, et al. Extracellular phospholipase A_2 in relation to systemic inflammatory response (SIRS) and systemic complications in severe acute pancreatitis. *Pancreas* 1999;18:385-391.

145. Kemppainen E, Sainio V, Haapiainen R, et al. Early localization of necrosis by contrast enhanced computed tomography can predict outcome in severe acute pancreatitis. *Br J Surg* 1996;83: 924-9.

146. Bradley EL III. Prediction of pancreatic necrosis by dynamic pancreatography. *Ann Surg* 1989;210: 495-503.

147. Bradley EL III. Clinically based classification system for acute pancreatitis. Summary of the International Symposium on Acute Pancreatitis, Atlanta, Georgia, September 11-13, 1992. *Arch Surg* 1992;128:586-590.

148. Brit Soc of Gastroenterology. United Kingdom guidelines for the management of acute pancreatitis. *GUT* 1998;42: S1-S13.

149. Carmona-Sanchez R, Uscanga L, Bezaury-Rivas P, et al. Potential harmful effects of iodinated intravenous contrast medium on the clinical course of mild acute pancreatitis. *Arch Surg* 2000;135:1280-1284.

150. Hwang TL, Chang KY, Ho YP. Contrast-enhanced dynamic computed tomography does not aggravate the clinical severity of patients with severe acute pancreatitis: Re-evaluation of the effect of intravenous contrast medium on the severity of acute pancreatitis. *Arch Surg* 2000;135:287-290.

151. Arvanitakis M, Delhaye M, DeMaetelaere V, et al. Computed tomography and magnetic resonance imaging in the assessment of acute pancreatitis. *Gastroenterology* 2004;126:715-723.

152. Ward J, Chalmers AG, Guthrie AJ, et al. T2-weighted and dynamic enhanced MRI in acute pancreatitis: Comparison with contrast enhanced CT. *Clin Radiol* 1997;52:109-114.

153. Liu TH, et al. The efficacy of magnetic resonance cholangiography for the evaluation of patients with suspected choledocholithiasis before laparoscopic cholecystectomy. *Am J Surg* 178: 480, 1999.

154. Balthazar EJ, Robinson DL, Megibow AJ, et al. Acute pancreatitis: Value of CT in establishing prognosis. *Radiology* 1990;174: 331-6.

155. Ranson JH. Etiological and prognostic factors in human acute pancreatitis: A review. *Am J Gastroenterol* 1998;77: 633-8.

156. Leese T, Shaw D. Comparison of three Glasgow multi-factor prognostic scoring systems in acute pancreatitis. *Br J Surg* 1988;75:460-462.

157. Porter KA, Banks PA. Obesity as a predictor of severity in acute pancreatitis. *Int J Pancreatol* 1991;10: 247-52.

158. Hynninen M, Valtonon M, Markkanen H, et al. Intramucosal Ph and cytokine release in severe acute pancreatitis. *Shock* 2000;13: 79-82.

159. Neoptolemos JP, Carr-Locke DL, London NJ, et al. Controlled trial of urgent endoscopic retrograde cholangiopancreatography and endoscopic sphincterotomy versus conservative treatment for acute pancreatitis due to gallstones. *Lancet* 1988; 2;979-983.

160. Folsch OR, Nitesche R, Ludtke R, et al. Early ERCP and papillotomy compared with conservative treatment for

acute biliary pancreatitis. The German Study Group on Acute Pancreatitis. *N Engl J Med* 1997;336;237-242.

161. Fan ST, Lai CS, Mok FP, et al: Early treatment of acute biliary pancreatitis by endoscopic papillotomy. *N Engl J Med* 1993;328:228-232.

162. Gullo L, Migiliori M, Olah A, et al. Acute pancreatitis in five European countries: Etiology and mortality. *Pancreas* 2002;24(3):223-227.

163. Banks PA, Gerzof SG, Langevin RE, Silverman SG, Sica GT, Hughes MD. CT guided aspiration of suspected pancreatic infection: Bacteriology and clinical outcome. *Int J Pancreatol* 1995;18(3);265-70.

164. Allordyce DB. Incidence of necrotizing pancreatitis and factors related to mortality. *Am J Surg* 1987;154(3): 295-299.

Chapter **11**

PANCREATIC EMERGENCY: ACUTE PANCREATITIS

Marc de Moya, MD, and Andrew L. Warshaw, MD

INTRODUCTION

Acute surgical emergencies of the pancreas usually result from complications of severe acute pancreatitis (SAP). This chapter will focus on the acute care surgical approach to SAP and its complications. Complications of chronic pancreatitis, eg, pain, pseudocyst, exocrine, and endocrine dysfunction will not be discussed. The basic tenets of surgical management will be emphasized to guide the acute care surgeon based on the evidence presented. The topics of biliary infections/obstructions will be discussed in the hepatobiliary chapter. A treatment algorithm for acute pancreatitis based on the current literature discussed in this chapter is provided at the end.

EPIDEMIOLOGY

In the United States, approximately 210,000 patients are admitted each year for acute pancreatitis, an incidence of 80/100,000.[1] The United States and Finland have the highest rates of acute pancreatitis. Most cases subside and heal without complication, but 20% of patients with acute pancreatitis progress to the severe form and incur a mortality of up to 30%.[2] The 1992 Atlanta classification was an attempt to standardize the definitions and nomenclature of acute pancreatitis. Since 1992, the understanding of the pathophysiology and natural history of pancreatitis has improved. The Atlanta classification is now under revision and the most current iteration will be used.

It has been recognized that the clinical manifestations of acute pancreatitis can be divided into early and late phases. The morphologic features of severe pancreatitis may not correlate with the clinical presentation, particularly in the early phase. The early manifestations of organ failure are related to the systemic inflammatory response to the tissue injury.

The clinical definition of acute pancreatitis requires two of the following three features: (1) abdominal pain strongly suggestive of acute pancreatitis, (2) serum amylase and/or lipase activity at least three times greater than the upper limit of normal, and (3) characteristic findings of acute pancreatitis on computed tomography (CT scan). If abdominal pain is strongly suggestive of acute pancreatitis, but the serum amylase or lipase activity is less than 3 times the upper limit of normal, characteristic findings of acute pancreatitis on CT scan are required to confirm the diagnosis of acute pancreatitis.

The definition of severe acute pancreatitis (SAP) is persistence of organ failure that exceeds 48 hours' duration. The modified Marshall score and the SOFA score define organ failure (Table 11-1). The acute care surgeon must have an understanding of the pathophysiology and treatment options for acute pancreatitis and its complications.

PREOPERATIVE MANAGEMENT

Pathophysiology

The most common causes of pancreatitis are gallstones and alcohol. Gallstone pancreatitis is most prevalent in Caucasian women over the age of 60 years[3,4] and in patients with small gallstones, or microlithiasis.[4,5] The association between alcohol consumption and pancreatitis is complex and seems to be multifactorial. In an effort to confirm a biliary origin of the pancreatitis serum biochemical markers may also be of use. In a meta-analysis, a threefold or greater increase in alanine aminotransferase had a positive predictive value of 95% in identifying pancreatitis with a biliary etiology.[6] Some other causes include metabolic aberrations (eg, hypertriglyceridemia and hypercalcemia), duct obstruction related to neoplasm (eg, intraductal papillary mucinous tumors) or pancreas divisum, medications (eg, azathioprine, thiazides, and estrogens), and trauma. A recent analysis of the underlying causes of necrotizing pancreatitis at the Massachusetts General Hospital is in Fig. 11-1.

Approximately 10-15% of patients have unknown causes. Recently, genetic polymorphisms have been

Table 11-1a Modified Marshall Scoring System

Organ system	Score				
	0	1	2	3	4
Respiratory (PO$_2$/FIO$_2$)*	> 400	301-400	201-300	101-200	≤ 101
Renal (serum creatinine, μmol/l)*	≤ 134	134-169	170-310	311-439	> 439
Cardiovascular (systolic blood pressure, mm Hg)*	> 90	< 90 Fluid responsive	< 90 Not fluid responsive	< 90, pH < 7.3	< 90, pH < 7.2
Coagulation (platelet count, × 10^3)	> 120	81-120	51-80	21-50	≤ 21
Neurologic (Glasgow coma score)	15	13-14	10-12	6-9	< 6

Table 11-1b SOFA Scoring System

	SOFA Score				
	0	1	2	3	4
Respiration (PO$_2$/FIO$_2$ torr)	> 400	≤ 400	≤ 300	≤ 200 with respiratory support	≤ 100 with respiratory support
Hematologic (platelet count) (× 10^3/mm^3)	> 150	≤ 150	≤ 100	≤ 50	≤ 20
Cardiovascular (hypotension)	No hypotension	MAP < 70 mmHg	Dopamine ≤ 5 or Dobutamine (any dose)	Dopamine > 5 or Epi ≤ 0.1 or Norepi ≤ 0.1	Dopamine > 15 or Epi > 0.1 or Norepi > 0.1
Neurologic (Glasgow coma score)	15	13-14	10-12	6-9	<6
Renal Creatinine (mg/dl) (μmol/l) Or urine output	< 1.2 < 110	1.2-1.9 110-170	2.0-3.4 171-299	3.5-4.9 300-440 Or < 500 ml/day	> 5.0 > 440 Or < 200 ml/day

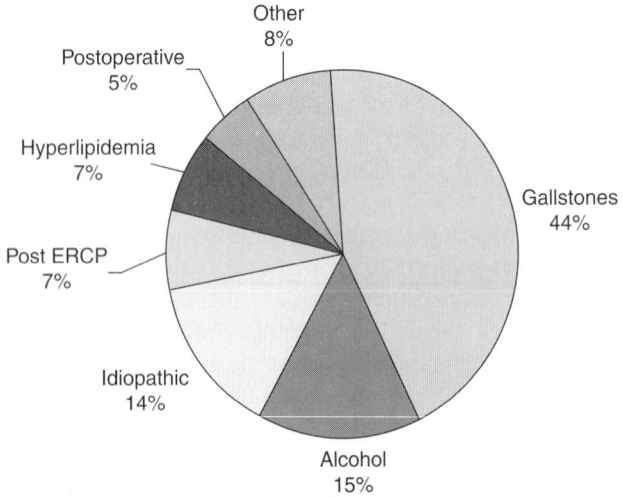

Figure 11-1 *Fifteen-year experience of 2449 patients with acute pancreatitis at Massachusetts General Hospital. ERCP = endoscopic retrograde cholangiopancreatography. (data from reference 60).*

implicated in the etiology of some of these instances. Single point mutations in cationic trypsinogen (PRSS-1), pancreatic secretory trypsin inhibitor (PSTI or SPINK-1), and cystic fibrosis transmembrane conductance regulator (CFTR) have been identified in some patients with recurrent pancreatitis. These polymorphisms are only just beginning to be characterized and may also be implicated in determining the severity of disease, particularly in those with alcohol-induced pancreatitis. The specific underlying cause of the "idiopathic cases" does not currently change treatment.

Acute pancreatitis is usually self-limited; however, in 10-20% of cases, there is a progression to complications. In this severe form, there are varying amounts of necrosis of pancreatic parenchyma and peripancreatic tissues, which, in turn, may become infected. Debridement and drainage may be required to control the damage and promote healing. Mortality in these patients can reach 30%.[7] In the early phase, the morphologic features of necrosis may not be present on the initial imaging. In the absence of these morphologic features, the severity may be underestimated on admission. Therefore, it cannot be overemphasized that continued scrutiny of the patient is warranted until recovery is assured.

The mechanism for the conversion or progression of mild interstitial edematous pancreatitis to necrotizing pancreatitis is not known, but it is now understood that activated pancreatic enzymes are liberated from the damaged acinar cells. The microcirculation of the pancreas is markedly reduced, leading to ischemic as well as enzymatic injury. Distant injury to the lungs, kidneys, and gut are mediated by the circulating activated enzymes, which in turn lead to neutrophil activation, upregulation of adhesion molecules (ICAM-1), chemokine monocyte chemotactic protein 1 (MCP-1), and endothelial injury.

DIAGNOSIS
Classification/Scoring
Acute pancreatitis is a progressive disease that can resolve with simple medical management or may deteriorate into a necrotic, infected, hemorrhagic devastation, necessitating surgical intervention. It is clear that morbidity and mortality rise in relation to degree of necrosis, with up to a 30% mortality in those admitted to an ICU. In our latest series, however, the overall mortality is approximately 12%.

It must be emphasized that although there are a number of scoring systems developed, none replace frequent and careful assessments of patients with acute pancreatitis. The first 72 hours of hospitalization often see a cascade of progressively worsening signs and symptoms requiring advancing levels of care. Scoring systems, however, may offer a more objective method of categorizing patients in an effort to predict outcomes. The currently accepted scoring systems are defined in Table 11-2.

The Atlanta classification and criteria were adopted in 1992 at the International Symposium on Acute Pancreatitis. The presence of any condition in the five main categories indicates SAP.[2] Ranson criteria are based on 11 clinical signs, 5 measured on admission and 6 in the 48 hours afterward.[8] The Acute Physiology and Chronic Health Evaluation (APACHE II) is based on 12 routine physiological measurements, age, and previous health status, with a score of 8 or more indicating SAP.[9,10]

In a study of 49 patients, Matos in 2000 reported that generic measures of disease severity such as the APACHE II or SOFA II scores were superior to disease-specific scoring systems for predicting mortality.[11] In 2002, however, Buter reported that evolution of organ dysfunction is a better predictor of outcome, suggesting that dynamic scores may be a better way of predicting outcomes.[12]

Patients with SAP who meet conventional criteria for ICU admission should in general be admitted to an ICU.[13] However, these criteria do not take into account the additional factors of advanced age, obesity (BMI > 30 kg/m^2), patients requiring ongoing volume resuscitation, and patients with evidence of > 30% pancreatic necrosis. When patients have these additional criteria, consideration should be given to admit to ICU or a step-down setting.

Biomarkers
Biomarkers fall into two categories: diagnostic and prognostic. Those discussed are the most commonly used and those with the most promise.[14]

Diagnostic
Serum amylase level is the most commonly used index for diagnosis of acute pancreatitis. The amylase level rises in the first 12 hours after the onset of symptoms and generally returns to normal in 3-5 days in uncomplicated pancreatitis.[15] However, up to 32% of cases of pancreatitis may have normal amylase levels at presentation as a consequence of timing or exocrine pancreatic insufficiency (underlying chronic pancreatitis), or occasionally because of massive pancreatic necrosis. Markedly elevated triglyceride levels, generally in excess of 2000 mg/dL may competitively interfere with the amylase assay, resulting in a false negative test. If lactescent plasma is present, serial dilutions will improve the accuracy of the test.[16] Hyperamylasemias are also associated with nonpancreatitic conditions as well, including salivary gland inflammation, diminished renal function, intestinal ischemia, and macroamylasemia. Choledocholithiasis may cause marked elevations of serum amylase even in the absence of pancreatitis (pseudopancreatitis). The sensitivity and specificity of elevated amylase if greater than three times normal are 61% and 95%, respectively, for diagnosis of acute pancreatitis.[12]

Serum lipase activity may remain above normal for up to 14 days. Pancreatic lipase production is typically four times greater than amylase and less likely to be affected by chronic pancreatic insufficiency. Lipase, like amylase, may be elevated in other acute abdominal disease states or in the presence of renal insufficiency. High triglyceride levels do not interfere with the assay. Serum lipase activity may be elevated with use of some drugs, including furosemide. With a cutoff of 600 IU/L, most studies report specificities > 95% and sensitivities 55% to 100%.[12]

Prognostic
Serum amylase and lipase are poor predictors of the severity of acute pancreatitis. Serum markers that target the systemic inflammatory response may better predict the extent of the insult. These novel markers include TAP, serum IL6, procalcitonin, polymorphonuclear elastase, serum amyloid A, and C-reactive protein.

The duodenum secretes enterokinase, which cleaves proenzyme trypsinogen to form the active

Table 11-2   Clinical Scoring Systems for Pancreatitis

Atlanta Criteria , 1992	Threshold Value
Ranson score	≥ 3
APACHE II score	≥ 8
Organ failure	
Shock	SBP < 90 mm Hg
Pulmonary insufficiency	$PaO_2 \leq 60$ mm Hg on room air
Renal failure	Creatinine > mg/dl after hydration
Systemic complications	
Disseminated intravascular coagulopathy	PLT $\leq 100,000/mm^3$
	Fibrinogen level of < 1 g/l
	Fibrin split products > 80 µg/ml
Metabolic disturbance	Calcium level of ≤ 7.5 mg/dl
Local complications	
Pancreatic necrosis	Present
Pancreatic abscess	Present
Pancreatic pseudocyst	Present
Ranson Score	SAP indicated by score > 3, with each criteria below counting as 1
At presentation	
Age	> 55 years
Blood glucose level	> 200 mg/dl
White-cell count	$> 16,000/mm^3$
Lactate dehydrogenase level	> 350 IU/l
Alanine aminotransferase level	> 250 IU/l
Within 48 hours	
Hematocrit	> 10% decrease
Serum calcium	< 8 mg/dl
Base deficit	> 4 mEq/l
Blood urea nitrogen	> 5 mg/dl increase
Fluid sequestration	> 6 l
PaO_2	< 60 mm Hg on room air
CT severity index	SAP indicated by ct-grade + necrosis score > 6
CT grade	
Normal pancreas (grade A)	0 points
Focal or diffuse enlargement (grade B)	1 point
Intrinsic change; fat stranding (grade C)	2 points
Single, ill-defined collection of fluid (grade D)	3 points
Multiple collections of fluid or gas in or adjacent to pancreas (grade E)	4 points
Necrosis score	
No pancreatic necrosis	0 points
Necrosis of one-third of pancreas	1 point
Necrosis of one-half of pancreas	4 points
Necrosis of > one-half of pancreas	6 points
APACHE II score	
Initial values of 12 routine physiological measurements, age, and previous health status	SAP is indicated by a score ≥ 8

24-kDa protease trypsin and trypsinogen activation peptide (TAP). TAP is not reabsorbed in the GI tract. A prospective European multicenter study investigated the level of urinary TAP as an early predictor in 176 patients with acute pancreatitis. Twenty percent of those patients had severe pancreatitis. At 24 hours after admission, the negative predictive value of a urinary TAP concentration greater than 35 nmol/l was only marginally better than a serum C-reactive protein level > 150 mg/l for predicting a severe course (89% vs 84%).

They were both similar to the APACHE II score (88%). The sensitivity of urinary TAP was 68%, compared with 63% for APACHE II and 47% for C-reactive protein. Other studies have also concluded that TAP and C-reactive protein have mediocre utility overall as prognostic markers.

Interleukin 6: The proinflammatory cytokine IL6 is one of the main inducers of C-reactive protein synthesis in the liver, and peaks earlier than C-reactive protein. A study of 38 patients with acute pancreatitis (15 with SAP) measured daily IL6, IL8, B2-microglobulin, and C-reactive protein values for 5 days. At 24 hours after admission, the sensitivity of IL6 for detecting SAP was 100% with a specificity of 86% with a cut off concentration of 2.7 ng/l.[17] Other series[18,19] have supported this finding but its use is limited by the complexity of the assay and the fact that its levels decrease rapidly.

Procalcitonin: Procalcitonin is an acute phase reactant that has been investigated extensively as an early marker of severity in SIRS and sepsis.[20] One study specifically employed a semiquantitative serum strip test in 162 patients with acute pancreatitis (38 SAP). At 24 hours after admission, the test had a 97% NPV for identifying those after admission and a 97% NPV for identifying those patients who later developed organ failure (cut off 0.5 pg/l), with a sensitivity of 92% and a specificity of 84%.[21] A Slovakian study of 101 patients with acute pancreatitis reported an NPV of 83% for severity when procalcitonin was measured within 12 hours after admission.[22] The clinical utility of procalcitonin is feasible and necessitates further prospective evaluation, but it is a promising marker for SAP.

Polymorphonuclear Elastase: Activated polymorphonuclear leucocytes release an enzyme that degrades the extracellular matrix—polymorphonuclear elastase. In a study of 182 patients with acute pancreatitis (28 SAP), serum polymorphonuclear elastase activity at 24 hours postadmission differentiated between a mild and severe course, with an NPV of 98% and a sensitivity of 93%, using a cutoff value of 300 μg/l.[23] However, there have been conflicting data presented and the utility of polymorphonuclear elastase as a prognostic biomarker has yet to be determined.

Carboxypeptidase B: Carboxypeptidase B (CAPB) is an exoprotease synthesized by acinar cells as an inactive proenzyme procarboxypeptidase B. It has at least three different molecular and immunoreactive forms: the proenzyme, the active enzyme, and the activation peptide. Measurement of the proenzyme was useful for the diagnosis of acute pancreatitis, but levels did not correlate with later development of pancreatic necrosis.[24] In a study of 85 patients with acute pancreatitis and 53 patients with acute abdominal pain of nonpancreatic origin, measurement of the activation peptide levels on admission correlated with the later development of pancreatic necrosis with an accuracy of 92%. In

a comparative study of measurement of serum CAPB and urinary TAP in 52 patients with acute pancreatitis, both were excellent prognostic markers, but within the first day of admission urinary TAP was superior.[25]

Radiographic Evaluation

There are a variety of imaging modalities; the most common ones will be discussed. Ultrasonography is a useful test when evaluating the gallbladder for gallstones in an effort to determine the cause of the pancreatitis. The sensitivity and specificity for cholelithiasis is 93% and 87%.[26] Ultrasonography of the pancreas may be limited by overlying bowel particularly in the setting of an ileus.

The preferred radiologic imaging modality is nonionic intravenous contrast-enhanced computed tomography (CECT).[27] Pancreatic necrosis may not be apparent until 48-72 hours after onset of symptoms after microvascular ischemia occurs. Although CECT provides clear images of the pancreas and surrounding inflammation, some have proposed that the contrast medium may induce a conversion of ischemic, but potentially recoverable regions, to frank necrosis. The potential mechanism of this conversion is unclear. Therefore, the early use of CECT, rather than CT without contrast, which may serve the purpose of confirming pancreatic inflammation, needs to be cautiously considered particularly given the unlikely change in treatment during this early phase.

CECT does enable the practitioner to stage the severity of the pancreatitis (Table 11-1). The extent of necrotic pancreas is helpful as a prognosticator and may be used as a map for necrosectomy. In the later phase, the CECT also allows the surgeon to recognize complications of pancreatitis such as peripancreatic or pancreatic fluid collections, perforated viscus, pseudoaneurysm, or gastrointestinal obstruction.

MRI is an alternative imaging modality when evaluation of the pancreas is necessary but contrast dye is contraindicated. It accurately characterizes the extent of the necrosis and can distinguish pancreatic inflammation and peripancreatic debris from the intestinal tract.[28] In addition, it is useful for visualizing the pancreatic and common bile ductal anatomy in select cases to demonstrate injury or a leak.

Fine Needle Aspiration (FNA)

After the first week of pancreatitis, the morphologic characteristics of necrosis become more apparent. During the second week, the necrosis incurs increasing rates of superinfection. FNA has a high sensitivity/specificity for infected necrosis (90% and 99%, respectively) after the first week. The current indications for an FNA hinge on the patient's clinical course. In patients with new-onset organ failure, new increase WBC, or new elevation of body temperature after initial conservative management, one should obtain a CT-scan guided FNA of areas of necrosis.

If a patient develops SAP and on CT scan has peripancreatic fluid collections/necrosis, there is no indication in the first 72 hours to conduct a fine-needle aspiration. If the patient is not improving after this time frame and has or develops pancreatic necrosis/peripancreatic fluid collections, a fine-needle aspiration can determine whether or not the collection is infected. If the collection is sterile, supportive therapy continues. If the Gram stain/culture is positive, the patient will need drainage and debridement.

There is a high correlation between positive Gram stains and operative cultures. The use of prophylactic antibiotics does not appear to affect accuracy. In patients with "persistent unwellness" or sepsis syndrome, repeat FNAs may be indicated to detect developing infection. Up to 43% of patients with sepsis syndrome will have positive operative cultures despite negative FNAs. Ashley et al, describing his group's experience with necrotizing pancreatitis, found in the series of 30 patients with positive FNA that the first FNA positive in 57%, the second FNA positive in 23%, and the third or more FNA results positive in 20% of the patients with infected pancreatic necrosis.[29] The failure to prove infection at first may be related to sampling error, given the heterogeneity of this disease, or to subsequent development of infection, possibly introduced by contamination from the needle.

PHASES OF TREATMENT

Treatments parallel the three phases of pancreatitis: inflammatory, necrotic, and infectious. A number of issues that arise in the subsequent days have been discussed and outlined in numerous reviews and guidelines. The International Association of Pancreatology developed evidence-based guidelines in 2002 that have been the basis for therapy since.[30] These guidelines, however, were subsequently reassessed by the American Thoracic Society, the European Respiratory Society, the European Society of Intensive Care Medicine, the Society of Critical Care Medicine, and the Societe de Reanimation de Langue Francaise. In 2004, changes were made, given new data and the focus on critical care issues.[31] There are also two recent reviews of the current literature, one in the Annals of Surgery, the other from the Japanese in the Journal of Hepatobiliary Pancreatic Surgery in 2006.[32,33] The evidence-based treatment regimen outlined below derives from these guidelines and reviews.

Inflammatory Phase (Acute)

The keys to immediate resuscitation are judicious fluid resuscitation, pressor therapy, ventilatory support, and ICU monitoring, if necessary. The hallmark of the initial phase of SAP is the associated systemic inflammatory response. As such, the focus of the initial treatment is on optimizing the physiologic status of the patient.

After the initial cardiopulmonary stabilization of the patient, several questions remain regarding treatment and are discussed later in this chapter.

Medical Treatment

The use of medications to curb the inflammatory response or to curb further stimulation of the pancreas is an area of active research. The most commonly used medications will be discussed.

Octreotide: In a meta-analysis of 4 randomized prospective trials,[34-37] octreotide did not significantly reduce surgical interventions (23.3% vs 16.3%, p = .09), sepsis (28.7% vs 21.1%, p = 0.25), mortality (20.6% vs 17.7%, p = .34), or overall complication rates (70.6% vs 63.2%, p = 0.2). In addition the route of administration, intravenous vs subcutaneous, made no detectable difference. There is not adequate level I data to support use of octreotide in patients with SAP.

Gabexate Mesilate: A protease inhibitor used in an effort to inhibit the inflammatory cascade and pancreatic necrosis. In an meta-analysis using the randomized prospective trials of Buchler et al[38] and Chen et al[39] there was no change either in the need for surgery (26.9% vs 22.7%, p = 0.46) or in mortality rates (17.9% vs 14.2%, p = 0.46). The evidence does not support the use of gabexate mesilate in SAP.

Aprotinin is a nonspecific serine protease inhibitor. Evaluated in a double-blind randomized trial comparing intraperitoneal versus saline administration, it failed to find any clinically significant difference.[40] A second randomized study, comparing intravenous aprotinin to gabexate mesilate, again failed to support the use of aprotinin.

Lexipafant is a platelet-activating factor (PAF) antagonist that significantly reduced pancreas activity in preclinical trials. It has been evaluated in two randomized, double-blind, placebo-controlled studies.[41,42] Johnson et al found a lower incidence of sepsis, but MOF and local complications remained unaffected. McKay et al demonstrated a significantly higher reduction in the MOF score during lexipafant treatment. However, the incidence of MOF, length of hospital stay, and mortality rates were not improved by lexipafant treatment. At this point, there does not seem to be a role for lexipafant in SAP.

Endoscopic Retrograde Cholangiography (ERC) with Sphincterotomy

All patients presenting with acute pancreatitis should be evaluated for gallstones with ultrasonography. Endoscopic ultrasound provides a more sensitive determination of choledocholithiasis in acute pancreatitis. There is no level I evidence to support the use of urgent ERC and endoscopic sphincterotomy (ES) in patients with severe gallstone pancreatitis. For those patients with evidence of obstructive jaundice or cholangitis, however, ERC and ES are beneficial if the obstruction does not clear within the first 48 hours of supportive care and antibi. A meta-analysis by Heinrich and others suggested that the overall complication rate (57.1% vs 18.2%, P = 0.0001, k = 2) and mortality rate (17.9% vs 3.6%, P = 0.03, k = 2) in patients with severe biliary pancreatitis was decreased. Earyl ERC and ES in patients with severe pancreatitis and biliary obstruction within the first 48 hours after presentation may improve both morbidity and mortality.

Nutrition (When and how to feed?)

The philosophy regarding alimentary feeding in SAP has changed during the last two decades. With the understanding that early postoperative nutrition in critically ill patients lowers the risk of infection, there has been reevaluation of early feeding in patients with acute pancreatitis, despite the earlier belief that "resting the pancreas" was important for recovery in patients with SAP.[43] In preclinical and clinical trials, the intestinal mucosa atrophies during fasting periods but returns to baseline with enteral nutrition.[44,45] It stands to reason that if the mucosal barrier could be kept intact by introduction of enteral nutrition, the incidence of infectious complications involving the necrotic pancreas might diminish.

There are eight trials comparing enteral nutrition to parenteral nutrition.[46-53] All of the studies used nasojejunal feeding except one, the Eatock study, which used nasogastric feeding. A systematic review of the literature by the Cochrane Collaboration in 2002 found a reduced relative mortality risk in patients receiving enteral nutrition, but this difference did not reach statistical significance.[54] Nonetheless, in these trials there were advantages for both feeding enterally versus parenterally and early versus late, as shown by fewer infections, fewer operative interventions, and decreased length of stay.

The specific formulations of feedings and supplements have also been investigated. There is no compelling evidence to support the use of immune-enhancing formulas, but the use of glutamine in parenteral feeding appears to help in patients with SAP who are not tolerating enteral feeding.

Necrosis (Intermediate Phase)

Within the initial 72 hours, necrosis may begin to develop, as supportive care continues. With imaging evidence of pancreatic tissue necrosis the treatment with antibiotics should be considered. There is no justification for use of antibiotics in the absence of necrosis. It is this necrotic tissue that provides a culture medium for microbes.

Prophylactic Antibiotics (Who Gets Antibiotics and Which One Do You Give?)

Infection occurs at some point in 30%-50% of patients with pancreatic and peripancreatic necrosis. The onset of infection has been found most often after the first week of the attack, thereby providing a potential window of opportunity for prophylaxis. There are six randomized prospective trials that investigated this possibility (Table 11-3). Unfortunately, these trials differ in their inclusion criteria and in the antibiotic used. Two studies demonstrated a reduced number of infections; however, only one of them was adequately powered to demonstrate a statistically significant outcome. Even so, the reduction of infections did not lead to lower

Table 11-3	Studies Evaluating the Use of Prophylactic Antibiotics					
Reference	N	Treatment	Infected Necrosis	Surgery	Sepsis	Mortality
Pederzoli et al	41	Imipenem	12.2%*	29.3%	26.8%	7.3%
	33	Control	30.3%	33.3%	78.8%	12%
Sainio et al	30	Cefuroxim	30%	23.3%	13.3%	3.3%
	30	Control	40%	46.6%	26.6%	23.3%
Schwarz et al	13	Oflox/Metro (proph)	62%	X	31%	0%
	13	Oflox/Metro (on demand)	54%	X	46%	15%
Nordback et al	25	Imipenem (proph)	8%*	8%*	X	8%*
	33	Imipenem (on demand)	42%	42%	X	15%
Isenmann et al	37	Cipro/Metro	18.9%	21.6%	X	8.1%
	33	Placebo	15.2%	15.2%	X	9.1%
Luiten et al	50	Selective	18%*	32%*	X	22%
	52	Decon Control	38%	46%	X	35%

risk of requiring operative debridement, incidence of organ failure, or rate of mortality.

The other four did not show that prophylaxis with antibiotics caused a significant reduction in the development of infected necrosis. The study by Sainio et al is the only study that shows a reduction in mortality, but, with a large number of deaths in the control group, the comparative cohort may have been skewed. The fifth study, the most methodically sound with a double-blinded, placebo-control design, did not find any differences in outcome of treatment.

Clearly the data is conflicting. For example, a recent meta-analysis of the Level II trials, referenced in Table 11-3, shows that antibiotic prophylaxis significantly reduced sepsis and mortality but did not prevent infection of pancreatic necrosis. This may mean that other associated infections, eg, ventilator-associated pneumonia, were treated more effectively or earlier. A subgroup analysis demonstrated a significant reduction in infected necrosis for patients receiving prophylactic imipenem (36.4% vs 10.6%, p = 0.002) in contrast with those receiving quinolones + metronidazole. There was no significant difference in efficacy between imipenem and meropenem. These data suggest that it is appropriate to treat patients who have > 30% necrosis of the pancreas with prophylactic imipenem or meropenem.

Some have suggested that the use of broad spectrum antibiotics has increased the incidence of fungal infections.[55] However, in a meta-analysis done by the Cochrane Collaboration, there was no significant difference in fungal infections between those treated with broad-spectrum antibiotics and controls. There is currently no indication for prophylactic antifungal treatment for necrotizing pancreatitis.

One study showed that selective gut decontamination resulted in a lower incidence of infected necrosis.[56] The finding has not been reproduced but merits prospective randomized trials to validate the role of gut decontamination.

There is rarely a need for FNA or exploration in the first several days of acute pancreatitis, even for acute fluid collections or evolving necrosis. However, failure to improve or secondary deterioration merits investigation with FNA to determine whether or not the collection is sterile. Infection is widely considered the sine qua non for intervention to debride and drain.[57-59] Symptomatic sterile collections remain a focus of debate.

Necrosis (Late Phase)
Debridement for Infection, Persistent Unwellness, or Sepsis Syndrome

In a review of the most recent 167 patients with necrotizing pancreatitis (of 2449 patients admitted to the Massachusetts General Hospital during this period with acute pancreatitis), the preoperative indications for surgery were (a) proven infected necrosis 50.1%, (b)

persistent unwellness 32.3%, and (c) persistent sepsis syndrome 16.8%.[60] In those patients with proven infection, 34% were diagnosed by FNA and 17% by presence of gas on CECT. Of those with persistent unwellness (patients in whom infected necrosis was not proven but whose symptoms and signs failed to resolve with prolonged conservative management alone[61]), half had an FNA but 20% had a false negative finding. Of those with sepsis syndrome (patients who progressively deteriorated beyond the first week with progressive failure of one or more organs, usually with leukocytosis and fever but without infection proven by culture or Gram stain), 43% had FNAs but again the false negative rate was 25%. Overall, 72% of the entire cohort was proven to be infected at operation. These findings emphasize that (a) infection may be present but remain undetected by FNA or CT scan, and (b) some patients will have sufficient clinical indications to warrant debridement even if infection has not been preoperatively proven.

Approximately 30% of patients required a postoperative IR drain for recurrent or residual infected collections and debris. The overall mortality was 11.4%. The median postoperative length of stay was 19 days with a mean of 29.5 days. The significant predictors of mortality were (a) preoperative APACHE II > 10, (b) multiple organ failure, (c) early surgery (< 21 days), and (d) female gender. Predictors that were not significant were (a) the presence of infection (bacterial or fungal), (b) hemorrhage, or (c) reoperation.

The optimal timing for the debridement seems to be approximately 21-27 days after the onset of symptoms.[60] It appears that earlier intervention is more likely to lead to incomplete clearance as a result of the lack of demarcation of the necrosis and the consequent need for further debridement to complete the removal of dead tissues which serve as a bacterial culture medium. The method of debridement and closed packing used at the Massachusetts General Hospital has achieved the lowest reported mortality, fewest reinterventions, and shortest length of hospitalization reported.[60]

The role of percutaneous drainage prior to definitive operation has not been established. With the advent of better drains, there may be a role for preoperative percutaneous drains in an infected pancreatic or peripancreatic fluid collection during the early phase of the disease.[66] This may allow the surgeon to temporize, stabilize an unstable patient, and allow sufficient time to pass to facilitate a successful single-stage debridement. However, the need for this tactic is uncommon. In contrast, percutaneous drains placed postoperatively to treat additional collections are often useful in avoiding the need for difficult reoperations.[66]

There is a group of patients who appear to have sterile pancreatic necrosis but who continue to manifest signs of inflammation and toxicity, a state that has been termed persistent unwellness. Despite the failure to find infection on preoperative testing, 25% of them have been to harbor infected necrosis at the time of debridement. Because most truly sterile necrosis, even if producing signs of inflammation, can be successfully treated with intervention, the indication and timing of debridement for persistent unwellness remains a matter of judgment.

Operative Management

Surgical Exposure of the Pancreas

The most common method for gaining access to the pancreas is via the gastrocolic omentum and the lesser sac. Inflammation may obscure the colon and stomach walls and lead to inadvertent injury and subsequent fistulas. The dissection to reach the pancreas may similarly be difficult and uncertain. The approach is made by dividing the gastrocolic omentum parallel to the gastric greater curvature, caudal to the gastroepiploic artery, which runs approximately 1-2 cm away from the greater curvature of the stomach. A wide exposure is desirable in order to clear the dead tissues as completely as feasible and also to be able to control bleeding vessels if encountered in the cavity.

The authors' preferred route for pancreatic debridement is via the transverse mesocolon. The pancreas lies immediately cephalad to this thin membrane and the collection to be accessed is easily seen, palpated, or demonstrated by needle aspiration through an avascular section of the mesocolon. The middle colic vessels are avoided and an incision is made to the left or right of them. The body and tail of the pancreas can be accessed to the left of the middle colic vessels and ligament of treitz. The head of the pancreas can be accessed to the right of the vessels. The entire pancreatic debridement and drainage can be performed via this route or the gastrocolic omentum can be safely opened with a hand in the cavity to indicate the space between the stomach and colon. There are three generally accepted techniques for accomplishing the debridement:

Debridement and Closed Packing

We utilize an upper midline incision. The cavity containing fluid and necrotic tissues is entered through the transverse mesocolon usually to the left of the mesenteric vessels. Access to the right side of the pancreas may require an incision to the right of the vessels. The hole in the mesocolon is sufficiently enlarged to facilitate the debridement by blunt dissection with fingers, instruments and swabs. Following the completion of the necrosectomy, stuffed penrose drains are placed to fill the cavity along with a few closed suction drains, as previously described[60,62,63] (see Figs. 11-2 A and B). The purpose of the stuffed penrose drains is to occupy the space, tamponade ooze from granulations, and provide egress for particulate matter that may still cling to the walls of the cavity.

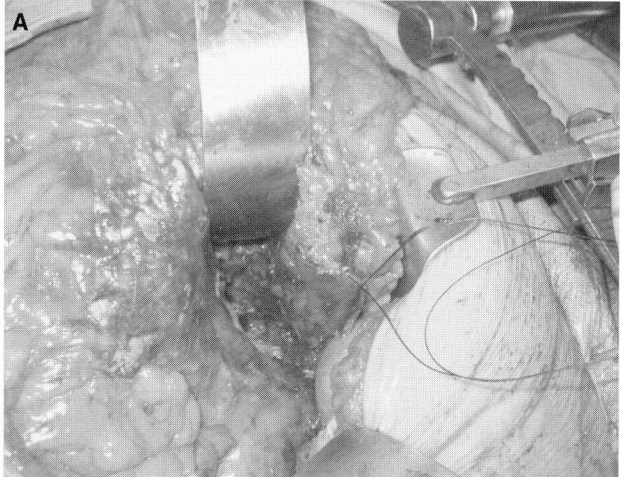

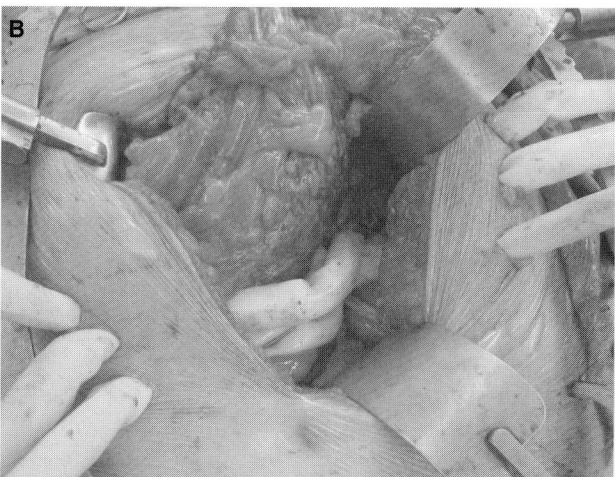

Figure 11-2 **A.** *Opening into lesser sac via transverse mesocolon;* **B.** *Placement of stuffed penrose drains into debrided cavity.*

The penrose drains are brought through the lateral abdominal wall through separate openings to minimize the risk of herniation. They are removed, one at a time beginning at a week after the operation, to allow the cavity to collapse and heal. The closed suction drains are left in place until the penrose drains have been removed and the drainage is minimal. If a pancreatic fistula becomes evident, the drains are left in as long as necessary for healing. In our experience about 15% of patients will require a second operation for further clearance of infected tissues or other complications. The mortality with use of this technique has been only 11.4%.[60]

Debridement and Open Packing

Various authors have recommended either a transverse, chevron, or midline incision. The gastrocolic omentum is opened and the lesser sac entered. As much as possible of the peripancreatic debris and

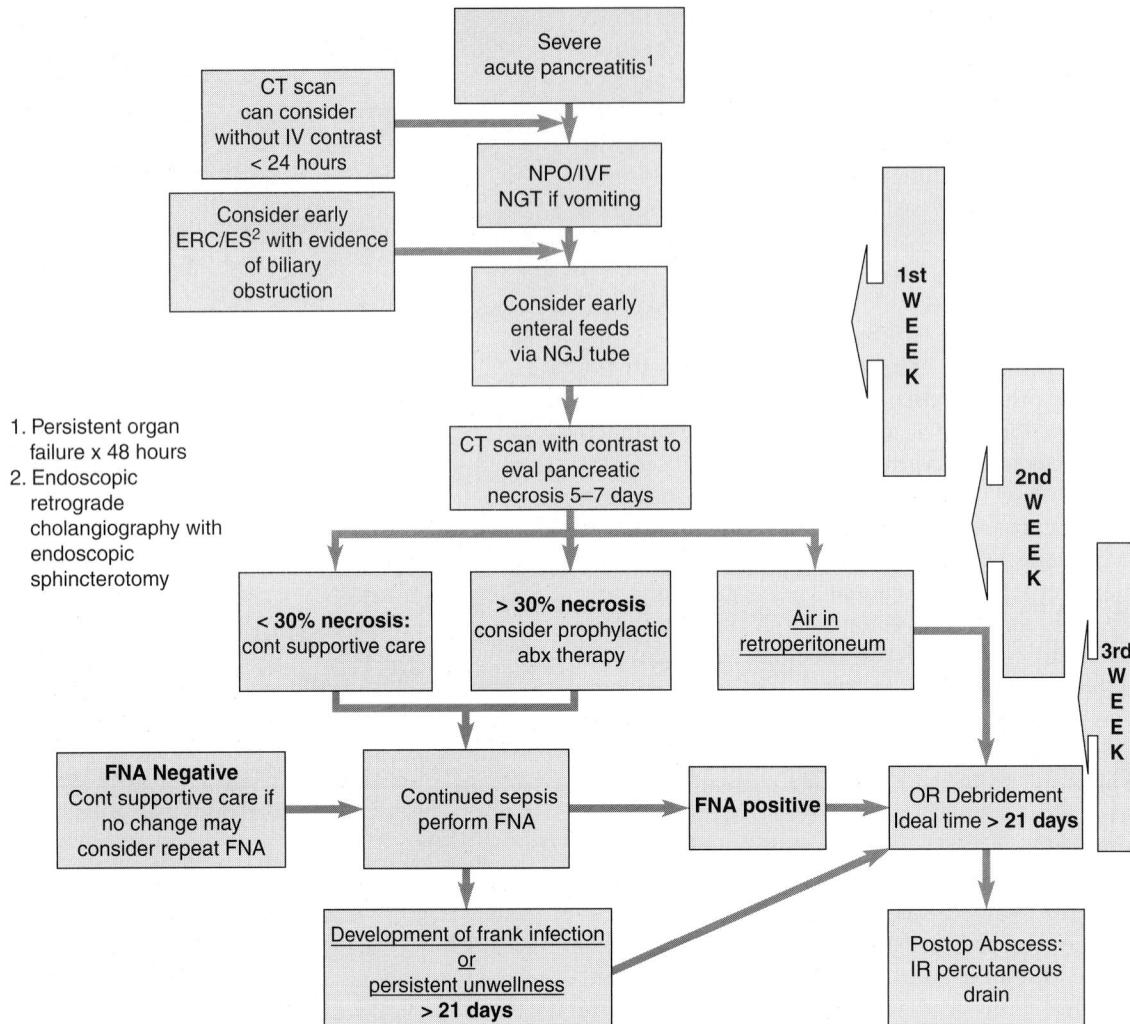

Figure 11-3   *Acute pancreatitis: Treatment algorithm. FNA = fine needle aspiration; IR = interventional radiology.*

pancreatic necrosis is bluntly removed. The cavity is lined with a nonadherent gauze layer, packed, and the abdomen left open. The packing is removed every 48 hours, the debridement extended as necessary, and the packing replaced until the bed is lined with granulation. In some cases, dressing changes can be safely accomplished at the bedside in the ICU. Later, the abdomen can be closed with drains left in the cavity or allowed to heal by secondary intention and split-thickness skin grafts. The reported mortality using this technique is 18% and the enteric fistula rate is 15%-20%.[60]

Debridement and Closed Continuous Lavage of the Lesser Sac

This technique also involves entry into the lesser sac via the gastrocolic omentum. After the debridement, the opening through the omentum and the abdominal wall are closed around lavage catheters and drains in order to isolate the space for lavage. The cavity is vigorously lavaged with isotonic fluid (7 to 48 L/day has been described) with the intent to wash out residual

adherent debris. The lavage persists until the effluent is clear. The drains are then sequentially removed. The median duration of lavage in one series was 25 days.[64] This technique is labor intensive for nursing and has a 31% rate of reexploration.

Endoscopic Drainage

In an effort to potentially avoid a laparotomy some have advocated endoscopic approaches. Transgastric, transgastrocolic, transmesocolic, and retroperitoneal approaches have been described in small series.[65,66] However, it is difficult at present to espouse a preference for one or the other (Fig. 11-3).

IV POSTOPERATIVE MANAGEMENT: COMPLICATIONS

A. Abdominal Compartment Syndrome

This phenomenon occurs uncommonly in SAP but must be recognized promptly to allow for abdominal decompression. Progressively rising intra-abdominal pressure may lead to renal, pulmonary, and cardiac compromise. In some cases, a paracentesis removing the exudates produced by the pancreatic inflammation may provide sufficient decompression to avoid a laparotomy. If unsuccessful, laparotomy is required. It may be impossible or inadvisable to try to reclose the abdomen following decompression. In such cases the open abdomen is controlled with a vacuum-seal dressing until the edema and distention of the abdominal contents subsides sufficiently to allow delayed closure of the abdominal wall. Patients should be returned to the operating room every 48 hours to wash out the abdomen and assess for abdominal approximation.

B. Visceral Infarction
Infarction of areas of neighboring viscera including the small and large bowel, stomach, and duodenum can occur in up to 15% of cases. Visceral infarction is more common in those with infected pancreatic necrosis. The resulting fistula may heal with appropriate drainage but some will require enteric diversion or resection.

C. Postoperative Hemorrhage
Life-threatening hemorrhage is usually the product of enzymatic erosion of a major artery, uncommonly a vein. Surgical access and control can be challenging and dangerous. Angiographic localization of the bleeding site and control by embolization is worth the effort and is effective in the majority of cases, at least for initial control and stabilization. If the bleeding is too massive to allow the time to attempt angiographic treatment, expeditious surgical exploration for hemostasis is unavoidable. Packing alone will usually be inadequate for definitive control but may be the only expedient way to allow for subsequent embolization of a vessel which cannot be directly accessed.

D. Persistent or Recurrent Infection
Infection after debridement and drainage of pancreatic necrosis, whether sterile or infected, most commonly is the consequence of necrotic tissues which were incompletely debrided or fluid collections which were inadequately drained. These postoperative collections are usually true abscesses with little or no semisolid tissues that would be difficult to remove through percutaneous drains. The success rate of percutaneous drainage for postoperative abscesses approaches 100%.[67]

E. Postoperative Fistula
Pancreatic fistulae may occur in up to 44% of patients, but most will heal with adequate drainage. Fewer than 10% will eventually require either excision of an isolated remnant pancreatic tail or internal drainage into a Roux-Y jejunal loop. Enteric fistulas can occur in up to 15% of patients, more frequently found in those with infected pancreatitis. Their natural history and treatment are complex and beyond the scope of this chapter.

F. Endocrine and Exocrine Insufficiency
Surprisingly, pancreatic insufficiency after debridement is uncommon, probably because much of the necrotic tissues, while impressive in volume, is devitalized peripancreatic and retroperitoneal fat, not pancreas. In our series of major debridements, only 16% of patients became diabetic and only 20% required supplementary pancreatic enzymes after recovery.

REFERENCES

1. Banks PA. Epidemiology, natural history, and predictors of disease outcome in acute and chronic pancreatitits. *Gastrointest Endosc* 2002;56(6 Suppl):S226-30.
2. Bradley EL III. A clinically based classification system for acute pancreatitis. Summary of the International Symposium on Acute Pancreatitis, Atlanta, Ga, Sept 11-13, 1992. *Arch Surg* 1993;128(5):586-590.
3. Chwistek M, Roberts I, Amoateng-Adjepong Y. Gallstone pancreatitits: a community teaching hospital experience. *J Clin Gastroenterol* 2001;33:41-44.
4. Levy P, Boruchowicz A, Hastier P, et al. Diagnostic criteria in predicting a biliary origin of acute pancreatitis in the era of endoscopic ultrasound: multicentre prospective evaluation of 213 patients. *Pancreatology* 2005;5:450-456.
5. Venneman NG, Buskens E, Besselink MG, et al. Small gallstones are associated with increased risk of acute pancreatitis: potential benefits of prophylactic cholecystectomy? *Am J Gastroenterol* 2005;100:2540-2550.
6. Tenner S, Dubner H, Steinberg W: Predicting gallstone pancreatitis with laboratory parameters: A meta-analysis. *Am J Gastroenterol* 1994;89:1863.
7. McKay CJ, Imrie CW. The continuing challenge of early mortality in acute pancreatitis. *Br J Surg* 2004;91:1243-1244.
8. Ranson JH, Rifkind KM, Turner JW. Prognostic signs and nonoperative peritoneal lavage in acute pancreatitis. *Surg Gynecol Obstet* 1976;143:209-219.
9. Knaus WA, Draper EA, Wagner DP, Zimmerman JE. APACHE II: a severity of disease classification system. *Crit Care Med* 1985;13:818-829.
10. Larvin M, McMahon MJ. APACHE-II score for assessment and monitoring of acute pancreatitis. *Lancet* 1989;2:201-205.
11. Matos R, Moreno R, Fevereiro T. Severity evaluation in acute pancreatitis: The role of SOFA score and generl severity scores. *Crit Care Med* 2000;4:S138-S139.
12. Buter A, Imrie CW, Carter CR, et al. Dynamic nature of early organ dysfunction determines outcome in acute pancreatitis. *Br J Surg* 2002;89:298-302.
13. Guidelines for intensive care unit admission, discharge, and triage. Task Force of the American College of Critical Care Medicine, Society of Critical Care Medicine. *Crit Care Med* 1999;27:633-638.

14. Matull WR, Pereira SP, O'Donohue JW. Biochemical markers of acute pancreatitis. Downloaded from jcp.bmj.com on November 26, 2006.

15. Smotkin J, Tenner S. Clinical reviews: pancreatic and biliary disease: laboratory diagnositic tests in acute pancreatitis. *J Clin Gastroenterol* 2002;34:459-462.

16. Yadav D, Agarwal N, Pitchumaoni CS. A critical evaluation of laboratory tests in acute pancreatitis. *Am J Gastroenterol* 2002;97:1309-1318.

17. Pezzilli R, Billi P, Miniero R, et al. Serum interleukin 6 interleukin 8, and [beta]2-microglobulin in the early assessment of severity of acute pancreatitis. Comparison with serum C-reactive protein. *Dig Dis Sci* 1995;40:2341-2348.

18. Pezzilli R, Morselli-Labate AM, Miniero R, et al. Simultaneous serum assays of lipase and interleukin-6 for early diagnosis and prognosis of actue pancreatitis. *Clin Chem* 1999;45:1762-1767.

19. Chen CC, Wang SS, Lee FY, et al. Proinflammatory cytokines in early assessment of the prognosis of acute pancreatitis. *Am J Gastroenterol* 1999;94:213-218.

20. Reinhart K, Carlet J. Procalcitonin—a new marker of severe infection and sepsis. *Intensive Care Med* 2000;26(suppl2):145.

21. Kylanpaa-Back ML, Takala A, Kemppainan E, et al. Procalcitonin strip test in the early detection of severe actue pancreatitis. *Br J Surg* 2001;88:222-227.

22. Pindak D, Parrak V, Pechan J, et al. The clinical value of the procalcitonin in prediction of severity and outcome in acute pancreatitis. *Hepatogastroenterology.* 2003;50:ccviii-ix, (suppl 2).

23. Dominguez-Munoz C, Carballo F, Garcia MJ, et al. Clinical usefulness of polymorphonuclear elastase in predicting severity of acute pancreatitis: results of a multi-center study. *Br J Surg* 1991;78:1230-1234.

24. Muller CA, Appelros S, Uhl W, et al. Serum levels of procarboxypeptidase B and its activation peptide in patients with acute pancreatitis and non-pancreatic diseases. *Gut* 2002;51:229-235.

25. Saez J, Martinez J, Trigo C, et al. Comparative study of the activation peptide of carboxypeptidase B and of trypsinogen as early predictors of the severity of acute pancreatitis. *Pancreatology* 2002;2:167-187.

26. Parys BT, Barr H, Chantarasak ND et al. Use of ultrasound scan as a bedside diagnostic aid. *Br J Surg* 1987;74: 611-612.

27. Silverstein W, Isikoff MB, Hill MC, Barkin J. Diagnostic imaging of acute pancreatitis: prospectivew study using CT and sonography. *AJR Am J Roestgenol* 1981;137:497-502.

28. Piironen A, Kivisaari R, Kemppainen E, et al. Detection of severe acute pancreatitis by contrast-enhanced magnetic resonance imaging. *Eur Radiol* 2000;10: 354-361.

29. Ashley SW, Perez A, Pierce EA, et al. Necrotizing pancreatitis: Contemporary analysis of 99 consecutive cases. *Annals of Surgery* 2001;234(4):572-580.

30. Uhl W, Warshaw A, Imrie C, et al. IAP Guidelines for the surgical management of acute pancreatitis. *Pancreatology* 2002;2:565-573.

31. Nathens AB, Curtis JR, et. al. Management of the critically ill patient with severe acute pancreatitis. *Crit Care Med* 2004;32(12): 2524-2536.

32. Takada T, Kawarada Y, Hirata K, et al. JPN Guidelines for the management of acute pancreatitis: cutting-edge information. *J Hepatobiliary Pancreat Surg* 2006;13:2-6.

33. Heinrich S, Schafer M, Rousson V, Clavien P. Evidence-based treatment of acute pancreatitis, a look at established paradigms. *Annals of Surgery* 2006;243(2): 154-168.

34. Uhl W, Buchler MW, Malfertheiner P, et al. A randomized, double blind, multicenter trial of octreotide in moderate to severe acute pancreatitis. *Gut* 1999;45: 97-104.

35. McKay C, Baxter J, Imrie C. A randomized, controlled trail of octreotide in the management of patients with actue pancreatitis. *Int J Pancreatol* 1997;21:13-19.

36. Planas M, Perez A, Igleasia R, et al. Severe acute pancreatitis: treatment with somatostatin. *Intensive Care Med* 1998;24:37-39.

37. Paran H, Mayo A, Paran D, et al. Octreotide treatment in patients with severe actue pancreatitis. *Dig Dis Sci.* 2000;45:2247-2251.

38. Buchler M, Malfertheiner P, Uhl W, et al. Gabexate mesilate in human aacute pancreatitis: German Pancreatitis Sutdy Group. *Gastroenterology* 1993;104: 1165-1170.

39. Chen HM, Chen JC, Hwang TL, et al. Prospective and randomized study of gabexate mesilate for the treatment of severe acute pancreatitis with organ dysfunction. *Hepatogastroenterology* 2000;47:1147-1150.

40. Berling R, Genell, Ohlsson K. High-dose intraperitoneal aprotinin treatment of acute severe pancreatitis: a double-blind randomized multi-center trial. *J Gastroenterol* 1994;29:479-485.

41. Johnson CD, Kingsnorth AN, Imrie CW, et al. Double blind, randomized, placebo controlled study of a platelet activating factor antagonist, lexipafant, in the treatment of and prevention of organ failure in predicted severe acute pancreattis. *Gut* 2001;48:62-69.

42. McKay CJ, Curran F, Sharples C, et al. Prospective placebo-controlled randomized trial of lexipafant in predicted severe acute pancreatitis. *Br J Surg* 1997;84:1239-1243.

43. Braunschweig CL, Levy P, Sheean PM, Wang X. Enteral compared with parenteral nutrition: a meta-analysis. *Am J Clin Nutr* 2001;74:534-542.

44. Alscher KT, Phang PT, McDonald TE, et al. Enteral feeding decreases gut apoptosis, permeability, and lung inflammation during murine endotoxemia. *Am J Physiol Gastrointest Liver Physiol* 2001;281:G569-G576.

45. Hadfield RJ, Sinclair DG, Houldsworth PE, et al. Effects of enteral and parenteral nutrition on gut mucosal permeability in the critically ill. *Am J Respir Crit Care Med* 1995;152:1545-1548.

46. McClave SA, Greene LM, Snider HL, et al. Comparison of the safety of early enteral vs parenteral nutrition in mild acute pancreatitis. *J Parenter Enteral Nutr* 1997;21:14-20.

47. Olah A, Pardavi G, Belagyi T, et al. Early nasojejunal feeding in acute pancreatitis is associated with a lower complication rate. *Nutrition* 2002;18:259-262.

48. Powell JJ, Murchison JT, Fearon KC, et al. Randomized controlled trial of the effect of early enteral nutrition on markers of the inflammatory response in predicted severe acute pancreatitis. *Br J Surg* 2000;87:1375-1381.

49. Windsor AC, Kanwar S, Li AG, et al. Compared with parenteral nutrition, enteral feeding attenuates the acute phase response and improves disease severity in acute pancreatitis. *Gut* 1998;42:431-435.

50. Kalfarentzos F, Kehagias J, Mead N, et al. Enteral nutrition is superior to parenteral nutrition in severe acute pancreatitis: results of a randomized prospective trial. *Br J Surg* 1997;84:1665-1669.

51. Abou-Assi s, Craig K, O'Keefe SJ. Hypocaloric jejunal feeding is better than total parenteral nutrition in acute pancreatitis: results of a randomized comparative study. *Am J Gastroenterol* 2002;97:2255-2262.

52. Eeatock FC, Brombacher GD, Steven A, et al. Nasogastric feeding in severe acute pancreatitis may be paractical and safe. *Int J Pancreatol* 2000;28:23-29.

53. Olah A, Belagyi T, Issedutz A, et al. Randomized clinical trial of specific lactobacillus and fibre supplement to early enteral nutrition in patients with acute pancreatitis. *Br J Surg* 2002;89:1103-1107.

54. Al-Omran M, Groof A, Wilke D. Enteral versus parenteral nutrition for acute pancreatitis. *Cochrane Database Syst Rev* 2002:CD002837.

55. Isenmann R, Schwarz M, Rau B, et al. Characteristics of infection with Candida species in patients with necrotizing pancreatitis. *World J Surg* 2002;26:372-376.

56. Luiten EJT, Hop WCJ, Lange JF, et al. Controlled clinical trial of selective decontamination for the treatment of severe acute pancreatitis. *Ann Surg* 1995;222:57-65.

57. Whitcomb DC. Clinical practice. Acute pancreatitis. *N Engl J Med* 2006;354(20):2142-2150.

58. Buchler MW, Gloor B, Muller CA, et al. Acute necrotizing pancreatitis: treatment strategy according to the status of infection. *Ann Surg* 2000;232(5):619-626.

59. Bradley EL III, Allen K. A prospective longitudinal study of observation versus surgical intervention in the management of necrotizing pancreatitis. *Am J Surg* 1991;161(1):19-24.

60. Rodriguez JR, Razo AO, Targarona J, et al. Debridement and closed packing for sterile or infected necrotizing pancreatitis: insights into indications and outcomes in 167 patients. *Ann Surg.* 2008 Feb;247(2):294-9

61. Warshaw AL. Pancreatic necrosis: to debride or not to debride—that is the question. *Ann Surg* 2000;232(5): 627-629.

62. Warshaw AL, Jin GL. Improved survival in 45 patients with pancreatic abscess. *Ann Surg* 1985;202(4):408-417.

63. Fernandez-del Castillo C, Rattner DW, Makary MA, Mostafavi A, McGrath D, Warshaw AL. Debridement and closed packing for the treatment of necrotizing pancreatitis. *Ann Surg* 1998;228(5):676-684.

64. Beger HG. Operative management of necrotizing pancreatitis: necrosectomy and contineuous closed postoperative lavage of the lesser sac. *Hepatogastroenterology* 1991;38:129-133.

65. Connor S, Ghaneh P, Raraty M, et al. Minimally invasive retroperitoneal pancreatic necrosectomy. *Dig Surg* 2003;20(4):270-277.

66. Connor S, Raraty MG, Howes N, et al. Surgery in the treatment of acute pancreatitis—minimal access pancreatic necrosectomy. *Scand J Surg* 2005;94(2):135-142.

67. Mithofer K, Mueller PR, Warshaw AL. Interventional and surgical treatment of pancreatic abscess. *World J Surg* 1997;21:162-168.

Chapter **12**

THE SPLEEN

Gary A. Vercruysse, MD, and David V. Feliciano, MD

INTRODUCTION

In ancient times, the spleen was thought to be responsible for a plethora of actions. It was the source of black bile, the heart of human emotion, responsible for melancholy, and thought to slow the average runner.[1] The word spleen in Greek is loosely translated as "ill temper." Early splenectomies performed on animals by surgeons demonstrated that the spleen is not essential for life. The first splenectomies performed on humans were for trauma and had a mortality rate of approximately 90%.[2] Interestingly, Berger reported that conservative management of splenic trauma had a mortality rate of approximately 90-100% during the same era.[3] Since then, advances in transport, diagnosis, resuscitation, anesthesia, and operative technique have lessened this mortality rate considerably. Recent laparoscopic data on elective splenectomy documents mortality rates of less than 1%.[4]

ANATOMY

The spleen is a solid organ located on the left side of the upper abdomen lateral to the stomach and pancreas, anterior to the left adrenal gland and kidney, and is protected beneath the 9th to 11th ribs. Average size and weight of the normal spleen approximates 7 to 11 cm in greatest dimension and 100-250 grams. The spleen has peritoneal attachments to the diaphragm (splenophrenic ligament), splenic flexure of the colon (splenocolic ligament), left kidney and adrenal gland and tail of the pancreas (splenorenal ligament), and the stomach (splenogastric ligament). Blood flow to the spleen averages between 250 and 300 ml/min and comes primarily from the splenic artery, a branch of the celiac axis. A secondary supply comes from the short gastric vessels between the stomach and spleen. Venous drainage is mainly via the splenic vein which joins the superior mesenteric vein to become the portal vein in the retroperitoneum directly behind the pancreas. Secondary venous drainage is via the short gastric vessels as well. The spleen is the source of the most frequent congenital anomaly, the secondary spleen, seen in approximately 20% of all individuals.[5]

FUNCTION

The spleen has four key functions, including the following: (1) filtration, (2) immunologic, (3) reservoir, and (4) hematopoietic. In adults, filtering of the blood and removal of aged or damaged red blood cells and microorganisms is the dominant function of the spleen. In addition, it is responsible for removal and destruction of antibody-antigen complexes, lymphocyte activation, and lymphokine production and release. The spleen is a reservoir in that it holds approximately 25% of the platelets in the body at any given time as well as a large portion of the granulocytes in reserve. The spleen is a major hematopoietic organ in the developing human, but is a minor contributor to production of blood products except in times of extreme stress in the adult.[6]

LAPAROSCOPIC VERSUS OPEN SPLENECTOMY

Traditionally, all splenectomies were performed through an open technique. Over the past 15 years, techniques have been developed for performing splenectomy laparoscopically. Initially, this was reserved for only the small spleen undergoing elective splenectomy. More recently, surgeons have had success with laparoscopic splenectomy for massive (600-1600 g) and even supermassive (> 1600 g) spleens.[7] There have been case reports describing laparoscopic splenectomy for emergent (trauma) indications, as well.[8,9] It is generally agreed that laparoscopic splenectomy should be reserved for elective cases and done only by qualified surgeons with advanced laparoscopic training and proven competence at this time. The laparoscopic emergent splenectomy is not recommended.

INDICATIONS FOR EMERGENT SPLENECTOMY

TRAUMA

The spleen is the most frequently injured solid organ in trauma and accounts for the majority of cases of splenectomy in the adult. If iatrogenic injury is added to this total, the vast majority of splenectomies are done for trauma of one form or another. A separate section of this book (Chapter 30) is devoted to the management of the patient with trauma to the spleen and other solid organs.

IMMUNE THROMBOCYTOPENIC PURPURA (ITP)

Also known as idiopathic thrombocytopenic purpura, this disease afflicts both children and adults equally. ITP occurs as a result of IgG autoantibodies to platelets which cause opsonization by macrophages and premature removal of platelets within the spleen and liver.[10] Symptoms include thrombocytopenia, ecchymoses and petechiae, and, sometimes, hemorrhage. The severity of bleeding is related to the platelet count, with minimal symptoms at counts around 50,000/mm^3 and major bleeding at counts below 10,000/mm^3. The mainstay of treatment in children with minimal symptoms is observation. Patients will show improvement with time in approximately 80% of cases.[11] In most adults, counts are low at presentation, and they seek treatment due to symptoms. For those who require treatment, intravenous immunoglobulin (IVIG) and corticosteroids significantly increase platelet counts in most patients.[12] Those who do not respond to IVIG or corticosteroids are candidates for elective splenectomy, while those who have life-threatening hemorrhage require emergent splenectomy. Whenever splenectomy is being performed for a hematologic disorder, a thorough search for accessory splenic tissue and removal of any accessory spleens is necessary to effect a cure.

SPLENIC VEIN THROMBOSIS AND LEFT-SIDED PORTAL HYPERTENSION

Splenic vein thrombosis is a rare event. It occurs most commonly in patients with a pancreatic neoplasm or chronic pancreatitis.[13] Even when patients present with these entities, left-sided (sinistral) portal hypertension is only seen in approximately 4%-8% of patients but has an associated mortality from bleeding exceeding 20%.[14] Mass effect from either cause listed leads to stasis of flow and eventual thrombosis of the splenic vein. In addition, the hypercoagulable state associated with cancer may enhance this phenomenon.

Left-sided portal hypertension results in normal portal and superior mesenteric venous pressures yet very elevated gastrosplenic pressures. In this condition, the left gastroepiploic vein and short gastric vessels become significant sources of collateral flow. Eventually, large gastric varices develop with occasional erosion and voluminous bleeding.

When acutely bleeding, patients should be resuscitated in an intensive care unit. In this situation, contrary to treatment for other sources of variceal bleeding, there is no role for transjugular intrahepatic portosystemic shunting (TIPS) as there is no intrahepatic portal hypertension. Unfortunately, there is no easy way to ensure that bleeding is due to isolated left-sided portal hypertension. Patients with esophageal and gastric varices due to portal hypertension may bleed to hypotension from gastric variceal erosion and have decompressed (invisible) esophageal varices during endoscopy. Upper gastrointestinal endoscopy is recommended as first line treatment for bleeding, because it is effective for both gastric and esophageal varices. Once temporary hemostasis has been accomplished, endoscopic or transabdominal ultrasound may be used to visualize the splenic vein and diagnose or rule out splenic vein thrombosis. If this technology is unavailable, Computed Tomographic Venography, Magnetic Resonance Imaging, or even Splanchnic Venography is an alternative.

Once diagnosed, splenic vein thrombosis should prompt splenectomy to avoid recurrence of this life-threatening bleeding. Although hemostasis during acute bleeding may be accomplished endoscopically, if there is delay or endoscopy is unavailable, splenectomy is curative.

SPLENIC ARTERY ANEURYSM

This aneurysm is the most common visceral aneurysm. It occurs most often in the distal splenic artery but can occur at any location along its tortuous course. Four times more common in women than men, asymptomatic aneurysms of the splenic artery come to the attention of surgeons as an anomalous finding on radiologic studies done for another reason. The overall risk of rupture is between 3% and 9%.[15]

In most patients, the risk of rupture is related to a size > 2 cm. Patients with persistent left upper quadrant pain or the presence of any inflammatory conditions such as pancreatitis should be considered to be at risk, as well. If any of these indications are present, treatment is warranted.

Traditionally, treatment consists of splenic artery ligation with excision of the aneurysm. If the aneurysm is distal, splenectomy is also performed as is the case in the vast majority of aneurysmectomies.

Recently, nonsurgical alternatives have been proposed with some level of success. Angiographic coiling of splenic artery aneurysms or pseudoaneurysms has been performed on several dozen patients with technical success; however, approximately 40% of the time splenic infarction was noted. Recently, splenic artery stenting has been proposed as an alternative to embolization. This has the advantage of excluding the aneurysm while preserving splenic blood flow. Technical advances are still necessary to allow this strategy to be employed in the often tortuous splenic artery.[16] Endovascular therapy is time-consuming and probably should be limited to use in an elective setting and not on ruptured aneurysms.

In pregnant patients, it is felt that elevated estrogen levels are an added risk factor for rupture. In cases of rupture, maternal and fetal demise occurs in approximately 70% and 95% of cases, respectively. Given their propensity for rupture and the significant maternal and fetal mortality rate associated with rupture, a pregnant patient or a woman who intends to become pregnant should have intervention to eliminate the aneurysm.[17] A gravid patient who presents with shock in the absence of vaginal bleeding and free fluid on abdominal ultrasound has a ruptured splenic artery aneurysm until proven otherwise. These patients should receive immediate laparotomy and splenic artery aneurysmectomy and splenectomy, which is curative.

SPLENIC ABSCESS

Splenic abscess is uncommon but potentially deadly. It generally occurs in individuals with cancer, HIV/AIDS, diabetes mellitus, sickle cell anemia, or another immunocompromised state. It can be the result of bacteremia, an arterial embolic phenomenon, or abdominal trauma. Although rare, splenic abscess has a mortality of approximately 20%. Patients typically present with malaise, fever, leukocytosis, anorexia, and left upper quadrant abdominal pain. Symptoms come on gradually and may be present for a prolonged period of time before patients seek treatment.[18] Computed tomography or ultrasonography is usually diagnostic of this condition. Both open splenectomy and percutaneous aspiration or drainage procedures in combination with long-term (3-12 weeks) intravenous antibiotics have been advocated as treatments.[19] Patients with multiloculated abscesses, documented bacteremia, and infection with a gram-negative bacillus often require multiple aspirations/drainage procedures. In this cohort of patients, open splenectomy has been shown to result in the highest survival rate, the lowest number of procedures and complications, and quickest recovery.[20]

OPERATION

With the overwhelming number of trauma patients with splenic injuries being managed with nonoperative approaches including splenic angioembolization, the once routine trauma splenectomy has become a rare event. Several concepts are important to understand prior to attempting a splenectomy. Remember, if the patient is not in hemorrhagic shock at the time of splenectomy, take your time. Splenectomy for emergent reasons presents a hostile surgical environment, with unnamed large retroperitoneal veins and many thick, vascular, diaphragmatic adhesions being the norm rather than the exception. Careful, deliberate, and methodical dissection will lead to a more hemostatic field and less potential for injury to other organs.

The spleen can be approached through a standard midline laparotomy or a left subcostal incision. Once entrance into the peritoneum has been gained, laparotomy packs are used to gently pack away the lower viscera to gain a clear path to the spleen. Elevating the left side of the operating table much as in laparoscopic splenectomy is helpful, as well. The peritoneal attachments to the diaphragm and colon should be taken down with electrocautery or scissors to allow for mobilization toward the midline. Next, the short gastric vessels should be individually identified, clamped, and ligated to free the spleen from the stomach. The main splenic artery and vein are then identified at the hilum of the spleen and skeletonized. This allows for visualization of the tail of the pancreas and prevents injury, which can lead to a postoperative pancreatic fistula. The artery should then be doubly clamped, divided, and suture ligated. The spleen may noticeably decompress as venous blood is allowed to return to the general circulation after clamping the splenic artery. If the patient is severely thrombocytopenic, platelets can now be given without the possibility of splenic sequestration. The splenic vein is then doubly clamped, divided, and suture ligated. Packs are placed in the splenic bed, and retroperitoneal hemostasis obtained before closure of the incision. Drains are not routinely placed.

POSTOPERATIVE CARE AND COMPLICATIONS

Patients generally tolerate splenectomy well. Parenteral narcotics for pain control are the norm for the first postoperative day with transition to oral medication as diet allows. Oral intake is allowed starting on postoperative day zero if the patient desires, and the diet is advanced as tolerated. Strict adherence to a regimen of pulmonary toilet is essential in helping prevent postoperative atelectasis and pneumonia, which occur in up to 20% of patients. Subcutaneous heparin, sequential compression devices, and early ambulation are utilized in an effort to prevent deep venous thrombosis in the lower extremities.

Thrombocytosis and postoperative leukocytosis are a normal physiologic response to splenectomy. Elevations are usually self-limited and tend to normalize over several weeks. Thrombocytosis is not usually associated with thrombotic events unless the platelet count rises to over 10^6/ul. Should this occur, 81 mg aspirin daily is recommended to prevent unwanted thrombosis.

At times, postoperative leukocytosis may complicate the diagnosis of infection. It is often difficult to decide when an elevated white blood cell count (WBC) is indicative of early infection or a normal result of splenectomy. As patients after splenectomy are at greater risk for infection than the general population, early diagnosis of infection/sepsis is essential in decreasing morbidity. Recently, the absolute WBC count $> 15 \times 10^3$/ul and platelet/WBC ratio < 20 at or after the fifth postoperative day have been validated as markers predicting postoperative sepsis, leading to earlier diagnosis and treatment.[21]

Wound infection, although not common after splenectomy, is probably more common than for other "clean" cases due to the immunosuppressive effect of splenectomy. Therefore, strict adherence to a policy of parenteral antibiotic administration against skin flora is essential.

A left upper quadrant abscess is also a rare complication, in the postoperative period, occurring in fewer than 15% of splenectomies not done for trauma. The combination of the sudden increase in dead space in the left upper quadrant, immunosuppressive effect of splenectomy, and the presence of a hematoma contribute to the formation of an abscess. When fever is accompanied by ileus, leukocytosis, or increasing left upper quadrant pain, an ultrasound or computed tomography scan can aid in the diagnosis of such an abscess as well as its drainage via percutaneous closed suction devices. Systemic broad spectrum antibiotics should be started once the diagnosis is suspected, and these should be tailored to the organisms found within the abscess cavity as soon as Gram stain and culture information is available. Drains should be discontinued once output is less than 50 ml/day. Reimaging is not necessary prior to discontinuation of drains in the afebrile patient without leukocytosis.

An incisional hernia is infrequent with either midline or left subcostal approaches. Incisional hernias are more common, however, in obese patients, smokers with cough, individuals with prostatic hypertrophy, chronic steroid use, or in the face of wound infection, severe anemia, or an immunocompromised state.

Although rare, injury to the tail of the pancreas is a known complication of splenectomy. Haphazard clamping in the region of the splenorenal ligament with inadvertent crush injury to the tail of the pancreas is the cause of this complication. It is more likely to occur in an emergent setting when patients are in extremis during the procedure. Careful dissection in the hilum of the spleen with purposeful skeletonization and ligation and division of the main splenic artery and vein is essential to avoid this complication as previously noted. Should this complication occur, patients present with malaise and hyperamylasemia. CT-guided aspiration and drainage is helpful in managing the collections that follow. Administration of subcutaneous somatostatin analogue, total parenteral nutrition, or feedings beyond the ligament of Treitz can aid in lowering the output of these fistulae.[22] ERCP with stenting of the pancreatic duct across the sphincter of Oddi is a relatively recent innovation to help lower intraductal pressure and allow for earlier resolution of a pancreatic fistula.[23] Very recently, several centers have reported success in treating distal pancreatic fistulas in outpatients with a simple oral diet and bulb

suction drainage. Drains were removed when less than 50 ml was collected daily.[24,25]

OVERWHELMING POSTSPLENECTOMY SEPSIS (OPSI)

Splenectomy, although done for necessary reasons, leaves individuals at an increased risk of infection, especially from bacteremia with encapsulated organisms. With a lifetime risk of 1%-5% in individuals after splenectomy, overwhelming postsplenectomy sepsis is relatively rare and has a mortality rate of approximately 25%-50%. Given this fact, patients should be vaccinated against encapsulated organisms several weeks prior to surgery if splenectomy is done on an elective basis. If splenectomy is done on an emergent basis, vaccination should be accomplished 2-3 weeks after surgery in reliable patients. Many surgeons, however, delay vaccination only several days and recommend vaccination just prior to discharge in an effort to avoid the early postoperative state of the immunosuppression. A study done approximately 10 years ago showed that of those trauma patients vaccinated at 1, 7, or 14 days post splenectomy, titers were highest in those vaccinated at 14 days.[26] Consideration should be given to the fact that many trauma patients are lost to follow-up, and cannot afford the costs associated with vaccination as an outpatient, prior to determining an optimal vaccination schedule. Standard vaccinations confer protection against meningococcal, pneumococcal, and *Haemophilus* species. Patients will need to receive annual influenza vaccine and pneumococcal boosters every 5 years. In the past, prophylactic antibiotics were recommended for children and for adults for the first 3-5 years after splenectomy; however, long-term antibiotics present a risk factor for selection of resistant organisms, efficacy is reduced with noncompliance, and there are not data to indicate that the risk of OPSI declines with time.[27,28]

In addition to vaccinations, patients should routinely be given prophylactic antibiotics by medical and dental professionals prior to any invasive procedures such as elective surgery, dental work, upper or lower gastrointestinal endoscopy, or cardiac catheterization. An antibiotic with gram-positive coverage is a suitable choice for most dental, vascular, and upper gastrointestinal surgery, with additional gram-negative and anaerobic coverage for colonoscopy or colon surgery.

Some physicians have recommended patients have a supply of antibiotics on hand should they become acutely ill. When the antibiotics are taken, patients should proceed to the nearest hospital immediately. The combination of a relatively short shelf life for antibiotics and patient noncompliance make this an impractical policy. Rather, patients should be taken immediately to the hospital where they can be resuscitated, cultured, and placed on broad spectrum antibiotics on an emergent basis.

REFERENCES

1. Upadhyaya P. Conservative management of splenic trauma: history and current trends. *Pediatr Surg Int* 2003;19:617.
2. Moynihan B. The surgery of the spleen. *Br J Surg* 1920;8:307.
3. Berger F. Die Verletzungen der milz und ihre chirurgische behandlung. *Arch Kin Chir* 1902;68:56.
4. Katkhouda N, Hurwitz MG, Rivera RT, et al. Laparoscopic splenectomy: Outcome and efficacy in 103 consecutive patients. *Ann Surg* 1998;228:1.
5. Park AE and McKinlay R. Spleen. In: Brunicardi FC, ed. *Schwartz's Principles of Surgery*, 8th ed. New York: McGraw-Hill; 2005:1297-1299.
6. Lefor AT and Phillips EH. Spleen. In Norton JA, ed. *Surgery—Basic Science and Clinical Evidence*, 1st ed. New York: Springer; 2001:764.
7. Grahn SW, Alvarez J, Kirkwood K. Trends in laparoscopic splenectomy for massive splenomegaly. *Arch Surg* 2006;141:755.
8. Huscher CG, Mingoli A, Sgarzini G et al. Laparoscopic treatment of blunt splenic injuries: initial experience with 11 patients. *Surg Endosc* 2006;20:1423.
9. Allran CF, Weiss CA, Park AE. Urgent laparoscopic splenectomy in a morbidly obese pregnant woman: case report and literature review. *J Laparoendo Adv Surg Tec* 2003;12(6):445.
10. Cines DB, Bussel JB, McMillan RB et al. Congenital and acquired thrombocytopenia. *Hematology Am Soc Hematol Educ Program* 2004;390-406.
11. Downs LA, Thomas NJ, Comito MA, et al. Idiopathic thrombocytopenic purpura complicated by an intracranial hemorrhage secondary to an arteriovenous malformation. *Ped Emerg Care* 2005;21(5):309.
12. Bayry J, Misra M, Latry V, et al. Mechanisms of action of intravenous immunoglobulin in autoimmune and inflammatory diseases. *Transfus Clin Biol* 2003;10:165.
13. Han DC, Feliciano DV. The clinical complexity of splenic vein thrombosis. *The American Surgeon* 1998;64(6):558.
14. Sakorafas GH, Sarr MD, Farley DR, et al. The significance of sinistral portal hypertension complicating chronic pancreatitis. *Am J Surg* 2000;179:129.
15. Piffaretti G, Tozzi M, Lomazzi C, et al. Splenic artery aneurysms: postembolization syndrome and surgical complications. *Am J Surgery* 2007;193:166.
16. Tulsyan M, Kashyap VS, Greenberg RK, et al. The endovascular management of visceral artery aneurysms and pseudoaneurysms. *J Vasc Surg* 2007;45:276.
17. Parangi S, Levine D, Henry A et al. Surgical gastrointestinal disorders during pregnancy. *Am J Surg* 2007;193:223.
18. Tung CC, Chen FC, Lo CJ. Splenic abscess: an easily overlooked disease? *The American Surgeon* 2006;72(4):322.
19. Choudhury RS, Chadha R, Sonker P et al. Management of splenic abscess in children by percutaneous drainage. *J Ped Surg* 2006;41:E53.
20. Chang KC, Chuah SK, Changchen CS, et al. Clinical characteristics and prognostic factors of splenic abscess: A review of 67 cases in a single medical center of Taiwan. *World J Gastroenterol* 2006;12(3):460.
21. Toutouzas KG, Belmahos GC, Kaminski A, et al. Leukocytosis after posttraumatic splenectomy. *Arch Surg* 2002;137:924.
22. Qin JL, Su AD, Zou Y, et al. Effect of parenteral and enteral nutrition combined with octreotide on pancreatic exocrine secretion of patients with pancreatic fistula. *World J Gastroenterol* 2004;10(16):2419.
23. Cohen SA, Siegel JH. Enodotherapy for pancreatic fistulae: inside out or outside in? *Am J Gastroenterol* 2007;102:525.
24. Pannegeon V, Pessaux P, Sauvent A, et al. Pancreatic fistula after distal pancreatectomy. *Arch Surg* 2006;141:1071.
25. Aranha GV, Aaron JM, Shoup M, et al. Current management of pancreatic fistula after pancreaticoduodenectomy. *J Surg* 2006;140:561.
26. Shatz DV, Schinsky MF, Pais LB, et al. Immune responses of splenectomized trauma patients to the 23-valent pneumococcal polysaccharide vaccine at 1 versus 7 versus 14 days after splenectomy. *J Trauma* 1998;44(5):760.
27. Davidson RN, Wall RA. Prevention and management of infections in patients without a spleen. *Clin Microbiol Infect* 2001;7:657.
28. Brigden ML, Pattullo AL. Prevention and management of overwhelming postsplenectomy infection—an update. *Crit Care Med* 1999;27:836.

Chapter 13

THE ACUTE CARE SURGEON'S APPROACH TO HERNIA REPAIR

Jay S. Jenoff, MD, and Vicente H. Gracias, MD

The modern term "hernia," derived from the Latin "to rupture," is defined as the protrusion of an organ or tissue through an abnormal opening.[1] The majority of abdominal wall hernias arise in the groin.[2] Each year, it is estimated that over 750,000 inguinal hernia and 100,000 inguinal hernia repairs are performed.[3,4] Given the ubiquitous nature of the problem, it is clear that the acute care surgeon will require a strong knowledge of the anatomy, physiology, evaluation, and treatment of abdominal wall hernias. William S. Halstead understood this in the 19th century. In his 1892 paper "The Cure of Inguinal Hernia in the Male," Halstead states in reference to inguinal hernia repair, that "There is, perhaps, no operation which, by the profession at large, would be more appreciated than a perfectly safe ... cure for rupture."[5]

DEMOGRAPHICS

The exact incidence of abdominal wall hernias in the general population is unknown, as many asymptomatic hernias may exist and remain undiagnosed. However, hernias are a common problem, with an estimated 5% of the population developing an abdominal wall hernia during their lifetime. Approximately 75% of these will arise in the groin (indirect inguinal, direct inguinal, femoral), with the rest composed of epigastric, umbilical, incisional, or "unusual" hernias (obdurator, spigelian, lumbar, etc).[4] Recent statistics list herniorrhaphy as one of the most common procedures performed by general surgeons today.[6]

The indirect inguinal hernia is the most prevalent regardless of age or gender. Overall, men are more predisposed to hernia formation with an estimated incidence of 25 to 1 compared with their female counterparts. Femoral and umbilical hernias are more common in women than men, although women are still more likely to develop an indirect inguinal hernia than any other sort. More hernias will develop on the right side compared with the left. This is thought to be

due to the delayed obliteration of the processus vaginalis on the right and slower descent of the right testis as compared with the left in males. With regard to femoral hernias, it is hypothesized that the sigmoid colon may have a protective effect on the left femoral canal.[3,4]

With increasing age, there is an overall increase in the prevalence of abdominal wall hernias. Likewise, the incidence of complications related to hernias, most notably strangulation, as well as the need for hospitalization, is also higher. With the overall aging of the population, one may extrapolate that the overall prevalence of abdominal wall hernias will increase over time. It is the aim of this chapter to discuss the issues surrounding the emergent repair of abdominal wall hernias. It is the urgent/emergent care of the incarcerated and or strangulated hernia that most concerns us.

HISTORY

The earliest written document known to mention hernias is the Egyptian Papyrus of Ebers (circa 1552 B.C.).[7] Through the ages, anatomical descriptions as well as surgical repair was described by the likes of Hippocrates, Celsus, Albucasis, Pare, Scarpa, Cooper, and Richter. Hernia surgery was revolutionized in the late 1800s by Edoardo Bassini (1844–1924). Noting a high rate of recurrence following high ligation alone, Bassini pioneered the concept of reconstructing the floor of the inguinal canal. Edoardo Bassini is credited as the creator of modern hernia surgery, with most current techniques being modifications of his basic tenets. These advances would be made by the likes of Halstead, Lotheisen, Cushing, McVay, and Shouldice. These anatomic tissue repairs would dominate until the 1980s.[2] Regardless of the method of repair, recurrence was still unacceptably high, with series reporting rates as high as 20%.[3] Understanding that recurrence was often due to excessive tension on the suture line, the search for a suitable prosthetic material to alleviate such strain was begun. With the advent of prosthetics in the 1950s, surgeons began experimenting with different materials to improve outcomes in hernia repair. In 1958, Horwich used elasticated nylon in his repair of large or recurrent hernias. That same year, Usher et al. began using Marlex. Most surgeons reserved prosthetics for the repair of large, sliding, or recurrent hernias, the fear of infection limiting its use.[2,3]

In contemporary times, the most impactful contribution has been the tension-free repair, first described in 1989 when Lichtenstein reported 1000 consecutive herniorrhaphies repaired with prosthetic materials. Lichtenstein was not the first to use mesh in inguinal hernia repair, but was the first to use it in all inguinal herniorrhaphies. His cohort was followed for greater than 1 to 5 years with no reported recurrences. Lichtenstein is credited with coining the phrase "tensionfree" repair.[8] Shortly thereafter, Dion and Martin were credited with the development of the transabdominal preperitoneal laparoscopic hernia repair (TAPP) whereas McKernan and Laws developed the totally extraperitoneal repair (TEP).[9,10]

CLASSIFICATION

The traditional classification of groin hernias as indirect, direct, or femoral has stood the test of time. Over the past 50 years, several classification schemes have been proposed to create a common nomenclature, and have been utilized around the world. The goal has been to more critically appraise and compare different operative approaches in an attempt to determine the optimal approach given the type of hernia. In the late 1950s, Harkins proposed a four grade classification scheme for hernias.[11] In 1958, McVay et al proposed their own classification, later expanding upon this in 1970.[12,13] Casten developed a three grade system of his own, publishing this in 1967.[14] The late 1980s saw the addition of two new taxonomies by Lichtenstein and Gilbert, respectively.[15,16] Rutkow and Robbins would later modify Gilbert's work.[17] In 1993, Nyhus et al published the Nyhus classification to "aid in the surgical decision-making best matching the type of hernia with specific operations."[11] The Nyhus classification may be the most widely used in the United States and Europe today, the details of which are listed here.

Nyhus Classification of Groin Hernias
Type I: Indirect inguinal hernia, small
Type II: Indirect, medium
Type III: A. Direct
           B. Indirect, large
           C. Femoral
Type IV: Recurrent
           A. Direct
           B. Indirect

C. Femoral
D. Combination of A, B, C

Modifications of the Nyhus Classification scheme has been proposed by Stoppa, allowing for "aggravating" factors that essentially upstage the hernia by one grade. These include patient comorbidities (age, pulmonary disease, obesity), size of hernia, abdominal distension, collagen vascular disease, infection, or technical difficulty.[18] Finally, a unified classification, drawing from the many existing schema already in publication, has been devised.[19] It is important to remember that these classification schemes, although extensive, were created to compare outcomes of repair. The one taxonomy that has remained throughout the years is the description of groin hernias as being indirect, direct, or femoral.[2]

Several classification schemes have also been devised to describe ventral hernias. In the strictest sense, the term "ventral hernia" would include groin hernias as described above, by convention, it usually is used to refer to anterior abdominal wall hernias excluding those of the inguinal region. Several classification and subclassification schemes have been developed. Functionally, division into congenital and acquired hernias has been widely used. Likewise, the anatomic location is usually used in this description. For acquired ventral hernias, the differentiation between incisional and traumatic is often made.[2]

PREOPERATIVE MANAGEMENT

DIAGNOSIS
As stated earlier, a hernia refers to the protrusion of an organ or tissue through an abnormal opening. A thorough working knowledge of anatomy is essential in both the accurate diagnosis of a hernia, as well as the operative intervention, maximizing successful repair and minimizing complications. A palpable bulge is the mainstay of presentation of a hernia. The patient may experience pain, tenderness, or obstructive symptoms; however, this is usually suggestive of incarceration or strangulation. Abdominal wall hernia should always be included in the differential diagnosis of abdominal pain, bowel obstruction, groin pain, and groin mass. The majority of the time, the diagnosis of abdominal wall hernia may be ascertained based on history and physical exam alone. In such cases, no further evaluation is necessary. In the incarcerated or strangulated hernia, unnecessary testing may delay operative intervention and affect outcome.

The hernia exam should be performed with the patient in both the supine as well as the standing position. Visual inspection and palpation of the inguinal region as well as the anterior abdominal wall may provide the diagnosis. Physical exam alone may not detect some hernias, especially small hernias and those in female and obese patients. Adjunctive imaging, such as ultrasonography, computed tomography (CT), and magnetic resonance imaging (MRI) are helpful in establishing the presence of a hernia. It has been found that all three modalities are helpful in overall diagnosis, however, ultrasound often does not differentiate the type of hernia (direct space, indirect) when compared with CT or MRI. Likewise, these modalities help differentiate abdominal wall hernias from benign, malignant, and inflammatory masses such as abscesses, aneurysms, lymphadenopathy, varicose nodules, hematoma, and soft tissue tumors. When ultrasound is nondiagnostic, CT or MRI may prove more useful. CT has the advantage of being quickly obtainable and lower in cost than MRI, whereas MRI does not expose the patient to ionizing radiation and provides greater definition of the abdominal wall.

TIMING OF REPAIR

The acute care surgeon must determine the urgency with which an abdominal wall hernia must be treated. Much of the data on hernia repair relates to the elective population. This affords the surgeon time for operative planning as well as risk-factor modification. The easily reducible hernia evaluated in the emergency department may be fixed on an elective basis, time permitting during the current hospital visit or later arranged as an outpatient. This is not the case for the patient presenting to the emergency department with an incarcerated or strangulated hernia at any anatomic location. Patient comorbidities, regardless of severity, must be managed quickly, and the patient aggressively resuscitated so as not to delay definitive operative intervention. Optimal patient monitoring with invasive arterial, central venous, and pulmonary artery catheters are rare occurrences but should be employed where indicated. The relationship between the surgeon and anesthesiologist is paramount in successful navigation of the quickly formulated operative course. Meticulous postoperative care is essential, and when necessary, management in an ICU setting.

When evaluating a patient with an abdominal wall hernia, strict attention to the patient interview and physical exam is the first step in operative planning. The surgeon must differentiate between an incarcerated hernia (trapped) as opposed to a strangulated hernia (ischemic), as the first is a surgical urgency while the second is a surgical emergency. The acuity of hernia formation also places contents at greater risk. More chronic larger hernias may exist for extended periods of time without compromising the hernia contents.

Eliciting a history of acute pain or obstructive symptoms such as nausea, vomiting, or obstipation are suggestive of incarceration and existing or impending strangulation. Laboratory evaluation including leukocytosis and indicators of hypoperfusion such as lactate are also indicative of compromised intra-abdominal contents. Physical signs such as tenderness and erythema of the overlying skin are concerning for ischemia and possible necrosis of the hernia contents consistent with strangulation. Doppler ultrasound can at time aid in ascertaining the presence of blood flow within the contents of a hernia sack. An irreducible hernia is incarcerated and demands urgent attention and operative intervention. A high index of suspicion is necessary as it will influence the operative plan.

ANESTHESIA

Throughout the history of herniorrhaphy, every mode of anesthesia has been employed from physical restraint during "cauterization" procedures, to deep general anesthesia. In 1898, Harvey Cushing first proposed hernia repair using local anesthesia.[20] He used local infiltration of cocaine as made popular by Halstead. The choice and administration of anesthetic truly need to be a collaborative effort between the surgeon, anesthesiologist, and patient. Although local anesthesia has become the preferred route for many individuals, it relies heavily on the surgeon having a greater knowledge of anesthetic principles as well as better technical abilities in anesthetic administration. It also demands greater cooperation from the patient, requiring them to comprehend, have no underlying language barrier, and be able to cooperate with the operating room staff. Recent studies in both the surgery and anesthesia literature has shown that > 90% of inguinal hernia repairs can be performed under local anesthesia.[21] Patients reported lower intraoperative and early postoperative pain when compared to regional and general anesthesia. Results at 8 and 30 days were unchanged. Likewise, local anesthesia had a lower postoperative rate of urinary retention and need for urinary catheter placement when compared to regional anesthesia.[21]

Today, much of the decision in choosing the route of anesthetic administration is determined by the anatomic and physiologic status of the patient. Age, body habitus, mental status, cardiac disease, pulmonary disease (including difficult airway), and hernia size all dictate the type of anesthetic to be employed. A thorough preoperative evaluation by the anesthesia staff is necessary to identify all comorbid conditions that may affect the intended procedure.

Patients with preexisting, severe cardiovascular disease benefit from herniorrhaphy under local anesthesia with or without sedation as opposed to general anesthesia as this should reduce perioperative risk. Likewise, repair of inguinal, umbilical, and small ventral hernias in patients with underlying pulmonary disease should successfully maintain normal respiratory mechanics if local anesthesia is used as opposed to general anesthesia (Fig. 13-1).[22]

Morbid obesity often presents a problem with regard to anesthetic administration. Often, these patients are

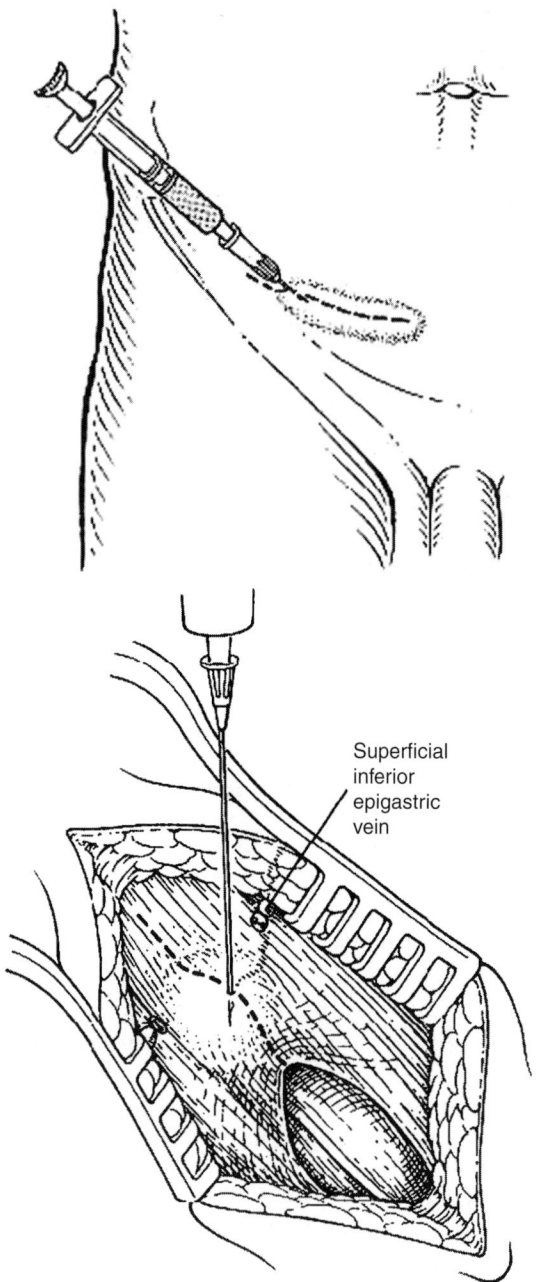

Superficial
inferior
epigastric
vein

Figure 13-1 *Administration of anesthetics. (Reproduced with permsision from Kurzer M et al. The Lichtenstein repair for groin hernias.* Surg Clin N Am *2003;83:1099-1117.)*

prone to aspiration and may be difficult to ventilate in the operating room. Likewise, they may have a predisposition to difficult airways based on anatomical considerations. Local anesthetics may diffuse through an expanded tissue mass, diluting the local concentration and impairing the surgeon's ability to adequately achieve anesthesia. Also, the necessary administered dose may exceed the limit based on the patient's lean body mass.

In the setting of elective hernia repair, the American Society for Anesthesiologists (ASA) classification would characterize patients designated as class I, II, or III as suitable candidates for outpatient procedures, with any class of anesthetic a possible option.[23] In the practice of acute care surgery, the patient presenting with groin pain and an easily reducible hernia that might fit this criteria and be scheduled for elective surgery is often the exception, not the rule. Likewise, ventral hernias and giant hernias of any location will require general anesthesia.

OPERATIVE MANAGEMENT

NONOPERATIVE OBSERVATION

Elective repair of asymptomatic, nonincarcerated, nonstrangulated abdominal wall hernias can be considered in patients with multiple comorbid conditions placing them at high surgical risk. In the acute care surgical population, this is a luxury rarely afforded to the surgeon. Although the same comorbidities are prevalent, the patient presenting with acute pain or obstructive symptoms necessitates operative intervention. The high risk during both the intraoperative and postoperative periods underscores the ideal role of the surgical critical care physician as acute care surgeon.

REPAIR OF GROIN HERNIAS

A discussion of groin hernia repair must touch on both inguinal as well as femoral herniorrhaphy. Inguinal hernias may be addressed in either an open or laparoscopic fashion. Likewise, open herniorrhaphy may be pursued by either an anterior or posterior approach.

Anterior Repair

The most common operative approach today is the open anterior repair (Fig. 13-2). Most anterior tissue repairs are a variation of the Bassini repair. These include the Cooper ligament or McVay repair, the Marci repair, the nylon darn repair, Shouldice (Canadian) repair, and the iliopubic tract repair. Tension-free repair may be of an anterior or posterior approach, with the Lichtenstein, Gilbert, and "plug and patch" approaches being performed anteriorly. Tension-free herniorrhaphy is the most common anterior approach, with anatomic tissue repair being reserved for small hernias. In 2003, Rutkow reported that 37% of all hernia repairs performed were accomplished by the Lichtenstein method, making it the most utilized approach. This was followed closely by the "plug" method at 34%, and laparoscopic repair at a distant 14%.[24]

Posterior Repair

Nyhus et al first introduced the pre-peritoneal approach in 1960.[25] The proposed benefit was in the repair of incarcerated and strangulated hernias. When feasible, Nyhus et al were proponents of polypropylene mesh to be placed as a buttress. Overall, their recurrence rate for indirect, direct, and femoral hernias was 3%, 6%, and 1%, respectively.[26,27] In 1969, Stoppa et al described the

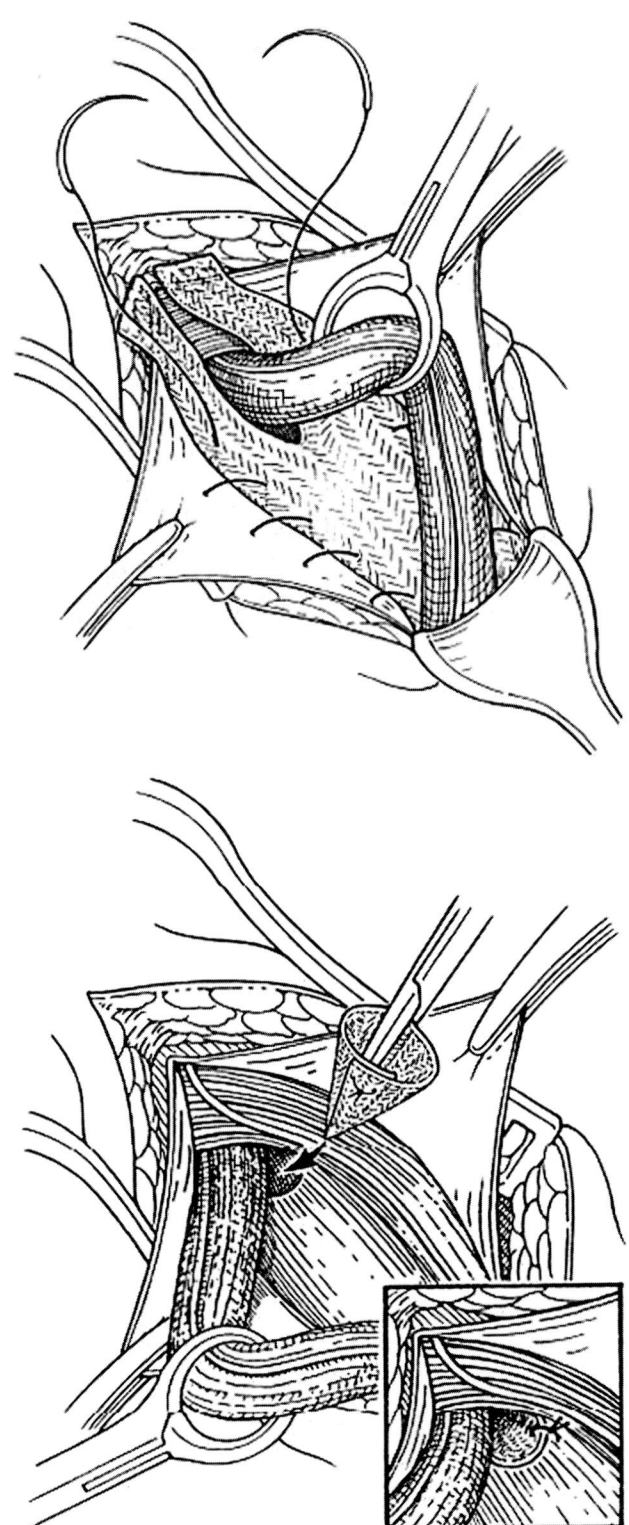

Figure 13-2 *Inguinal hernia repair. (Reproduced with permission from Kurzer M et al. The Lichtenstein repair for groin hernias.* Surg Clin N Am *2003;83:1099-1117.)*

use of a giant piece of mesh placed in the preperitoneal space, reporting an overall recurrence rate of 1.4%.[28,29] The open preperitoneal repair using the Kugel Patch (Davol, Cranston, Rhode Island), involves placement of a self-expanding polypropylene mesh placed

through a muscle-splitting incision without any attempt at tissue repair. Kugel reports a 0.4% recurrence rate; however, other studies have published recurrence up to 27%.[30-32]

Laparoscopic Inguinal Hernia Repair

Two main techniques of laparoscopic inguinal hernia repair are employed today. The first, transabdominal preperitoneal (TAPP) approach employs laparoscopic techniques to enter the abdomen, create a peritoneal flap, and enter the preperitoneal space. The totally extraperitoneal (TEP) approach creates a preperitoneal potential space through which the hernia is repaired, never entering the peritoneum. Laparoscopic inguinal hernia repair has been shown to have a lower recurrence rate compared to tissue repair (3% vs 6%).[33,34] Comparisons to tension-free open repairs has not been as clear cut. Proponents cite lower postoperative pain, shorter hospital stay, ability to interrogate and repair the contralateral side as well as femoral canal, and quicker return to work as evidence for its implementation. Detractors point to a higher complication rate during the early, steep learning curve, initially longer operative times, and equipment cost to the hospital, and potential difficulty with future pelvic surgery.[3] Importantly, the role of laparoscopic hernia repair has yet to be ascertained in the acute care surgery setting.

Femoral Hernia Repair

Although not as prevalent as inguinal hernias, femoral hernias are a major contributor to the morbidity and mortality of groin hernias. They account for 2% to 8% of all groin hernias, occur four to five times more commonly in females, and usually occur between ages 40 and 70.[35]

There are three common approaches to repairing femoral hernias. The first is the femoral approach (Fig. 13-3). First described in 1879 by Socin, the hernia sac was reduced through an incision over the femoral canal. Modifications of this were made by Bassini, Marcy, and Cushing, closing the femoral ring. However, these repairs were plagued by a high recurrence rate and thus, this approach was abandoned for many years. It was revived by Lichtenstein, creating a tension-free repair by placing a rolled polypropylene mesh in the femoral ring through this approach. Modifications of this were made by Gilbert and Rutkow and Robbins.[16,17]

The second approach is the inguinal approach, first attempted by Annandale in 1876. This was modified several times with poor results. Finally, in 1942, Chester McVay demonstrated that the transverses abdominus and transversalis fascia need to be reapproximated to Cooper's ligament, thus developing the Cooper's ligament (McVay) repair.[35]

The third approach is the preperitoneal approach. Cheatle's original work in 1921 was expanded upon by Nyhus in 1960, with a reported 1% recurrence

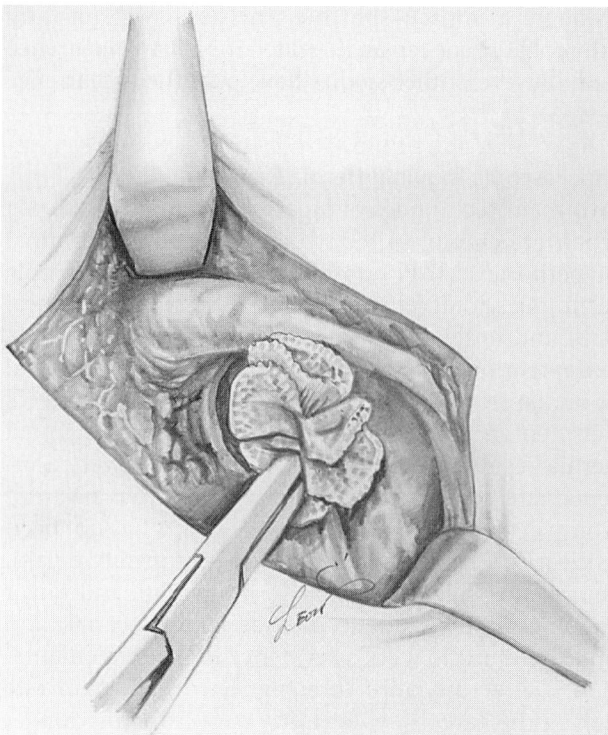

Figure 13-3 *Femoral hernia repair. (Reproduced with permsision from Hachisuka T. Femoral Hernia Repair.* Surg Clin N Am *2003;83:1189-1205.)*

rate.[36,37,38] Stoppa modified this in 1973, showing a 3% recurrence rate with his technique.[39] Finally, in 1990, Phillips applied laparoscopic principles to Stoppa's approach, using the TEP technique.[40]

Ventral Hernia Repair

Ventral hernia repair includes a vast array of anatomic locations. Incisional, epigastric, umbilical, and parastomal sites may all be involved. Overall, the principles of successful repair are the same, including a healthy blood supply, good tissue approximation, and a lack of tension. Each year, 2 million laparotomies are performed in the United States. Studies show that 2% to 11% of laparotomies will be complicated by incisional hernias, resulting in approximately 100,000 incisional herniorrhaphies performed each year. The recurrence rate from this procedure has been reported at 10% to 50%.[41]

Ventral hernias tend to enlarge over time. As they become symptomatic, pain with movement and straining is often encountered. Similar to groin hernias, symptoms of nausea, vomiting, and obstipation usually accompany incarceration and/or strangulation. No gold-standard repair has been developed for ventral hernia repair. Techniques include primary closure, primary closure with relaxing incisions, primary closure with onlay/inlay mesh, onlay/inlay mesh alone, retrorectus mesh placement, and intraperitoneal mesh placement. Laparoscopic techniques are also employed.

Primary closure is reserved for defects < 5 cm in diameter. Even at this small size, recurrence rates can approach 50%. With the variety of mesh reinforced closure methods, recurrence rates have been reported as low as 5% to 10%.[41]

SPECIAL CONSIDERATIONS

There is an old surgical adage that you cannot reduce dead bowel. This, however, has potential false security as reduction en masse has been described where hernia and hernia sac are reduced in entirety into the abdomen, and hernia content remains strangulated and ischemic. Also, it is not uncommon that upon induction of general anesthesia, the hernia spontaneously reduces. Preoperative marking of the hernia site and standard landmarks before induction will make operative exploration easier and is highly recommended. Regardless, the surgeon is left with the dilemma of determining the viability of the contents of the hernia sac. In the case of a larger ventral hernia, the abdomen may be explored through the pre-existing defect. For groin hernias, the surgeon has several options. If the peritoneal fluid is clear, it is reasonable to repair the hernia and observe the patient with a high index of suspicion and a low threshold for returning to the operating room for formal exploration. If the peritoneal fluid is at all turbid or sanguinous, or the surgeon is concerned about visceral compromise, three approaches exist. The first is to attempt abdominal exploration through the given groin incision. This may be accomplished by running the bowel through the existing incision, potentially enlarging it to facilitate doing so. The second would be to place a laparoscope through the hernia sac and perform abdominal exploration in this manner. The final approach would be to perform a separate midline laparotomy or diagnostic laparoscopy. An objective assessment regarding presentation signs and symptoms must be performed regardless of timing in order to choose the correct treatment option. If unsuccessful in full exploration through the given incision or the inability to systematically run the bowel laparoscopically, a separate incision should be employed.

Dilemmas also revolve around abdominal hernia repair in the setting of known or suspected compromised bowel. Permanent mesh is the mainstay of tension-free repair. In the setting of strangulated bowel and possible resection, most surgeons are hesitant to implant such mesh due to the fear of infection and the need for explantation. In 2006, Wysocki et al reported their results using polypropylene for Lichtenstein inguinal hernia repair in the setting of incarcerated bowel. They observed no infectious complications in 51 of 55 patients, although contamination was not graded.[42] If a grossly contaminated operative field is encountered, the results could be different.

POSTOPERATIVE MANAGEMENT

COMPLICATIONS

Several complications following abdominal hernia repair are well described. Recurrence, although greatly reduced in the era of tension-free repair, is still a concern. In the acute care surgery population, this may be greater, as acutely compromised bowel may lead to overall higher infection rates and subsequent failure of the repair. Also, the subset of patients requiring anatomic tissue repairs is likely higher in this population where gross contamination precludes the use of prosthetic mesh.

Local wound infection continues to be a problem following hernia repair. Cellulitis should be treated accordingly. When present, the presence of prosthetic mesh compounds this problem, and a determination of its necessity in the repair must be made. Abscesses should be drained with care not to expose the mesh if possible. Redundant areas of mesh may be locally removed with the greater whole left intact if not exposed. If necessary, the entire mesh may need to be removed. Other local complications such as hematoma and seroma formation may be observed expectantly. Complications involving the testes, spermatic cord, and neurologic structures may also occur. Overaggressive dissection of the spermatic cord structures may lead to ischemic orchitis or frank necrosis. The ilioinguinal and genitofemoral nerves may be injured. Finally, posthernior-rhaphy pain is an extensive topic, and one deserving of more detail than will be provided here, as it is not specific to the acute care surgical population.

CONCLUSION

As the field of acute care surgery continues to evolve, it is intuitive that those involved will be faced with the challenge of addressing complex abdominal wall hernias. With a firm knowledge of anatomy and physiology, as well as sound surgical judgment and technique, the acute care surgeon sits poised to successfully care for these problems.

REFERENCES

1. *Dorland's Illustrated Medical Dictionary.* 26th ed. Philadelphia, PA: W.B. Saunders Company; 1985.
2. Fitzgibbons Jr. RJ, Greenburg AG. *Nyhus and Condon's Hernia.* 5th ed. Philadelphia, PA: Lippincott, Williams, & Wilkins; 2002.
3. Reuben B, Neumayer L. Surgical management of inguinal hernia. *Adv. Surgery* 2006;40:299-317.
4. Townsend et al, ed. Hernias. In: *Sabiston Textbook of Surgery: The Biological Basis of Modern Surgical Practice,* 17th ed. Philadelphia, PA: Elsevier Saunders; 2004.
5. Halsted WS. *Surgical Papers by William Stewart Halsted: The Operative Treatment of Inguinal Hernia,* vol 1. Baltimore, MD: Johns Hopkins Press; 1924.
6. Rutkow IM. Epidemiologic, economic, and sociologic aspects of hernia surgery in the United States in the 1990s. *Surg Clin North Am* 1998;78(6):941-951.
7. Lyons AS, Petrucelli RJ II. Medicine: An Illustrated History. New York: Harry N. Abrams Publishers; 1987.
8. Lichtenstein IL, Shulman AG, Amid PK, et al. The tension-free hernioplasty. *Am J Surg* 1989;157:188-193.
9. Dion YM, Martin J. Laparoscopic inguinal herniorrhaphy. *Can J Surg* 1992;35:209-212.
10. McKernan JB, Laws H. Laparoscopic preperitoneal prosthetic repair of inguinal hernias. *Surg Rounds* 1992; 595-607.
11. Nyhus LM. Individualization of hernia repair: a new era. *Surgery* 1993; 114:12.
12. McVay CB, Chapp JD. Inguinal and femoral hernioplasty. *Ann Surg* 1958;148:499512.
13. Halverson K, McVay C. Inguinal and femoral hernioplasty. *Arch Surg* 1970;101:127-135.
14. Casten DF. Functional anatomy of the groin area as related to the classification and treatment of groin hernias. *Am J Surg* 1967;114:984-989.
15. Lichtenstein IL. Herniorrhaphy. *Am J Surg* 1987;153: 553-559.
16. Gilbert AI. An anatomic and functional classification for the diagnosis and treatment of inguinal hernia. *Am J Surg* 1989;157:331-333.
17. Rutkow IM, Robbins AW. Classification systems and groin hernias. *Surg Clin North Am* 1998;78:1122–1124.
18. Stoppa R. In: Chevrel JP, ed. *Hernias and Surgery of the Abdominal Wall.* Berlin: Springer; 1998:175-178.
19. Zollinger RM Jr. A unified classification for inguinal hernias. *Hernia* 1999;3:195-200.
20. Cushing H. Cocaine anesthesia in the treatment of certain cases of hernia and in operations for thyroid tumors. *Johns Hopkins Hosp Bull* 1898;9:192.
21. Amado WJ. Anesthesia for groin hernia surgery. *Surg Clin N Am* 2003;83:1065-1077.
22. M Kurzer et al. The Lichtenstein repair for groin hernias. *Surg Clin N Am* 83;2003:1099-1117.
23. Dripps RD. Preanesthetic consultation and choice of anesthesia. In: Dripps RD, Eckenhoff JE, Vandam LD, eds. *Introduction to Anesthesia: The Principles of Safe Practice.* Philadelphia, PA: WB Saunders; 1988:13-21.
24. Rutkow I. Demographic and socioeconomic aspects of hernia repair in the United States in 2003. *Surg Clin North Am* 2003;83:1045-1051.
25. Nyhus LM, Condon RE, Harkins HN. Clinical experiences with the preperitoneal hernia repair for all types of hernia of the groin: with particular reference to the importance of transversalis fascia analogues. *Am J Surg* 1960;100:234-244.
26. Nyhus LM, Pollak R, Bombeck CT. The preperitoneal approach and prosthetic buttress repair for recurrent hernia: the evolution of a technique. *Ann Surg* 1988;208:733-737.

27. Nyhus LM. Iliopubic tract repair of inguinal and femoral hernia: the posterior (preperitoneal) approach. *Surg Clin North Am* 1993;73:487-499.

28. Stoppa RE, Quintyn M. Les deficiencies de la poroi abdominale chez le suget age: colloque avec le praticien. *Semin Hop (Paris)* 1969;45:2182-2184.

29. Stoppa RE. The giant prosthesis for the reinforcement of the visceral sac in the repair of groin and incisional hernias. In: Nyhus LM, Baker RJ, Fischer JE, eds. *Mastery of Surgery.* Boston, MA: Little Brown; 1997.

30. Kugel R. The Kugel repair for groin hernias. *Surg Clin North Am* 2003;83:1119-1139.

31. Schroder DM, Lloyd LK, Boccaccio JE, et al. Inguinal hernia recurrence following preperitoneal Kugel patch repair. *Ann Surg* 2004;70:132-136.

32. Reddy KM, Humphreys W, Chew A, et al. Inguinal hernia repair with the Kugel patch. *ANZJ Surg* 2005;75:43-47.

33. Tschudi J, Wagner M, Klaiber C, et al. Controlled multicenter trial of laparoscopic transabdominal preperitoneal hernioplasty vs Shouldice herniorrhaphy: early results. *Surg Endosc* 1996;10:845-847.

34. Liem MS, van der Graaf Y, van Steensel CJ, et al. Comparison of conventional anterior surgery and laparoscopic surgery for inguinal-hernia repair. *N Engl J Med* 1997;336:1541-1547.

35. Hachisuka T. Femoral hernia repair. *Surg Clin N Am* 2003;83:1189-1205.

36. Cheatle GL. An operation for the radical cure of inguinal and femoral hernia. *BMJ* 1920;2:68-69.

37. Nyhus LM, Condon RE, Harkins HN. Clinical experiences with preperitoneal hernia repair for all types of hernia of the groin. *Am J Surg* 1960;100:234-244.

38. Nyhus LM. Iliopubic tract repair of inguinal and femoral hernia; the posterior (preperitoneal) approach. *Surg Clin N Am* 1993;73:487-499.

39. Stoppa RE et al. The preperitoneal approach and prosthetic repair of groin hernias. In: Nyhus LM, Condon RE, eds. *Hernia.* 4th ed. Philadelphia: JB Lippincott Co.; 1995:188-206.

40. Phillips EH, Carroll BJ, Fallas MJ. Laparoscopic preperitoneal inguinal hernia repair without peritoneal incision. *Surg Endosc* 1993;7:159-162.

41. Millikan KW. Incisional hernia repair. *Surg Clin N Am* 2003;83:1223-1234.

42. Wysocki A, Kulawik J, Pozniczek M, Strzalka M. Is the Lichtenstein operation of strangulated groin hernia a safe procedure? *World Journal of Surgery* 2006;30(11):2065-2070.

Chapter 14

SOFT TISSUE INFECTIONS

Sharon Henry, MD, and Thomas Scalea, MD

INTRODUCTION

Skin and soft tissue are among the most frequent sites of bacterial infection. They account for nearly 10% of hospital admissions in the United States and represent the most common indication for antibiotic treatment.[1] Soft tissue infections are extremely varied in their presentation and etiologies. The clinical range in presentation is from superficial and innocuous to deep-seated and life threatening. Trivial infections are thankfully much more common than are life threatening infections. However, the potential lethality of more severe infections, mandate familiarity with the diagnosis and treatment.

EPIDEMIOLOGY

CLASSIFICATION

The terminology used to describe soft tissue infections can be quite confusing. Much written work utilizes terminology that is archaic and not commonly used in clinical practice thus adding to the confusion. A useful classification mechanism is based on anatomic skin structure (Fig. 14-1). This simplifies classification enormously. Classification by etiology also offers some advantage. It is sometimes useful to recognize infections that occur primarily are distinctive from those that occur secondarily. Secondary skin infections usually occur as a complication of a chronic skin problem (Table 14-1). Another scheme to classify infections involves recognition of the severity of the infection and the likely necessity of surgical intervention.

Uncomplicated infections are likely to respond to nonsurgical treatment and may frequently be treated in an outpatient setting with or without antibiotic therapy (Table 14-2). Complicated infections, by contrast, more frequently require in patient treatment, antibiotics, and surgical intervention. Finally, infections can be grouped by their pathophysiology such as into necrotizing and nonnecrotizing types. This is probably least helpful, as this may not become apparent until surgical intervention is carried out.

PREOPERATIVE

Uncomplicated soft tissue infections include impetigo, ecthyma, erysipelas, cellulitis, folliculitis, furuncles, abscess, and carbuncle. Impetigo, usually diagnosed in children is characterized by vesicles that rupture producing yellow crusted exudates. These lesions are usually caused by streptococcus, but may result from a combination of streptococcus and staphylococcus. The lesions are superficial, limited to the epidermal layer and are not painful, but may be pruritic. Treatment with oral antibiotics effective against the causative organisms is appropriate. When these lesions are associated with a shallow ulceration, ecthyma should be diagnosed. Treatment with appropriate antibiotics and topical care is curative.

Erysipelas is typically superficial cellulitis, accompanied by streaky lymphangitis. The skin is erythematous, raised, well demarcated and may be tender. Fever is frequently present. Group A streptococcus is often the causative organism and it occurs most frequently on the lower extremities. It can produce lymphatic obstruction, often occurs in sites of previous infection, and may be recurrent. Treatment with antibiotics effective against staphylococcus and streptococcus is recommended.

Cellulitis is a spreading infection affecting the dermis and subcutaneous tissue. Unlike the erythema of erysipelas, raised skin edges and sharp demarcation are not usually seen with cellulitis. The causative organisms are usually the same. Group A streptococcus can cause an aggressive infection, that rapidly advances. Lymphatics may become involved, causing tense edema. Significant constitutional symptoms may accompany cellulitis. Cellulitis is frequently associated with a dermatologic condition, a surgical site or impaired lymphatic drainage. The findings of cellulitis are clinically nonspecific and may mimic other more deep seated infections that require surgical treatment.

Folliculitis, furuncles, carbuncles, and abscesses represent suppurative soft tissue infections that affect the dermis and subcutaneous layers. Folliculitis is usually most superficial, associated with a hair follicle. The lesions occur on hair bearing areas as erythematous mildly painful nodules. In dark pigmented individuals, the lesions may not appear particularly erythematous. This

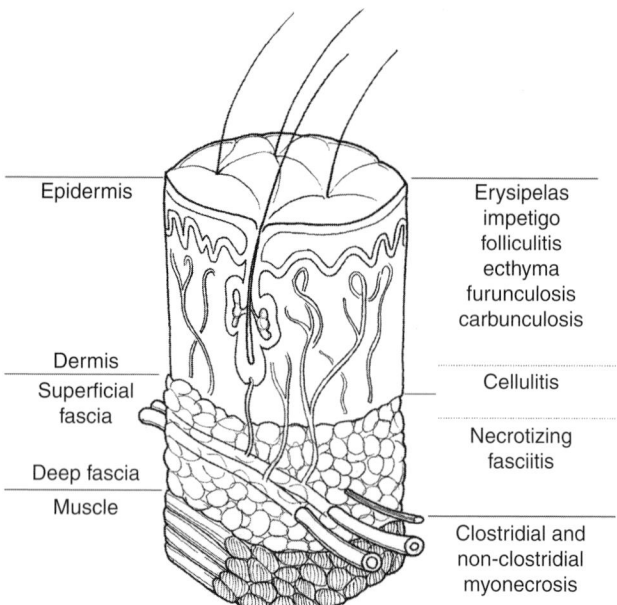

Figure 14-1 *Skin anatomy and corresponding infections. From* Current Therapy in Trauma Surgery and Critical Care. *ed Asensio, JA and Trunkey. DD Mosby Elesevier; Philadelphia PA: 2008 (chapter Soft Tissue Infections) pp 579-583.*

Table 14-2 Uncomplicated Skin Infections
Uncomplicated Skin Infections
■ Impetigo
■ Pyoderma
■ Ecthyma
■ Infected epidermal cysts
■ Erysipelas
■ Erythasma
■ Folliculitis
■ Superficial abscess
■ Cellulitis
■ Hidradenitis supprativa

lesion is usually adequately treated with topical therapy, including warm soaks and topical antimicrobial agents. Staphylococcus is the usual causative pathogen. Furuncles may develop from folliculitis. The lesion becomes a red, raised indurated nodule and may ultimately become fluctuant with a yellow center. It may rupture spontaneously draining white creamy pus. A carbuncle is an area of multiple furuncles, which develop multiple draining sinuses. The overlying skin is thick and indurated and the borders are poorly demarcated.

Pyomyositis is an infection of skeletal muscle. The most common offending organism is SA, although *Streptococcus pyogenes*, *Escherichia coli*, mycobacteria, fungi, and parasites can also cause this disease. It can occur after injury, with vascular insufficiency, and usually spreads contiguously. Bacteremic spread is possible but not common. Most patients have predisposing illness including diabetes mellitus, alcohol liver disease, steroid use, and immunosuppressive illness. Patients usually complain of achy or crampy feelings in their muscles. Induration may be apparent on physical examination. This may progress to fluctuance and bogginess. Surgical or in selected cases percutaneous drainage can be used to treat the infection.[2]

Necrotizing fasciitis (NF) is a soft tissue infection that is invasive and requires early recognition and surgical debridement. There have been multiple terms used to describe this infection including gas gangrene, Fournier gangrene, streptococcal hemolytic gangrene, Meleney synergistic gangrene, and the flesh-eating bacteria (Table 14-3). This infection may present innocuously with signs and symptoms that mimic cellulitis. At other times, it presents with pain, swelling, frank skin necrosis, blistering, and crepitance.

The pathophysiology of these infections involves with vascular thrombosis, which produces the advancing tissue necrosis. The bacteria produce proteases and collagenases, which aids their progress along tissue planes.[3] A thin watery (dishwater) pus often accompanies superficial fat and fascial necrosis. The fluid may be quite foul-smelling. Thrombosis of the skin's nutrient vessels produces the skin necrosis that may be seen with NF. Microscopically, severe subcutaneous fat necrosis, severe inflammation of the dermis and subcutaneous fat, vasculitis, endarteritis, and local hemorrhage are usually seen.[4] Edema, suppuration, and thrombosis of vessels may be seen. Myonecrosis may also be seen in advanced cases.

The infections affect the subcutaneous tissues and superficial fascia while sparing the more superficial layers until late in the presentation. The infection may

Table 14-1 Causes of Secondary Infections
Secondary Skin Infections
■ Chronic venous ulcers
■ Chronic diabetic ulcers
■ Psoriatic lesions
■ Varicella lesions
■ Eczematous lesions
■ Decubitus ulcers

Table 14-3 Necrotizing Soft Tissue Infections
Complicated Skin Infections
■ Gangrenous cellulitis
■ Progressive bacterial synergistic gangrene
■ Synergistic necrotizing cellulitis
■ Fournier gangrene
■ Gangrenous balaniti
■ Streptococcal gangrene
■ Meleny ulcer
■ Clostridial myonecrosis (gas gangrene)

be rapidly progressive or more indolent in its course. Although treatment includes antibiotic therapy, surgical therapy is mandatory.

Type I infections are polymicrobial including anaerobes, facultative anaerobes and/or aerobic bacteria and most commonly occur in diabetic patients.[5] Type II infections involve group A Streptococcus (GAS) either alone or in combination with *Staphylococcus aureus*.[6] These infections may occur anywhere throughout the body, including the face, head, and neck; extremities, torso, and perineum. The clinical appearance may be of swelling, erythema, and tenderness. These seemingly benign symptoms may progress to worsening pain, swelling, blistering, violaceous skin discoloration, and skin necrosis. These symptoms can progress over hours to days to weeks. Systemic symptoms may also be present. Fever, chills, malaise, and mental status changes are often present.

Organ system dysfunction may be manifested by elevated blood urea nitrogen (BUN) and serum creatinine (CR). Coagulopathy and anemia may also be seen. Leukocytosis is frequently found.

Necrotizing fasciitis affects the same demographic population as cellulitis. Like cellulitis, it occurs more commonly in patients who have comorbidities (Table 14-4). Diabetes mellitus, morbid obesity, alcohol abuse, injection drug use, or immunosuppression is commonly associated with the development of both cellulitis and NF. However, an epidemiological study from a tertiary referral center found that 61% of patients with invasive GAS infections had no comorbid conditions.[7]

Cellulitis and NF may also be associated with underlying skin abnormalities. Chronic venous stasis ulcers, diabetic foot ulcer, ulcers associated with arterial insufficiency, chronic decubitus ulcers, and skin abrasions from eczema and skin fissures associated with tenia pedis may be the setting for the development of NF. Traumatic or surgical wounds are another common

stage for NF. Poorly or under treated abscesses may also account for the development of NF.

NF may represent a diagnostic challenge. The findings may be nonspecific and the clinical setting may be common. An accurate diagnosis is nonetheless imperative. Mortality rates as high as 76% have been reported but most recently mortality statistics seem to be closer to 15% in patients with the disease.[8] The mortality of NF seems to relate directly to the initiation of timely and appropriate treatment.[9] Several studies have sought to develop diagnostic criteria to improve the ability to diagnose the disease accurately. Wall retrospectively compared admission vitals, physical examination, and radiologic studies in consecutive patients with NF and compared them with a matched control without NF.[10] Patients with NF more commonly had elevated white blood cell counts (WBC) and low serum sodium (Na) levels. A follow-up study retrospectively compared consecutive patients with and without necrotizing fasciitis. A model using WBC > 15.4×10^9 and Na < 135 mmol/L had a sensitivity of 90%, a positive predictive value of 76% and a negative predictive value of 99% in diagnosing necrotizing fasciitis. In these patients, physical findings were much less predictive. Only 38% of patients with NF had tense edema, 24% had bullae, 5% had skin necrosis, and none had crepitance.[11]

A 2004 article retrospectively reviewed cases of NF over a 7-year period in two hospitals in Japan and Belgium.[12] It was found that creatinine phosphokinase (CPK) levels were higher in patients with NF due to GAS than in non GAS infections. Wong et al created a unique scoring system based on hematologic and biologic markers on admission. Univariate and multivariate analysis identified WBC, hemoglobin (HGB), Na, glucose (GLU), CR, and C reactive protein as factors associated with NF.[13] A multiple logistic regression model created a scoring system based on these variables. A level of 6 was associated with a positive predictive value of 92% and a negative predictive value of 96%. A prospective evaluation of cytokine levels in 35 patients department with suspected necrotizing fasciitis measured while in the emergency department found statistically significantly lower Il–1β levels in patients whom NF was confirmed.[14]

Although none of these offers diagnostic certainty, combining these factors with clinical examination may help to increase the specificity of the diagnosis of NF and lead to earlier surgical intervention. A novel study by Wilson modified the Fine Scoring System developed to identify patients with community acquired pneumonia with a low risk of death to create a severity scoring system for soft tissue infection.[15]

This soft tissue severity score is derived from the patient's age added to points accrued from four physical examination findings, six laboratory tests, the size and depth of wound involvement and presence of a surgical wound infection, bacteremia, or comorbid

Table 14-4   Factors and Etiologies
Comorbidities and Factors
■ Diabetes mellitus
■ Alcoholism
■ Age > 60
■ Immunosuppressive medications
■ Immunosuppressed states (HIV/AIDS)
■ Intravenous drug use
■ IV/IM/SC injections
■ Peripheral vascular disease
■ Obesity
■ Venous disease
Etiologies
■ Trauma
■ Post-op
■ Chronic wound
■ Intravenous drug use

conditions (Table 14-5). Higher scores were associated with increased antibiotic failure. The authors propose a use of the system to identify those patients that require aggressive support and urgent debridement.

DIAGNOSIS

Several radiographic studies may be indicated to assist with correctly demonstrating when surgical intervention may be needed to treat soft tissue infections. Plain x-ray may demonstrate air in the soft tissues. In patients who are injection drug users, needle fragments may be seen. This is important to the surgeon, so that they may avoid injury from these embedded foreign bodies when performing debridement or draining an abscess. In the case of the diabetic patients with neuropathy, it is often prudent to look for foreign bodies, as it is easy for such patients to suffer injury by stepping on tacks, nails, or fragments without being aware of it. Not all foreign bodies are radio opaque. Wood splinters, for example, would not be expected to be demonstrable by x-ray. Plain x-rays may also show an unsuspected fracture or evidence of osteomyelitis.

Table 14-5 Disease Severity Scoring System		
Patient characteristic	Score (points)	Independent predictors of treatment failure
Demographic		BUN > 30 mg/dL
Age		Na < 130 meq/L
Comorbid Condition		HCT < 30%
Cancer	+30	Skin lesion = 150 cm^2
Cardiac	+10	Surgical wound infection
Diabetes	+10	
Hepatic	+20	
Immunologic	+30	
Renal	+10	
Respiratory	+30	
Transplantation	+30	
Vascular	+10	
Physical examination		
Respiratory rate > 30	+20	
Systolic BP < 90 mm Hg	+20	
Temperature < 35°C or > 40°C	+15	
Pulse > 125 beats/min	+10	
Laboratory		
BUN > 30	+20	
Na < 130 meq/L	+20	
Glucose > 250 mg/dL	+10	
HCT < 30%	+10	
WBC < 4.5 or > 10 × 10^3 cells/mm^3	+10	
Bands > 15%	+10	
Other		
Bacteremia	+20	
Degree of involvement (deep)	+10	
Skin lesion > 150 cm^2	+10	
Surgical wound	+10	

Modified from Wilson SE, et al. *Am J Surg* 2001;185:369-375.

This is especially important in patients who have chronic skin wounds, such as diabetic ulcers, venous ulcers, and decubitus ulcers.

Ultrasound evaluation of the affected area may be useful when a deep-seated abscess is suspected, but fluctuation is not appreciated on physical examination. False negative exams can occur when there is significant debris and semisolid material present in the abscess cavity. Fluid appears echogenic, but the more solid components will be isoechoic and will appear to be solid.[16] Air may also be apparent on this evaluation. Diffuse thickening of the skin and underling subcutaneous fat may be seen in cellulitis. This is however, a nonspecific finding.

Computed tomography (CT) has become the most commonly utilized adjunctive study to aid in the diagnosis of soft tissue infection. CT, like ultrasound is capable of demonstrating fluid collections and does so with higher resolution. When intravenous contrast is administered, the abscess wall may enhance demonstrating its increased vascularity. Gas collections are demonstrated with a higher sensitivity than with either plain x-ray or ultrasonography. Bony changes and abnormalities are easily seen using CT. CT scanning allows the visualization of contiguous structures and is therefore very helpful when constructing a surgical plan. Intraperitoneal or retroperitoneal extension of infection is not uncommon and should be looked for. Joint effusions and infections can also be demonstrated. Swelling and rim enhancing fluid collections in the muscle may be seen with pyomyositis.

Magnetic resonance imaging (MR) is felt to give improved resolution of muscle and soft tissue. It may demonstrate muscular involvement that is not seen on CT scan. Abnormal signal intensity along the fascial plane can be seen with cellulitis and necrotizing fasciitis. MR has been thought to be a better test to use in the patient with renal failure, although this may not be certain. A retrospective review of patient with stage 3 and 4 (glomerular filtration rates 59–15) renal failure found 12.1% developed acute renal failure after receiving intravenous gadolinium.[17] Patients are frequently critically ill, which may limit their ability to be transported to MR for evaluation. Patients with radio-opaque hardware are usually better candidates for MR than CT scan because of distortion and scatter produced by CT.

The results of diagnostic studies must be evaluated with full knowledge of the patient's clinical condition. A patient who is clinically very ill, such as with hypotension and end organ dysfunction like renal failure, who has a CT scan or MR that is equivocal usually is best served by surgical exploration for definitive diagnosis. Frozen section pathologic evaluation may be required to establish the diagnosis. Fine needle aspiration biopsy may aid in identifying the pathogen associated with the infection. In a study from Australia bacteria where cultured from 81% of aspirates obtained before initiation of antibiotics and 30% of aspirates obtained after initiation of antibiotics.[18]

BACTERIOLOGY

The bacteriology of soft tissue infections is changing to include many more cases of community-acquired methicillin resistant *Staphylococcus aureus* (MRSA). Risk factors have classically been prior antibiotic use, being a health care worker, or nursing home resident, recent hospitalization, intravenous drug abuse, indwelling vascular devices, long-term hemodialysis, recent surgical procedures, and underlying chronic illness or immunosuppression. Between 36% and 92% of patients with soft tissue infections from community acquired MRSA (CAMRSA) will require surgical treatment.[19] Many strains of CAMRSA are sensitive to clindamycin, trimethoprim sulfamethoxazole, and quinolones. Hospital-acquired MRSA is only sensitive to vancomycin, linezolid, and daptomycin. Clinicians must be aware of the sensitivity pattern of these bacteria in their community. It is also important to be aware of the prevalence of CAMRSA in a community, so that intelligent antibiotic choices can be made.

Most commonly, necrotizing soft tissue infections are polymicrobial (type 1). The gram negatives, *E. coli*, pseudomonas aeruginosa, *Klebsiella pneumonial*, *Acinetobacter*, and *Enterobacter* are common isolates. Anaerobes are frequently present as well, although they are less frequently cultured. Therefore, in addition to gram-positive coverage for SA and streptococcus, empiric therapy for severe soft tissue infections should include gram-negative coverage. When MRSA or CAMRSA are not suspected, single agent coverage with extended spectrum penicillins may be adequate. Penicillin allergic patients are generally adequately treated with clindamycin in combination with a quinolone or an aminoglycoside. Once culture data is available, these broad antibiotics can be tailored to fit the sensitivities of the organism grown. Yeasts are present in patients who have altered immune systems, such as diabetics, patients with HIV or AIDS, or those who are receiving chemotherapy. Yeast may be present in soft tissue infections resulting from operative procedures or from hollow viscous rupture. Critically ill patients require empiric treatment for yeast and fungal cultures should be obtained.

Marine Vibrio soft tissue infections may occur in patients exposed to salt water. These patients may present with severely compromised physiology and be critically ill. This occurs most commonly in patients with underlying liver disease. These patients may even develop infection from ingestion of raw seafood. Patients infected with vibrio require treatment with doxycycline, cefotaxime, or ceftazidime.[20]

Type 2 necrotizing soft tissue infections are due to GAS either alone or in combination with SA. Thankfully, these organisms are quite sensitive to penicillins. Alternatively clindamycin may be used. Vancomycin, daptomycin, or linezolid should be added if the risk for MRSA exists. Patients can often be critically ill with hypotension resulting from exotoxin exposure. In these cases, heroic supportive care along with prompt and wide debridement is required. Immunoglobulin (IVIG) can be administered in some severe cases.[21] Other therapies aimed at removal of toxins have been advocated. Continuous venovenous hemofiltration/dialysis and plasmaphoresis have been used with anecdotal success.

Clostridial species may cause severe soft tissue infections. These organisms usually gain access through traumatic or surgical wounds. They also are notorious for releasing exotoxin and causing severe systemic manifestations. These organisms may progress at alarming rates similarly to GAS, with skin changes advancing in minutes. Wide, radical debridement or possibly amputation is necessary to control this infection. Clostridia septicum is associated with underlying gastrointestinal malignancy.[22] Thus, when clostridial infections are diagnosed outside the setting of trauma or postoperative wound infection, workup for malignancy is wise. Clostridial infections are best treated with clindamycin in combination with penicillin. Erythromycin and ceftriaxone are alternatives. Clindamycin has the added advantage of decreasing bacterial toxin production.[23]

OPERATIVE MANAGEMENT

Surgical treatment of deep-seated or necrotizing fasciitis is mandatory. When the diagnosis is in doubt, surgical exploration may also be warranted. Generally, the incision is planned to encompass the area of maximal skin change. The infection frequently extends beyond the area of skin change. Vertical incisions on extremities are usually superior to transverse. When doubt exists as to the appropriate incision for the extremities, fasciotomy type incisions are an excellent choice. Exploration in postoperative or trauma-associated infections should begin via the initial incision and can be extended based on the intraoperative findings.

Control of the infection is primary. Thoughts of eventual reconstruction should be secondary to control and eradication of necrotic and infected tissue. When intraoperative findings are minimal, the tissue planes should be tested. Blunt exploration with a finger or a clamp to determine if the planes are intact and resist penetration. Loss of the integrity of the soft tissue plane may be the only finding in early cases. If the diagnosis of NF is still questioned, then tissue biopsy for pathologic evaluation is warranted. Tissue culture should also be obtained. Frozen section evaluation has been discussed as a possibility to aid in the diagnosis.[24]

More often, the diagnosis is obvious on exploration. Frankly necrotic tissue is often encountered in the subcutaneous plane. It may extend to the deep fascia and to the muscle. Muscle and fascia may require partial or complete excision. The surgeon must beware of the location of critical blood vessels and nerves in order to protect them from injury. This ensures the best functional outcome for the patient and may spare an amputation. Cases of abdominal wall involvement may require laparotomy to exclude intra-abdominal involvement. When extensive debridement is required, creation of colostomies and placement of feeding tubes may be challenging, but it should be deferred until follow-up exploration verifies the viability of the remaining abdominal wall.

Nearly all wounds require early reexploration to assure adequate control of the infection. This exploration usually occurs between 24 and 72 hours after the initial debridement. Once control of the infection is achieved, reconstruction may proceed as long as the systemic response to the infection has also abated. Delayed primary closure is sometimes possible, although frequently the volume of tissue removal precludes this. Skin grafting is commonly needed. A clean vascularized base is essential. Similar to the burn patient, when involvement is extensive finding an appropriate donor site may be a challenge. When extensive muscle and soft tissue deficits exist, leaving exposed bone rotation or free myocutaneous or fasciocutaneous flaps may be required.

POSTOPERATIVE

Systemic considerations are paramount in these patients. Adequate nutritional repletion is a must. In many instances, reconstruction may need to be delayed until the patient is nutritionally replete and occur at another admission.

Wound care for these large and complex wounds may be a challenge. For years, gauze dressings have been the mainstay of treatment. They are inexpensive and are universally familiar. They require frequent change in the case of highly exudative wounds and they are labor-intensive. Foam dressings are now available that have superior absorptive qualities. Nearly every variety of dressing is now also available in a silver ion impregnated format. This offers the advantage of being antimicrobial, thereby offering topical suppression of bacterial growth. The VAC (Kinetic Concept Incorporated) is an open cell foam dressing that is connected to machine to generate negative pressure and remove tissue fluid. This device offers the advantage of removing excess tissue fluid and allowing quantification of the fluid loss, removing the guess work from calculating daily fluid losses. It may also remove bacteria that would ordinarily remain on the wound. The expense of the dressing and machine rental seem to be off set by the decrease in wound care labor by nurses and physicians. It can be used in almost any body area. Care must be exercised in the cases of exposed bone, tendon, bowel, or blood vessels.

Topical antiseptic solutions are generally avoided unless the wounds are grossly infected, which should not be the case after an adequate debridement. It should be remembered that hydrogen peroxide, acetic

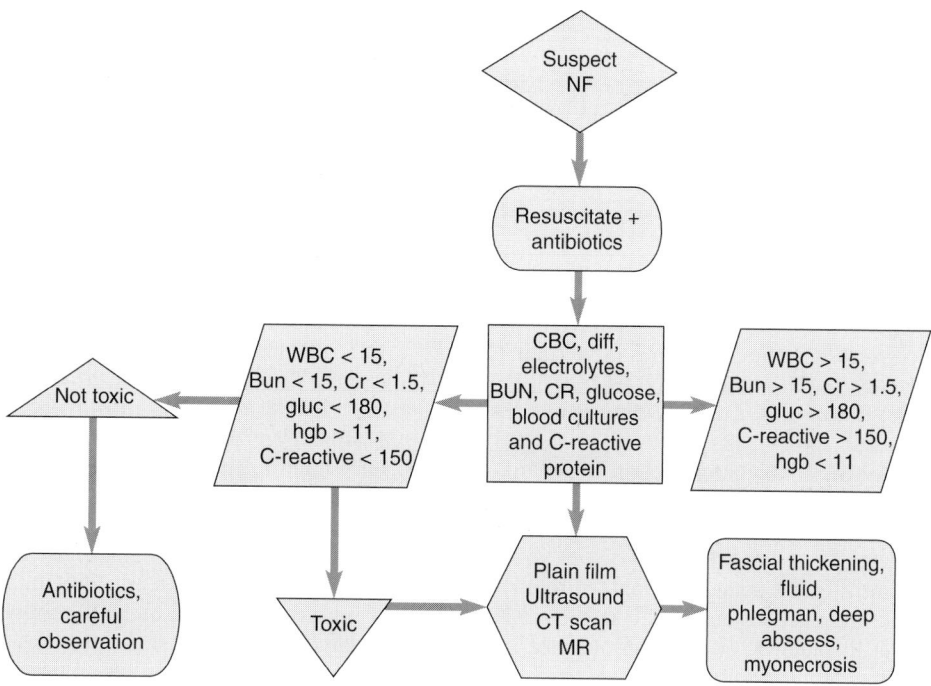

Figure 14-2 *Algorithm for suspected necrotizing fasciitis.*

acid, dacon solution, and clorpactin (oxyclorasene) solution are all toxic to healing tissue and may in fact delay wound healing. These solutions should be diluted adequately to be safely used on wounds.

Edema reduction usually plays an important role in care of extremity soft tissue infections. A mechanism to elevate the affected part must be created. It may be necessary to hang the arm from an IV pole to assure proper elevation. Pillows are usually inadequate. Similarly the leg may need to be elevated from an orthopedic frame. Pressure redistribution for dependent areas should not be overlooked. A variety of mattress overlays and specialty beds are available for rental to accomplish this sometimes overlooked, but vitally important, task.

Hyperbaric oxygen (HBO) treatments can be used as an adjunct to the treatment of severe soft tissue infections. It is currently recommended and reimbursed for cases of NF due to clostridia. Reimbursement is also available for NF from other etiologies as well, although the data supporting its use is less compelling. There are several theoretic and proven mechanisms by which it could offer potential improvements in outcome. It produces an environment of hyperoxia. Normal tissues require 60 ml oxygen/L blood flow for adequate cellular metabolism. At atmospheric pressure the dissolved oxygen content of plasma is 3 ml/L. At 3 atmospheres, the dissolved oxygen content increases to 70 ml/L, exceeding resting metabolic requirements. This alone may be lethal to facultative aerobes and anaerobic bacteria. At increased oxygen levels the leukocytes ability to kill aerobic bacteria is improved. This also improves the efficacy of antibiotics. The

superoxygenated tissue may present a barrier to further spread of infection.[25]

Animal studies suggest that HBO may decrease plasma levels of tumor necrosis factor alpha. Collagen formation is stimulated in the hyperoxic environment. Superoxide dismutase is increased, which may protect tissues from damage from free oxygen radicals.[26]

Treatments with HBO have not been standardized. The depth is generally 2 to 3 atmospheres; however, the length or duration of treatment varies from center to center. Most studies suffer from small numbers, retrospective format, and nonstandardized treatment protocols. There are several reports that document an improvement in survival in patients treated with HBO.[27] Other studies have shown no such benefit.[28] There is also data that suggests that HBO allows for fewer and more limited debridement.[29] Another report found closure could be attained more commonly in patients treated with HBO versus control.[30] Use as an adjunct seems a reasonable consideration. Surgery however, remains the mainstay of treatment.

SUMMARY

Soft tissue infections represent a spectrum of presentations. They may be self-limited or treatable with short course of antibiotics and uncomplicated local wound care. Neglected infections or those occurring in a compromised host or with high bacterial load or virulence, may develop into deep-seated complex infections. These infections, although uncommon, need to be identified quickly as time to treatment affects outcome.

Unfortunately, signs and symptoms of these infections are nonspecific until advanced.

It is important to remember to maintain a high degree of vigilance when treating what appears to be a routine soft tissue infection in a high-risk population (Fig. 14-2). If a patient fails to respond to or worsens on what should be appropriate therapy, consider the possibility of a deeper, more complicated, infection. The clinical situation should guide treatment decisions, as radiographic studies do not have 100% negative predictive value. Exploration for diagnosis may be the wisest strategy.

REFERENCES

1. DiNubile MJ, Lipsky BA. Complicated infections of skin and skin structures: when the infection is more than skin deep. *J Antimicrob Chemother* 2004;53: S2: ii37.
2. Caro I, Thomas VD. Myositis. *Current Treatment Options in Infectious Diseases.* 2002;4:233.
3. Stone DR, Gorbach SL. Necrotizing fasciitis: the changing spectrum. *Dermatologic Clinics* 1997;15:213-220.
4. Green R, Dafoe D, Raffin T. Necrotizing fasciitis. *Chest* 1996;110:219-229.
5. Stevens DL. Necrotizing soft tissue infections: current treatment options in infectious diseases 2000;2:359-368.
6. Giuliano A, Lewis F, Hadley K, et al. Bacteriology of necrotizing fasciitis. *Am J Surg* 1977;134:52-57.
7. Ben-Abraham R, Keller N, Vered R, et al. Invasive Group A streptococcal infections in a large tertiary center: epidemiology, characteristics and outcome. *Infection* 2002;30:81-85.
8. McHenry CR, Piotrowski JJ, Petrinic D, et al. Determinants of mortality for necrotizing soft-tissue infections. *Ann Surg* 1995;221:558.
9. Wong CH, Chang HC, Pasupathy S, et al. Necrotizing fasciitis: clinical presentation, microbiology, and determinants of mortality. *J Bone Joint Surg* 2003;85A:1454.
10. Wall DB, de Virgilio C, Black S, et al. Objective criteria may assist in distinguishing necrotizing fasciitis from Nonnecrotizing soft tissue infection. *Am J Surg* 2000; 179:17.
11. Wall DB, Klein SR, Black S, et al. A simple model to help distinguish necrotizing fasciitis from Nonnecrotizing soft tissue infection. *J Am Coll Surg* 2000;191:227.
12. Simonart T, Nakafusa J, Narisawa Y. The importance of serum creatine phosphokinase level in the early diagnosis and microbiological evaluation of necrotizing fasciitis. *J Eur Acad Dermatol and Venereol* 200;418:687.
13. Wong CH, Khin LW, Heng KS, et al. The LRINEC (laboratory risk indicator for necrotizing fasciitis) score: a tool for distinguishing necrotizing fasciitis from other soft tissue infections. *Crit Care Med* 2004;32:1535.
14. Anaya DA, McMahon K, Nathens AB, et al. Predictors of mortality and limb loss in necrotizing soft tissue infections. *Arch Surg* 2005;140:151.
15. Wilson SE, Solomkin JS, Le V, et al. A severity score for complicated skin and soft tissue infections derived from phase III studies of linezolid. *Am J Surg* 2003; 185:369.
16. Loyer EM, DuBrow RA, David DL, et al. Imaging of superficial soft-tissue infections: sonographic findings in cases of cellulitis and abscess. *American Journal of Radiology* 1996;166:149.
17. Ergun I, Keven K, Uruc I, et al. The safety of Gadolinium in Patients with Stage 3 and 4 renal failure. *Nephrology Dialysis Transplantation* 2006;21:697.
18. Pik-Chuen L, Turnidge J, McDonald P. Fine-needle Aspiration biopsy in diagnosis of soft tissue infections. *J Clin Microbiol* 1985;22:80.
19. Cohen PR, Grossman ME. Management of cutaneous lesions associated with an emerging epidemic: community-acquired methicillin-resistant *Staphylococcus aureus* skin infections. *Journal American Academy of Dermatology* 2004;51:132.
20. Elko L, Rosenbach K, Sinnott J. Cutaneous manifestations of waterborne infections. *Curr Infect Dis Rep* 2003;5:398.
21. Norrby-Teglund A, Low D. Group A streptococcal toxic shock syndrome and necrotizing fasciitis. *Current Treatment Options in Infectious Diseases* 2003;5:419.
22. Chapnick EK, Abter EI. Necrotizing soft-tissue infections. *Infect Dis Clin North Am* 1996;10:835.
23. Stevens DL. Streptococcal toxic-shock syndrome: spectrum of disease, pathogenesis, and new concepts in treatment. *Emerg Infect Dis* 1995;1:69.
24. Majeski JA, John JF. Necrotizing soft tissue infections: a guide to early diagnosis and initial therapy. *South Med J* 2003;96:900.
25. Jallali N, Withey S, Butler PE. Hyperbaric oxygen as adjuvant therapy in the management of necrotizing fasciitis. *Am J Surg* 2005;189:462.
26. Luongo C, Imperatore F, Cuzzocrea S, Filipelli A, et al. Effects of hyperbaric oxygen exposure on a zymosan-induced shock model. *Crit Care Med* 1998;26:1972.
27. Wilkinson D, Doolette D. Hyperbaric oxygen treatment and survival from necrotizing soft tissue infection. *Arch Surg* 2004;139:1339.
28. Shupak A, Shoshani O, Goldberg I, Barzilai A, et al. Necrotizing Fasciitis: An indication for hyperbaric oxygenation therapy? *Surgery* 1995;118:873-878.
29. Riseman JA, Zamaboni WA, Curtis DR, Konrad FR, Ross DS. Hyperbaric oxygen therapy for necrotizing fasciitis reduces mortality and the need for debridements. *Surgery* 1990;108:847-850.
30. Elliott DC, Kufera JA, Meyers RA. Necrotizing soft tissue infections risk factors for mortality and strategies for management. *Ann Surg* 1996;224:672.

Chapter **15**

TRAUMATIC AORTIC RUPTURE

Thomas Abbruzzese, MD, Christopher J. Kwolek, MD, and Michael T. Watkins, MD

OVERVIEW

Traumatic aortic rupture is a devastating clinical problem, which is difficult to manage due to the need to approach aortic repair in concert with management of complex associated injuries to nonvascular organ systems. The purpose of this chapter is to delineate current concepts in the management of traumatic rupture of the thoracic and abdominal aorta. Management of nontraumatic aortic rupture (due to dissection and infected or degenerative aortic pathology) is outside the scope of this review.

The natural history of aortic transection is relatively self selective—ie, the majority of the patients exsanguinate at the scene. Of those who make it to the hospital alive, up to 38% die largely as a result of associated injuries.[1] Review of outcomes following rupture of the thoracic aorta dates back to an analysis of Korean War victims with blunt aortic trauma. In this early analysis, only 15% of patients survived and most died without surgical intervention.[2] In a number of retrospective clinical series, it is clear that patients requiring repair of thoracic aortic disruptions are considerably younger (mean 43 ± 14 years) than patients undergoing repair of degenerative thoracic aortic aneurysms and dissections.[3] Prospective analysis of the results of treatment is difficult because of the relatively low numbers of the annual cases treated by any particular institution. Fabian et al estimate that approximately 7500 to 8000 traumatic aortic disruptions occur in the United States annually, and that about 1000 to 1500 patients arrive at hospitals alive.[4] It took 50 centers 2.5 years to generate 274 patients for this prospective report. This averages just over two patients per year per center. Despite the low numbers, contemporary analysis reveals that of the 9%-19% who can now expect to survive to reach the hospital,[5] approximately 30% will die within the next 6 hours, rising to 50% within 24 hours.[6] Until recently, open operative intervention for these traumatic injuries required thoracotomy, anticoagulation, and application of an aortic cross clamp. These operative maneuvers had the potential to exacerbate associated injuries and cause spinal cord injury.[4,7,8] Proximal to distal aortic bypass using a Gott Shunt, left heart bypass with heparin bonded circuits and cardiopulmonary bypass may all significantly reduce the likelihood of paraplegia.[9,10] Thus, the current status of traumatic aortic disruption and traditional repair is not ideal. Compounding the complexity of the problem is the fact that patients with aortic rupture often have concurrent injuries such as head and neck damage, pulmonary contusions, lacerations of visceral organs, pelvic fractures, and extremity fractures. These concomitant injuries also contribute to the overall mortality rate and contraindicate open surgery, heparinization, delay operative solution, and cause a shift toward "medical management." In this scenario, blood pressure may be reduced and closely monitored in the hope of decreasing risk of rupture; however, total rupture occurs in 2%-5% of patients within a week of the injury. The introduction of endovascular repair for traumatic rupture has resulted in a major change in the approach to treatment of this devastating clinical entity.[11-13] This change in approach is based on reduction in mortality associated with repair by endovascular versus open techniques in patients with multiple traumas.[14]

INITIAL APPROACH TO THE PATIENT

Optimal care of the patient with ruptured aorta begins with appropriate resuscitation, recognition of the problem and detailed history of the mechanism of injury. Most often, the mechanism of injury involves a motor vehicle (automobile or motorcycle) accident, where patients are exposed to sudden deceleration due to collision with other vehicles or stationary objects. Treatment should proceed in accordance with advanced trauma life support (ATLS) protocols, with the initial focus on airway patency, breathing, and circulation. It is important to avoid excessive administration of intravenous crystalloid as controlled hypotension is preferred to avoid blood pressure increases and decrease the likelihood of aortic rupture. Maintaining systolic blood pressure less than 120 mm Hg or mean arterial pressure less than 80 mm Hg has been shown to significantly reduce the risk of rupture.[15,16] β-Blockade and antihypertensive medications can be used to modulate the systolic blood pressure.

IMAGING STUDIES

Findings on chest radiography, such as a widened mediastinum, deviation of the esophagus to the right or a left apical cap resulting from hematoma are important clues suggesting the presence of aortic rupture. Aortic rupture should then be confirmed by spiral computed tomographic angiography (CTA), which is part of ATLS protocols. Technologic advances from helical and multirow detector CT were associated with improved multiplanar reformations. CT has become the usual definitive screening test for major thoracic vascular injury. Arteriography or transesophageal echocardiography may be required only when CTA is equivocal or technically inadequate.[17] CT findings associated with blunt traumatic aorta include mediastinal hematoma, aortic pseudoaneurysm, variation in aortic contour, intimal flap, and thrombus.[18] Mediastinal hemorrhage is believed to arise from the vaso vasorum of the aorta itself. When mediastinal hemorrhage is isolated to the anterior mediastinum and not in contact with the aorta, major arterial injury is unusual. Intimal dissection, or intraluminal clot can diminish blood flow into the descending aorta, and the aortic lumen below the injury may be atypically small in caliber. In some patients, this effect provides an anatomic representation similar to coarctation, which is rarely appreciated on physical examination. Displacement of the esophagus (or nasogastric tube) or trachea are important secondary signs or aortic injury. Anatomic variants such as the ductus diverticulum may simulate aortic injury. The ductus diverticulum is the term applied to a focal, convex bulge along the anterior undersurface of the isthmic region of the aortic arch. The ductus typically has a smooth contour forming obtuse angles with the aortic lumen without intimal flaps. In contrast, the typical pseudoaneurysm forms an irregular outpouching from the lumen displaying acute margins and intimal irregularity at its base. In certain individuals, a narrow and dilated area of the aorta between the left subclavian and the ductus arteriosus—the aortic spindle, may be mistaken for aortic trauma on CT scanning. In addition, common congenital anomalies may lead to aortic injuries in atypical locations. The most common anomalies include aberrant left subclavian artery, coarctation, vascular slings, and variant origins of branch vessels. Traumatic aortic rupture has been associated with a retroesophageal right subclavian artery. Schneider et al report such a patient who underwent a two-staged operative procedure where the aberrant right subclavian artery was reimplanted into the right common carotid artery, followed by distal aortic arch replacement and reimplantation of the left subclavian.[19] Mediastinal hemorrhage can certainly occur in the absence of major arterial injury. Sternal fractures or cervico thoracic spine injuries can cause bleeding confined to the anterior or posterior mediastinum. Bleeding from venous structures or small arteries can cause hematoma into the periaortic mediastinum. In 10% of the cases, aortic injury may occur in atypical locations such as the peridiaphragmatic aorta, the ascending aorta, and the aortic arch.

ASSOCIATED INJURIES

Patients with aortic rupture often have concurrent injuries such as head and neck damage, pulmonary contusions, lacerations of visceral organs, pelvic and extremity fractures (Table 15-1). These associated injuries often make open emergent surgical repair risky. Blunt disruption of the diaphragm visualized on plain films of the chest in trauma patients should mandate interrogation of the abdominal and thoracic aorta, as these injuries may coincide.[20] In a series of 52 patients treated for traumatic aortic rupture at the University of Cincinnati, the average Injury Severity Score was 40.[21] In this series, patients underwent repair of their thoracic aortic tear within 6 days of injury. Seven of thirteen patients underwent operation for chest, abdominal, or orthopedic injuries in the interval before endovascular stent repair without obvious compromise to the injured aortic segment. In these patients, blood pressure was kept less than 140 mm Hg using β-blockade and other antihypertensive medications. No patient in this study became unstable or died of ruptured aorta while awaiting endovascular repair. The authors of this study suggest that in select patients, immediate repair of traumatic aortic tears is not necessary as long as there is no CT scan evidence of extravasation and the patient's blood pressure can be controlled. At our institution, we usually repair these injuries as soon as they have been identified, so as to eliminate the possibility that these injuries might contribute to any subsequent hemodynamic instability. At present, there is no means of predicting who will remain stable and who will progress to uncontrolled

Table 15-1 Common Associated Injuries with Traumatic Thoracic Transection
Closed Head Injury
Pelvic Fractures
Visceral Fracture
Pulmonary Contusions
Cervical Spine Fracture
Cardiac Contusion

hemorrhage.[22] Potential reasons to delay intervention include obvious life-threatening hemorrhage from a source other than the thoracic aorta, severe respiratory insufficiency, or a patient in whom an endovascular device might be appropriate, is commercially available, but is not present on the shelf. Usually, these devices can be made available within 24 hours; thus, some delay in treatment is feasible.

OPEN SURGICAL APPROACH

The procedure may be performed either with direct cross-clamping alone or with circulatory assistance (left-sided heart bypass with heparin-coated conduits, cardiopulmonary bypass, or femoral-femoral bypass).[10,23,24] The thoracic aorta is optimally approached through a posterolateral thoracotomy, with an incision in the fourth intercostal space. The aortic arch may be controlled either with clamping between the left common carotid and left subclavian, or just distal to the left subclavian artery. The descending thoracic aorta is controlled distally immediately after the traumatic injury to avert sacrifice of the intercostal arteries. The aorta may be repaired with direct suturing or graft interposition.

ENDOVASCULAR APPROACH
Optimally, the operating room in a trauma center should be equipped with radiographic fixed or mobile C-arm and angiographic equipment. In this way, the patients can be treated for the vascular injury via open cut down or percutaneously in a setting where surgical interventions for associated injuries may also be pursued if indicated by the patient's overall condition.[3] Although there are no specifically designed commercially available devices used to treat thoracic aortic transections, the use of endoluminal abdominal aortic extension cuffs has been shown to be technically feasible in several small series.[3,25,26] This is particularly so in young individuals with normal sized aortas. Patients need to be prepped and draped widely, so that emergent intervention for associated abdominal or thoracic injuries can be pursued while the patient is intubated and anesthetized. Patients should be placed supine on the appropriate x-ray table with slight rotation to a decubitus position. This positioning provides access not only to the femoral vessels but also the iliac vessels and abdominal aorta if needed. The diameter of the stent grafts should be oversized at least 20% based on sizing obtained from CT angiography. Unlike treatment of patients with degenerative aneurysms, the aortic diameter proximal to the injured aorta is most often in the 18-26 mm range. Generous oversizing can lead to collapse of a stent graft.[27] Grafts are placed under fluoroscopic control over stiff guide wires parked in the aortic root. At times, the turn radius in the arch of young patients may be too tight for the Lunderquist wire. The smallest thoracic endograft available

commercially in the United States is the 26-mm diameter Gore TAG device. In our institution, we have used proximal and distal Zenith TX2 thoracic endograft extensions, Gore TAG thoracic endografts, and Medtronic extensions from aortic endografts. Precise placement of the stent graft can be facilitated by adjusting the mean arterial pressure to 70 mm Hg during implantation. Depending on the patient's heart rate, the device being implanted, and associated injuries, intravenous administration of adenosine to induce transient bradycardia/asystole may be used immediately prior to deployment of the graft. Completion angiography should be performed after the stent graft has been deployed to ensure that the false aneurysm has been properly excluded. After removing the introducer delivery systems, femoral arteriotomy is repaired. After implantation of the thoracic endograft, CT scans are performed prior to discharge, at 3 and 6 months, then yearly thereafter. Systemic anticoagulation should be used selectively to avoid thromboembolic complications associated with transient occlusion of the femoral vessels and wire/catheter manipulations in the aortic arch. This is often a major issue in patients with extensive associated injuries, particularly in patients with associated head trauma.

Figure 15-1 demonstrates a CT scan representation of a traumatic aortic disruption localized to the isthmus in a 42-year-old male victim involved in an airplane crash. Coronal and sagittal images of the thoracic aortic tear in the preoperative (panel A white arrow, B black arrow) and postoperative appearance of an aortic tear are evident (panels C and D).

COMPLICATIONS
A recent review of 61 publications related to endovascular treatment of traumatic rupture of the aorta revealed a 14.4% overall complication rate.[14] Interestingly, procedure related paraparesis or paraplegia was not mentioned in any of these papers. In contrast, rates of paraplegia associated with open repair of these injuries range from 0 to 37%. In the four largest series, the overall complication rate for endovascular repair was 9%. When open versus endovascular repair were compared, the overall mortality for open repair was 18.9% versus 4% for endovascular repair. Type I endoleak was detected most often, followed by arm ischemia (Table 15-2). Procedure-related mortality included a more proximal rupture, missed on initial CT, stroke, endoleaks associated with hemorrhage, and intraoperative respirator failure during deployment of the graft. Another frequent complication includes arterial injury at the graft insertion site. These complications are often avoided by serial dilation of the femoral vessels prior to graft insertion, placement of a prosthetic conduit, or transabdominal direct puncture of the aorta.

REPAIR OF ABDOMINAL AORTIC INJURIES
Endovascular repairs have been reported for traumatic aortic transection in a pediatric patient,[28] and in

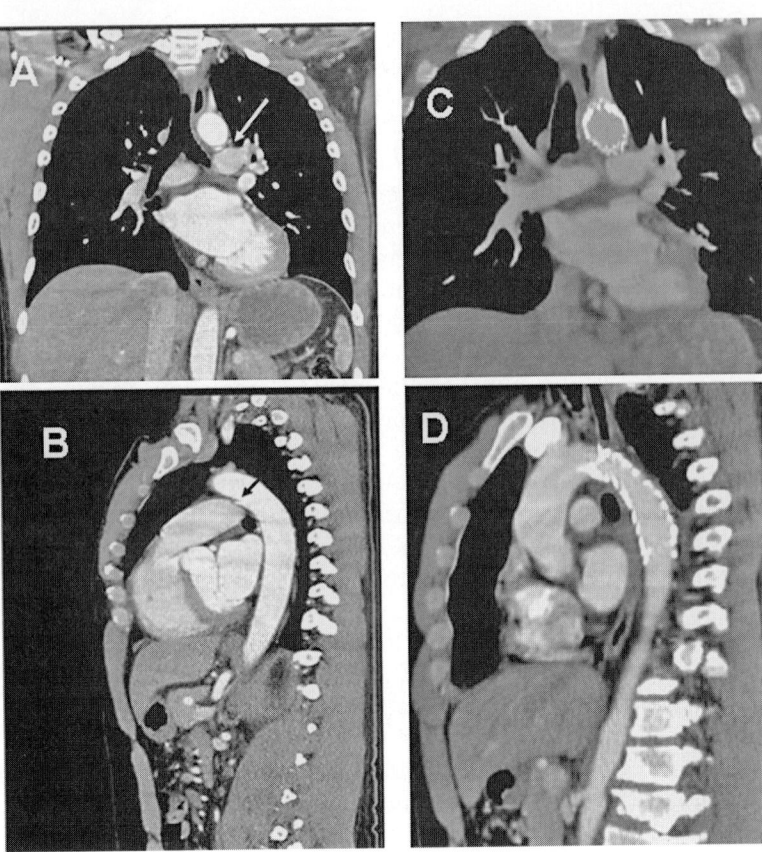

Figure 15-1 *Pre- and postoperative CT scan images of thoracic aortic tear. Coronal (Panel A, white arrow) and Sagittal (Panel B, black arrow) views of the thoracic aorta demonstrate a significant tear on the proximal descending thoracic aorta. The respective postoperative views (C, D) demonstrate apposition of a 34 mm x 10 cm Gore TAG device.*

patients with traumatic dissection of the abdominal aorta.[29,30] In one report, the abdominal aortic graft was placed after repair of multiple intra-abdominal intestinal injuries.[31] Blunt traumatic disruption of the aorta is more common after falls[32] and motor vehicle accidents.[33] Traumatic disruption of the abdominal aorta is associated with an overall mortality rate (73%) that approaches that of trauma to the thoracic aorta.[34] In a recent review where 20% of the injuries to the abdominal aorta were blunt, patients resuscitated in the operating room had lower mortality (40%) than those resuscitated in the trauma room (78%). Thus, unlike the management of patients with thoracic aortic injuries, patients with abdominal aortic injuries need urgent transport to the operating room for resuscitation. None of the patients in this series were candidates for endovascular repair because of hemodynamic instability.

SUMMARY

Endovascular treatment for traumatic aortic rupture is promising, but current results should be interpreted with caution (Table 15-3).[35] The long-term durability of endovascular grafts implanted in relatively young trauma patients, who, having survived a life-threatening event, potentially have several decades of life expectancy. It is possible that young patients with normal aortas may eventually develop increased aortic diameters as they age and develop cardiovascular risk factors such as hypertension, hyperlipidemia, and chronic obstructive pulmonary disease. Thus, serial CT scanning is essential for these individuals. The effect of the cumulative radiation dose associated with serial CT angiography must also be considered.[36] Magnetic Resonance Imaging is only suitable for devices with a nitinol skeleton. Technologic advances that will create more suitable grafts for repair of thoracic aortic disruption include a proximal end, which may have a smaller articulation to better appose the inner wall in the turn of the aortic arch. To date, the reduction in mortality and morbidity justifies endovascular repair, but ongoing follow-up over many years will be necessary before the technique is clearly superior over the long term.

Table 15-2 Complications of Repair Thoracic Aortic Rupture	
Endovascular	Open Repair
Type I Endo Leak	Paraplegia
Access Site Injury	Prolonged Intubation
Left Arm Ischemia	Exacerbate Associated Injuries
Device Collapse	
Device Migration	

Table 15-3 Pros and Cons of Open Versus Endovascular Repair of Traumatic Aortic Rupture

| Open | | Endovascular | |
Pros	Cons	Pros	Cons
Durable Repair	Worsen lung injury	No paraplegia	Arm ischemia
Rare 2° Operations	Paraplegia	Durability uncertain	2° Operations common
	Prolonged hospital Stay	Decreased mortality	Follow-up requires radiation exposure

REFERENCES

1. Camp PPC, Shackford SR. Outcome after blunt traumatic thoracic aortic laceration: identification of a high-risk cohort: Western Trauma Association Multicenter Study Group. *J Trauma* 1997;43(3):413-422.

2. Parmley LF, Mattingly TW, Manion WC, Jahnke, EJ Jr. Nonpenetrating traumatic injury of the aorta. *Circulation* 1958;17(6):1086-1101.

3. Peterson BG, Matsumura JS, Morasch MD, West MA, Eskandari MK. Percutaneous endovascular repair of blunt thoracic aortic transection. *J Trauma* 2005;59(5):1062-1065.

4. Fabian TC, Richardson JD, Croce MA, et al. Prospective study of blunt aortic injury: multicenter trial of the American Association for the Surgery of Trauma. *J Trauma* 1997;42(3):374-380; discussion 380-383.

5. Richens D, Kotidis K, Neale M, Oakley C, Fails A. Rupture of the aorta following road traffic accidents in the United Kingdom 1992-1999: the results of the co-operative crash injury study. *Eur J Cardiothorac Surg* 2003;23(2):143-148.

6. Jamieson WR, Janusz MT, Gudas VM, Burr LH, Fradet GJ, Henderson C. Traumatic rupture of the thoracic aorta: third decade of experience. *Am J Surg* 2002;183(5):571-575.

7. Cowley RA, Turney SZ, Hankins JR, Rodriguez A, Attar S, Shankar BS. Rupture of thoracic aorta caused by blunt trauma: a fifteen-year experience. *J Thorac Cardiovasc Surg* 1990;100(5):652-660; discussion 660-661.

8. von Oppell UO, Dunne TT, De Groot MK, Zilla P. Traumatic aortic rupture: twenty-year metaanalysis of mortality and risk of paraplegia. *Ann Thorac Surg* 1994;58(2):585-593.

9. Jahromi AS, Kazemi K, Safar HA, Doobay B, Cina CS. Traumatic rupture of the thoracic aorta: cohort study and systematic review. *J Vasc Surg* 2001;34(6):1029-1034.

10. Weiman DS, Gurbuz AT, Gursky A, Valaulikar G, Pate JW. Comparison of spinal cord protection utilizing left atrial-femoral with femoral-femoral bypass in patients with traumatic rupture of the aortic isthmus. *World J Surg* 2006;30(9):1638-1641; discussion 1641-1643.

11. Kato N, Dake MD, Miller DC, Semba CP, Mitchell RS, Razavi MK, et al. Traumatic thoracic aortic aneurysm: treatment with endovascular stent-grafts. *Radiology* 1997;205(3):657-662.

12. Lebl DR, Dicker RA, Spain DA, Brundage SI. Dramatic shift in the primary management of traumatic thoracic aortic rupture. *Arch Surg* 2006;141(2):177-180.

13. Dake MD, Miller DC, Semba CP, Mitchell RS, Walker PJ, Liddell RP. Transluminal placement of endovascular stent-grafts for the treatment of descending thoracic aortic aneurysms. *N Engl J Med* 1994;331(26):1729-1734.

14. Lettinga-van de Poll T, Schurink GW, De Haan MW, Verbruggen JP, Jacobs MJ. Endovascular treatment of traumatic rupture of the thoracic aorta. *Br J Surg* 2007;94(5):525-533.

15. Fabian TC, Davis KA, Gavant ML, et al. Prospective study of blunt aortic injury: helical CT is diagnostic and antihypertensive therapy reduces rupture. *Ann Surg* 1998;227(5):666-676; discussion 676-677.

16. Wahl WL, Michaels AJ, Wang SC, Dries DJ, Taheri PA. Blunt thoracic aortic injury: delayed or early repair? *J Trauma* 1999;47(2):254-259; discussion 259-260.

17. Downing SW, Sperling JS, Mirvis SE, et al. Experience with spiral computed tomography as the sole diagnostic method for traumatic aortic rupture. *Ann Thorac Surg* 2001;72(2):495-501; discussion 501-502.

18. Mirvis SE, Shanmuganathan K. Diagnosis of blunt traumatic aortic injury 2007: Still a nemesis. *Eur J Radiol* 2007;64(1):27-40.

19. Schneider J, Baier R, Dinges C, Unger F. Retroesophageal right subclavian artery (lusoria) as origin of traumatic aortic rupture. *Eur J Cardiothorac Surg* 2007;32(2):385-387.

20. Rizoli SB, Brenneman FD, Boulanger BR, Maggisano R. Blunt diaphragmatic and thoracic aortic rupture: an emerging injury complex. *Ann Thorac Surg* 1994;58(5):1404-1408.

21. Reed AB, Thompson JK, Crafton CJ, Delvecchio C, Giglia JS. Timing of endovascular repair of blunt traumatic thoracic aortic transections. *J Vasc Surg* 2006;43(4):684-688.

22. Lachat M, Pfammatter T, Witzke H, et al. Acute traumatic aortic rupture: early stent-graft repair. *Eur J Cardiothorac Surg* 2002;21(6):959-963.

23. Pate JW, Fabian TC, Walker WA. Acute traumatic rupture of the aortic isthmus: repair with cardiopulmonary bypass. *Ann Thorac Surg* 1995;59(1):90-98; discussion 98-99.

24. Benckart DH, Magovern GJ, Liebler GA, et al. Traumatic aortic transection: repair using left atrial to femoral bypass. *J Card Surg* 1989;4(1):43-49.

25. Amabile P, Collart F, Gariboldi V, Rollet G, Bartoli JM, Piquet P. Surgical versus endovascular treatment of traumatic thoracic aortic rupture. *J Vasc Surg* 2004;40(5):873-879.

26. McPhee JT, Asham EH, Rohrer MJ, et al. The midterm results of stent graft treatment of thoracic aortic injuries. *J Surg Res* 2007;138(2):181-188.

27. Idu MM, Reekers JA, Balm R, Ponsen KJ, de Mol BA, Legemate DA. Collapse of a stent-graft following treatment of a traumatic thoracic aortic rupture. *J Endovasc Ther* 2005;12(4):503-507.

28. Saad NE, Pegoli W, Alfieris G, Waldman DL, Davies MG. Endovascular repair of a traumatic aortic transection in a pediatric patient. *J Vasc Interv Radiol* 2007;18(3):443-446.

29. Berthet JP, Marty-Ane CH, Veerapen R, Picard E, Mary H, Alric P. Dissection of the abdominal aorta in blunt trauma: endovascular or conventional surgical management? *J Vasc Surg* 2003;38(5):997-1003; discussion 1004.

30. Teruya TH, Bianchi C, Abou-Zamzam AM, Ballard JL. Endovascular treatment of a blunt traumatic abdominal aortic injury with a commercially available stent graft. *Ann Vasc Surg* 2005;19(4):474-478.

31. Halkos ME, Nicholas J, Kong LS, Burke JR, Milner R. Endovascular management of blunt abdominal aortic injury. *Vascular* 2006;14(4):223-226.

32. Marti M, Pinilla I, Baudraxler F, Simon MJ, Garzon G. A case of acute abdominal aortic dissection caused by blunt trauma. *Emerg Radiol* 2006.

33. Katsoulis E, Tzioupis C, Sparks I, Giannoudis PV. Compressive blunt trauma of the abdomen and pelvis associated with abdominal aortic rupture. *Acta Orthop Belg* 2006;72(4):492-501.

34. Deree J, Shenvi E, Fortlage D, et al. Patient factors and operating room resuscitation predict mortality in traumatic abdominal aortic injury: a 20-year analysis. *J Vasc Surg* 2007;45(3): 493-497.

35. Starnes BW, Arthurs ZM. Endovascular management of vascular trauma. *Perspect Vasc Surg Endovasc Ther* 2006;18(2):114-129.

36. Plurad D, Green D, Demetriades D, Rhee P. The increasing use of chest computed tomography for trauma: is it being overutilized? *J Trauma* 2007;62(3):631-635.

Chapter 16

ARTERIAL AND VENOUS OCCLUSION

Benjamin M. Jackson, MD, and Edward Y. Woo, MD

INTRODUCTION

Among the most common vascular surgical emergencies is acute lower extremity ischemia. Likewise, sudden-onset occlusion of any major artery presents with symptoms and signs that must be recognized and acted on to salvage the organs supplied. Meanwhile, slowly progressive occlusion of arteries does not cause acute ischemia but can nevertheless bring patients to seek emergent surgical care for the resulting chronic or subacute symptoms. Venous thrombosis and occlusion are also frequent problems encountered in the urgent and emergent setting; appropriate and expeditious medical and surgical interventions are essential.

EVALUATION AND DIAGNOSIS OF ACUTE LIMB ISCHEMIA

The incidence of acute limb ischemia is approximately 1.7/10,000 per year.[1] Patients presenting with a pulseless extremity suffer amputation rates as high as 10%, and mortality rates of 5%-15%.[2,3] These patients are characteristically at high risk for perioperative complication and are medically fragile (Table 16-1).

CLASSIFICATION OF ETIOLOGY

Table 16-2 catalogues the various etiologies of acute limb ischemia. Sudden onset acute pain is indicative of an embolic event, whereas a history of chronic pain or claudication prior to the acute ischemic episode is suggestive of a thrombotic etiology. Graft occlusions are slightly more common than thromboses of native arteries. Thrombotic occlusions are approximately six times more common than embolic events.

Native artery thrombosis occurs at sites of atherosclerotic lesions, where there is flow disturbance resulting in turbulence and a thrombogenic surface for platelet aggregation. Thrombosis causing complete occlusion can occur in even mildly stenotic atherosclerotic vessels. In cases of native artery occlusion without underlying luminal lesion, consideration must be given to other causes of thrombosis, including hypovolemia, hypercoaguable states including malignancy, and blood dyscrasias.

Bypass graft thrombosis has become the leading cause of acute lower extremity ischemia. Intimal hyperplasia and valvular hyperplasia are the most common causes of thrombosis in native conduit bypasses. In prosthetic grafts, acute thrombosis is most commonly due to kinking across joints or to the thrombogenicity of the graft material itself.[4]

GRADING OF SEVERITY

Since 1997, the Rutherford criteria have been used to grade the clinical severity of acute limb ischemia.[5] These categories, as summarized in Table 16-3, are indicative both of whether emergent surgical intervention is indicated and of whether the limb is salvageable. Most commonly, category I represents an acute occlusion in a chronically narrowed artery, with well-formed collaterals. Category II represents a limb that is salvageable with immediate therapy or intervention. In the case of irreversible ischemia, category III, the patient will present with profound vascular and neurologic deficits; the limb may be in a state of *rigor mortis*, and will require amputation. Ouriel has described a useful management algorithm depending on the class of ALI (Fig. 16-1).[3]

CLINICAL MANIFESTATIONS

Patients commonly present within hours of the onset of pain. Muscle and nerve tissues are able to tolerate no more than 6 hours of profound ischemia. Lower extremity ischemia presents with six "Ps"—pain, pallor, paresthesias, paralysis, pulselessness, and poikilothermia. A thorough history and physical will frequently elucidate both the nature and the etiology of the ischemic event. In general, limb ischemic symptoms and signs will be present at a level one joint below the acute occlusive phenomenon; thus, common femoral artery occlusion will result in foot and calf pain.

The patient will experience a variable sensory deficit—in extreme cases, the affected limb will be insensate to even penetration of a needle into the muscles of the foot or calf; use of a sterile 19-gauge needle

Table 16-1   Incidence of Medical Comorbidities in Patients Presenting with ALI

Comorbidity	Incidence (%)			
	Rochester Trial (N = 114)	TOPAS-1 Trial (N = 213)	TOPAS-2 Trial (N = 544)	Total (N = 871)
Cerebrovascular disease	NR	15.4	11.5	11.6
Congestive heart failure	NR	15.5	12.5	13.3
Coronary artery disease	56.1	47.1	42.5	45.4
Diabetes mellitus	28.1	36.7	29.0	30.8
Hypercholesterolemia	31.6	29.6	23.5	26.0
Hypertension	63.2	60.9	69.6	60.3
Malignancy	NR	11.9	11.5	11.6
Tobacco history	51.8	79.3	77.5	74.6

NR–not reported TOPAS–Thrombolysis or Peripheral Arterial Surgery.
From Ouriel K. Acute ischemia and its sequelae. In: Rutherford RB, ed. *Vascular Surgery*, 5th ed. Philadelphia, PA: WB Saunders; 2000.

may allow the clinician to objectively determine whether any sensation remains.

Paralysis is a poor prognostic sign, indicating relatively profound ischemia. Deficits in dorsiflexion and plantarflexion of the foot—which are accomplished by the muscles of the leg—are indicative of more extensive ischemia and a more proximal occlusive arterial lesion than are weakness or paralysis of the intrinsic muscles of the foot.

Normal proximal and contralateral pulse exam is indicative of an embolic event, in an otherwise normal vascular tree. In contrast, evidence of diffuse chronic atherosclerotic disease suggests a thrombotic etiology of the acute ischemia.

ANATOMIC DISTRIBUTION
Aortic Bifurcation
In the case of acute aortic occlusion, the patient will complain of sudden onset of bilateral buttock and lower extremity pain. Mottling of the lower extremities and lower abdomen, sometimes up to the umbilicus will be evident on physical exam. The diagnosis in these patients is too frequently missed, owing probably to the bilateral nature of the ischemic insult. Even in the setting of absent femoral pulses, patients are often evaluated for possible neurologic or neurosurgical

problems, resulting in a delay of diagnosis and appropriate therapy.

Common Femoral Artery
The most common site of clinically significant embolism in the lower extremity is the common femoral artery (CFA) bifurcation.[6] Patients with CFA embolism will experience foot and calf pain.

Popliteal Artery
An embolus to the popliteal artery will result in absent pedal pulses, and weak or absent popliteal pulse. In contrast, in the setting of a thrombosed popliteal artery aneurysm, the popliteal artery pulse may be prominent, or there may be a thrombosed pulseless mass palpable posterior to the knee joint.

EVALUATION AND DIAGNOSIS
Studies
A complete blood count, serum electrolytes, and coagulation profile should be checked. In particular, and in anticipation of imaging studies using nephrotoxic contrast agents, a serum creatinine should be obtained. If a hypercoaguable state is suspected, a hypercoaguable profile should be sent prior to institution of any anticoagulation. An electrocardiogram will aid in the diagnosis of atrial fibrillation, a possible etiologic factor in thromboembolic disease, and will provide some information as to the patient's cardiac status. Similarly, assessment of the patient's cardiac risk for general anesthesia using the Goldman index or other scale may be useful.[7]

Doppler examination of the lower extremity should be undertaken, with attention both to arterial and venous signals. When arterial signals are present in the ankle—at either the dorsalis pedis (DP) or the posterior tibial (PT) arteries, the ankle-brachial index (ABI) should be measured. First, the systolic blood pressure is measured in

Table 16-2   Causes of Acute Limb Ischemia

Embolism (often to an arterial bifurcation)

Thrombosis
    at site of preexisting atherosclerotic lesion
    of a preexisting aneurysm
    in normal artery as a result of hypercoagulability

Bypass graft occlusion
    anastomotic stenosis due to intimal hyperplasia

Table 16-3   Clinical Categorization of Acute Limb Ischemia

Category	Description/Prognosis	Findings		Doppler signals	
		Sensory loss	Muscle weakness	Arterial	Venous
I. Viable	Not immediately threatened	None	None	Audible	Audible
IIa. Marginally threatened	Salvageable if promptly treated	Minimal (toes) or none	None	Inaudible	Audible
IIb. Immediately threatened	Salvageable with immediate revascularization	More than toes, associated with rest pain	Mild, moderate	Inaudible	Audible
III. Irreversible	Major tissue loss or permanent nerve damage inevitable	Profound, anesthetic	Profound, paralysis (rigor)	Inaudible	Inaudible

From Rutherford RB, Baer JD, Ernst C, et al. Recommended standards for reports dealing with lower extremity ischemia: revised version. *J Vasc Surg* 1997;26:517.

each arm, and the higher is taken as the brachial pressure. The cuff is then placed on the calf, inflated, and then slowly deflated; the highest pressure at which the Doppler signal—at either the PT or DP—becomes audible again marks the ankle pressure. A ratio of 1.0 is normal; an ABI of less than 0.7 usually signifies a hemodynamically significant occlusive process. The absence of venous "hums" indicates more severe ischemia.

Duplex ultrasonography can be a valuable adjunctive study in the setting of acute limb ischemia. It can localize the site of occlusion, especially in bypass grafts. If the equipment and a capable operator are available in the emergency room setting, duplex ultrasound can identify and localize stenoses, dissections, thrombi, emboli, and atherosclerotic plaques.

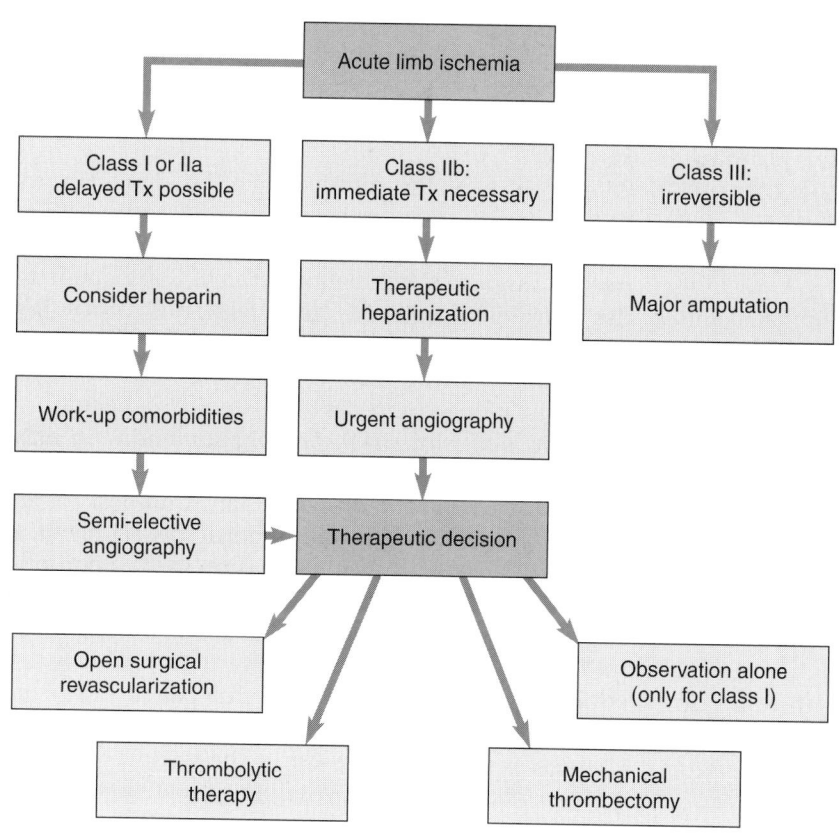

Figure 16-1   *Management of patients with acute limb ischemia. From Ouriel K. Acute limb ischemia. In: Rutherford RB, ed. Vascular Surgery. 6th ed. Philadelphia, PA: Elsevier Saunders; 2005.*

Imaging

Arteriography is the gold standard for diagnosis and anatomic evaluation of acute limb ischemia. However, a patient suffering from limb ischemia should not undergo a separate diagnostic angiogram if any delay in revascularization might result in limb loss. Access for diagnostic arteriography should be established at a site distant from the presumed occlusion, so as to avoid any future need for thrombolytic delivery in the region of the arteriotomy. Arteriography is often performed intraoperatively in the setting of a pulseless extremity. In patients allergic to iodinated contrast dye or with renal insufficiency, CO_2 or gadolinium may be used as contrast agents; these, however, yield poorer quality suprainguinal arteriograms. In all cases, digital subtraction angiography is preferred, because it provides satisfactory images with the use of smaller amounts of intravenous contrast.

The arteriogram should include examination of both inflow and outflow anatomy, as well as study of the runoff vessels into the foot. In the case of embolic ischemia, arteriography will demonstrate minimal atherosclerotic disease, a sharp cutoff of the artery at the site of occlusion, and few collateral vessels. Meanwhile, if the acute event is thrombotic in nature, angiography will most often reveal diffuse atherosclerotic disease, irregular and tapered cutoffs, and a well-developed collateral circulation.

Other imaging studies are often useful and indicated in the setting of class I and IIa acute limb ischemia. Magnetic resonance angiography (MRA) excels at identifying patent tibial arteries as potential bypass targets; in addition, intravenous gadolinium is much less nephrotoxic than iodinated contrast. Computed tomography angiography (CTA) is also capable of identifying occlusive disease and arterial anatomy for operative planning, but requires the administration of intravenous contrast.

TREATMENT

Initial Therapy

Maintenance intravenous fluids should be initiated and the patient kept *nil per os*, given the likely need for surgical intervention. A Foley catheter should be inserted to monitor urine output. Consideration should be given to either oral acetylcysteine[8] or bicarbonate infusion[9] if the patient has chronic renal insufficiency or diabetes, because diagnostic or completion angiography will likely be indicated.

Temperature extremes and fluctuations should be avoided: cold temperatures cause vasoconstriction and heat causes increased tissue metabolic demands. Transfusion and optimization of cardiac output should be accomplished whenever these might result in improved oxygenation of the affected limb.

Anticoagulation

Immediate anticoagulation by systemic heparinization—first bolus and then continuous infusion—should be instituted in any patient experiencing acute limb ischemia. This measure will prevent clot propagation and extension, thereby minimizing the risk of the development of more profound ischemia and potentially facilitating surgical embolectomy. In the setting of limb ischemia from an embolic source, systemic anticoagulation will also minimize the risk of further embolic events. However, heparin is not a fibrinolytic agent, and so does not lyse existing clot.

Thrombolysis

Intra-arterial or catheter-directed thrombolysis or fibrinolysis has proved effective and beneficial in a variety of clinical scenarios involving acute limb ischemia. However, in a number of situations, thrombolytics are absolutely contraindicated: these include recent surgery or trauma, recent stroke, an active bleeding diathesis, and a recent history of gastrointestinal bleeding.

Three prospective randomized clinical trials have compared early catheter-directed thrombolysis with early surgery for acute limb ischemia.[10,11,12] These data suggest that thrombolytic therapy is effective as an initial therapeutic measure in patients with acute arterial and graft occlusions. Its use is favored in patients who do not have any sensimotor deficits, and in patients with occluded bypass grafts.

In some cases, percutaneous aspiration or mechanical thrombectomy is utilized prior to and in conjunction with thrombolysis. It is essential that any stenoses revealed on arteriography following thrombolysis be treated with angioplasty, bypass graft revision, or revascularization. In the interim from completion of thrombolysis until intervention directed at flow-limiting lesions, heparin infusion must be continued.

Surgery

Prior to 1963 and the introduction of Thomas J. Fogarty balloon embolectomy catheter (Fig. 16-2), only 23% of patients suffering embolic vascular occlusion were treated surgically with embolectomy. Subsequent to the introduction of his catheter, and continuing today, the vast majority of these patients undergo surgical embolectomy, which now—along with systemic anticoagulation—comprises the mainstay of therapy.

Aortic occlusion is a rare phenomenon. It may result from aortic saddle embolus, *in situ* thrombosis of an atherosclerotic abdominal aorta, thrombosis of an abdominal aortic aneurysm, or aortic dissection. It is essential to recognize aortic occlusion in the appropriate clinical setting: bilateral lower extremity weakness and sensory loss can be confused with a primarily neurologic disorder. It is also important to establish the etiology of aortic occlusion, because balloon catheter embolectomy via a femoral cut down (see later in this chapter) is usually successful in the setting of saddle embolus, but infrequently helpful in patients with *in situ* thrombosis of a chronically diseased abdominal aorta. In the latter scenario, the limbs are usually not

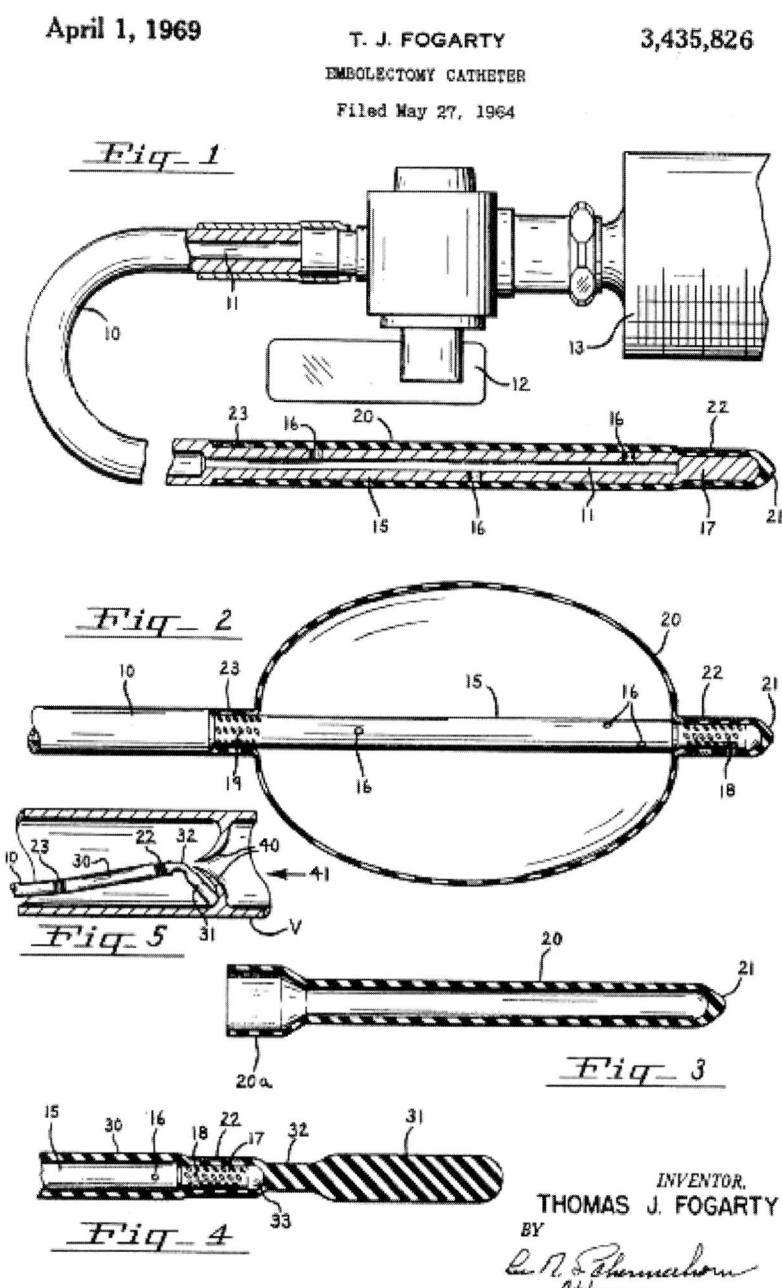

April 1, 1969   T. J. FOGARTY   3,435,826

EMBOLECTOMY CATHETER

Filed May 27, 1964

Fig. 1

Fig. 2

Fig. 5

Fig. 3

Fig. 4

INVENTOR.

THOMAS J. FOGARTY

BY

Attorney

Figure 16-2 *Original patent application for Fogarty embolectomy catheter. From archives of U.S. Patent and Trademark Office, with permission.*

profoundly ischemic owing to the chronic nature of the disease and resulting extensive collateralization; these patients may require aortobifemoral grafting to reestablish lower extremity perfusion.

Acute unilateral iliac occlusion can occur in patients having undergone prior aortic aneurysmorrhaphy with a bifurcated graft, prior aortobifemoral reconstruction, or prior abdominal aortic stent grafting. In these situations, the surgeon may be able to restore patency of the graft limb with balloon thrombectomy performed from a groin incision, but a technical problem in the affected limb and graft stenosis must be suspected and subsequently addressed (Fig. 16-3).[13] If limb patency cannot be reestablished, femoral-femoral or axillofemoral bypass is indicated.

Symptomatic popliteal aneurysms generally present with limb ischemia—from aneurysm thrombosis or distal thromboembolism—rather than rupture. The diagnosis should be suspected in any patient with acute or chronic ischemia of the leg and a palpable firm pulseless (in the case of thrombosis) or pulsatile mass behind the knee. Duplex ultrasound can confirm the diagnosis. Angiography, MRA, or CTA are useful for operative planning. Treatment of a popliteal aneurysm presenting with acute limb ischemia consists of emergent catheter-directed thrombolysis to reestablish distal arterial patency[14] and subsequent surgical exclusion and bypass; resection of the aneurysm is not necessary. The aneurysm is ligated proximally and distally and a bypass is fashioned from normal caliber

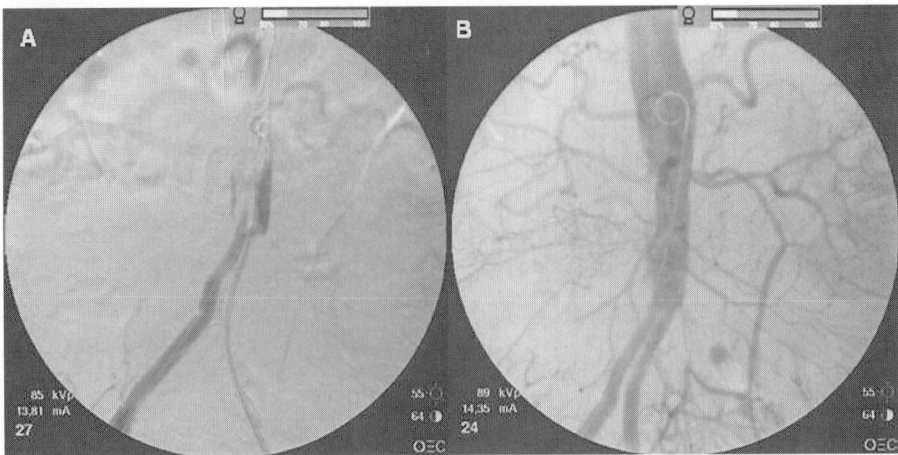

Figure 16-3 *A. Occluded left limb of an abdominal aortic stent graft. Wire access to the aorta was accomplished from the patient's groins bilaterally. Stents were placed in the newly patent left iliac limb to displace residual thrombus and treat any stenoses that might have contributed to the thrombosis.* **B.** *Completion angiogram.*

popliteal artery above the knee to normal popliteal artery below the knee. If the superficial femoral artery is aneurysmal or ectatic, it may be bypassed as well, via construction of a common femoral-to-distal popliteal artery bypass. Saphenous vein conduit is preferred, but in a patient without available autologous conduit, prosthetic may be necessary. Finally, there is an emerging experience with covered stents for treatment of popliteal aneurysms.[15]

In patients presenting with local symptoms from popliteal aneurysm, including compression of adjacent nerves or veins, a posterior approach to resection or endoaneurysmorrhaphy is preferred. Arterial reconstruction is then performed in an end-to-end fashion using reversed saphenous vein. It should be recognized that one-half of patients will have bilateral popliteal aneurysms, and that one-third of patients with a popliteal aneurysm will have a coincident abdominal aortic aneurysm; therefore, these patients should be screened for coexisting aneurysmal disease.

In patients suffering thrombotic arterial occlusions, and those whose thromboembolism cannot be extracted or lysed, arterial bypass grafting may be necessary to treat stenotic or occluded vascular segments.

Intraoperative management

Reperfusion of an ischemic limb is a potentially dangerous period. It has been posited that up to one-third of deaths from arterial thromboembolism result from the metabolic consequences of revascularization.[16] The ischemic limb has very high concentrations of potassium, lactic acid, myoglobin, and cellular enzymes, which are released into the systemic circulation upon reestablishing perfusion to the limb, resulting in "reperfusion syndrome." Acutely, the patient may become severely acidemic and hyperkalemic, resulting in consequences as severe as cardiac arrest. Toxic oxygen radicals are systemically circulated upon reperfusion, and can cause depression of cardiac

function, cardiac arrhythmias, and a loss of vascular tone resulting in profound hypotension. Finally, myoglobin from injured muscle (rhabdomyolysis) can contribute to acute renal failure. Treatment is supportive, but the clinical entity must be anticipated by the surgeon and anesthesiologist. The surgeon must remain vigilant for these potential problems in the operating room and the early postoperative period.

ARTERIAL EMBOLISM—FURTHER CONSIDERATIONS

Because of its acuity, and thus the absence of adequate preformed collateral arteries, arterial embolization is the classic situation resulting in acute arterial occlusion and organ-threatening ischemia. The absence of a palpable pulse—even if Doppler signals are present—in the symptomatic limb in the setting of a corresponding palpable pulse in the unaffected limb, is highly suggestive of acute embolic disease.

SOURCES
Cardiac
Approximately 90% of the time, arterial emboli arise in the heart.[17] Most commonly, atrial fibrillation results in a dilated, noncontractile left atrial appendage, which predisposes to thrombus formation and—upon spontaneous or therapeutic cardioversion—thromboembolism. Left ventricular (LV) thrombus may also form, for instance, adjacent to a noncontractile segment of LV following myocardial infarction, in a LV aneurysm, or in the setting of dilated cardiomyopathy. Saddle emboli, which lodge at the aortic bifurcation and cause bilateral lower extremity ischemia, are most commonly the result of LV thrombus.

Thromboembolism from heart valves is less common today than in the past, as a result of the relative decrease in prevalence of rheumatic heart disease.

Bacterial endocarditis can result in septic emboli, which may cause both acute ischemia and infection of the distal vessel wall, which in turn results in mycotic aneurysm. Atheroemboli may arise from either the thoracic or the abdominal aorta. Finally, in some 5% of cases, the source of embolism is never identified.

ANATOMIC DISTRIBUTION

The anatomic distribution of arterial embolism is depicted in Fig. 16-4. The embolus most frequently lodges at an arterial bifurcation. In the patient with bilateral lower extremity ischemia and absent femoral pulses, the most common clinical scenario is saddle embolus to the bifurcation. This disease can carry with it a poor prognosis, with a 27% mortality in one modern series.[18] The most common site of clinically significant embolism in the lower extremity is the common femoral artery (CFA) bifurcation. Patients with CFA embolism will experience foot and calf pain. Finally, an embolus to the popliteal artery will result in absent pedal pulses.

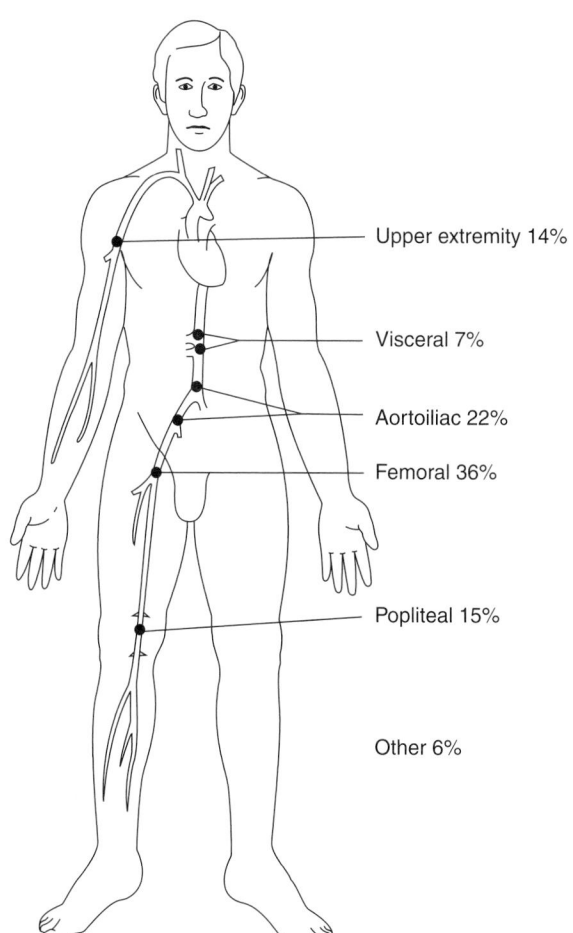

Upper extremity 14%

Visceral 7%

Aortoiliac 22%

Femoral 36%

Popliteal 15%

Other 6%

Figure 16-4 *The most common sites of arterial embolic occlusions. From Fecteau SR, Darling RC III, Roddy SP. Arterial thromboembolism. In: Rutherford RB, ed.* Vascular Surgery. *6th ed. Philadelphia, PA: Elsevier Saunders; 2005.*

TREATMENT

In most clinical situations, embolectomy—along with systemic anticoagulation—is the treatment of choice for arterial embolism. As discussed previously, thrombolysis and percutaneous mechanical thrombectomy devices can be valuable therapies, but their roles and indications for use are not well-defined.

Balloon catheter embolectomy via a femoral cutdown is indicated in the setting of saddle embolus to the aortic bifurcation. It is essential that embolectomies be performed through both groins. Number 5 or 6 Fogarty catheters are usually used. The contralateral femoral artery should be occluded during the passage of each catheter, to prevent further distal embolism. If perfusion cannot be restored, then transperitoneal or retroperitoneal access to the aorta and common iliacs is required; alternatively, extra-anatomic bypass with axillobifemoral reconstruction may be considered.

For embolism to the iliac bifurcation or common femoral artery, the preferred therapy is Fogarty balloon catheter embolectomy through a groin incision (Fig. 16-5). This should be considered an emergent surgical procedure, for which general anesthesia is indicated regardless of the patient's cardiac status and other comorbidities. Most often a transverse arteriotomy is utilized, allowing closure without narrowing the artery. However, in the setting of significantly diseased femoral artery or anticipated need for a bypass graft during the procedure, a longitudinal arteriotomy

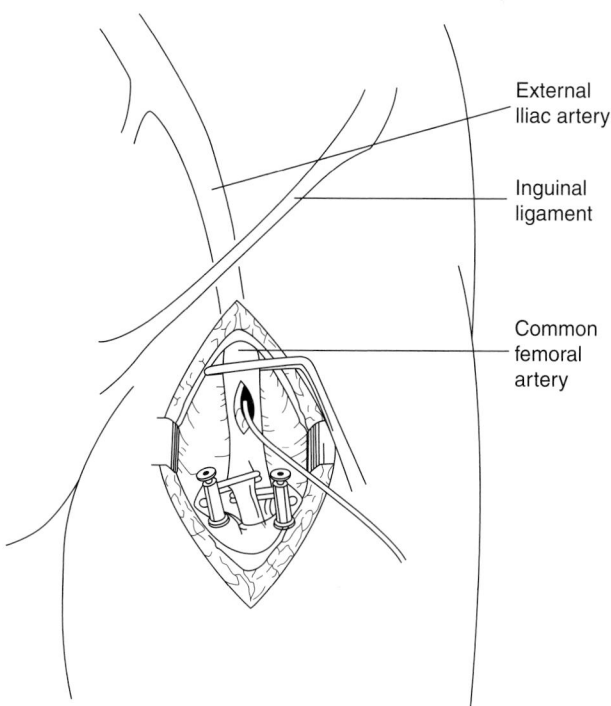

External Iliac artery

Inguinal ligament

Common femoral artery

Figure 16-5 *Femoral approach to embolectomy. From Khatri VP, Asensio JA.* Operative Surgery Manual. *Philadelphia, PA: Saunders; 2003.*

may be used. If a longitudinal arteriotomy is subsequently to be closed primarily, a vein or prosthetic patch should be used to prevent narrowing. Balloon catheter thromboembolectomy can be performed with fluoroscopic guidance, and—using over-the-wire balloon catheters—using wire and catheter access. Number 5 balloon catheters are generally appropriate for iliac vessels; number 4 catheters are used for the common femoral and superficial femoral arteries; numbers 3 or 4 catheters may be appropriate for the profunda femoris artery and the popliteal artery; finally, number 2 or 3 catheters are typically used for tibial vessels. Several passes of the catheter are necessary, and should be continued until no additional thrombus is extracted. Completion angiography is required to assess for completeness and success of the procedure; often, occlusive disease and vasospasm can mislead one's clinical exam of the reperfused distal circulation. For further details of the procedure, please refer to a surgical manual and atlas, for example, Dr. Fogarty's chapter in *Mastery of Surgery*.[19]

In cases of popliteal artery embolism, the clot can usually by extracted via balloon catheters passed from the groin. However, in the case of distal embolization or involvement of the trifurcation vessels with thromboembolism, a separate incision may be necessary to expose the popliteal artery and isolate its branches. This is because catheters passed blindly from the femoral artery enter the peroneal artery preferentially in 90% of patients.[20] Using an infrageniculate approach to the popliteal artery and its branches allows selective catheterization of the tibial vessels, normally with a number 2 Fogarty catheter. This can be performed from a preexisting femoral arteriotomy, with manual compression of the branches of the popliteal trifurcation to select each sequentially. Alternatively, a popliteal arteriotomy may be performed and embolectomy catheters passed from the infrageniculate site.

Occasionally, residual thrombus will be present in the tibial vessels on angiography following thrombectomy performed from a popliteal approach. In this setting, exploration of the posterior or anterior tibial arteries just above the ankle may be attempted. However, arteriotomies in these locations are often subject to rethrombosis after closure in the setting of ALI. Catheter-directed or direct injection of thrombolytics may be considered in the situation of residual occlusive distal tibial and pedal vessel thromboembolus.[21]

POSTOPERATIVE CARE

Postoperatively in the patient with acute thromboembolic limb ischemia, full anticoagulation—initially with heparin infusion and subsequently with oral warfarin therapy—should be considered. If indicated, warfarin anticoagulation should be continued for at least 6 months.

Measures to identify the embolic source should be undertaken once limb survival has been assured. Transthoracic echocardiography should be performed. If the etiology is still in doubt, transesophageal echocardiography and contrast CT of the thoracic and abdominal aortas should be considered. Finally, bubble echocardiography and venous duplex ultrasound of the lower extremities will identify the relatively unusual case of "paradoxical emboli" of venous thrombus through a patent foramen ovale.

COMPARTMENT SYNDROME

In limbs ischemic for 4-6 hours, significant reperfusion injury may occur. Swelling may result in increased compartment pressures, typically presenting earliest in the anterior compartment of the leg, which has both a significant mass of slow twitch red muscle fibers and a strong encasing fascial envelope. The contents of the anterior compartment include the deep peroneal nerve, the tibialis anterior muscle, and the anterior tibial artery; compartment syndrome with accompanying tissue necrosis in this distribution classically results in foot drop.

Although some surgeons will elect to observe a transiently ischemic limb for signs of compartment syndrome postoperatively, in the setting of greater than 6 hours of profound ischemia many would perform four-compartment fasciotomies at the time of revascularization. If one elects to observe the patient's leg, any increased pain, especially with passive plantarflexion of the foot, or loss of sensation in the first web space of the foot (sensory distribution of the deep peroneal nerve), should prompt reevaluation by the surgeon. There should be a low threshold to measure compartment pressures, using a Stryker needle (Stryker Instruments, Kalamazoo, MI) or other device. Compartment pressures greater than 30 mm Hg can result in tissue ischemia and necrosis. Patients demonstrating hypotension or shock, those requiring pressors, those with absent flow through the popliteal artery at presentation, and younger patients with greater muscle mass and fewer arterial collaterals are at increased risk of developing compartment syndrome.

Four compartment fasciotomy is usually performed through both a medial and a lateral incision (Fig. 16-6). The incisions are left open for subsequent delayed primary closure or skin grafting.

Compartment syndromes of the thigh, forearm, and upper arm do occur; however, usually these are related to bleeding or infusions into a compartment, or traumatic and crush injuries. Regardless, if there is concern for compartment syndrome in one of these anatomic locations in the setting of ischemia-reperfusion, fasciotomies should be performed.

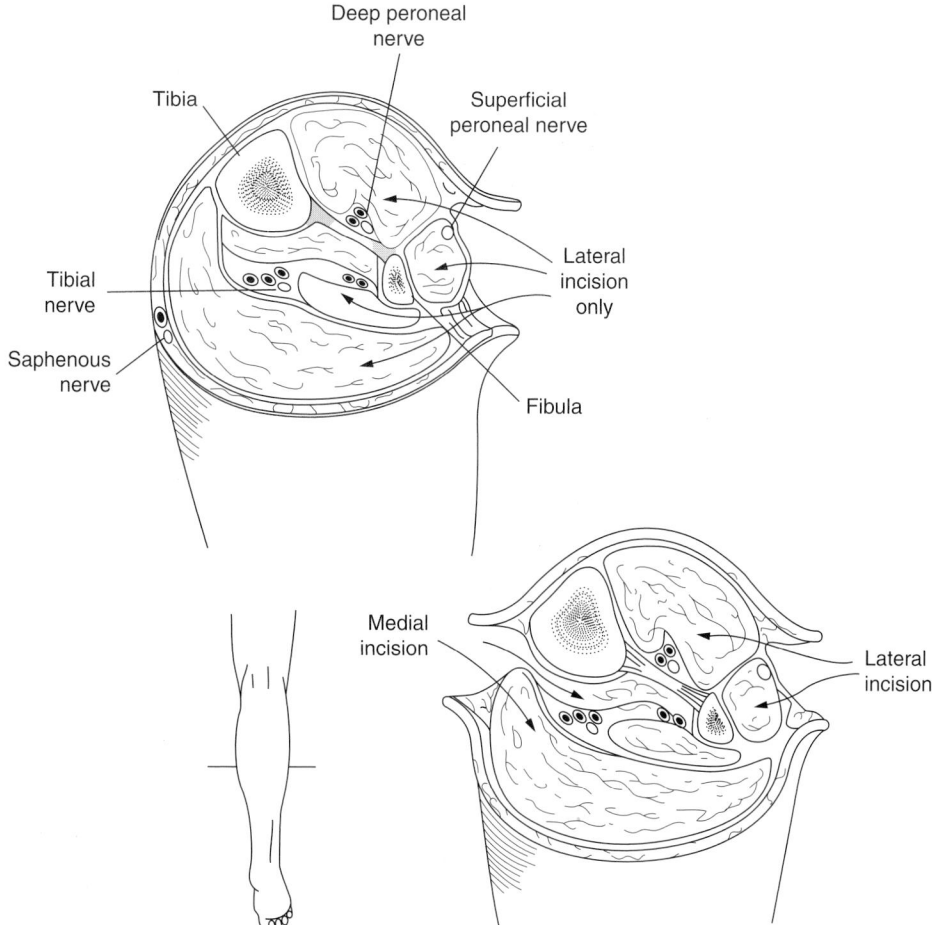

Figure 16-6 *Four-compartment fasciotomy of the leg is usually performed through both a medial and lateral incisions, but can be performed through a lateral incision only. From Velmahos GC, Toutouzas KG. Vascular trauma and compartment syndromes.* Surg Clin N Amer *2002;88:1.*

RHABDOMYOLYSIS

In any clinical scenario in which compartment syndrome is a concern, the possibility of rhabdomyolysis should also be considered. In patients whose limbs have suffered significant ischemia reperfusion from arterial occlusion, rhabdomyolysis can occur and should be suspected in patients demonstrating increased muscle pain and weakness, renal failure, or hyperkalemia. Laboratory tests that aid in the diagnosis are urinalysis and serum creatinine phosphokinase. The urine dip will be positive for blood, whereas the microscopic urinalysis will not demonstrate significant numbers of red blood cells; urinalysis will also demonstrate casts and myoglobin. Treatment consists of volume expansion (with goal urine output of 1 to 2 ml/kg/hr) and alkalinization of the urine with sodium bicarbonate infusion. Renal compromise in those patients suffering rhabdomyolysis generally resolves in time, if the patient does not succumb to their primary illness and the acute renal failure.

ATHEROEMBOLISM

In atheroembolism, microscopic cholesterol-laden debris is showered from atherosclerotic or aneurysmal vessels into the distal-most arteries. Patients most often present with "blue toe syndrome," ischemic toes in the setting of palpable pedal pulses. Vital internal organs—including the kidneys and intestines—may also be affected if the source of emboli is the proximal aorta. This problem commonly presents following surgical manipulation—either clamping or balloon occlusion—of the atherosclerotic or aneurysmal artery.

Treatment of atheroembolism consists of antiplatelet therapy. If the patient is not already taking aspirin, it should be initiated immediately. If the patient is already on aspirin therapy, consideration should be given to the addition of clopidogrel. Ischemic digits should be treated expectantly; necrotic digits will require amputation.

If atheroemboli recur on antiplatelet therapy, consideration may be given to surgical management.

Options include excision or bypass of the responsible artery, or exclusion of the source of atheroemboli with covered stents.

ACUTE UPPER EXTREMITY ISCHEMIA

Acute ischemia of the arm is usually caused by embolism, most commonly from a cardiac source. Rare causes include subclavian artery aneurysms, arteriovenous fistulae, and iatrogenic manipulation of the arterial tree. The bifurcation of the brachial artery is the most common site of embolism. Antecubital approach to the brachial artery for catheter embolectomy is appropriate in this setting.

DEEP VENOUS THROMBOSIS

Surgeons play important roles in the diagnosis and treatment of deep venous thrombosis (DVT). Unfortunately, surgery confers a significantly increased risk of DVT formation on our patients. Meanwhile, we are asked to evaluate patients with acute DVT for surgical thrombectomy, for management of anticoagulation, for vena caval interruption, and, in the case of complications arising as a result of DVT, such as phlegmasia cerulea dolens and pulmonary embolism. Finally, DVT—especially in the upper extremity—occurs often as a consequence of an existing central venous catheter, and surgeons have expertise and experience in managing venous access.

EPIDEMIOLOGY
Estimates of the yearly incidence of symptomatic diagnosed DVT in the United States range from 71 to 117 per 100,000 population.[22,23] However, autopsy data indicate that up to 80% of DVT are undiagnosed. Meanwhile, most studies have demonstrated an incidence of pulmonary embolism, the most catastrophic sequelae of DVT, which is approximately one-half that of DVT.

PATHOPHYSIOLOGY AND RISK FACTORS
The classic model of pathogenesis of venous thrombosis invokes Virchow's triad: damage to the vessel wall, venous stasis, and hypercoaguability. Vessel wall damage abrogates the endothelium's influence toward anticoagulation and fibrinolysis. Venous stasis prevents the expedient removal of activated clotting factors and platelets. Thrombophilia—whether acquired or congenital—promotes clot formation.

The risk factors for VTE are legion, and one or more are present in most hospitalized patients. They include age, pregnancy, estrogens and other medicines, recent surgery, malignancy, hematologic hypercoaguability (Table 16-4).

Table 16-4   Risk Factors for Venous Thromboembolism

Risk Factor	Estimated Relative Risk
Inherited conditions[†]	
Antithrombin deficiency	25
Protein C deficiency	20
Protein S deficiency	10
Factor V Leiden mutation	
Heterozygous	5
Homozygous	50
G20210A prothrombin-gene mutation (heterozygous)	2.5
Dysfibrinogenemia	18
Acquired conditions	
Major surgery or major trauma	5–200[‡]
History of venous thromboembolism	50
Antiphospholipid antibodies	
Elevated anticardiolipin antibody level	2
Nonspecific inhibitor (e.g., lup us anticoagulant)	10
Cancer	5
Major medical illness with hospitalization	5
Age	
> 50 years	5
> 70 years	10
Pregnancy	7
Estrogen therapy	
Oral contraceptives	5
Hormone-replacement therapy	2
Selective estrogen-receptor modulators	
Tamokifen	5
Ralokifene	3
Obesity	1–3
Hereditary, environmental, or idiopathic conditions	
Hyperhomocysteinemia[§]	3
Elevated levels of factor VIII (> 90th percentile)	3
Elevated levels of factory IX (> 90th percentile)	2.3
Elevated levels of factor XI (> 90th percentile)	2.2

Data are from Rosendaal[14] and Kearon.[15] Relative risks are for patients with the specified risk factor, as compared with those without the risk factor.

[†]The definition of deficiency of antithrombin, protein C, or protein S varies among studies; it is usually defined as a functional or immunologic value that is less than the 5th percentile of values in the control population.

[‡]The risk varies greatly, depending on the type of surgery, the use and type of prophylaxis, and the method of diagnosis.

[§]The definition of hyperhomocysteinemia varies among studies; it is usually defined as a persistent elevation of fasting plasma homocysteine levels or plasma homocysteine levels after methionine loading that are greater than the 95th percentile of the control population or more than 2 SD above the mean for the control population. From Bates SM and Ginsberg JS: Treatment of Deep-Vein Thrombosis. N Engl J Med 2004;351:3.

CLINICAL MANIFESTATIONS

Patients with occlusive DVT usually present with swelling of the involved limb, and pain or tenderness overlying the affected veins. Patients with nonocclusive DVT will often be asymptomatic and demonstrate minimal or no signs of venous thrombosis.

DIAGNOSIS

The gold standard for detection of DVT has been ascending venography; however, given the invasive and cumbersome nature of this procedure, it is currently seldom used in the clinical arena. Intravascular thrombosis can be detected by measurement of D-dimer, a product of fibrinolysis. This laboratory measurement is often useful to eliminate an entertained diagnosis of DVT or PE, and can aid in the diagnosis of DVT in outpatients and those presenting to the emergency room. However, its utility in inpatients is limited because of coincident medical and surgical conditions that also tend to increase D-dimer levels.

Duplex ultrasonography has the capability to directly visualize thrombus within calf and thigh veins, and has become the test of choice to diagnose DVT.[24] The presence of a filling defect in the venous lumen, of deranged Doppler color flow in the vein, or failure of the deep vein to compress with directed pressure exerted with the ultrasound probe are findings indicative of DVT.

In outpatients presenting with DVT, the physician or surgeon must determine the cause. Spontaneous venous thrombosis in patients without evident predisposing features often heralds a heretofore undiagnosed malignancy or a congenital clotting disorder. Inpatients diagnosed with new DVT most often have easily identified predisposing risk factors, related to their illness and hospitalization.

TREATMENT

Unless contraindicated, therapy for DVT consists of anticoagulation. Bed rest and elevation of the affected limb are recommended for symptomatic DVT.

Unfractionated heparin has traditionally been used as the initial anticoagulant in the treatment of DVT. Heparin binds with antithrombin III to increase that molecule's affinity for thrombin. It is delivered as a continuous intravenous infusion. Therapy is initiated with a bolus of 80 μ/kg and then maintained with and infusion of 18 μ/kg/hr titrated to maintain an activated partial thromboplastin time (aPTT) of 2.0 to 3.0 times the patient's baseline aPTT. Unfractionated heparin therapy requires periodic monitoring of aPTT because the dose-response relationship is not predictable, as a result of the drug's nonspecific binding to plasma and cellular proteins. Beyond bleeding, the feared complication of unfractionated heparin is heparin-induced thrombocytopenia, occurring in 1%-2% of patients having undergone cardiac surgery.[25] Alternative intravenous anticoagulants appropriate for use in patients with HIT or a history thereof include the direct thrombin inhibitors lepirudin and argatroban.

Low-molecular weight heparins—including enoxaparin—are effective in treating DVT and have more predictable dose response than unfractionated heparin because of less nonspecific protein binding. They are administered subcutaneously in once or twice daily doses and are dosed based on patient weight, without the need for laboratory monitoring of coagulation parameters. Therefore, they are suitable for use in the outpatient setting. However, outpatient treatment is not appropriate for patients with massive venous thrombosis, serious coexisting illnesses, or increased risk of hemorrhage.

Long-term anticoagulation is customarily accomplished with oral warfarin therapy, initiated while the patient is therapeutically anticoagulated using heparin or an analogue. The goal international normalized ratio (INR) is 2.0 to 3.0 for patients being treated for DVT. Duration of therapy is determined based on the etiology of DVT and existing risk factors for VTE, generally ranging from 3 months for uncomplicated DVT in a patient with recognized transient risk factors for their development to lifelong therapy in patients with hereditary thrombophilias.

Thrombolysis is an attractive modality of therapy for patients with acute DVT. It can potentially remove the thrombus and restore venous patency more quickly and completely than anticoagulation alone. Early removal of thrombus has been postulated to reduce the chronic sequelae of DVT, including post-thrombotic syndrome. Thrombolytics can be given systemically or by catheter-directed infusion, allowing a higher local concentration of the agent at the thrombus. Thrombolysis causes more bleeding complications than anticoagulation alone; in addition, there is an attendant risk of hemorrhagic stroke. It is most often reserved for patients who have extensive symptomatic DVTs and those with limb-threatening ischemia. Anticoagulation is required following thrombolysis, to prevent rethrombosis.

In those patients with extensive venous clot burden or a threatened limb, and either contraindication to thrombolysis or following unsuccessful thrombolysis, surgical venous thrombectomy can be considered, although clinical success and long-term iliac vein patency are variable.[26] This is performed through a femoral incision and venotomy for iliofemoral DVT, and via a transperitoneal approach for IVC thrombus. In either case, general anesthesia is required in order that positive end-expiratory pressure can be administered via the ventilator, to assist in the prevention of PE. Distal thrombus in the leg can be removed through the femoral venotomy by external compression using a rubber bandage. The endothelium subject to thrombectomy and the sutured venotomy sites are thrombogenic, so a temporary arteriovenous fistula is fashioned in an end-to-side fashion by ligating the saphenous vein and anastamosing its proximal end to the side of the femoral artery.

If anticoagulation is contraindicated, or the patient has failed anticoagulant therapy, inferior vena cava filter are indicated to prevent PE in the setting of diagnosed DVT. If anticoagulation is not contraindicated, patients undergoing IVC filter placement should nevertheless be therapeutically anticoagulated in order to treat the DVT.

COMPLICATIONS

Pulmonary embolism (PE) is the most feared and devastating consequence of DVT. There are approximately 700,000 cases of PE in the United States yearly, resulting in 200,000 deaths. PE is the most common preventable cause of death in hospitalized patients. Investigations of the deep veins in patients having suffered PE may reveal occlusive, nonocclusive, or no deep vein thromboses. Diagnosis of PE requires a high index of suspicion and significant clinical acumen, aided by measurement of D-dimer (to detect DVT as a marker of PE), arterial blood gases, electrocardiogram, chest x-ray, ventilation-perfusion (VQ) lung scanning, spiral computed tomography pulmonary arteriography, echocardiography, and pulmonary angiography. Treatment algorithms include anticoagulation, thrombolysis, and pulmonary thromboendarterectomy.

Phlegmasia alba dolens results from occlusion of the major deep veins of an extremity. This progresses to phlegmasia cerulea dolens (PCD) when the venous collaterals are also thrombosed and occluded. PCD occurs most often in the cachectic, dehydrated patient with a coincident critical illness. It more often involves the lower extremity than the arm. The iliac, common femoral, and superficial femoral veins are most often occluded. The limb is swollen, bluish, and mottled from the complete venous outflow obstruction. The limb becomes acutely ischemic, and the patient goes into shock, in part from the fluid loss into the affected limb. PCD should be suspected in a patient presenting with the triad of limb edema, severe pain, and cyanosis. The diagnosis is made on clinical grounds, supplemented by either duplex ultrasonography or venography to diagnose or confirm the presence of DVTs and venous obstruction. Treatment consists of aggressive isotonic fluid resuscitation, limb elevation, anticoagulation, thrombolysis, and—if those are unsuccessful—surgical venous thrombectomy performed through a femoral incision. The disease may result in compartment syndrome of the limb, in which fasciotomies may be required.

Up to 50% of people may have chronic symptoms following an acute DVT: pain, edema, hyperpigmentation, varicosities, and ulceration. This post-thrombotic syndrome is a consequence of ambulatory venous hypertension, caused by persistent venous obstruction and valvular incompetence. There is evidence that treatment of the acute DVT with thrombolysis or surgical venous thrombectomy can reduce the incidence of subsequent post-thrombotic syndrome. Studies have suggested reduced severity and incidence of post-thrombotic syndrome in patients treated with compression stockings early after acute DVT.[27]

UPPER EXTREMITY DVT

Only 1%-4% of DVTs present in the upper extremity; these may involve the axillary, subclavian, or innominate veins. The superior vena cava is rarely involved except in circumstances of long-term central venous catheterization or external compression (as with tumor). Two etiologic circumstances are frequently encountered in patients with upper extremity DVT's: central venous catheters and thoracic outlet compression.

In patients with arm swelling or tenderness and an indwelling central line, removal of the catheter may be sufficient treatment. If the patient also exhibits fever or bacteremia, or if the symptoms do not resolve with removal of the catheter, then duplex ultrasonography or venous angiography should be performed. If a DVT is identified, anticoagulation is indicated, as are antibiotics in the case of septic thrombophlebitis.

Effort thrombosis, or Paget-Schroetter syndrome, is characterized by swelling and cyanosis of the arm, which frequently progresses to pain. The syndrome is caused by venous obstruction near the junction of the axillary and subclavian veins at the entrance to the thorax in proximity to the first rib. Occasionally, a cervical rib is the causative factor. In most patients, the anterior scalene muscle is believed to compress the vein. It is two times more common in men, and characteristically presents in the dominant arm of young active patients. Treatment includes catheter-directed thrombolysis and anticoagulation; however, rethrombosis is the norm unless operative decompression of the thoracic outlet is performed. This is accomplished by first rib resection.

SUMMARY

Patients presenting emergently with limb ischemia have a variety of etiologies of either arterial of venous occlusion. Signs and symptoms must be recognized and acted on rapidly to salvage the ischemic tissues. Appropriate and expedient surgical management and—frequently—operation are essential to limb salvage and patient survival.

REFERENCES

1. Davies B, Braithwaite BD, Birch PA, et al. Acute leg ischaemia in Gloucestershire. *Br J Surg* 1997;84:504.
2. Dormandy J, Heeck L, Vig S. Acute limb ischemia. *Semin Vasc Surg* 1999;12:148.
3. Kasirajan K, Ouriel K. Acute limb ischemia. In: Rutherford RB (ed.) *Vascular Surgery*. 6th ed. Philadelphia, PA: Elsevier; 2005: 959-971.
4. Ouriel K, Shortell CK, Green RM, et al. Differential mechanisms of failure of autogenous and non-autogenous bypass conduits: an assessment following successful graft thrombolysis. *Cardiovasc Surg* 1995;3:469.
5. Rutherford RB, Baer JD, Ernst C, et al: Recommended standards for reports dealing with lower extremity ischemia: revised version. *J Vasc Surg* 1997;26:517.
6. Pfeiffer RB III and O'Mara CS. Peripheral arterial embolus. In Cameron JL (ed.) *Current Surgical Therapy*. 8th ed. Philadelphia, PA: Elsevier; 2004.
7. Goldman L, Caldera DL, Nussbaum SR, et al. Multifactorial index of cardiac risk in noncardiac surgical procedures. *N Engl J Med* 1977;297:845-850.
8. Tepel M, van der Giet M, Schwarzfeld C, et al. Prevention of radiographic-contrast-agent-induced reductions in renal function by acetylcysteine. *N Eng J Med* 2000;343(3):180-184.
9. Merten GJ, Burgess WP, Gray LV, et al. Prevention of contrast-induced nephropathy with sodium bicarbonate: a randomized controlled trial. *JAMA* 2004;291:2328-2334.
10. Ouriel K, Shortell C, DeWeese JA, et al. A comparison of thrombolytic therapy with operative revascularization in the initial treatment of acute peripheral arterial ischemia. *J Vasc Surg* 1994;19:1021.
11. Weaver FA, Camerota AJ, Youngblood M, et al. Surgical revascularization versus thrombolysis for non-embolic lower extremity native artery occlusions: results of a prospective randomized trial. *J Vasc Surg* 1996;24:513.
12. Ouriel K, Veith FJ, Sasahara AA. Thrombolysis or peripheral arterial surgery: phase I results. TOPAS investigators. *J Vasc Surg* 1996;23:64.
13. Milner R, Golden MA, Velazquez OC, et al. A new endovascular approach to treatment of acute iliac limb occlusions of bifurcated aortic stent grafts with an exoskeleton. *J Vasc Surg* 2003;37:1329-1331.
14. Carpenter JP, Barker CF, Roberts B, et al. Popliteal artery aneurysms: current management and outcome. *J Vasc Surg* 1994;19(1):65-72.

15. Mohan IV, Bray PJ, Harris JP, et al. Endovascular popliteal aneurysm repair: are the results comparable to open surgery? *Eur J Vasc Endovasc Surg* 2006;32: 149-154.
16. Haimovici H. Muscular, renal, and metabolic complications of acute arterial occlusions: myonephropathic-metabolic syndrome. *Surgery* 1979;85:461.
17. Abbott W, Maloney R, McCabe C, et al. Arterial embolism a 44 year perspective. *Am J Surg* 1982;143:460.
18. Woratyla S, Darling RC III, Lloyd W, et al. Acute and chronic aortic occlusion: analysis of outcome. *Proceedings of the Eastern Vascular Society* 1998;12:82.
19. Fogarty TJ, Hill BB, Zarins CK. Fogarty catheter thromboembolectomy. In: Baker RJ, Fischer JE (eds.) *Mastery of Surgery*. 4th ed. Philadelphia, PA: Lippincott; 2001: 1991-2001.
20. Short D, Vaughn GI, Jachimcyzk J, et al. The anatomic basis for the occasional failure of transfemoral balloon catheter thromboembolectomy. *Ann Surg* 1979;190:555.
21. Comerota A, White J. Intraoperative intraarterial thrombolytic therapy for salvage of limbs in patients with residual and distal arterial thrombosis. *Semin Vasc Surg* 1992;5:110.
22. Silverstein MD, Heit JA, Mohr DN, et al. Trends in the incidence of deep vein thrombosis and pulmonary embolism: a 25-year population-based study. *Arch Intern Med* 1998;158:585-593.
23. White RH. The epidemiology of venous thromboembolism. *Circulation* 2003;107(23 Suppl 1):1-4.
24. Bates SM and Ginsberg JS. Treatment of deep-vein thrombosis. *N Engl J Med* 2004;351:3.
25. Arepally GM and Ortel TL. Heparin-induced thrombocytopenia. *N Engl J Med* 2006;355:8.
26. Eklof B and Rutherford RB. Surgical thrombectomy for acute deep venous thrombosis. In: Rutherford RB (ed) *Vascular Surgery*. 6th ed. Philadelphia, PA: Elsevier Saunders; 2005.
27. Kahn SR, Ginsberg JS. Relationship between deep venous thrombosis and the postthrombotic syndrome. *Arch Intern Med* 2004;164(1):17-26.

Chapter 17

THE EXTREMITIES

Aaron Bransky, MD, Heidi Frankel, MD, and Larry Gentilello, MD

INTRODUCTION

The acute care surgeon may be asked to handle ischemic, infectious, and traumatic lesions of the extremities. In this chapter, we will discuss management of pressure ulceration and compartment syndrome and describe various amputations that may be required for these conditions. Vascular repairs and treatment of necrotizing soft tissue infections will be handled in the chapter on soft tissue infections.

DECUBITUS ULCERS VERSUS PRESSURE ULCERS

Prevention and treatment of decubitus ulcers is far from a new endeavor. Egyptian mummies have been unwrapped revealing pressure ulcerations. The word decubitus comes from the Latin word "decumbere" that means "to lie down." Although the majority of decubitus ulcers develop in a dependent position, it is more appropriate to describe these lesions as pressure ulcerations or sores to account for those that develop while in other positions. Pressure ulcer prevalence rates vary widely, ranging from 10% to 20% in acute care and up to 30% and higher in long-term care.

EPIDEMIOLOGY

Pressure ulceration occurs in patients with some form of physiological derangement. In patients with normal mobility, nutrition, sensation, and mental status, these ulcers are uncommon. Among patients who are neurologically impaired, pressure sores occur with an annual incidence of 5-8%, with lifetime risk estimated to be 25%-85%. Moreover, pressure sores are listed as the direct cause of death in 7-8% of all paraplegics. Two-thirds of pressure sores occur in patients older than 70 years. Pressure ulcers in the elderly result in a five-fold increase in mortality with an in-hospital mortality of 25%-33%. Over 80% of hospitalized patients with pressure ulcers develop them within 5 days of admission, many on the day of operation. Recurrence rates, despite adequate medical and surgical therapy, have been reported as high as 90%.

The Agency for Healthcare Research and Quality (AHRQ) recommends the use of risk-assessment tools for pressure ulcer development. One such tool is the Braden Scale that has six risk factor categories: sensory perception, moisture, activity, mobility, nutrition, and friction and shear. A total score is derived that should trigger interventions to prevent pressure ulcer formation. The score should be frequently reassessed as patient condition changes.

Pressure ulcers form as a result of localized tissue ischemia and malnutrition. A nutritional assessment is crucial for identifying patients at high risk for malnutrition and subsequent pressure ulcer formation. Adequate nutrition high in protein and micronutrients is vital. Other contributory endogenous factors to pressure ulcer formation include hyperglycemia, anemia, and endothelial dysfunction with microvascular disease. Pressure lasting 2 hours exceeding that of the capillary bed pressure (~30 mm Hg) is sufficient to promote ulcer formation. The combination of ischemia and accumulation of toxic metabolites increases the rate of cell death.

The National Pressure Ulcer Advisory Panel was established in 1987 in an effort to assist health care professionals in reducing the incidence and prevalence of pressure ulcers. Staging of pressure ulcers is based on the depth of tissue destruction (Fig. 17-1). Stage 1 ulcerations have minor skin color, whereas Stage 4 ulcerations penetrate the fascia with bone and deep tissue destruction. There is neither a continuous progression from stage 1 to stage 4 nor a regression systematically from stage 4 to stage 1.

Stage 1 pressure ulcers may be protean with subtle changes in skin temperature (warmth or coolness), tissue consistency (firm or boggy feel), or sensation (pain, itching). The ulcer appears as a defined area of persistent redness in lightly pigmented skin, whereas in darker skin tones, the ulcer may appear with persistent red, blue, or purple hues.

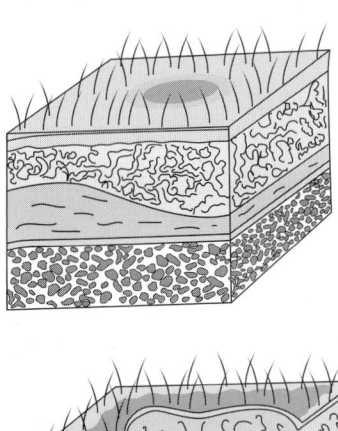

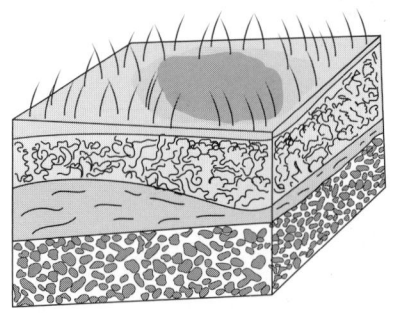

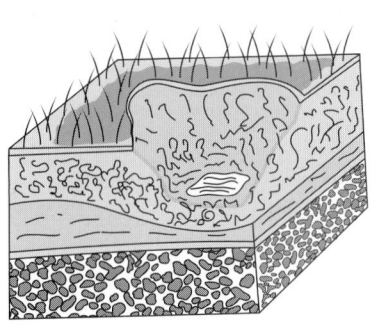

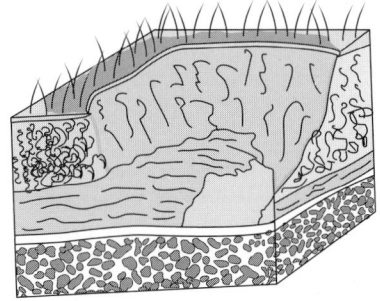

Figure 17-1 *Stages of pressure ulcers. See text for further details.*

Stage 2 ulcers have partial thickness skin loss involving epidermis, dermis, or both. The ulcer is superficial and presents clinically as an abrasion, blister, or shallow crater.

Stage 3 ulcers involve full thickness skin loss involving damage to, or necrosis of, subcutaneous tissue that may extend down to, but not through, underlying fascia. The ulcer presents clinically as a deep crater with or without undermining of adjacent tissue past the edge of the ulceration.

Stage 4 pressure ulcers have full thickness skin loss with extensive destruction, tissue necrosis, or damage to muscle, bone, or supporting structures (eg, tendon, joint, capsule). Undermining and sinus tracts also may be associated with Stage IV pressure ulcers. Although the bone may be involved, any extension beyond fascia is consistent with Stage IV pressure ulceration.

LOCATION

Pressure ulcerations develop in areas of the body that are susceptible to continuous forces necessary to create local tissue ischemia. The most common sites of pressure ulceration in descending order are sacral, trochanteric, and heel ulcerations. However, inappropriately applied or ill-fitting cervical collars may cause chin breakdown. Nasogastric tubes may cause nasal alar necrosis.

TREATMENT

PREVENTION
In order to reduce the pressure on the wound, a variety of techniques can be employed. Frequent repositioning

is the cornerstone of pressure ulceration prevention. Topical barriers include hydrocolloid barriers (DuoDerm) and hydrogels. A variety of contact barriers are available to reduce the pressure on a given site for both mattresses and wheelchairs. The barriers range from foam and gel pillows/overlays to specialty mattresses.

The next level of pressure-relieving therapy is use of low air loss mattresses. Air is pumped into the mattress through air permeable pillows to reduce pressure points and therefore tissue ischemia. Air fluidized therapy beds further reduce pressure. These beds pump air within a mattress containing microspheres of silicon to provide an increased supporting surface while reducing pressure; however, they can increase fluid loss.

The reduction of spasticity may reduce pressure points and allow healing of pressure ulcers. Spasticity may be relieved with diazepam, cyclobenzaprine, baclofen, dantrolene sodium, or dimethothiazine.

MEDICAL TREATMENT
Medical therapy of pressure ulcers is appropriate for the care of Stage 1 and 2 ulcers. Medical debridement can be performed in several ways, including mechanical, chemical, autolytic, and biologic. The method used depends on the urgency, setting, and amount of necrotic tissue present. The exception to this principle may be those with heel pressure ulcers in the presence of critical ischemia where a dry eschar may be maintained in the absence of drainage or obvious infection.

First and foremost, the wound should be kept clean. Some pressure ulcerations, especially sacral and trochanteric, are prone to be soiled with urine and feces. With good hygiene come lower bacterial counts, leading to improved healing. Newer time-release antimicrobial wound dressings such as cadexomer iodine and silver decrease the bioburden of pressure ulcers. The decision to use parenteral antibiotic therapy is indicated for invasive or systemic infection.

Mechanical debridement includes the use of wet-to-dry dressings and hydrotherapy (whirlpool). Both have largely fallen out of favor due to the nonselective nature of debridement and their slow speed. Handheld whirlpool therapy devices, by contrast, have been used more extensively of late. Ultrasound-assisted wound therapy is a variant of this strategy. Whirlpool therapy cleans the wound bed directly, stimulates angiogenesis, and reduces pain at the site of the ulceration. *Chemical debridement* uses enzymes to remove devitalized tissue. This method of debridement is slow and does not harm healthy tissue. *Autolytic topical therapy* uses the body's own enzymes to accomplish debridement. Panafil is an ointment containing urea, papain, and chlorophyllin copper complex sodium that cause *enzymatic debridement*. In 2004, the FDA gave clearance to produce and market medical maggots for *biologic debridement* of pressure ulcers. Maggots feed on necrotic tissue, debriding the wound and leaving the healthy tissue alone. Debridement results from proteolytic digestive enzymes liquefying the necrotic tissue and from the physical action of the mouth hooks on the tissues that pierce and tear the necrotic tissue, allowing the digestive enzymes to reach the depths of the necrotic tissue.

Surgical treatment is appropriate for Stage 3 and 4 ulcers. Sharp debridement is the most efficacious way of removing necrotic tissue quickly.

Coverage after debridement provides the next challenge. The use of negative pressure wound therapy has increased dramatically over the past several years, markedly diminishing the reliance on myocutaneous flaps for coverage. Recurrent pressure ulcers after flap coverage are common, occurring in up to half of all patients, arguing for the more liberal use of negative pressure wound therapy after all necrotic tissue has been removed.

Negative pressure wound therapy by Vacuum-Assisted Closure (VAC Therapy, KCI USA, Inc, San Antonio, TX) was developed at the Wake Forest University School of Medicine and has been available since 1995. This therapy consists of a specialized foam dressing, evacuation tubing, a fluid-collection canister, and a vacuum therapy pump with adjustable settings. Black foam (polyurethane) dressing stimulates granulation tissue whereas white foam (PVA) dressing assists in wound contraction. The latter is helpful for tunneled and undermined wounds and those with underlying structure that need protection (tendon). It causes less pain than the black foam dressing. Negative pressure therapy converts an open wound to a controlled closed system. Depending on the nature of the wound, the pump delivers continuous or intermittent subatmospheric pressures ranging from –50 to –200 mm Hg. Typically, pressure ulcers receive –125 (black foam) to –175 (white foam) mm Hg. This may be lowered if pain is an issue. Application of topical negative pressure removes chronic wound exudates, infectious materials, and assists in the formation of granulation tissue. Average daily closure of pressure ulcers occurs at 0.23 cm compared to 0.09 cm for more traditional therapy. Contraindications to negative pressure wound therapy include chronically malnourished patients, patients in whom a seal cannot be achieved, patients with bleeding disorders, an inadequately prepared wound bed or one with poor circulation, eschar or fibrosis, and very small wounds.

COMPARTMENT SYNDROME

Compartment syndrome is characterized by excessive pressure on the neurovascular bundles and soft tissues occupying a closed space. Excessive pressure results in critical ischemia to muscles, veins, arteries, and nerves. Although this can happen in any closed space including the skull and the abdomen, focus will remain on compartment syndrome in the extremities.

In 1881, Richard von Volkmann published an article describing contractures of the forearm flexor compartment (felt to be associated with tight bandages following supracondylar fracture) leading to arterial insufficiency and poor venous return. It was 25 years before Hildebrand coined the phrase Volkmann's ischemic contracture to describe the endpoint of an untreated ischemia from compartment syndrome.

It is interesting to note that whereas most will think of compartment syndrome in the lower leg (it is most common after tibial fractures with prevalence as high as 10%), the early descriptions by Volkmann and others were almost exclusive to the upper extremity and the forearm in particular.

A variety of different compartment syndromes have been described in the upper and lower extremities. Compartment syndrome has been documented in the shoulder, arm, forearm, hand, buttock, thigh, leg, and foot. Causes of compartment syndrome include open or closed fracture, gunshot wound, crush injury, snakebite, and thermal injury. Further causes include tight dressings, casts, or excessive fluid resuscitation after shock/reperfusion.

PATHOGENESIS

Compartment syndrome develops as a result of a reduction of venous outflow. This can be correlated with local tissue edema directly compressing on venous outflow channels or direct injury to vessels as well. Reperfusion injury after vascular injury also causes tissue edema leading to the development of compartment syndrome. In the case of a fracture, a bleeding long bone and the development of a space occupying hematoma can exacerbate this situation.

DIAGNOSIS

It is of great importance to examine a patient regularly for compartment syndrome in the presence of poly-trauma. Without the ability to verbalize pain, the unconscious patient may be at greater risk for developing an unrecognized compartment syndrome. A complete tertiary examination of patients at risk is required.

There are, however, limited data from which to define the usefulness of clinical findings for the diagnosis of compartment syndrome. Pain on passive stretch may be the most sensitive clinical finding of compartment syndrome. This pain is out of proportion to the suspected injury. However, the clinician should not wait for the development of further signs before establishing the diagnosis of compartment syndrome, as significant ischemia is present once paresthesias and pulselessness are present. Ischemia of underlying structures may occur as quickly as 30 minutes after symptoms present. Irreversible Wallerian degeneration occurs after 8 hours of symptoms.

The critical compartment pressure that mandates surgical intervention is a point of much controversy. Mubarak et al (1997) recommend surgical intervention for compartment pressures greater than 30 mm Hg. This recommendation is based on the fact that normal capillary pressure is 30 mm Hg; thus, any pressure in excess of this value will lead to tissue ischemia. Matsen et al (1980) recommend 45 mm Hg of compartment pressure as a cutoff. This is based on the theory that as compartment pressure increases so must the capillary pressure. They feel that normal physiologic capillary pressure is not representative of the clinical situation of compartment syndrome. McQueen and Court-Brown showed that there is a high correlation with the development of compartment syndrome and a difference between diastolic pressure and compartment pressure of less than 30 mm Hg.

There are four main techniques to measure compartment syndrome: needle manometer, wick catheter, slit catheter, or STIC catheter system. The needle manometer utilizes an 18-gauge needle attached to a three-way stopcock. A saline filled syringe is attached to the stopcock to which a transducer is also attached. The pressure required to infuse the fluid is recorded. A disadvantage of this technique is that it is not suitable for continuous pressure monitoring and it is not as reproducible as other techniques.

Scholander et al developed the wick catheter. It has a piece of polyglycolic acid suture within a piece of polyethylene tubing. It does not rely on continuous infusion. The catheter is introduced into the compartment through a large trocar. Once in place, the

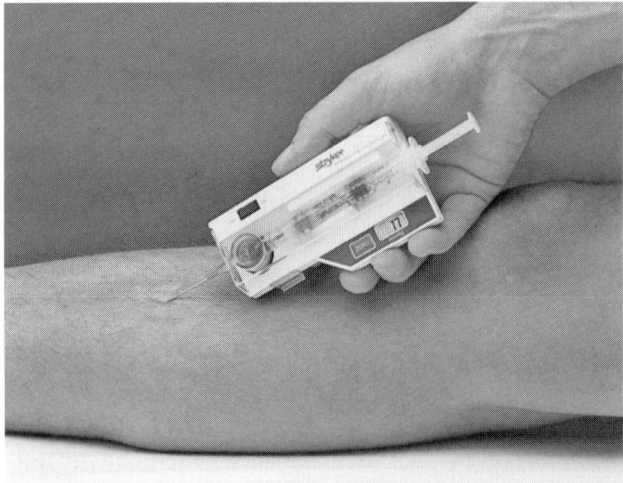

Figure 17-2 *The STIC catheter system by Stryker used to measure intracompartmental pressures.*

catheter is taped in position. It will function well to monitor continuous intracompartmental pressures. Its main disadvantage is that the tip of the catheter may become obstructed with blood clot, rendering it inaccurate. Also, over time, the polyglycolic wick may become hydrolyzed.

The slit catheter technique employs a piece of poly-ethylene tube with five 3 mm slits in the end of the tube. The slit catheter is connected to a three-way stopcock similar to the other techniques. Similar to the wick catheter, it is vital not to let air bubbles into the system, as this will falsely dampen the readings. The catheter is introduced into the muscle of the compartment in question through a 16-gauge needle at an oblique angle. The needle is removed when the catheter is in place.

Stryker manufactures the STIC catheter system (Fig. 17-2). It is a hand-held self-contained pressure monitoring system. The device is very easy to use and is portable. Once the device is charged, the one-time use disposable syringe that is preloaded with fluid is connected to the measuring instrument. At the other end, a disposable needle-catheter is attached. The device is flushed with fluid and zeroed. The needle is then inserted into the compartment in question. The measured compartment pressure is displayed on the device screen.

CHRONIC COMPARTMENT SYNDROME

Compartment syndrome may still develop without an acute fracture or reperfusion injury. In a study by Byrk et al, 3% of all patients that present to sports medicine clinics had chronic exertional compartment syndrome. The patients describe pain or a deep ache in the anterior and/or lateral compartments of the lower leg. Symptoms usually occur simultaneously in both lower extremities and usually occur after sustained exercise.

Chronic exertional compartment syndrome is diagnosed with a resting compartment pressure of greater that 12 mm Hg and pressures after exertion and a one-minute recovery period of greater than 30 mm Hg. One can also see an inability for the compartment pressure to drop below 20 mm Hg after 5 minutes of rest. Treatment is targeted at the cause. Therefore, the patient should use periods of rest and cross training throughout their exercise regime. Furthermore, proper shoe attire, physical therapy, massage therapy, and stretching may all be used. If unsuccessful with less invasive therapy, elective fasciotomy should be considered.

ACUTE COMPARTMENT SYNDROME

Acute compartment syndrome usually follows trauma. The treatment is to decompress the compartment as soon as is feasible. This may simply involve removing circumferential dressings or pneumatic trousers or bivalving casts. More often, surgery is necessary. In order to eliminate a compartment syndrome, all compartments within an anatomical region should be decompressed. For example, in the lower leg, a four-compartment fasciotomy is typically necessary even if only one of the compartments has elevated pressures. After completion of the fasciotomy, many surgeons will staple vessel loops interwoven on the skin to synch the skin closed over the subsequent days as pressures and swelling decrease.

ARM

The arm or brachium is divided into an anterior and posterior compartment. Compartment syndromes of this region are rare. A single longitudinal incision along the length of posterior-medial aspect of the biceps brachii will allow for access into both compartments with adequate decompression (Fig. 17-3A). The basilic vein and medial brachial cutaneous nerves should be identified and preserved if possible.

FOREARM

Compartment syndrome of the forearm is usually associated with a fracture, often involving a crushing injury or a gunshot wound to the forearm. It may also be seen associated with infection, infiltration of fluid, or attempted closure of a tight surgical wound after internal fixation.

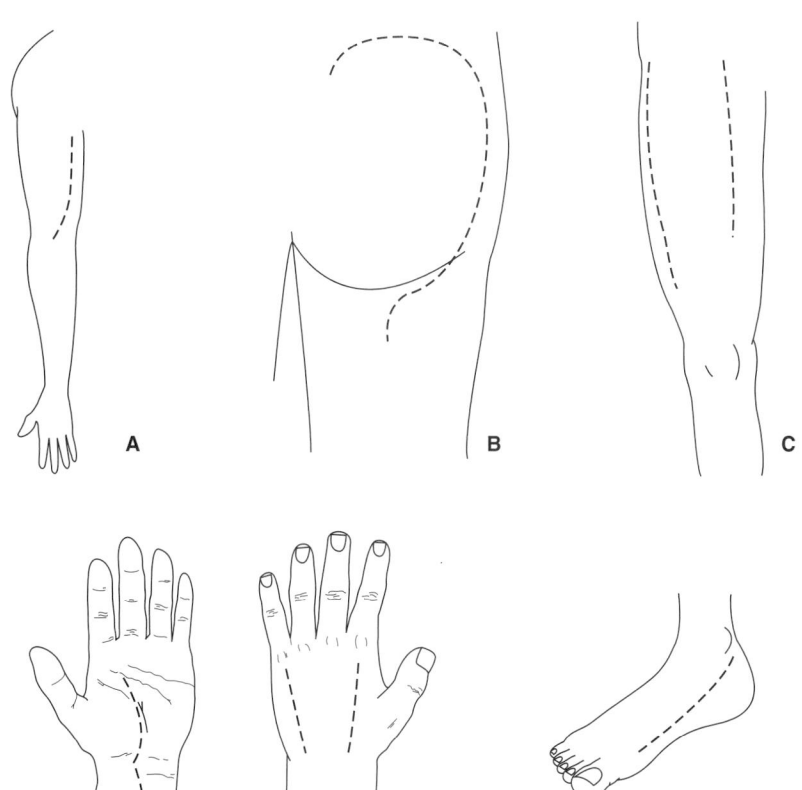

Figure 17-3 *Incisions used for more atypical locations of compartment syndrome. See text for further details. A. Arm. B. Buttock. C. Thigh. D. Hand. E. Foot.*

The forearm is composed of three fascial compartments: superficial flexor, deep flexor, and extensor. In order to completely decompress the forearm, two incisions should be made (Fig. 17-4). A longitudinal incision is first made over the dorsal aspect of the forearm. This dorsal incision should begin at the lateral epicondyle of the humerus and extend to the wrist. The skin and subcutaneous tissues are opened exposing the fascia. The fascia is then incised longitudinally as well for the length of the incision. This will provide access to the extensor compartment and the mobile wad.

The volar incision is carried out slightly differently. Proximally, it starts on the brachial side of the antecubital crease. The crease should be crossed slightly obliquely. An S-shaped incision is continued passing laterally around the common flexor tendon then extending down the volar forearm. The skin incision should extend onto the hand on the medial aspect of the thenar eminence. Attention should be paid to preservation of the palmar branch of the median nerve. Once the skin and subcutaneous tissues are incised, the fascia overlying the superficial compartment is opened. A space can be created between the superficial radial nerve and brachioradialis laterally and the flexor carpi radialis and radial artery medially. This will expose and decompress the deep compartment. Completion of the fasciotomy includes a carpal tunnel release by incising the transcarpal ligament as well as division of the bicipital fascia (lacertus fibrosus) proximally.

BUTTOCK

Compartment syndrome of the gluteal region is relatively rare. Most commonly, it is associated with immobility although it has been described from trauma as well as vascular causes. Three separate nondistensible gluteal compartments exist, ie, (1) the gluteus maximus compartment, enveloped by its own fascia, (2) the gluteus medius-minimus compartment, surrounded by the gluteal fascia and a deep ileal boundary, and (3) the tensor fascia lata, enveloped by the gluteal fascia and the lateral fibrous coverings of the hip. Ultimately, it is the nondistensible gluteal fascia and aponeurosis anchored to the sacrum, coccyx, ilium, and iliotibial tract that confine these three compartments. The inferior gluteal artery and nerve travel out from beneath the inferior border of the pyriformis muscle and over the superior gemellus into the gluteus maximus. The sciatic nerve, posterior femoral cutaneous nerve, pudendal nerve, and nerve to the obturator internus and superior gemellus muscles also arise from beneath the inferior edge of the pyriformis. This location predisposes to compression and loss of function, particularly of the very large sciatic nerve.

A single "question mark" incision over the posterior margin of the iliotibial tract is usually adequate for complete decompression (Fig. 17-3B). This incision is made from the posterior superior iliac spine, approximately 10 cm superolaterally along the iliac crest, then continuing over the greater trochanter to the level of the inferior gluteal fold. The incision is extended medially beneath the buttocks to the midline of the upper thigh and down a few centimeters over the mid-posterior thigh. The superolateral edge of the gluteus maximus is separated from the iliotibial tract, enabling exposure of the underlying muscles while protecting the neurovascular bundles. In particular, the gluteus maximus must be reflected carefully to avoid the superior gluteal artery. Furthermore, the gluteus maximus is reflected medially to expose the gluteus medius.

THIGH

The thigh is divided into three anatomical compartments: anterior, adductor, and posterior. Within the anterior compartment are the rectus femoris, vastus lateralis, vastus medialis, and vastus intermedius muscles. The femoral neurovascular bundle traverses the

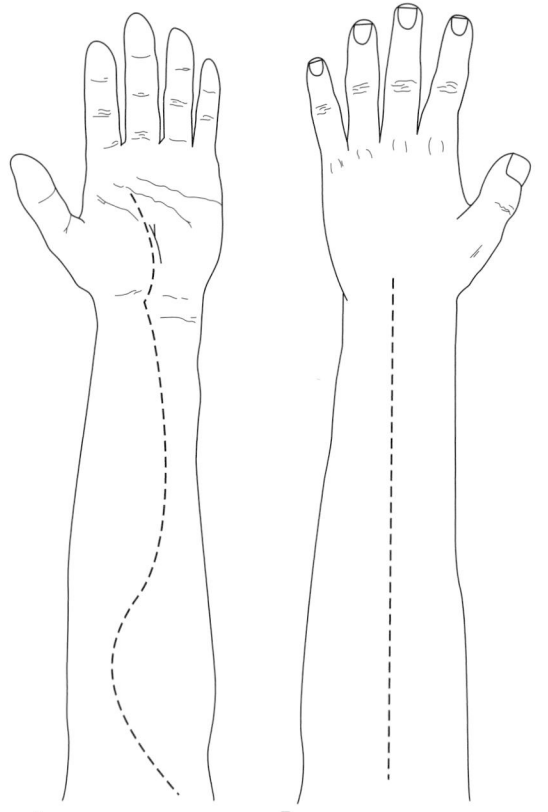

Figure 17-4 *Incisions used in forearm for (suspected) compartment syndrome. A. Extensive opening of fascia of anterior forearm in forearm compartment syndromes. B. Incision used for dorsal forearm compartment syndromes in which skin and underlying fascia are released completely throughout the length of the incision.*

anterior compartment until it passes through the adductor canal and eventually the adductor hiatus to enter the popliteal space. The adductor compartment contains the adductor magnus, adductor longus, adductor brevis, pectineus, and gracilis muscles. It also contains the anterior and posterior division of the obturator nerve as well as the femoral neurovascular bundle. The posterior compartment contains the biceps femoris, semimembranosus, and semitendinosus muscles as well as the sciatic nerve.

There are two main intermuscular septa, medial and lateral. In order to reduce pressures in the thigh, all three compartments need to be opened. This can be done with two generous longitudinal skin incisions (Fig. 17-3C). The anterior and posterior compartments can be reached through an anterior-lateral incision. The incision should be carried down through the iliotibial band. This exposes the anterior compartment. The fascia over the vastus lateralis should be divided. Next the intermuscular septum is divided, opening the posterior compartment. The adductor compartment should be addressed through a longitudinal incision over the anterior-medial thigh.

LEG

A compartment syndrome of the lower leg is the one that surgeons are likely to encounter most frequently. Anatomically, the leg is divided into four fascial compartments: anterior, lateral, superficial posterior, and deep posterior. The three neurovascular bundles reside in the anterior (one) and deep posterior compartments (two neurovascular bundles).

Other than the tibia and fibula, the stiff interosseous membrane, the anterior intermuscular septum dividing the anterior from the lateral compartment, and the transverse intermuscular septum dividing the superficial from the deep posterior compartments bind the compartments. As with any anatomical region, the goal is to fully release all compartments within the anatomic space.

There are three main techniques to accomplish that goal in the lower leg. They include a fibulectomy, a single lateral incision technique, and a two-incision technique. While a fibulectomy would clearly open all four compartments by dividing the interosseous membrane and intermuscular septa, it causes significant morbidity without added benefit. Currently it is only of historical interest and rarely performed at this time. The leg can also be decompressed using a single skin incision with a technique popularized by Matsen et al (1980), called the perifibular fasciotomy. The skin incision extends distally from the fibular head to the ankle along the contour of the fibula.

The most popular technique for decompression of the lower leg is a two-incision four-compartment fasciotomy (Fig. 17-5). The lateral incision extends from the fibular head to the ankle. It is centered over the border of the anterior and lateral compartments. The skin and subcutaneous tissues are separated from the overlying fascia. Care must be taken to identify and preserve the superficial peroneal nerve. Next, a fasciotomy of the fascia overlying the anterior compartment 1 cm anterior to the intermuscular septum is performed followed by a fasciotomy 1 cm posterior to the intermuscular septum on the fascia overlying the lateral compartment. The fasciotomies should be generous, extending

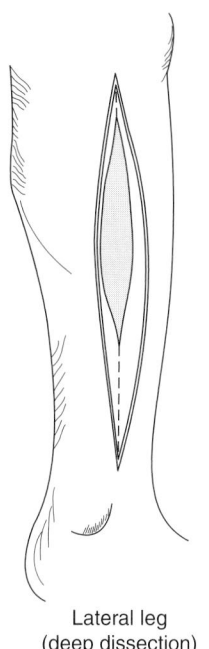

Lateral leg
(deep dissection)

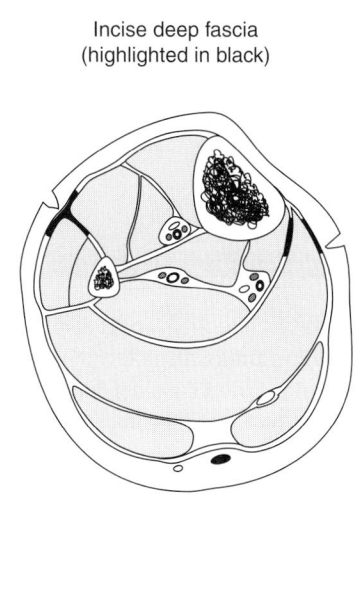

Incise deep fascia
(highlighted in black)

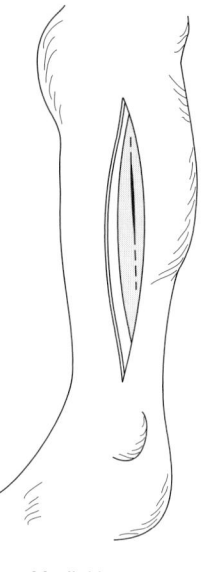

Medial leg
(deep dissection)

Figure 17-5 *Illustration showing the cross-section of the leg as well as the medial and lateral views of the superficial and deep dissections for a two-incision fasciotomy.*

the length of the skin incision. A medial incision is fashioned approximately 2 cm posterior to the posterior-medial border of the tibia. The greater saphenous vein along with the saphenous nerve should be identified and preserved. A fasciotomy should be performed along the full length of the compartment. The soleal bridge should be removed from the posterior tibia for adequate exposure to the deep posterior compartment.

FOOT/HAND

Both the hand and the foot are rare locations for compartment syndrome and they are treated very similarly. Diagnostically, pain on passive stretch is a much more reliable sign of compartment syndrome in the hand than it is in the foot. The most common compartment involved in compartment syndrome of the hands or feet are the interossei. Dorsal longitudinal incisions can be made over the interossei to decompress these compartments (Fig. 17-3D). In the foot the medial, central, and lateral compartments must also be opened. This can be accomplished with a medial incision to expose the deep flexor muscles (Fig. 17-3E).

POSTOPERATIVE CARE

After completion of a fasciotomy, careful follow-up is required (Fig. 17-6). The surgeon should consider return to the OR at 48 hours to debride any devitalized tissue. Additionally, it is usually at this point that the skin can begin to be reapproximated. At the time of operation, many surgeons will place vessel loops interlaced through skin staples at the skin edge. Over subsequent days, an attempt is made to close the wound. For those wounds that ultimately do not close, a split thickness skin graft should be used.

Attention need also be directed to diagnosing rhabdomyolysis and preventing resultant renal failure. Delayed recognition of compartment syndrome may result in significant cell death with markedly elevated CPKs. Involvement of large muscle groups or occurrence in small patients or those with volume deficits may pose an increased risk for the development of myoglobinuric renal failure. Adequate volume resuscitation is key to prevention of renal compromise; the added role of alkalinization of the urine is controversial.

AMPUTATIONS

Approximately 60,000 amputations are performed annually in the United States. In the context of a comprehensive acute care surgery service, the trauma

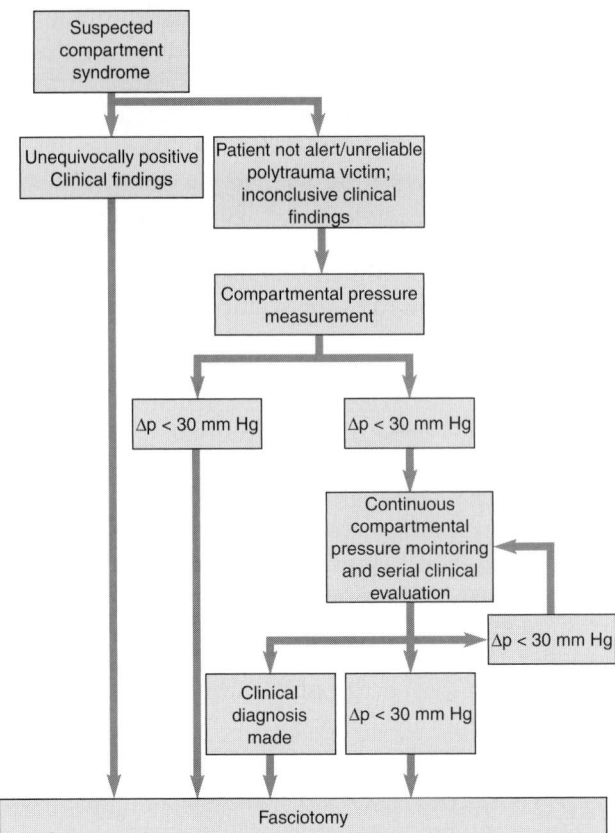

Figure 17-6 *An algorithm for management for a patient with suspected compartment syndrome. Δp is defined as the difference between the diastolic pressure and the measured compartment pressure in mm Hg as documented by McQueen and Court-Brown.*

surgeon may be asked to perform amputations on patients with vascular disease and gangrene, diabetes, and infections in addition to those in injured patients. Ninety percent of amputations occur for ischemia or infected gangrene; 70% are related to diabetes complications. Mortality for all lower limb amputations is around 10%, most commonly due to associated cardiovascular disease.

BASIC PRINCIPLES OF THERAPY

Several basic principles apply to amputations of all levels. The maximum length of bone possible should be maintained. The skin length should be maximized to allow for a tension free closure over the wound. Named arteries and veins should be individually isolated and ligated. Tying vessels together may contribute to the development of arteriovenous fistulae. Nerves are transected under tension to allow for retraction of the severed end. This will lessen associated pain when the cut nerve end comes to rest within an amputation stump.

DETERMINATION OF AMPUTATION LEVEL

It can be difficult to determine the proper level of amputation in the face of ischemia. Clinical assessment is the most accurate way to determine the level of amputation. Angiography is helpful in patients with peripheral vascular disease. Although it is impossible to determine that an amputation level is appropriate purely by looking at an angiographic image, it is reasonable to use it as an adjunct to help determine surgical level of resection. A surface electrode monitoring system may be placed to establish the oxygen tension of the subcutaneous tissue ($TcpO_2$). If the Tcp_{O2} less than 20 mm Hg, healing is unlikely. If the Tcp_{O2} is >40 mm Hg this represents a level that will likely heal well. Blood pressure by Doppler may also be used to assess for healing potential. A Doppler systolic blood pressure greater than 60 is preferred to assume an incision that will heal. Xenon 133 clearance is another adjunct to help determine amputation level. The Xenon is injected transdermally and the clearance is calculated. The most distal site followed by more proximal potential amputation levels is checked until a capillary skin blood flow rate greater than or equal to 2.6 mL/min/100 g of tissue is found. A level greater than 2.4 ml/min/100 g of tissue has as much as 95% sensitivity.

TOE AMPUTATION

Toes are amputated for gangrene, infection, neuropathic ulcers that fail to heal, and osteomyelitis of the distal or middle phalanx. Toes with dry gangrene may auto-amputate. A circular skin incision is made at the base of the digit to perform a transphalangeal amputation. Dorsal and plantar skin flaps may either be of equal length or the plantar flap may be longer. Hemostatis is usually easily obtained either through electrocautery or direct ligation of the digital vessels. The wound is left open and packed loosely with moist to dry dressing sponges. Contraindications to toe amputations include osteomyelitis of the metatarsal heads, dependent rubor, and forefoot ischemia. Ray amputation removes the phalanx and the metatarsal head of the contiguous digit (Fig. 17-7A). A longitudinal incision is made at the dorsum of the shaft of the metatarsal head. A circular incision is made distally on the phalanx. Multiple transphalangeal amputations are functionally well tolerated. If, however, ray amputation of the great toe or more than one small toe is required, it may be preferable to perform a transmetatarsal amputation.

TRANSMETATARSAL AMPUTATION

The next level of amputation is the transmetatarsal amputation or TMA (Fig. 17-7B). This amputation is appropriate for a patient with a palpable pulse in the foot or functional infrainguinal bypass. It is

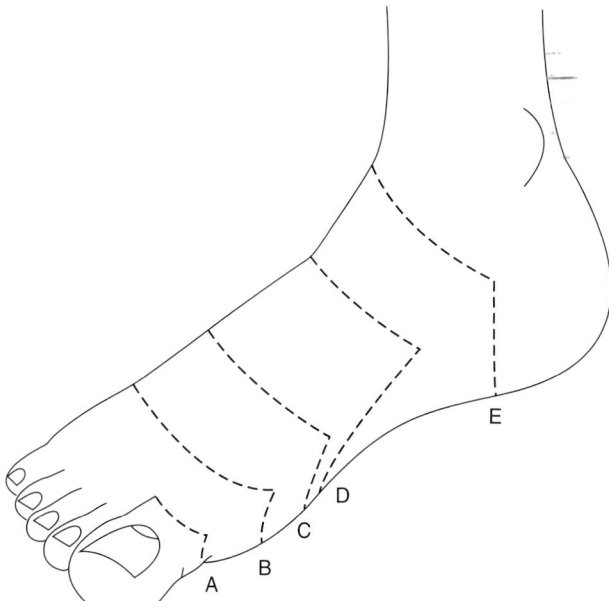

Figure 17-7 *A. Ray amputation. B. Transmetatarsal amputation C. Lisfranc amputation. D. Chopart amputation. E. Syme's amputation. See text for further details.*

contraindicated with a preexisting foot drop. The skin incision uses a long plantar flap to afford wound closure. The individual digital vessels are located and ligated. The digital nerves are separated, placed under tension, and divided. The metatarsals are stripped of their periosteum using a periosteal elevator. The bones are divided using a power saw or a manual saw. The wound is closed in two layers using interrupted sutures. The first layer approximates the fascia with the skin closure being the second layer. A Lisfranc or Chopart amputation can be used when the forefoot ischemia extends slightly more proximally (Fig. 17-7C, 17-7D). The dorsal skin incision is made over the tarsal-metatarsal junction and the plantar incision is made parallel to but just proximal to the metatarsal heads. The bone incision is made at a 45° angle through the cuboid and cuneiform bones.

Syme's amputation is a modified ankle disarticulation with removal of the calcaneus (Fig. 17-7E). The blood supply to this amputation is via the posterior tibial vessels. It may be used in ischemia but is most often used in traumatic foot crush injury. It should not be used with spreading foot infections or in the face of neuropathy resulting in loss of heel sensation. The procedure can be performed in a two stage or a single stage technique. Many authors advocate the single stage method thereby resecting the distal malleoli followed by forward rotation of the heal pad with closure. Because bony union is not an issue, ambulation can be initiated within 4 weeks of the procedure.

Below knee amputation is a common procedure (Fig. 17-8). The length of the amputation is critical for a proper fitting and functioning prosthesis. A minimum

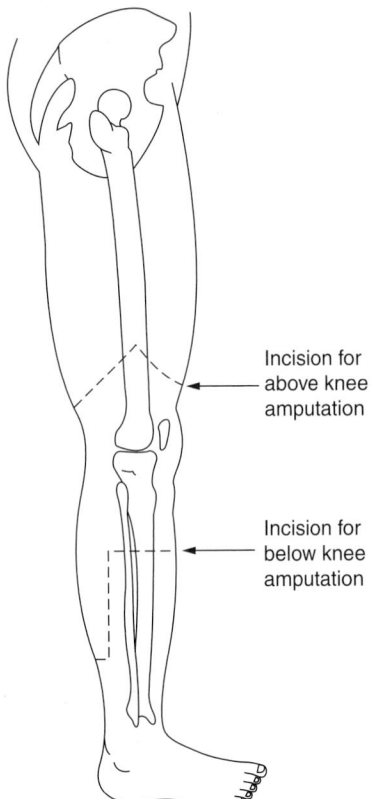

Incision for
above knee
amputation

Incision for
below knee
amputation

Figure 17-8 *The levels and relative shape of the incisions used for above knee amputation as well as below knee amputation.*

of 7 cm of tibial length is necessary for a proper amputation. A more appropriate amputation will be 10-12 cm below the tibial tuberosity. A tourniquet may be inflated to 250 mm Hg (or higher in diabetics with calcified vessels). Two-thirds of the circumference is used to make a horizontal incision over the anterior and lateral portions of the leg. The remaining one-third is used for the myocutaneous flap. The flap should extend for a distance no less than one-third the circumference. The three neurovascular bundles are individually identified. The artery and vein of each bundle are individually ligated. The tibia is then divided in the location described previously after elevating the periosteum circumferentially. The anterior surface of the tibia should be beveled at a 60° angle. The fibular length should be slightly shorter than the tibia. All rough edges should be excised and a bone rasp should be used to smooth the contour of the bone.

The wound is closed in two layers using interrupted suture. The wound is dressed with generous gauze padding and most authors will suggest a posterior cast or splint to prevent flexion contractures. At approximately 6 weeks, the amputation is ready for a prosthesis. The presence of a below knee amputation increases energy expenditure by 40-60% over baseline.

In the event of an uncontrolled infection a need for nondefinitive amputation arises. A guillotine amputation should be performed at the lowest level possible (usually 2-3 cm proximal to the malleoli). After several days of aggressive wound care, a definitive below knee amputation can be performed.

ABOVE KNEE AMPUTATION

When a below knee amputation is not possible secondary to ischemia or infection, an above knee amputation is performed (Fig. 17-8). Length of the femoral shaft is critical to proper postoperative function. Longer femoral shafts result in lower energy expenditure secondary to a longer lever arm to distribute force. Unlike the below knee amputation, the skin incisions are symmetric anteriorly and posteriorly in an above knee amputation. A tourniquet may be used. A "fish mouth" incision is made. The greater saphenous vein, femoral artery and femoral vein are suture-ligated. The tissue over the femur is removed proximally using a periosteal elevator. The femur is divided using a power saw or manual saw. At this point, it is helpful to place a "bump" of towels under the extremity to flex the soft tissue posterior to the femur. The sciatic nerve is isolated, placed under tension and divided. This allows it to retract into the soft tissues. The remainder of the soft tissues is divided. The tourniquet is released and additional hemostasis is obtained. The wound is dressed with gauze fluff followed by an elastic stocking or compressive bandage.

Hip disarticulation may be used in the face of sarcomas, trauma, or infections. The surgical technique is similar to the above knee amputation in that a fish mouth incision is placed at the level of the base of the femoral triangle. The femoral vessels are isolated and suture ligated. The medial and lateral thigh musculature is transected above the level of the greater trochanter. The adductor attachments of the muscles are removed from their origin along the ischium and pubic rami. The hip is then flexed to make the posterior incision. The sciatic nerve is placed under tension and divided high. The superior and inferior gluteal vessels are individually ligated and divided. The joint capsule is entered and the ligamentous attachments are divided. After assuring hemostasis, the wound is closed in two layers using interrupted sutures.

Complications associated with amputations include wound breakdown, infection, joint contracture, swelling, pain, and phantom limb sensation. Additionally, there is a deep venous thrombosis and pulmonary embolism risk of approximately 15% and 2%, respectively. Small areas of wound breakdown may be treated with moist to dry dressings. Larger areas may require flap coverage or revision of the amputation. Postoperative edema or swelling is common. Prior to prosthesis, swelling may be associated with a tight proximal surgical dressing. This can lead to venous congestion and swelling. Joint contracture can be avoided with a splint while in the acute healing phase followed by range of motion exercises. Phantom pain, or the sensation that an amputated portion of the body is still present, is common complication of amputations. The cause for phantom pain is multifactorial. A neuroma may develop in the cut end of a nerve that tethers to the amputation skin. Furthermore, if the neurovascular bundle is taken and ligated *en masse*, the pulsations from arterial blood flow on the nerve is thought to act in a similar fashion. If phantom pain persists, medications including gabapentin are used with mixed results. Sympathectomy may be necessary to minimize or eliminate the sensation.

AFTERCARE OF THE AMPUTATION PATIENT

An amputation is a life-altering procedure. Physical and occupational therapy are the cornerstones of care. Adaptation to balance, transfers, locomotion, as well as psychological adjustments are required. Clearly a multifactorial, multiple team approach is necessary to achieve the best outcome in these patients.

SUGGESTED READINGS

Asgari M, Spinelli H. The vessel loop shoelace technique for closure of fasciotomy wounds. *Ann Plast Surg* 2000;44:225.

Bleicher RJ, Sherman HF, Latenser BA. Bilateral gluteal compartment syndrome. *J Trauma* 1997;42:115-122.

Braden BJ, Maklebust J. Preventing pressure ulcers with the Braden scale: An update on this easy-to-use tool that assesses a patient's risk. *Am J Nurs* 2005;105:70-72.

Chang BB, Jacobs RL, Darling RC III, et al. Foot amputations. *Surg Clin North Am* 1995;75:773-782.

Gupta S, Baharestani M, Bararoski S, et al. Guidelines for managing pressure ulcers with negative pressure wound therapy. *Advances in Skin and Wound Care* 2004;17:1-16.

K C Young, Railton R, Harrower ADB, and Brookes RW, "Transcutaneous oxygen tension measurements as a method of assessing peripheral vascular decease" *Clin Phys Physiol Meas* 1981;2:147-152.

Klitzman BKC, Glasofer SL, et al. Pressure ulcers and pressure relief surfaces. *Clin Plast Surg* 1998;25(3):443-450.

Lee B, Brancato RF, Park IH, Shaw WW. Management of compartmental syndrome: Diagnosis and surgical considerations. *Am J Surg* 1984;148:383.

Matsen FA III, Winquist RA, Krugmire RB. Diagnosis and management of compartmental syndromes. *J Bone Joint Surg Am* 1980;62:286.

McQueen MM, Court-Brown CM. Compartment monitoring in tibial fractures. *J Bone Joint Surg Br* 1996;78:99.

Mittal R, Gupta V. Compartment syndrome of the thigh and the role of skin scars: case report and review of the literature. *J Trauma* 1998;45:395-6.

Moed BTK. Measurement of intracompartmental pressure: A comparison of the slit catheter, side-ported needle, and simple needle. *J Bone Joint Surg Am* 1993;75:231.

Mubarak SJ, Owen CA. Double-incision fasciotomy of the leg for decompression in compartment syndromes. *J Bone Joint Surg Am* 1997;59A:184-187.

Niezgoda JA, Mendez-Eastman S. The effective management of pressure ulcers. *Advances in Skin and Wound Care* 2006;19:3-15.

Pandian GKK. Daily functioning of patients with an amputated lower extremity. *Clin Orthop* 1999;361:91-97.

Panel NPUA. Pressure ulcers prevalence, cost and risk assessment: Consensus development conference statement. *Decubitus* 1989;2:24-28.

Pedowitz RA, Hargens RA, Mubarak SJ. Modified criteria for the objective diagnosis of chronic compartment syndrome of the leg. *Am J Sports Med* 1990;18(1):35-40.

Sørensen J. Surgical treatment of pressure ulcers. *Am J Surg* 2004;188(1A Suppl):42-51.

Stal S, Serure A, Donovan W, et al. The perioperative management of the patient with pressure sores. *Ann Plast Surg* 1983;11:347-356.

Ulmer T. The clinical diagnosis of compartment syndrome of the lower leg: Are clinical findings predictive of the disorder? *J Orth Trauma* 2002;16:572-577.

Waters RL, PJ, Antonelli D, Hislop H. Energy cost of walking of amputees: The influence of level of amputation. *J Bone Joint Surg Am* 1976;58(1):42-46.

Chapter 18

PEDIATRIC SURGERY

Nikunj K. Chokshi, MD, and Henri R. Ford, MD, and Jeffrey S. Upperman, MD

INTRODUCTION

BRIEF HISTORY

Pediatric surgery is a relatively new subspecialty of general surgery. As late as the 1950s, the fathers of contemporary pediatric surgery still operated on more adult than pediatric patients. In 1937, the first Pediatric Surgery training program was started at the Boston Children's Hospital, under the leadership of Dr William E. Ladd. His dedication to the training of surgeons specializing in pediatric surgery attracted surgeons from all over the globe, and included notable pediatric surgeons such as Robert E. Gross, Jesus Lozoya-Solis, and Orvar Swenson. Dr Gross succeeded Ladd as Chief at Boston Children's in 1945, and continued his legacy of teaching. Over the next 23 years, he would train 69 pediatric surgeons. Today, two-thirds of all pediatric surgeons can trace an educational line of descent from Dr Ladd.[1] There are currently 35 accredited Pediatric Surgery training programs in the United States, and approximately 995 American Board of Surgery certified pediatric surgeons. The American Pediatric Surgery Association has 940 members, 282 of them being senior members.

Why do we need pediatric surgery as its own separate specialty? Initially, there was substantial resistance to this development. The American College of Surgeons refused to recognize pediatric surgery as a specialty originally, believing it would lead to the further fragmentation of general surgery. It was not until 1966, when an oversight committee was formed from the Surgical Section of the American Academy of Pediatrics (AAP), that Pediatric Surgery gained credibility. In 1972 following the AAP's adoption of internal oversight, the American Board of Surgery and the Residency Review Committee were approached, and pediatric surgery was recognized with its own certificate.[2]

ROLE OF THE PEDIATRIC SURGEON

Pediatric surgeons treat patients with a broad disease spectrum that not only vary in age, but also in developmental physiology and pathophysiology. Pediatric surgeons treat fetuses still in the womb, and young adults who continue to have issues related to childhood diseases. Pediatricians, pediatric intensivists, and neonatologists consult pediatric surgeons. Pediatric surgeons are trained to diagnose and treat infants and children afflicted with disease processes that can occur in vastly different clinical settings.[3]

The pediatric surgeon may also function as a trauma surgeon. Trauma is the most common cause of death and morbidity in children between the ages of 1 and 14 years old; intentional and unintentional injury accounts for over 50% of all childhood deaths.[4] Although childhood trauma is largely nonoperative in nature, the assessment and management of pediatric trauma patients still requires attention to detail and dedicated resources.

PEDIATRIC PHYSIOLOGY

Pediatric surgical care requires a unique fund of knowledge. Children are not little adults, and the pediatric physiology and psyche undergoes significant change from birth to adulthood. The first year of life is very dynamic. The neonate is undergoing rapid physiological change as they adapt from fetal to extrauterine life. In addition, neonates and infants have a physiology that is geared toward anabolic growth. The metabolic demands of growth supersede all other physiological demands.

In the following section, we review basic pediatric physiological concepts with particular attention to the neonate and young child. A fundamental understanding of pediatric physiology provides a foundation for discussing pediatric surgical diseases.

FLUID COMPARTMENTS

At term, the neonate's total body water (TBW) is 75% of body mass (BM). The TBW is increased if the infant is premature. For example, a 32-week gestational age neonate has a TBW of 80%. A newborn has a surplus of TBW, which diureses over the first few days of life. The percentage TBW falls rapidly during the first week of

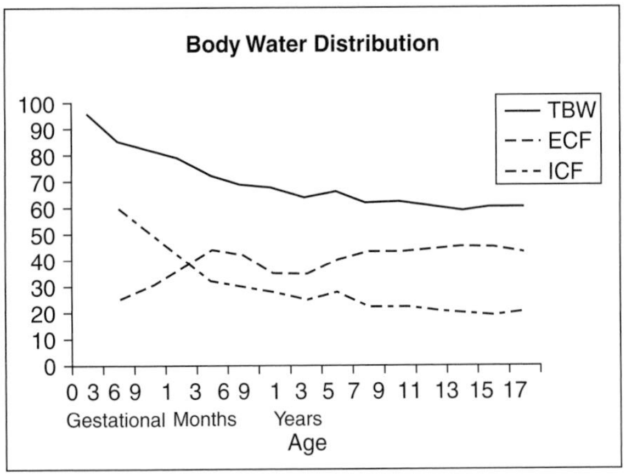

Figure 18-1 *Age-based changes in body water composition. Total body water (TBW), extracellular fluid (ECF), and intracellular fluid (ICF) change in relation to body mass over the course of gestation and into childhood. Data from Friis-Hansen B. Changes in body water compartments during growth.* Acta Pediatr Suppl *1957;46[suppl]:110.*

life, and then it decreases more gradually for the remainder of the first year, approaching 65% of BM. During childhood the TBW continues to trend down, approaching 60% by adolescence (similar to an adult). See Fig. 18-1.

The extracellular compartment makes up a higher percentage of TBW in the neonate. At birth, both the intracellular and extracellular compartments are approximately 40% of BM. The extracellular compartment is reduced during postnatal diuresis, and over the first year of life as adipose tissue and muscle are laid down, it decreases further to approximately 25% of BM. The intracellular compartment rises over this time, to approximately 45% of BM.

Intravascular volume is approximately 25% of the extracellular compartment; in the newborn this equates to about 90 ml/kg. The intravascular volume increases with prematurity, and decreases as the infant ages. In school-aged children, intravascular volume can be estimated as 75 ml/kg, and in adolescents 65 ml/kg. Intravascular fluid volume, as a percentage of total body weight, is lower in obese children.

MAINTENANCE FLUID

Early Developmental Fluid Changes

During the first day of life, neonates have low urine output regardless of fluid status; it is often less than 1 cc/kg per hour. Subsequently urine output increases during days 2 and 3, when they may produce as much as 5 cc/kg/hour. The increase in urine output is due to the mobilization of extracellular fluid stores. By day four, urine output is a relatively accurate reflection of volume status, if it is correctly measured.[5] In children less than 2 years of age, the kidneys differ in their relative abilities to excrete and conserve water and solute compared to older children and adults. Infants less than 2 years old do not concentrate urine well, and hence they have a low tolerance for dehydration.

Fluid Loss

Given the developmental changes and inability to conserve fluids in infants and young children, it is important to account for fluid loss when determining fluid needs. Similar to adults, obligate fluid losses include water lost in urine production, gastrointestinal losses, skin and respiratory tract losses, and water consumed in anabolic metabolism. Maintenance fluid replacement includes fluid and nutrient losses due to these processes. In children, in order to calculate the correct fluid needs, one must utilize a weight-based algorithm (see Table 18-1). Just as in adults, one must remember to account for any increases in obligate losses, because in these cases fluid requirements are increased. For example, a premature infant with nonkeratinized skin may have a higher transepithelial fluid loss, and therefore require higher maintenance fluid volumes.

Electrolyte Requirements

Nutrient requirements are also calculated by weight. The sodium requirements are 2-3 mEq/kg per day. Premature infants should get slightly more as they are

Table 18-1 Fluid Requirements		
	Fluids (cc/kg/day)	Fluids (cc/kg/hr)
Newborn		
< 1 day old	70	3
2 days old	80	3.5
3 days and older	100-150	4-6
Child		
0-10 kg	100	4
11-20 kg	First 10 kg = 1000 cc + 50 cc/kg thereafter	First 10 kg = 40 cc + 2 cc/kg thereafter
> 20 kg	First 20 kg = 1500 cc + 25 cc/kg thereafter	First 20 kg = 60 cc + 1 cc/kg thereafter

not able to conserve sodium. Potassium should be started after 48 hours of life, with a goal of 1-2 mEq/kg per day. In newborns, a 1/4 normal saline solution is appropriate. In premature infants unable to conserve sodium, 1/2 normal saline may be needed. The clinician must monitor serum electrolytes while newborns are receiving intravenous fluid.

Intravenous Fluids

Infants unable to feed will develop hypoglycemia. At birth, an infant's blood sugar is 70%-80% of the mothers'. Facilitative diffusion across the placenta maintains the glucose level throughout pregnancy. Once separated from the placenta, an infant can maintain blood glucose levels for 2 to 3 hours. However, hypoglycemia counter-regulatory mechanisms (ketogenesis and gluconeogenesis) are developmentally immature at birth. Enteral feeding may stimulate the pathways involved in ketogenesis. Hepatic gluconeogenesis is compromised by peripartum or neonatal stress. For these reasons, all intravenous fluids for infants should contain dextrose. During the first month of life, 10% dextrose in 1/4 normal saline is the intravenous fluid of choice. After 1 month, infants tolerate 5% dextrose solutions. After the second year of life, it is appropriate to use 5% dextrose in 1/2 normal saline, because their renal function is now similar to adults in the ability to excrete salt and conserve water. Even older children should receive dextrose in their maintenance fluids, especially when acutely ill, because they do not have adult level hepatic glycogen stores.[6]

METABOLISM

The demands of a high growth rate in the neonatal period translate to a high resting energy expenditure and basal metabolic rate. The infant's caloric need decreases over the course of the first year, and during childhood. The caloric needs settle at adult levels during the teenage years when growth is complete. Age-dependent caloric needs are important considerations when providing nutrition to pediatric surgical patients. In addition to the demands of growth, the added stress of surgery and the disease process itself must be calculated.

It is important to start nutrition early in the newborn. The fetus is exposed to a constant energy source, as discussed in the previous section. At delivery placental support is terminated and the neonate quickly becomes hypoglycemic. Relying on glycogenolysis, the neonate maintains blood glucose levels for 2-3 h before hepatic glycogen stores are depleted. If an outside source of glucose is not provided, the neonate can activate the gluconeogenesis pathways by utilizing adipose and muscle. These stores are limited, and quickly depleted. In the premature infant, who is more vulnerable to hypoglycemia as compared to the full-term newborn, the substrate stores are decreased. The time tolerated before the onset of hypoglycemia after birth is inversely related to the degree of prematurity, and in extreme prematurity administration must be within minutes rather than hours.

Table 18-2	Caloric needs by age and weight
Age	Caloric need (Kcal/kg/day)
0-1 year	90-120
1-7 years	75-90
7-12 years	60-75
12-18 years	30-60

The metabolic requirements are calculated by age, or are simplified to a weight-based calculation (see Table 18-2). Enteral feeding is always the goal in supporting newborns. When enteral feeding is not an option, the parenteral route is a valid means of providing nutritional support.

The calculations discussed in Table 18-2 provide baseline nutritional needs in an unstressed child. Stressed children have higher caloric needs. This may be due to energy needs for wound healing, burn injury-associated metabolism, or sepsis. In children, the increased caloric needs can be significant, approaching 50%-100% in patients with severe burns. Infants and neonates devote approximately 30%-40% of their caloric intake to growth and development. But in stress states, much of the infant's anabolic machinery shuts down, and the baby is in a catabolic state.[6] The calories that would be used for growth are diverted as the child deals with the stress state. The resting energy expenditure (REE) of infants does not increase during low stress states (routine post operative care), and these children do not have an increase in nutritional requirements.[7] In cases of sepsis however, the REE can increase 40%-70%, and thus increased nutrition must be provided.[8] It is best to follow trends in weight gain and head circumference to ensure adequate nutrition in premature and full-term infants.

METABOLIC SUBSTRATES

The metabolic substrate requirements for children are similar to adults. Children need diets consisting of 50% carbohydrates, 35% fat, and 15% protein. Carbohydrates and fats are the main sources of energy substrates, whereas amino acids are used for protein synthesis. The protein requirement in children decreases with age. In premature infants, the protein requirement is 3-4 g/kg per day, in full-term neonates 1 1/2 to 3 g/kg per day, and in older children 1-1 1/2 g/kg per day. All standard formulas contain a balance of amino acids, including the eight essential amino acids. Glutamine is added, as it is a necessary substrate for certain cells, including enterocytes.

PEDIATRIC SURGICAL DISEASES

Emergency pediatric surgical diseases are due to congenital and acquired conditions that vary according to age. At birth, surgical conditions include congenital diaphragmatic hernia, tracheo-esophageal fistula, intestinal atresia, and abdominal wall defects. Although usually requiring urgent management, they do not always require emergency surgery. Conditions, such as midgut volvulus and severe necrotizing enterocolitis, present commonly during the first month of life and may require immediate operations. Other surgical ailments occur more commonly in infants. For instance, infants with pyloric stenosis present from 2 weeks to 2 months of age and require urgent operations after resuscitation. During the first year of life, inguinal hernias are common and incarcerated inguinal hernias are surgical emergencies because of intestinal obstruction and possible bowel loss. Intussusception occurs commonly from 6 months to 3 years old. If radiographic-guided reduction fails to reduce the intussusception, these patients require urgent surgery. In older children, the incidence of appendicitis increases, as does the risk of symptomatic Meckel diverticulum or foreign body aspiration. In the following sections, we will discuss selected pediatric surgical emergencies, beginning with neonates and continuing into the pediatric age group.

NEONATAL SURGICAL EMERGENCIES

OMPHALOCELE AND GASTROSCHISIS
Epidemiology
The overall incidence of abdominal wall defects is approximately 0.4-3 per 10,000. The incidence rate for infants with omphaloceles is 1.5-3 per 10,000 and over the last several decades this incidence remains stable. However, the incidence for gastroschisis is about 0.4-3 per 10,000 but recent trends suggest that the incidence is increasing. There appears to be different risk factors for these abdominal wall defects. For instance,

gastroschisis appears to be associated with maternal age less than 20 years old, whereas omphalocele appears to occur in mothers greater than 30 years old. Gastroschisis is not commonly associated with other anomalies (between 10% and 20%, most commonly intestinal atresia), whereas omphalocele is more often associated with anomalies (between 50%-70%). Omphalocele-associated anomalies include anomalies of the intestinal tract, genitourinary system, bone structure, and the cardiopulmonary system. Cardiac anomalies occur in 30%-50% of infants with omphalocele and the heart anomalies are typically the most clinically significant abnormalities. In severe cases, such as those with ectopia cordis or pentalogy of Cantrell, the mortality rate is high.[9]

Pathophysiology
In normal development, the midgut elongates within the yolk sac, outside the coelomic cavity. During the 10th and 11th week of gestation, the midgut returns to the coelomic cavity, completing rotation and then beginning fixation. The aforementioned process occurs in conjunction with fusion of the cranial, caudal, and two lateral embryonic anterior body folds. Omphalocele and gastroschisis have distinct anatomical patterns based on failures at different points in normal intestinal development.

The omphalocele is a midline abdominal wall defect caused by a failure in the anterior abdominal wall closure process. Specifically, when the body folds fail to grow and fuse and the intestine fails to return to the body cavity, this results in omphalocele formation. Infants with omphaloceles have herniated bowel covered by a complex translucent membrane that consists of peritoneum on the internal surface, amnion on the external surface, and mesenchymal tissue, also known as Wharton jelly, in between these layers (see Fig. 18-2). This covering provides a valuable biological dressing;

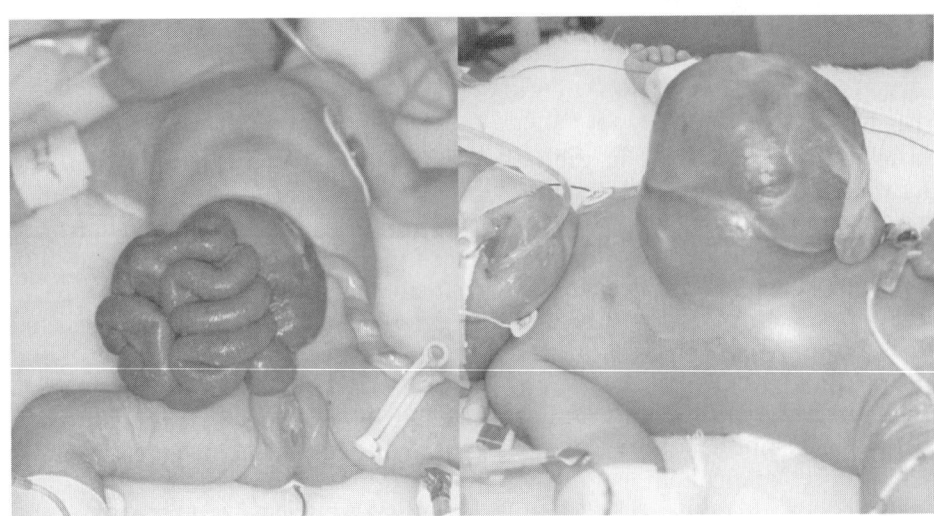

Figure 18-2 *Gastroschisis pictured on the left, with intestine herniating lateral to the umbilicus. Omphalocele pictured on the right, with an intact sac and eccentric umbilical cord.*

therefore, it is important not to rupture the membrane. Finally, the umbilical vessels attach to the membranous sac (apically or eccentrically), not to the body wall itself.

The gastroschisis anomaly derives from a different failed developmental mechanism, but the process is not completely understood. Normally, there are two umbilical veins in the developing fetus that are positioned on each side of the umbilicus. When the right umbilical vein is unexpectedly resorbed, some believe this area becomes ischemic and weak, leading to a site for potential herniation. If the thin hernia sac ruptures, gastroschisis may occur. Many believe that the herniated bowel passes to the right of the umbilicus through the ruptured hernia sac defect caused by ischemic insult. Finally, the herniated bowel is exposed to amniotic fluid because a membrane does not cover it. The exposed bowel undergoes inflammatory changes and these bowel loops may form adhesions.

Treatment

At birth, the initial goals of care are resuscitation and protection of the exposed viscera. Intubation should be considered if there is a prolonged transfer time, or if there is any question regarding the infant's cardiopulmonary status. There is increased insensible fluid loss due to exposed bowel in infants with gastroschisis or a ruptured omphalocele. Increased losses require increased intravascular replacement fluids. These neonates may need between 150-200 cc/kg/day in intravenous fluids. Clinicians should use an orogastric tube to decompress the gastrointestinal tract and prevent lung aspiration, broad-spectrum antibiotics to prevent sepsis, and an incubator to maintain body temperature.

In concert with fluid resuscitation, clinicians should cover the viscera, since it is a source of fluid and heat loss. For infants with gastroschisis, the surgeon should examine the intestine and mesenteric pedicle for proper alignment in order to ensure proper blood flow. If the infant needs to be transported to another facility for optimal care, the patient's lower body, including the gastroschisis, ought to be placed in a sterile plastic bag (eg, a bowel bag), with saline-soaked gauze loosely wrapped around the intestine. The infant should be placed with its left side down for transport to facilitate intestinal blood flow. Once the patient arrives at the destination for definitive care, the pediatric surgeon should reexamine the intestine. The next decision is whether to close in abdominal wall or place a silo device over the exposed intestine. In most cases, the choice hinges on the patient's hemodynamic stability, weight, and perceived intra-abdominal capacity. Silo placement is favored in most cases because the newer spring-based device may be placed fairly rapidly with appropriate sedation and lighting in the neonatal intensive care unit. Immediate definitive abdominal wall closure is rarely needed.

The omphalocele is handled in a slightly different manner because the intestine is usually covered by a sac. Clinicians should examine the sac to ensure that it is completely intact. It should then be covered with nonadherent gauze. If the sac is ruptured, then it is treated in a fashion similar to gastroschisis (see earlier). In the case of a large omphalocele, with liver herniation, placement of the infant in a supine position may lead to caval occlusion. These patients are positioned in a left lateral decubitus position, with proper support of the viscera to ensure blood flow.

Once the patient is resuscitated and the bowel appropriately dressed, the patient is transferred to a pediatric surgery center for definitive management. This will entail preoperative assessment for associated anomalies (chest radiograph, echocardiogram and renal ultrasound for omphaloceles). Surgical treatment can include either primary or staged abdominal wall closure. This decision is made based on the size of the abdominal compartment, the amount of viscera exposed, and the increase in intra-abdominal pressure caused by reduction of herniated viscera.

CONGENITAL DIAPHRAGMATIC HERNIA (CDH)
Epidemiology

The incidence of CDH is approximately 2.5-4 per 10,000 births. Clinicians that prenatally diagnose infants with CDH should arrange for delivery at a center that specializes in the treatment of surgical neonates. Infants with CDH have a mortality rate that remains quite high (10%-50%) even with the increasing use of new diagnostic and treatment modalities.[10,11]

Pathophysiology

In normal development the diaphragm fuses by the 8th week of development, separating the peritoneal and pleural cavities prior to the return of the midgut into the abdomen. If the diaphragm fusion is not complete prior to the reentrance of the midgut, the intestine may herniate into the thoracic cavity, preventing normal intestinal rotation and fixation. The CDH defect commonly occurs in the postero-lateral region, at the junction of the lumbar and costal muscle groups, and it is known as a Bochdalek hernia. Left diaphragmatic defects are more prevalent (80%) than right-sided lesions and defects are rarely bilateral. Nearly one-third of these children will have other major anomalies. The lung development is impaired by direct physical force from the herniated viscera and indirect pressure on the contralateral thoracic cavity, leading to bilateral lung hypoplasia. In addition to lung underdevelopment, infants with CDH may have reactive pulmonary hypertension, and this is the most significant management issue.[12]

Presentation

Infants with CDH can be very ill at birth due to respiratory distress secondary to lung hypoplasia and pulmonary hypertension. CDH disease severity depends on the degree of lung hypoplasia. On exam, the infant will have a scaphoid abdomen, and a plain chest radiograph will demonstrate abdominal viscera in the thoracic cavity. After assessing the infant's airway, breathing and circulation, clinicians should place an orogastric tube to decompress the gastrointestinal tract and limit abdominal pressure on the thoracic cavity.

Treatment

In some cases, infants with CDH and respiratory failure will require emergent endotracheal intubation. Clinicians ventilating with bag-valve or mechanical ventilation should maintain and monitor pressures that deliver adequate oxygenation while not causing a pneumothorax. Many suggest that reducing barotrauma by avoiding hyperventilation improves long-term morbidity.[5] One option in minimizing iatrogenic lung damage is using the gentle ventilation strategy.[13] The resuscitating physician should obtain an arterial blood gas to assess for metabolic and respiratory status. In many infants with CDH, acidosis is common, and this should be corrected. Once stabilized, the neonatologist should transport the infant to a tertiary care center that offers extracorporeal membrane therapy (ECMO).

Once the patient is transferred to a dedicated pediatric surgical center, pediatric surgeons and neonatologists should craft a strategy for addressing pulmonary hypertension. Clinicians have a number of ventilator techniques available to improve oxygenation including high frequency oscillators and inhaled nitric oxide (iNO). If these methods are not successful, pediatric surgeons should consider ECMO therapy. Pediatric surgeons should stabilize infants prior to CDH surgery. Stabilization includes conventional ventilation support or ECMO therapy. After the stabilization period, pediatric surgeons may proceed with open or minimally invasive surgical repair that generally entails reducing the herniated viscera from the thorax into the abdominal cavity and closing the diaphragmatic defect. If there is not enough muscle to close the defect, surgeons can use a prosthetic patch to perform a tension-free closure. In summary, the urgency in treating infants with CDH may involve urgent ECMO support and nonemergent closure of the diaphragmatic defect.

NECROTIZING ENTEROCOLITIS
Epidemiology

Necrotizing enterocolitis (NEC) is the most common neonatal gastrointestinal surgical emergency. NEC, a disease predominantly of premature neonates, has a high morbidity and mortality rate. Recent investigators demonstrate that NEC hospitalization rates nationwide are approximately 1 in 1000 live births, with 4500 admissions nationally per year. The in-hospital NEC mortality rate is approximately 16% for all infants and 20% for very low birth weight infants (< 1500 g).[14]

Pathophysiology

NEC is a severe inflammatory disorder of the intestines, leading to ischemia and necrosis that in some cases can involve the entire intestine. The etiology of NEC is multifactorial. Risk factors for developing NEC include enteral feeding, intestinal bacterial colonization, hypoxemia, respiratory disease, and cardiac defects. The disease progression includes an inflammatory response, enterocyte death, and bacterial dissemination that lead to a local and systemic inflammatory response. The immaturity of the neonatal immune system is thought to play a significant role in the propagation of NEC.[15]

Presentation

Clinically NEC may present with gastrointestinal and systemic signs and symptoms. Premature infants typically present at 2-3 weeks of age whereas the near-term infant may present within a few days of birth. Bell first described NEC disease staging in 1978.[16] Stage I NEC is characterized by feeding intolerance, mild abdominal distention, lethargy and temperature instability. An abdominal radiograph may show intestinal dilation or a nonspecific bowel gas pattern. In Stage II NEC, infants have more significant abdominal distention or even gastrointestinal bleeding. The radiograph may demonstrate pneumatosis intestinalis (a classic sign of NEC), portal venous gas, intestinal distention or bowel wall edema. In Stage III NEC or surgical NEC, the disease progresses to abdominal wall erythema, tenderness, and hemodynamic instability with evidence of shock. An abdominal radiograph may show pneumoperitoneum. Gestational age (GA) appears to impact NEC presentation; pneumatosis intestinalis or portal venous gas appear in older infants, whereas distention and pneumoperitoneum appear more commonly in younger neonates (23- to 26-week GA), and decreases in older infants (> 37 weeks).[17]

The diagnosis of NEC is based on the clinical findings, laboratory values and radiological studies. In NEC and suspected NEC, neonatologists should obtain serial abdominal radiographs every 6 to 8 hours. Laboratory studies include complete blood counts and blood gases. Neonates with NEC often have leucopenia, thrombocytopenia, and acidosis.

Treatment

Stage I and Stage II NEC are considered medical. In these infants, clinicians should discontinue enteral feeds, place an orogastric tube for stomach decompression and initiate broad-spectrum antibiotics. Prior to starting antibiotics, clinicians must initiate a sepsis evaluation to rule out other causes. These infants may also require fluid resuscitation, ventilator support, and blood product transfusion. Medical treatment can last up to 14 days for radiograph-proven medical NEC but less for suspected NEC. In Stage III NEC, surgery is performed to control intra-abdominal sepsis. In infants with abdominal films that do not show pneumoperitoneum, surgeons may perform a paracentesis to confirm the presence of stool or bacteria in the peritoneal cavity.[18]

In NEC surgery, the goal is to control intra-abdominal sepsis, preserve viable intestine and resect necrotic bowel. The overall approach is to perform damage control surgery by resecting bowel as necessary, constructing a diverting enterostomy, or leaving discontinuous bowel in the abdomen for a second-look exploration in 24-48 hours after the initial surgery. In unstable very low birth weight infants (< 1500 g), surgeons may consider an alternative strategy of placing a peritoneal drain as a temporizing measure prior to performing a formal operation in the next 24-48 hours after drain placement. Patients with signs of NEC should be transferred to a NICU with pediatric surgical coverage.

NEONATAL BOWEL OBSTRUCTION
Diagnostic Approach
Suspected neonatal bowel obstruction requires rapid assessment and diagnosis. Many conditions can present with signs of obstruction such as emesis including

congenital anatomic defects and inherited metabolic diseases or physiological disorders. A summary of the causes of neonatal intestinal obstruction can be found in Table 18-3.

Clinicians must obtain a complete history of the patient including prenatal findings and perinatal events. Prenatal ultrasound exams may detect intestinal anomalies. For instance, dilated bowel loops or polyhydramnios are associated with proximal intestinal atresias. Postnatal events such as early meconium passage or bilious emesis are useful in determining intestinal function. Bilious emesis requires prompt evaluation. Clinicians should complete a thorough physical examination when evaluating infants with potential bowel obstructions. Neonates with suspected intestinal obstruction might have a distended abdomen if the obstruction is distal but a flat abdomen if the blockage is more proximal. If the neonate has a tender abdomen, a surgeon must be consulted for a potential bowel perforation. Other genetic or congenital associations with intestinal obstruction include trisomy 21 and duodenal atresia; infants with cloacal anomalies or VACTERL association may have tracheoesophageal fistulas or an imperforate anus.[19] The

Table 18-3	Neonatal Mechanical Intestinal Obstruction				
Diagnosis	History	Physical Findings	Studies	Treatment	Concerns
Midgut Volvulus	Bilious Emesis	Abdominal distention	UGI	Ladd procedure (see text)	
Duodenal Atresia	Feeding Intolerance	Gastric distention	Plain radiographs	Duodenoduodenostomy	Down Syndtrome
Annular Pancreas	Feeding Intolerance	Gastric distention	Plain radiographs	Duodenoduodenostomy	
Intestinal Atresia	Feeding Intolerance, Bilious Emesis	Distention	UGI	Enteroenterostomy	Down Syndrome
Meconium Ileus	Distention, bilious emesis, no meconium passed	Possible mass, possible distention	Plain radiographs, Contrast enema	Dependent on severity, water soluble contrast enema if simple, laparotomy if perforated	Cystic Fibrosis
Meconium Plug	Distention, bilious emesis, no meconium passed	Possible distention	Plain radiographs, Contrast enema	Water-soluble contrast enema	Cystic Fibrosis
Hirschsprungs disease	Possible no meconium, constipation	Possible distention	Contrast enema, transanal mucosal biopsy	Leveling colostomy or primary pull-through	
Imperforate Anus	No meconium passed	Absent or ectopic anus	None preoperatively	Colostomy, PSARP at later time	VACTERL Syndrome
Necrotizing Enterocolitis	Feeding intolerance	Distention, abdominal skin changes	Plain radiographs	See text	

VACTERL mnemonic describes a nonrandom association of birth defects, including vertebral anomalies, anal atresia, cardiac defects, tracheoesophageal fistula, renal abnormalities, and limb deformities (most commonly a radial limb dysplasia).

Bilious emesis or gastric aspirates may help differentiate the level of intestinal obstruction and, therefore, help the clinician determine the diagnostic algorithm. If there is bile detected, an urgent surgical evaluation is usually required. The most worrisome cause of obstruction in the neonatal period is midgut volvulus. Suspected midgut volvulus requires emergent abdominal exploration in order to detorse the intestine and limit intestinal ischemia and possible bowel loss (see following section).

The clinician's initial evaluation should include a history, physical exam, routine laboratory tests such as complete blood count, blood cultures and abdominal radiographs with two views, anterior-posterior and left lateral decubitus. If the infant has a tender abdomen, the surgeon may elect to operate without any additional radiographic testing. However, in many cases, the plain films help localize the level of intestinal obstruction. For example, infants with duodenal atresia may demonstrate a double bubble radiological sign (see Fig. 18-3) and in this case no further radiological studies are typically required. If proximal atresia is not suspected on plain film, then upper and lower gastrointestinal contrast radiographic studies may help determine the anatomy.

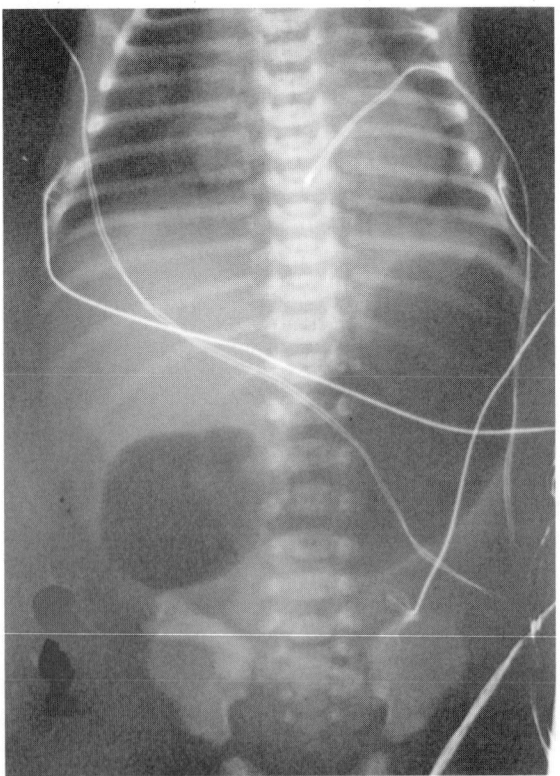

Figure 18-3 *Plain abdominal radiograph with the classic "double bubble" sign, seen in duodenal atresia.*

PEDIATRIC SURGICAL EMERGENCIES

MALROTATION AND MIDGUT VOLVULUS
Epidemiology
The incidence of malrotation in the general population is approximately 1:100 to 1:500 live births. Infants or children with bilious emesis are considered candidates for malrotation. Malrotation anomalies may present with midgut volvulus or bowel obstruction; however, some cases of malrotation are incidentally discovered on studies performed for other reasons such as gastroesophageal reflux disease. Most patients with malrotation (80%) present in the first month of life, and approximately 90% in the first year.[20]

Pathophysiology
To understand malrotation, one must understand the embryological development of the intestinal tract. The term malrotation is a misnomer, because it is not caused by "bad" rotation but instead by non- or incomplete rotation. Infants with malrotation are at risk for obstruction because in addition to the intestinal rotational errors, the intestine is abnormally fixed and possibly obstructed by malpositioned peritoneal attachments (Ladd bands). In the embryo, the gastrointestinal tract development begins as a straight tube. The maturation of the intestinal tract is complex. Briefly, intestinal development occurs in three stages, as described by Frazer and Robbins. Stage 1 occurs during weeks 5-10, with herniation of the rapidly elongating midgut through the umbilical defect. Stage 2 occurs during weeks 10-11, with return of the intestine into the coelomic cavity. Finally, stage 3 is the period of fixation, which lasts from the end of stage 2 until shortly after birth. During stages 1 and 2, the midgut undergoes elongation and rotation. The midgut divides into two portions, a cephalad midgut (duodenojejunal loop) and a caudad midgut (cecocolic loop), with the superior mesenteric artery (SMA) as the dividing line. The SMA is also the rotational axis for the intestinal development. During stages 1 and 2, the intestine rotates 180 degrees counterclockwise, and then the intestine returns to the abdomen at the end of stage 2 and it rotates for a final 90 degrees. Normally, the intestine undergoes 270 degrees of rotation. At the end of successful intestinal development, the cephalad midgut lies inferior to the SMA, while the caudad midgut lies superior to the SMA. The cecum elongates and descends into the right lower quadrant throughout the remainder of gestation, and for the first few months of life.[20]

During the cecal elongation phase, intestinal fixation occurs. The retroperitoneal duodenum attaches to the posterior and the ligament of Treitz extends from the area of the right diaphragmatic crus to the duodenojejunal junction. The ascending, descending, and sigmoid colon assume their partially retroperitoneal positions, whereas the transverse mesocolon fuses with the greater omentum. The cecum is not attached during this phase. Under normal circumstances, the small bowel mesentery extends from the ligament of Treitz in the left upper quadrant to the ileocecal junction in the right lower quadrant.[21] Malrotation can arise with any error in the rotational or fixation processes described above. Nonrotation is defined as failure of the cephalad or caudal portions of the intestine to rotate after the first 90-degree turn. This leaves the small bowel to the right of the SMA, and the cecum and colon to the left. In nonrotation, abnormal fixation of the cecum and ascending colon may happen with peritoneal bands crossing anterior to the duodenum to the right posterior abdominal wall. These aberrant bands (Ladd bands) may lead to duodenal obstruction. When there is failure during the final 180 degrees of rotation in the cephalad or caudal midgut, we describe this as an incomplete or mixed rotation anomaly. The small bowel and cecum location can vary in incomplete or mixed rotation cases. When mesenteric attachments develop abnormally, poor intestinal fixation leads to a high risk of volvulus. In cases with reversed rotation, the caudal midgut reenters the coelomic cavity before the cephalad midgut, leading to clockwise rotation of the duodenum. As a result, the duodenojejunal loop is now anterior to the SMA and the colon is posterior. This anatomical arrangement can lead to an internal hernia.

Presentation

Symptomatic malrotation occurs when the intestines are obstructed due to partial or complete twisting of the intestine, or volvulus. Volvulus may occur prenatally and the twisted bowel will die and lead to short gut at birth. After birth infants with malrotation typically develop volvulus within the first month of life. Symptomatic infants are irritable and feed poorly. Infants with volvulus may vomit bile and signs can progress to abdominal distention with tenderness. Infants with prolonged ischemia due to the twisted intestine may have worrisome signs such as hematemesis, hypotension, and metabolic acidosis.

Infants presenting with bilious emesis and other signs of intestinal obstruction need immediate attention for diagnosis and treatment considerations. Intestinal viability decreases with time and a missed or delayed diagnosis can lead to a catastrophic loss of intestine. Abdominal radiographs (two views) will show gastric and proximal duodenal distention and in some cases a paucity of small bowel gas. Surgeons use plain or contrast abdominal radiographs in order to differentiate between proximal and distal obstruction. Radiologists employ contrast gastrointestinal series to diagnose possible obstruction causes. The key initial finding on an upper gastrointestinal study is the depiction of the duodenal anatomy. If the duodenal course is abnormal, with a corkscrew or spiral course of the

distal duodenum and proximal jejunum, this usually suggests malrotation. If the upper gastrointestinal series is not diagnostic, a lower gastrointestinal series may detect distal anatomic changes that suggest malrotation such as a malpositioned cecum. Clinicians may consider using an ultrasound or computerized tomography study to determine the cause of obstruction. Key findings on these studies include an abnormal position of the superior mesenteric vessels in which the superior mesenteric vein lies to the left of the SMA.

Treatment

If the diagnosis of malrotation or volvulus is suspected or confirmed based on the clinical findings and the radiographic studies, the patient is resuscitated and emergently taken to the operating room for abdominal exploration. Resuscitation should occur in tandem with the diagnostic workup, so there is no delay in going to the operating room.

In the operating room, the patient is placed supine and undergoes nasogastric decompression and induction of general anesthesia. In infants, surgeons perform a laparotomy through a right upper quadrant transverse incision. The bowel is initially inspected for viability and position and then it is eviscerated and examined. If the intestine is volvulized or twisted, surgeons must detorse the intestine in order to restore blood flow. Volvulus occurs in a clockwise fashion; therefore, surgeons will detorse the intestine by untwisting it in a counterclockwise manner. Following this, the operator will fan out the small intestine over the lower abdomen to clearly identify mesenteric vessels. The peritoneal bands passing from the right colon across the duodenum (Ladd bands) are incised at the medial aspect of the duodenum, allowing visualization of the underlying mesentery. Avascular attachments are divided until the cecum and colon lie to the left, and the duodenum and small bowel lie to the right. By incising the anterior mesenteric leaf, the surgeon widens the mesenteric base thus broadening the pedicle on which the intestine sits. If the bowel is nonviable, the surgeon may consider complete resection but this will result in short bowel syndrome and TPN-dependence. If the bowel appearance is marginal, the surgeon should consider placing a silo over the intestine and reexamining the bowel in 24 to 48 hours. In order to complete the operation, surgeons perform an appendectomy, because the appendix may end up in an atypical position in the abdomen and thus confuse future clinicians in making the diagnosis of appendicitis.

Outcome

Patients treated for malrotation do well following the postoperative recovery period. Patients with bowel resections may require parenteral nutrition for a period of time, since the return of bowel function is often delayed. The recurrence of volvulus is rare. Postoperative small bowel obstruction secondary to adhesions is more common, occurring in up to 10% of patients. Patients who require a large resection often develop short bowel syndrome, with the subsequent complications such as sepsis, liver failure, and nutritional failure.

INFANTILE HYPERTROPHIC PYLORIC STENOSIS
Epidemiology
Infantile hypertrophic pyloric stenosis (IHPS) is commonly diagnosed in patients between the ages of 2 to 8 weeks. Nonbilious, forceful (projectile) vomiting is the most common presentation. The incidence in North America and Western Europe has consistently been between 2 and 5 per 1000 live born infants. There is also a link to birth order, as first-born children have the highest incidence.[18]

Pathophysiology
Normally, the pyloric muscle releases gastric contents into the duodenum after the requisite early digestion is completed in the stomach. Pylorus muscle hypertrophy leads to a functional gastric outlet obstruction, thus infants commonly present with nonbilious, forceful vomiting. Recent evidence suggests that pyloric muscle hypertrophy may be due to a lack of nitric oxide (NO) in the muscular layer. Investigators believe that low amounts of NO lead to poor circular muscular layer relaxation.[22,23] There appears to be no genetic predisposition to pyloric stenosis, although the condition appears to be clustered in some families.

Presentation
Infants suspected of having pyloric stenosis usually present with nonbilious emesis. Early in the course of the disease, parents attempt to feed the infant more often since they are not satiated. In some cases, pediatricians will recommend changing formulas because of the high prevalence of formula intolerance or physiological gastroesophageal reflux. However, as the disease, progresses, the infant can become dehydrated and even malnourished, with a loss of weight if the signs and symptoms are not recognized.

On exam, clinicians may detect signs of dehydration, lethargy, and weight loss. On abdominal exam, the clinician may detect the pylorus as an "olive" in the right upper quadrant region. If an experienced clinician finds a mass consistent with a hypertrophic pylorus then surgical consultation is recommended and no further studies are needed. In many cases, infants with excessive vomiting are sent for an abdominal ultrasound or an upper gastrointestinal contrast study. Radiologists interpret ultrasound findings for pylorus thickness and length. If the ultrasound results are not diagnostic, many clinicians order an upper gastrointestinal contrast study with barium to determine the gastrointestinal tract anatomy; in addition, the upper GI study is more sensitive than the ultrasound study and it will confirm the presence of pyloric stenosis.

Once the diagnosis is confirmed, the infant should be admitted to a center with a pediatric surgeon and a serum electrolyte panel must be ordered. Patients with pyloric stenosis who vomit for a prolonged period of time are dehydrated, hypochloremic, hypokalemic, and alkalotic secondary to emesis and excessive loss of hydrogen chloride. With dehydration, the aldosterone response accentuates the metabolic derangements already present and this leads to sodium retention and an increased loss of potassium. The blood flowing to the kidney has decreased chloride content, thus leading to increased tubular uptake of bicarbonate with the sodium, increasing alkalosis and resulting in paradoxical aciduria.

Treatment
The priority in patients with pyloric stenosis is to correct dehydration and electrolyte abnormalities. In most cases, surgeons should provide 10% dextrose in 0.45% normal saline intravenous fluids at 1.5 times the maintenance rate and monitor urine output. It is imperative to normalize bicarbonate and chloride levels prior to the operation. Failure to correct electrolytes may result in postoperative respiratory compromise.

Medical treatment of pyloric stenosis has growing interest but the preliminary findings are not proven in randomized control trial. Furthermore, patients have a prolonged hospital stay (> or = 12 days), and must be sent home on oral atropine for an additional amount of time (> or = 40 days).[24] Further study is needed to confirm early observations with medical therapeutic success.

Surgical approaches for pyloromyotomy are evolving. Over the last several years, surgeons introduced minimal invasive approaches to remedy this ailment. The following section will outline the open procedure and briefly describe the laparoscopic pyloromyotomy. Open pyloromyotomies are conducted through right upper quadrant or umbilical incisions. Surgeons dictate the abdominal incision choice but the condition of the umbilical stump is the prevailing factor in determining this choice. The traditional incision is a right upper quadrant transverse incision (Robertson muscle splitting grid-iron incision). The umbilical incision when feasible offers better cosmesis but it has an increased risk of infection.[25] In our hands, the umbilical approach is preferred. The operator makes a curvilinear incision in the skin and incises the midline fascia longitudinally, superior to the umbilicus. Once in the peritoneal cavity, the omentum is identified (Koop maneuver) and pushed down toward the pelvis. This maneuver displaces the transverse colon caudally and pulls the gastric antrum into the wound. The surgeon delivers the pylorus through the wound and then incises the seromuscular layer. The back end of the scalpel is used to bluntly open the circular muscle of the pylorus and the pyloric spreaders are used to split the muscular layer. Once the circular muscle is split, the two sides of the "olive" must move independently. In addition, the anesthesiologist instills air into the antrum via an orogastric or nasogastric tube, to assess mucosal integrity.

In many centers, pediatric surgeons perform laparoscopic pyloromyotomies. Recent evidence suggests that after an initial learning curve, the complication rates are similar to those of open pyloromyotomy. The laparoscopic approach has a considerable learning curve; therefore the procedure should only be performed by trained pediatric surgeons.

Outcomes

Following the pyloromyotomy, surgeons allow infants to recover for a few hours and begin feeds with small volume of clears and advance to a couple ounces of formula. Infants may continue to have emesis after surgery due to prolonged preoperative vomiting, gastroesophageal reflux disease and gastritis. Incomplete pyloromyotomy is rare, but it may be a reason for continued emesis. Wounds infections rarely occur but in general umbilical wounds have higher incidence of wound infection then other wounds. In summary, the short-term outcomes for pyloric stenosis depend on preoperative resuscitation and less on actual operative technique.

INTUSSUSCEPTION
Epidemiology

Intussusception is an invagination of a proximal portion of intestine (the intussusceptum) into the distal contiguous intestine (the intussuscipiens). In children 3 to 36 months old, intussusception is the most common cause of intestinal obstruction with most cases occurring before 12 months and rarely occurring after 5 years old. In the United States, the incidence of intussusception is between 1 and 4:1000 children. There is a slight male predominance, with a 3:2 male to female ratio.

Pathophysiology

Children with intussusception are believed to have a lead point that pulls the proximal portion of intestine into the distal portion with normal peristalsis. Over time the folded intestine becomes compressed because of inflammation and induration. There is no digestive flow through the compressed lumen, resulting in bowel obstruction. The intestinal vascular supply becomes compromised with time, and the intestine may become ischemic. This bowel is then prone to perforation.

In infants, there is usually no pathological lead point (eg, tumor); instead there may be local intestinal wall edema due to intestinal lymphoid tissue hypertrophy. Peyer Patch hypertrophy may be due to viruses or other ingested antigens. The ileocecal region is the most common area for intussusception, since there is an abundant amount of lymphoid tissue in the terminal ileum. In infants who have recurrent episodes of intussusception or older children (above the age of 12-18 months) with intussusception, clinicians should consider a pathological lead point in these cases.

Pathological lead points include polyps, hemangiomas, Meckel diverticulum, or intramural tumors.

Presentation

The infant or toddler with intussusception often presents with a previous episode of gastroenteritis, viral syndrome, or Henoch-Schonlein purpura (HSP) several days before the onset of abdominal pain. Infants may complain or exhibit signs of acute, colicky, severe, and episodic pain. The infant shows signs of lethargy and anorexia in between episodes. Clinicians considering intussusception in the differential diagnosis should inquire about a history of episodic pain in suspected cases. Infants may also vomit and have bloody diarrhea. The classic association of currant jelly stools (mucus and bloody stool intermixed) is not as common as the finding of occult blood during rectal exam. On exam, a mass may be appreciated in the right side of the abdomen with a sense of emptiness in the right lower quadrant, known as Dance sign. In rare cases of small bowel intussusception (jejunojejunal, as is seen in HSP), clinicians may detect a sausage-like mass in the epigastric region.

In suspected intussusception, the first step in management is IV line placement and resuscitation. An abdominal radiograph is performed to assess for free air. If a physician suspects intussusception then a surgical consultation may be important to assess for peritonitis. If the surgeon finds peritonitis, or if free air is present, the patient should be taken to the operating room for emergency laparotomy. If there are no signs of peritonitis or free air, the clinician should order an air or contrast enema to diagnose and treat intussusception. Ultrasounds and CT scans are useful in detecting intussusception; however, these modalities cannot treat the problem. In cases of suspected jejunojejunal intussusception, a CT scan or ultrasound may be preferred, because a contrast enema is not therapeutic with these lesions.

Treatment

Most clinicians give infants broad-spectrum antibiotic prophylaxis for the enema. Air or hydrostatic barium enemas are used to diagnose and attempt reduction. Intussusception reduction is marked by free flow of air or contrast into the small bowel. In dedicated pediatric centers, successful reduction is achieved in up to 95% of cases. If the radiologist fails to reduce the intussusception on the first attempt, the radiologist can repeat the reduction up to three times. It is important that a skilled radiologist perform this procedure, given that reducing strangulated bowel is less common in experienced hands. After reducing the lesion, the patient is admitted for 24 hours and fed about 12 hours after admission.

If reduction fails, the patient should be immediately taken to the operating room for exploration and manual reduction. At exploration, the intussusception is located and reduced by applying pressure to the lead point (rather than pulling on the proximal bowel).

If the intestine cannot be reduced or the bowel is nonviable, a resection is performed. The surgeon can perform a primary anastomosis or a diverting enterostomy if indicated. Diversion is appropriate if the patient is in shock or there is fecal peritonitis. Postoperative management is dictated by the operation performed, and there are no specific concerns, other than recurrence. Recurrent intussusception occurs in approximately 5% of infants; a nonsurgical reduction approach is still the preferred approach. If a second operation is needed, a more vigorous examination for a lead point is appropriate; however, an enterotomy is typically not necessary. Some surgeons employ a laparoscopic approach in diagnosing and treating intussusception.

Outcomes

Intussusception-related mortality is rare in developed countries, and is most commonly related to a delay in diagnosis, with strangulated intestine leading to systemic shock. Most patients with intussusception do well and rarely have recurrent disease. Recurrence is most likely to occur within days of the first episode of intussusception.

INCARCERATED INGUINAL HERNIA
Epidemiology

Inguinal hernias are a common surgical condition in infancy and childhood, thus hernia repair is the most frequently performed elective pediatric operation. Inguinal hernias occur in 1%-5% of term infants and the incidence increases with prematurity. The incidence rate in preterm neonates less than 28-weeks gestation approaches 35%. Males have more hernias than females; the male to female ratio is 6:1. Infant inguinal hernias are congenital and indirect. Infants can have direct or femoral hernias, but they occur infrequently with incidence rates of approaching 0.5% for each. Indirect inguinal hernias arise on the right side greater than the left (60% vs. 25%), with the remainder being bilateral. Many believe that females have more bilateral hernias than males.[19] Incarceration is the most common complication associated with an inguinal hernia, and it happens in approximately 12% of children with hernias. The incidence increases in infants less than the age of 1 yr.

Pathophysiology

The congenital inguinal hernia is due to a continuation of the peritoneum that descends with the testicle as it passes through the internal ring and inguinal canal. This process results in the formation of the patent processus vaginalis. The eventual development of hernias or hydroceles depends on the degree of processus vaginalis patency. Infant hernias are caused by the descent of viscera (intestine, omentum, or ovaries) into the inguinal canal. Hernia incarceration is defined as nonreducible viscera in the hernia sac; prolonged incarceration may lead to viscera vascular compromise. In infants, the risk of incarceration is high and since infants cannot adequately communicate, inguinal hernias are repaired soon after diagnosis. Indications for delaying repair sometimes include prematurity and congenital diseases that place the child under greater risk with general anesthesia. Infants with high-risk congenital disease are repaired under spinal, caudal, or local anesthetic blocks if general anesthesia is contraindicated. Premature infants with hernias may be repaired before discharge home. If a premature infant is not diagnosed with a hernia prior to discharge, then repair is generally scheduled per the local facilities practice regarding gestational age. Hospital age thresholds for elective surgery range from 44- to 50-weeks gestation in order to decrease anesthetic risks.

Presentation

Children with an incarcerated hernia present with an acute, tender mass in the inguinal canal, scrotum, or labia. Infants with prolonged incarceration can develop abdominal distention, emesis, and irritability and these are symptoms of bowel obstruction. In infants with advanced incarceration, the groin becomes edematous, erythematous, and tender. If the patient is in shock on arrival, and it appears that the cause is gangrenous bowel, the surgeon must take the patient directly to the operating room.

Treatment

For a nonreducible hernia, the clinician should elevate the child's lower extremities and place the child in slight Trendelenburg, in an attempt to trigger spontaneous reduction. If simple relaxation and positioning is unsuccessful, then a skilled clinician should attempt manual reduction with minimal sedation. The physician gently uses the forefinger and thumb of one hand to align the incarcerated mass transversely, in line with the canal, placing one digit on each side. Next, the physician applies pressure along the sides to decrease swelling. Following this, the clinician places gentle pressure at the lead point with the other hand to assist in the reduction manipulation.

If reduction is successful, monitor the patient overnight and repair the hernia during the same hospitalization. The rationale for keeping the patient hospitalized is to monitor for signs of bowel ischemia due to the bowel incarceration. If the hernia is irreducible, the surgeon should operate and repair the hernia. The patient should receive preoperative antibiotics and adequate resuscitation. The surgeon should resist the temptation to reduce the hernia once the patient is under general anesthesia because the surgeon should inspect the bowel or other hernia contents. For repair, the surgeon uses an inguinal incision to dissect the hernia sac. Next, the surgeon identifies the inguinal nerve and then opens the fascia over the hernia and separates the cremasteric muscle fibers. After that, the spermatic vessels and vas deferens, usually identified on the posterolateral aspect of the sac, are separated from the sac. Once the sac is completely isolated, the surgeon opens the sac and examines the incarcerated viscera. If the bowel is viable, the operator returns it to the peritoneal cavity, and continues the high ligation hernia repair. If the hernia sac extends into the scrotum, the surgeon divides it distally but does not remove the distal sac. If the internal ring is large, the surgeon places interrupted sutures at the opening to tighten it. Finally, the surgeon aligns the spermatic cord within the inguinal canal and checks to see that the testes are within the scrotum. The surgeon completes the operation by closing the fascia, subcutaneous tissue and skin in layers.

If there is purulent or bloody fluid within the sac or the bowel is not viable, the surgeon must perform a laparotomy to examine the bowel in more detail and perform a resection if necessary. Postoperative care in these patients will require increased pain medication and monitoring for bowel function return.

Outcomes
There is an increased complication rate in patients requiring emergency surgery for incarcerated hernia. Complications include injury to testicular vessels and the vas deferens, testicular atrophy, recurrent hernia, and wound infection.

APPENDICITIS
Epidemiology
Acute appendicitis is one of the most common causes of abdominal pain in children, and the most common cause for emergent abdominal surgery. Although appendicitis can affect close to 10% of people in the Western world, it is most common between the ages of 4 and 15 years. It is uncommon under the age of 3, and in this population can be very difficult to diagnose.

Pathophysiology
In appendicitis, there is obstruction of the appendiceal lumen by a fecalith, which prevents passage of mucus from the appendix. In other cases, the obstruction is due to lymphoid hyperplasia, helminthic infection (pinworm), or a carcinoid tumor. Obstruction leads to appendiceal distention, bacterial overgrowth, and eventually, abdominal pain and tenderness. If the obstruction is not relieved and the infection progresses, the appendix will perforate, leading to peritonitis and abscess formation.

Presentation
Children with appendicitis initially complain of periumbilical or epigastric pain. Following the onset of pain, children may be anorexic and their symptoms can progress to nausea and vomiting. The pain migrates most commonly to the right lower quadrant. The patient may have brief pain relief with perforation, but this is short-lived because free spillage of bacteria-laden fluid leads to peritonitis. In children, it is important to discuss the

history thoroughly with the patient and parents. Surgeons should ask the parents questions regarding ill contacts, past medical and surgical history, and previous episodes of similar pain. Other causes of abdominal pain in children include viral gastroenteritis, mesenteric adenitis, constipation, and referred pain from an intrathoracic process (eg, lower lobe pneumonia).

On physical exam, the clinician should also observe the child's body habitus and movements. Some children with peritonitis will prefer to lie still in their parent's arms or on the gurney. If the child has mild symptoms, the clinician should ask the older child to walk and jump in order to detect peritoneal irritation. The surgeon should perform the abdominal exam with the patient supine on the examination table, with knees slightly flexed. In patients in whom the history and exam are not convincing, but still suggestive, clinicians should order a white blood cell count and urine analysis. Based on clinical findings and preliminary laboratory findings, one can consider adjunctive imaging studies including computerized tomography or ultrasound to assist in making the diagnosis.

Treatment
If the diagnosis of appendicitis is made, the patient is taken to the operating room for an appendectomy. The patient should receive preoperative antibiotics, intravenous fluids, and analgesics. The surgical team must resuscitate the patient. If the patient has complicated appendicitis and is in shock, the patient should have adequate urine output prior to going to the operating room. The surgeon performs an appendectomy with an open or minimally invasive approach.

Outcomes
Children with appendicitis rarely die from this disease process, and mortality has steadily decreased over the last three decades. There is an increased risk of wound infection and abscess formation post operatively in patients with complicated or perforated appendicitis compared to nonperforated appendicitis. The rate of negative appendectomy has stayed fairly constant, approaching 9% in males and 15% in females.

TESTICULAR TORSION
Epidemiology
A patient who presents with acute scrotal pain must be evaluated immediately for testicular torsion. Conditions that can present with acute onset testicular pain or swelling include epididymitis/orchitis, torsion of the appendage testis, testicular torsion, fat necrosis, inguinal hernia, hydrocele, varicocele, trauma, or a tumor. Testicular torsion occurs most commonly in males between 12 and 19 years old. The incidence of testicular torsion between the ages of 10 and 19 years is 8.6 per 100,000. The median age of patients presenting with testicular torsion is 15 years. Of patients aged 1-9 years old with testicular torsion, 19% will require

orchidectomy, whereas in patients 10-19 years old, 33% will require orchidectomy. Viability of the testes is compromised with testicular torsion not treated within 4 to 8 hours, and for this reason there must be a high index of suspicion.

Pathophysiology

Testicular torsion occurs by two mechanisms, extravaginal or intravaginal torsion. Extravaginal torsion occurs primarily in the perinatal group, whereas intravaginal torsion is more common in older patients. The definition is based on whether the torsion occurs above or below the reflection of the tunica vaginalis from the spermatic cord. In extravaginal torsion, the twist develops because the tunica is not attached securely to the scrotum, and the entire complex, including the tunica and testis, rotates within the scrotum. In extravaginal torsion, the testicular twist is above the reflection. In cases of intravaginal torsion, twisting of the cord and testis occurs below the reflection and within the tunica, but does not involve the tunica. Anatomical abnormalities including the bell-clapper anomaly may play a role in intravaginal torsion. In these cases, the tunica attaches to the cord in a higher location, and the epididymal-testicular complex is not properly fixed posteriorly to the tunica. The abnormal attachment permits more mobility of the testis and this may lead to torsion.

Presentation

In perinatal torsion, the presentation varies based on when the torsion occurred. For instance, if it was antenatal, there is often no systemic effect and the infant has a nontender scrotal mass or swelling with overlying skin discoloration. However, in patients with postnatal torsion, there are commonly systemic symptoms, such as lack of appetite and increased irritability and scrotal tenderness. The parents may report redness and swelling in the scrotum.

In older patients, the presentation is often more acute. There is sudden onset of severe scrotal pain, often with swelling of the testicle. Some patients may have a history of preceding scrotal trauma, a recent episode of epididymitis, or torsion of the appendage testis. In cases of testicular torsion, the testis may rest in a retracted and horizontal position with associated loss of the cremasteric reflex.

Treatment

The diagnosis of perinatal and other suspected testicular torsion cases is based on the clinical assessment. In the perinatal period, the clinician must differentiate between antenatal and postnatal torsion. In antenatal torsion, surgery is required but it can be deferred until 44-60 weeks adjusted gestational age when anesthetic risks are decreased. In antenatal cases, the testis is usually not viable, so the surgeon should perform an orchidectomy with contralateral orchidopexy. In postnatal torsion, the surgeon must explore the scrotum emergently to detorse the testis. If it is truly not viable, the surgeon should perform an orchidectomy. If there is any chance the testis will be viable, the surgeon should perform an orchidopexy, with plans to return for an orchidectomy if symptoms progress. In addition, the surgeon should do an orchidopexy on the contralateral testis to prevent torsion.

With older children, the surgeon must explore any patient who presents with a history and exam strongly suggestive of testicular torsion. If the history and exam are equivocal, but 6 or more hours have elapsed, exploration is warranted. In cases where the history and exam are not suggestive, but torsion is still possible, the clinician can perform Doppler ultrasound or radioisotope imaging. Radioisotope imaging of the testis is more reliable than Doppler flow studies, and shows an absence of uptake in the nonperfused testis, surrounded by normal uptake in the scrotal tissue and contralateral testis.

Once the diagnosis is made, the clinician prepares the patient for the operating room. A skilled clinician can attempt manual detorsion, but this should not delay the operation. If attempting to manually untwist the cord, a spermatic cord nerve block may be helpful. The testis most commonly rotates inward, toward the midline, so to untwist the clinician should turn it outward.

Once the patient is in the operating room, the surgeon uses either an inguinal or trans-scrotal approach depending on the patient's age. In neonates, surgeons should use an inguinal incision because there may be an associated hernia or tumor present in the scrotum. The operator should correct the extravaginal torsion by rotating the testis into the proper orientation. If there is a question regarding viability, the surgeon can cover the testis with warm, moist gauze, leave it in place, then perform an orchidopexy on the contralateral testis via a scrotal incision. Once this is done, reexamine the questionable testis. If its viability is still unclear, nick the tunica albuginea to expose the seminiferous tubules. The surgeon should examine the color, in order to determine if the testis is viable. If viable, the surgeon should fix the testis to the scrotal wall in 2 to 3 places to prevent recurrent torsion. If it is not viable, the surgeon should perform an orchidectomy.

In older patients, the surgeon should examine the testis once the patient is anesthetized. If there is concern for a testicular tumor or incarcerated hernia, the operator should use an inguinal approach. If these pathologies are not evident, a trans-scrotal approach is used. The surgeon should make an incision in the midline scrotal raphe, dissect bluntly to the torsed testis and deliver it through the incision. The surgeon should manually detorse the testicle and examine it for viability, as outlined earlier. If it is viable, append the testis to the wall of the scrotum at two to three locations. Debate exists as to whether the tunica vaginalis should be everted at this point. To evert the tunica vaginalis, open it lengthwise, and suture it to itself after eversion. This prevents recurrent intravaginal torsion, and allows scar to form between the tunica and the dartos fascia. If the testis is not viable, perform an orchidectomy. If prosthetic testicles are available, they can be placed at the same time for a late adolescent, or at a later date. The surgeon should fix the contralateral testis through the same midline incision, to prevent contralateral torsion in the future.

Outcomes

Long-term sequelae may occur; therefore, these patients need to be followed. A testis that is left in place because it appears viable may undergo atrophy with time if the blood supply is not adequate. Contralateral testicular atrophy is also concerning since cases are documented in the literature. Finally, there are cases of torsion in previously fixed testicles.

Salvage rates in neonates have been documented as low as 5%, but these do not differentiate between antenatal and postnatal torsion. Aggressive management of postnatal torsion will likely result in improved salvage rates, whereas antenatal torsion will continue to be unsalvageable. In older patients, testicular salvage rates improve with early identification and prompt surgery. If less than 6 hours elapses, salvage rates are 83%-97%. Between 6 to 12 hours after onset, salvage rates are between 55%-85%, and after 24 hours, salvage rates fall to less than 10%. Long-term sequelae in these patients still occur, and testicular function is often decreased.

Summary/Conclusions

Children require special consideration because age, developmental changes, and congenital anomalies have direct impact on disease severity and end-organ salvage. Although care by a pediatric surgeon is the gold standard for surgical pediatric diseases, the general surgeon should acquaint themselves with this catalog of diseases and become comfortable with dealing with emergencies that develop in this population.

REFERENCES

1. Nance ML. The Halifax disaster of 1917 and the birth of North American pediatric surgery. J Pediatr Surg 2001;36(3):405-408.
2. Ziegler MM. Pediatric surgical training: an historic perspective, a formula for change. J Pediatr Surg 2004;39(8):1159-1172.
3. Grosfeld JL. World Federation of Associations of Pediatric Surgeons: declaration of pediatric surgery. J Pediatr Surg 2001;36(12):1743.
4. Fildes JJ. National Trauma Data Bank Pediatric Report 2004. In: Fildes JJ (ed.) National Trauma Data Bank, Version 4.3. Washington DC: American College of Surgeons; 2004:9-15.
5. Chahine AA, Ricketts RR. Resuscitation of the surgical neonate. Clin Perinatol 1999;26(3):693-715.
6. Parker MM, Hazelzet JA. Carcillo JA Pediatric considerations. Crit Care Med 2004;32(11 Suppl):S591-S594.
7. Lloyd DA. Energy requirements of surgical newborn infants receiving parenteral nutrition. Nutrition 1998;14(1):101-104.
8. Torine IJ, et al. Effect of late-onset sepsis on energy expenditure in extremely premature infants. Pediatr Res 2007;(5 Pt 1):600-603.
9. Ledbetter DJ. Gastroschisis and omphalocele. Surgical Clinics of North America 2006; 86(2):249-260.
10. Javid PJ, et al. Survival rate in congenital diaphragmatic hernia: the experience of the Canadian Neonatal Network. J Pediatr Surg 2004;39(5):657-660.
11. Colvin J, et al. Outcomes of congenital diaphragmatic hernia: a population-based study in Western Australia. Pediatrics 2005;116(3):e356-e363.
12. Adzick NS, Nance ML. Pediatric surgery: second of two parts. N Engl J Med 2000;342(23):1726-1732.
13. Boloker J et al. Congenital diaphragmatic hernia in 120 infants treated consecutively with permissive hypercapnea/spontaneous respiration/elective repair. J Pediatr Surg 2002;37(3):357-366.
14. Holman RC et al. Necrotising enterocolitis hospitalisations among neonates in the United States. Paediatr Perinat Epidemiol 2006;20(6):498-506.
15. Ford HR. Mechanism of nitric oxide-mediated intestinal barrier failure: insight into the pathogenesis of necrotizing enterocolitis. J Pediatr Surg 2006;41(2):294-299.
16. Bell MJ et al. Neonatal necrotizing enterocolitis. Therapeutic decisions based upon clinical staging. Ann Surg 1978;187(1):1-7.
17. Sharma R et al. Impact of gestational age on the clinical presentation and surgical outcome of necrotizing enterocolitis. J Perinatol 2006;26(6):342-347.
18. Lin PW, Stoll BJ. Necrotising enterocolitis. Lancet 2006;368(9543):1271-1283.
19. Hajivassiliou CA. Intestinal obstruction in neonatal/pediatric surgery. Semin Pediatr Surg 2003;12(4):241-253.
20. Applegate KE, Anderson JM, Klatte EC. Intestinal malrotation in children: a problem-solving approach to the upper gastrointestinal series. Radiographics 2006;26(5):1485-500.
21. Strouse PJ. Disorders of intestinal rotation and fixation ("malrotation"). Pediatr Radiol 2004;34(11):837-851.
22. MacMahon B. The continuing enigma of pyloric stenosis of infancy: a review. Epidemiology 2006;17(2):195-201.
23. Vanderwinden JM et al. The pathology of infantile hypertrophic pyloric stenosis after healing. J Pediatr Surg 1996;31(11):1530-1534.
24. Kawahara H. Medical treatment of infantile hypertrophic pyloric stenosis: should we always slice the "olive"? J Pediatr Surg 2005;40(12):1848-1851.
25. Leinwand MJ, Shaul DB, Anderson KD. The umbilical fold approach to pyloromyotomy: is it a safe alternative to the right upper-quadrant approach? J Am Coll Surg 1999;189(4):362-367.

Chapter 19

ENDPOINTS OF RESUSCITATION: WHAT HAVE WE LEARNED?

Frederick A. Moore, MD, and Bruce A. McKinley, PhD

INTRODUCTION

Shock resuscitation is an obligatory intervention. Its optimal application is dependent on many factors including type and severity of shock, competing priorities, and physical setting/monitoring capabilities. Our primary interest, which will be the focus of this chapter, has been in optimizing resuscitation of major torso trauma patients without serious concomitant head injuries who present with life-threatening hemorrhage. This discussion will address (a) initial management, (b) the rationale for optimizing oxygen delivery, (c) resuscitating to supranormal oxygen delivery, (d) evolving experience with this approach, (e) development of a computerized decision support resuscitation protocol, (f) lessons learned, (g) current algorithms, and (f) conclusions.

INITIAL MANAGEMENT

Initial care of severely injured patients presenting in shock is prioritized to ensure survival. Advanced trauma life support (ATLS) is a time-honored management approach that has saved many lives. Empiric volume loading with large volume isotonic crystalloids is an emphasized early intervention. The response of blood pressure (BP) and heart rate (HR) to volume loading defines stability, which is key in triage decisions. For those who do not respond appropriately, diagnostic testing is focused on identifying sources of uncontrolled hemorrhage that need prompt attention in the operating room (OR) or interventional radiology (IR) suite. A controversy exists whether BP and HR should be normalized at this point. One recent well known prospective randomized trial (PRT) in penetrating torso demonstrated worse survival in those patients who were volume loaded before definitive vascular control was obtained in the OR, although subgroup analysis confined significance to only those with pericardial tamponade.[1] Whether early hypotensive resuscitation should be applied to blunt trauma patients is not clear. It is being practiced in at least one major U.S. trauma center and is becoming the current battlefield standard of care for special operation medics.[2-4] One unresolved issue in our patient cohort is that 20% of major torso trauma patients will have a serious concomitant closed head injury (CHI) and, if under resuscitated, decreased cerebral perfusion pressure (CPP) may result in devastating secondary brain injury. Fortunately, in most patients, there is time to obtain additional information. An arterial blood gas (ABG) with base deficit (BD) determination indicates the severity of shock and serial hemoglobin measurements assess ongoing bleeding. Additional monitoring should include central venous pressure (CVP, via central venous catheter), urine output rate (via Foley catheter), and arterial hemoglobin O_2 saturation (via pulse oximetry.) Current endpoints in emergency department (ED) resuscitation are to normalize BP and HR, establish urine output while maintaining CVP in a moderate range (8 to 12 mm Hg).

RATIONALE FOR OPTIMIZING OXYGEN DELIVERY (DO_2)

Once patients have had their diagnostic studies and their hemorrhage control interventions successfully completed, they are transferred to the intensive care unit (ICU) where optimized resuscitation is the major early priority. The primary goal of shock resuscitation is the early establishment of "adequate" DO_2 to vital organs. The yet to be resolved controversy is what is "adequate." DO_2 is the product of cardiac output (CO) and arterial oxygen content (CaO_2). By convention, CO is indexed to body surface area and expressed as cardiac index (CI), which when multiplied by CaO_2 yields an oxygen delivery index (DO_2). Normal DO_2 is roughly 450 ml/min/m²; it will increase by as much as 30% in response to injury. CaO_2 and DO_2 are calculated as follows:

$$CaO_2 \text{ (ml/dl)} = [Hb] \text{ (g/dl)} \times 1.38 \times SaO_2 \text{ (\%)}$$
$$+ [PaO_2 \text{ (mm Hg)} \times 0.003]$$
$$DO_2 \text{ (ml/min-m}^2) = CI \text{ (L/min-m}^2)$$
$$\times CaO_2 \text{ (ml/dl)} \times 10$$

where [Hb] is the hemoglobin concentration, SaO_2 is oxyhemoglobin saturation, PaO_2 is arterial oxygen tension, and 0.003 is the solubility of O_2 in blood. Thus, there are four variables (ie, PaO_2, SaO_2, [Hb], and CI) that determine DO_2. The following is a brief discussion of these oxygen transport variables.

ARTERIAL PARTIAL PRESSURE OF OXYGEN (PaO₂)

PaO_2 is monitored by intermittent or continuous arterial blood gas (ABG) analysis. The amount of oxygen dissolved in plasma is dependent upon the partial pressure of oxygen in the alveolar air. At a PaO_2 of 100 mm Hg, the amount of O_2 dissolved in the plasma is 0.3 ml/dl. At normal [Hb], this accounts for only 1.5% total oxygen carried in the blood. Dissolved oxygen in plasma does not contribute substantially to DO_2 until [Hb] becomes very low (eg, [Hb] < 4 gm/dl) or when hemoglobin cannot carry oxygen (eg, carbon monoxide poisoning). With exception of these examples, attempting to increase DO_2 by increasing PaO_2 does not make sense.

ARTERIAL HEMOGLOBIN OXYGEN SATURATION (SaO₂)

SaO_2 is monitored by continuous pulse oximetry or intermittent lab oximetry or intermittently calculated based on ABG results. Of the three, pulse oximetry is preferred because it is a simple, reliable, and reasonably accurate monitor. The oxyhemoglobin dissociation curve depicts the relationship between SaO_2 and PaO_2. At high SaO_2 (above 95%), a large increase in PaO_2 is needed to cause significant increase in SaO_2 and, in critically ill patients, this will require increased FIO_2. SaO_2 less than 92% falls on the portion of the oxyhemoglobin dissociation curve where the slope is steepest. This improves the pulse oximeters sensitivity for identifying changes in oxygenation (ie, a small drop in PaO_2 results in a significant drop in SaO_2), but does diminish DO_2. During resuscitation, we strive to maintain $SaO_2 \geq 92\%$. In general, this is not difficult because resuscitation is complete before acute lung injury becomes severe.

HEMOGLOBIN CONCENTRATION [Hb]

The traditional recommended "optimal" [Hb] in a stressed surgical patient is 10 gm/dl. This number was derived from isovolumic hemodilution models that demonstrate that the body compensates for decreased [Hb] by increasing CI, This is a result of decreased blood viscosity, which decreases afterload and increases venous return to the heart. Laboratory models and clinical studies of shock resuscitation have supported this recommendation. Recently, however, the fear of (a) transmitting infections, (b) amplifying proinflammation, and (c) inducing immunosuppression

has prompted recommendation that [Hb] = 7 gm/dl is "acceptable." In fact, a recent PRT demonstrated that ICU patients randomized to restrictive blood transfusions (transfuse if [Hb] < 7.0 gm/dl and maintain [Hb] between 7 to 9 gm/dl) did as well and possibly better than patients who were liberally transfused (transfuse if [Hb] < 10 gm/dl and maintain [Hb] between 10 and 12 gm/dl).[5] It is important to note that to be entered into this study, the patients had to be "considered to be euvolemic after initial treatment by attending physician" and have no evidence of active blood loss. Thus, this now often cited study is most likely not applicable to patients who urgently require shock resuscitation after major trauma. During acute shock resuscitation, it is recommended to maintain [Hb] $\geq$ 10 gm/dl in patients with evidence of ongoing bleeding and [Hb] should be monitored more frequently (ie, q 1-2 hours). After the patient has stabilized a [Hb] = 7 gm/dl is acceptable unless the patient has persistent significant tachycardia.

CARDIAC INDEX

CI is the last important oxygen transport variable to consider. Unfortunately, it is the most difficult variable to monitor as well as to manipulate. Thermodilution (TD) is used to measure CI because it is more convenient than alternative indicator dilution methods (direct Fick, dye dilution). For many years, CI by TD used a manual intermittent thermal dilution technique[6] with thermal dilution washout curves calculated by computerized algorithm. Since the mid-1990s, PA catheters have been available that provide continuous cardiac index measurement. They incorporate a heater element that is placed in the right ventricle. This filament delivers known, safe amounts of heat into the blood and the resulting temperature changes measured at the distal tip of the catheter "downstream" in the pulmonary artery are used to determine CI continuously from multiple thermal dilution washout curves. This technology has proved to be sufficiently accurate and precise, and has the advantage of continuous trending of CI, which gives a "real time" response to resuscitative efforts and decreases nursing time. At present, continuous TD using the PAC remains the method of choice to measure CI, although it does require placement of this invasive device. A PAC also provides the pulmonary capillary wedge pressure (PCWP) or, more recently, the right ventricular end diastolic volume index (RVEDVI), which are needed to optimize preload. PACs are relatively expensive, time consuming, potentially hazardous and logistically limits its use to the ICU. Thus, there is a need for less invasive methods to assess cardiac performance. Transthoracic electrical bioimpedance, transesophageal echocardiography, and Doppler ultrasound are continuous noninvasive CO monitor technologies that have challenged the role of TD via PAC. Although these alternatives perform reasonably well in stable patients, they have questionable accuracy in unstable patients. In recent years, several new or improved methods of accessing CI have been introduced into the clinical arena. These include (a) the lithium dilution technique, (b) arterial pressure waveform analyses, and (c) esophageal Doppler. These are not well tested in trauma resuscitation and would not likely be accepted as a standard of care. If $SaO_2 \geq 92\%$ and $[Hb] \geq 10$ gm/dl, CI is the key variable to focus on. Thermodilution is the current standard of care and a PAC capable continuous cardiac output and mixed venous oximetry is recommended.

RATIONALE FOR RESUSCITATION TO SUPRANORMAL DO_2

The rationale for using DO_2 as an endpoint for resuscitation originated with the physiologic observations made by Shoemaker and colleagues starting in the 1970s.[7-14] In an analysis of a large cohort of surgical patients they demonstrated that "supranormal" DO_2 index (ie, $DO_2 \geq 600$ mL/min-m^2) was associated with improved survival. They proposed that this "survivor response" to stressful insults become the resuscitation hemodynamic performance goal for high-risk patients. They developed an organized algorithmic strategy of fluid, blood, and inotrope therapy to achieve this DO_2 goal. In subsequent clinical trials, they demonstrated that the use of this "goal oriented" resuscitation protocol improved the rate of survival.[15] For several reasons, the concept of goal-oriented ICU resuscitation gained popularity in the early 1990s. "Damage control" laparotomy was becoming the standard care in many U.S. trauma centers.[16] An implicit purpose of truncating the initial laparotomy was early ICU triage to correct acidosis, coagulopathy, and hypothermia, all of which occur with effective resuscitation. Additionally, PAC continuous cardiac output technology became widely available, and permitted routine ICU monitoring of oxygen transport variables. Trauma surgeons could witness the "survival response" in their own ICUs. In fact, in 1992, we reported that the failure to achieve this "survival response" within 12 hours of ICU admission was highly predictive of subsequent development of post-injury multiple organ failure (MOF).[17] These data were consistent with the enticing hypothesis that unrecognized flow-dependent oxygen consumption (VO_2) was an important cause of MOF. In the early 1980s, MOF was recognized to be the leading cause of late post postinjury death and prolonged ICU stays.[18] Early studies from U.S. trauma centers conclude that MOF was the "fatal expression of unremitting sepsis." However, reports from Europe in the mid-1980s provided convincing evidence that early MOF frequently occurred in blunt trauma patients in the absence of infection. Shock appeared to be the overriding risk factor. The concept of resuscitating to supranormal DO_2 to eliminate flow-dependent VO_2 was championed by a number of well-known surgical

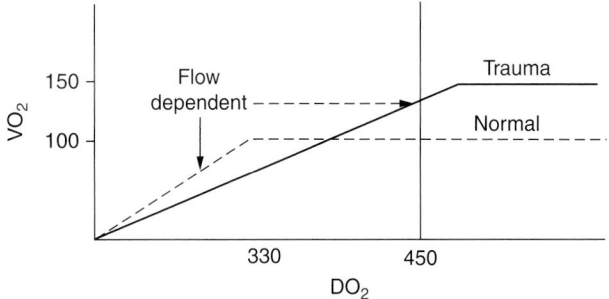

Figure 19-1 *Unrecognized flow-dependent VO_2. DO_2, oxygen delivery; VO_2, oxygen consumption.*

intensivists, and their explanation seemed sound physiologically. Figure 19-1 depicts the relationship between DO_2 and VO_2. Under normal conditions at a normal DO_2 of 450 mL/min-m^2, VO_2 is 100 mL/min-m^2. As DO_2 decreases VO_2 does not change. It is maintained by increasing O_2 extraction until DO_2 decreases below the critical level of 330 mL/min-m^2 after which VO_2 becomes flow dependent. This is normal physiology and a clinician recognizes that the patient is in shock because the patient has overt signs of shock (eg, tachycardia and hypotension). With conditions of severe traumatic shock, this relationship changes in several ways: (1) VO_2 increase from 100 to 150 mL/min-m^2, (2) Oxygen extraction is impaired (ie, the slope of the flow-dependent portion of the curve decreases), and (3) myocardial dysfunction is common. Thus, it is conceivable that a patient could have a normal DO_2 and have flow-dependent VO_2. This is not recognized by the clinician because the patient is not in overt shock as defined by traditional vital signs.

EVOLVING EXPERIENCE WITH RESUSCITATION TO SUPRANORMAL DO_2

Throughout the 1990s, a series of prospective randomized trials (PRTs) were performed to test the hypothesis that resuscitation to supranormal DO_2 improved survival.[19-23] These PRTs failed to find consistent outcome advantages with this approach. These disparate results may be explained by a number of confounding variables, the most important being (a) age and comorbid disease, (b) variable timing of resuscitation, (c) different interventions, and (d) responders versus nonresponders. Shoemaker's original studies were designed to optimize DO_2 prior to a major operative insult and to maintain it perioperatively.[14] Further reports focused on severe trauma patients, and demonstrated improved survival.[15] Other investigators have studied nonsurgical ICU patients with established sepsis, septic shock, or ARDS.[19] These patients already had organ failure, and it is not surprising that outcome was not improved.

In the most recent PRT from Velmahos, Shoemaker, and colleagues, trauma patients who achieved supranormal goals, spontaneously or through intervention (ie, the responders) had improved survival rate (100 vs 70%), and less organ failure (29 vs 70%) compared to those patients who did not achieve supranormal goals (ie, the nonresponders).[24] However, in contrast with their previous PRTs, the intent to treat to $DO_2 \geq 600$ mL/min-m^2 was not associated with increased survival (85 vs 89%), or decreased organ failure (38 vs 57%). A criticism of this study is that the supranormal (experiment) and normal (control) resuscitated patients were managed by a trauma team with an established practice pattern of supranormal resuscitation, and there was no difference the average volume of fluid (~14 vs 13 L) or blood (~11 vs ~11 units) given to either group. The only apparent difference was the fraction of patients in each group to receive inotrope support during the first 24 hours after hospital admission (32 vs 17%). DO_2 versus time data are not reported, but are likely not significantly different between groups. Resuscitation to "supranormal" goals as described by Shoemaker and colleagues has been the subject of hundreds of reviews, editorials, and meta analyses and remains controversial.[25-29] Based on our recent experience (described later in this chapter), we do not advocate aggressive application of this concept.

DEVELOPMENT OF COMPUTERIZED DECISION SUPPORT FOR SHOCK RESUSCITATION

In 1993, our group became a test site for assessing the feasibility of computerized bedside decision support of mechanical ventilation of ARDS. This PRT was completed in 1998, and demonstrated that the cohort managed with computerized decision support received much more consistent care.[30] Recognizing that this technology could be applied to other aspects of care, we pursued development of a decision support tool for shock resuscitation. Development of clinical logic was done by a consensus group of trauma surgeon/intensivists, ICU nurses, and biomedical engineers/informaticists. Initial tasks were to identify the essential variables and thresholds for intervention required to drive a logical algorithm. These variables and thresholds were evidence based or, if unavailable, local expert opinion. The required variables were determined to be [Hb], CI, SaO_2, PCWP, base deficit (BD), and lactate concentration. We later added urinary bladder pressure as an index of intra-abdominal pressure (IAP) and gastric tonometry to measure regional gastric mucosal PCO_2 as index of gut perfusion. Requirement for a PAC was justified with knowledge that cardiac dysfunction is difficult to recognize by standard clinical criteria sund, if monitoring is delayed until obvious, dysfunction is often irreversible. Controversy notwithstanding,[31,32] PACs were used liberally in most U.S. trauma centers in patients with evidence of ongoing hemorrhagic shock. The PAC incorporating continuous cardiac output thermodilution and mixed venous oximetry technology became the clinical standard for monitoring the hemodynamically unstable major trauma victim.[6] Our next task was to identify specific criteria that would identify high-risk patients on ICU admission who would benefit from resuscitation. Our basic premise is that shock is the major modifiable risk factor for the postinjury MOF. Based on previous work we identified early risk factors for MOF.[33,34] A checklist to meet specific criteria consistently was developed: (1) severe torso trauma (≥ 2 abdominal organ, ≥ 3 rib fractures, major vascular injury, complex pelvic fracture, or ≥ 2 long bone fractures), (2) anticipated need for ≥ 6 units packed red blood cell (PRBC) transfusion, and (3) early $BD \geq 6$ mEq/L.

The resulting protocol directed $DO_2 \geq 600$ mL O_2/min-m^2 for 24 hours as the goal using four sequential algorithms for interventions: (1) transfusion of packed red blood cells (PRBC) if [Hb] < 10 g/dL and volume loading with lactated Ringer solution (LR) if PCWP < 15 mm Hg, (2) CI-PCWP optimization ("Starling curve") if [Hb] ≥ 10, PCWP ≥ 15 and DO_2 < 600, (3) inotrope (dobutamine) if [Hb] ≥ 10, PCWP ≥ 15, DO_2 < 600, and (4) vasopressor (norepinephrine) if mean arterial pressure (MAP) < 65 mm Hg.[30-33] With this standardized, data driven protocol, we found the incidence of therapies to be consistent with the hierarchical design, that is fluid and blood used predominantly, inotrope agent used less frequently.[35] The protocol was implemented at bedside in the ICU using paper logic flow diagrams and text description through mid-2000. Since mid-2000, the protocol has been implemented using computerized logic. The algorithms were developed as described originally by Morris and colleagues.[36,37] This has offered the unique opportunity to prospectively record how patients respond to various interventions. A software application was developed in-house and used at bedside using a portable laptop workstation and touch-screen display. This technology has proven reliable to guide decision making for nurses and physicians. A standardized, data-driven process is guided by logical responses to requested measurements that are compared to thresholds. In our experience, over 95% of the computerized instructions are accepted and implemented by the bedside clinicians. The ICU nurses were initially resistant to accepting this as standard care. However, once they gained experience they liked it for several reasons. The trauma surgeon identified the high-risk candidates prior to ICU admission. A special cart was designed that contained all essential equipment and supplies necessary to implement the protocol. The protocol was a proactive logical plan in which the nurses had ownership. Nursing representatives were part of the multidisciplinary team, which designed and refined the protocol. They witnessed continued improvement in the protocol through process review and data analysis. An example of the precision of controlling the process with this computerized technology is described in the section Decreasing DO_2 Goal Reduced Incidence of ACS.

WHAT WE HAVE LEARNED

ELDERLY TRAUMA PATIENTS

Whereas the ICU nurses became protocol advocates, they questioned the wisdom of doing this in elderly patients. Shock is not well tolerated in the elderly trauma patient, but these patients are also vulnerable to complications from aggressive preload-directed intervention. Therefore, one of our first studies was to determine how the elderly patients responded to the protocol.[38] Typically, elderly patients start resuscitation with pathologically low DO_2 ~ 260 mL O_2/min-m^2. They respond well to volume loading, but are much more likely to require inotrope support. Their maximum DO_2 response (~550 mL O_2/min-m^2) is less than that of the younger patients (~700 mL O_2/min-m^2). Similar to previous reports from Scalea et al[39] and Yu et al,[23] our elderly patients appeared to benefit from resuscitation and had minimal complications attributable to the process. With their limited DO_2 response and need for inotrope support to achieve this, however, we decreased the endpoint/goal to $DO_2 \geq 500$ mL O_2/min-m^2 for elderly trauma patients (ie, age $\geq$ 65).

Preload-Directed Intervention to Optimize Cardiac Performance

In our experience, volume loading is the first and most efficacious approach to improve cardiac function following severe injury.[40,41] The traditional variable used to assess volume status is the PCWP. It is important to recognize that significant hypovolemia can exist despite reasonable PCWP. Peripheral vasoconstriction of less essential organs (eg, kidney, gut, muscle, and skin) results in blood volume shift to maintain the central circulation and perfusion of more essential organs (eg, heart and brain). With initial volume resuscitation, peripheral vasodilation can result in a paradoxical decrease in PCWP. Consequently, with relatively low PWCP (ie, < 12 mm Hg), volume loading should be undertaken. After PCWP increases to $\geq$ 15 mm Hg, the benefits of increasing myocardial performance by the Frank Starling mechanism must be weighed against the potential risk of increased hydrostatic pressure leading to increased pulmonary edema in patients with endothelial cell damage. Here an assessment should be done concerning whether additional CI is needed and if so, then proceed in a stepwise fashion to identify the optimal PCWP. Because the shape and position of the Frank Starling curve is

dependent on left ventricular contractility, compliance and afterload, it is difficult to identify optimal or plateau levels during volume loading without frequent sequential measurements during volume loading. A precipitous increase in PCWP during volume loading signals that the limit of stretch of the myocardium has been reached.

Therefore, for patients who do not respond to initial volume loading and PRBC transfusion, we developed an algorithm to optimize cardiac performance using the "Starling curve" concept. We have found "Starling curve" generation to be feasible and to reliably improve cardiac performance (Fig. 19-2).[41] However, a subset of this cohort of patients is "nonresponders." These patients do not vasodilate with initial volume loading. Additional volume loading in the setting of persistent high systemic vascular resistance (SVR) sets the stage for problematic tissue edema. We have restricted the use of the "Starling curve" intervention in our protocol. The computer instructs the bedside clinician to consult the in-house trauma attending before implementing this intervention. We avoid using it in patients with pulmonary contusions, acute lung injury and significant intra-abdominal hypertension (described later in this chapter).

Our experience is very similar to that of the Wake Forest group. They have extensively studied optimization of cardiac performance in this cohort of patients. They, instead, use a right ventricular ejection fraction (RVEF) PAC that incorporates a rapid response thermistor at the tip that allows the analysis of beat-to-beat temperature changes in the pulmonary artery.[6] The computer calculates the right ventricular ejection fraction by analyzing the temperature decay curve over consecutive beats. This has been promoted to reflect right ventricular contractility. The stroke volume index is calculated by dividing the CI by the HR. The right ventricular end diastolic volume index (RVEDVI) is calculated by dividing the stroke volume index by the ejection fraction. This has been promoted

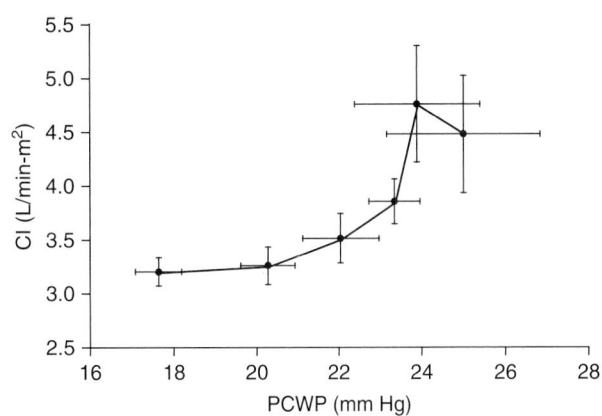

Figure 19-2 *CI, cardiac index; PCWP, pulmonary capillary wedge pressure.*

to reflect right ventricular preload and several investigators have provided reasonably convincing data that the RVEDVI is a better reflection of preload than PCWP. The Wake Forest group uses RVEDVI as their index of pre preload. In a study by Miller et al, high-risk patients were volume loaded to euvolemia (defined as a RVEDVI of 90-100 mL/m^2). They then randomized the nonresponders to additional volume loading to a RVEDVI of 120 mL/m^2 or treatment with inotrope support (dopamine or epinephrine). They demonstrated that the best response for improving visceral perfusion was achieved with the additional volume loading.[42]

Our Experience Resuscitation with Afterload Reduction

Patients who have sustained blunt thoracic aortic injury (TAI) and undergo early operative repair frequently require postoperative ICU resuscitation. These patients are admitted to the Shock Trauma ICU and, if indicated, are resuscitated by the standardized protocol. Early in our experience, the cardiothoracic surgeons were adamant that blood pressure needed to be controlled and would write a standing order for sodium nitroprusside (Nipride). Hypertension was rarely a problem upon ICU admission, but with progressive volume loading, it would occur and Nipride titration would be started. To our surprise, no adverse events occurred. In fact, the hemodynamic response was quite favorable.[43] Analysis of data from 11 TAI patients over a 9-month period in whom sodium nitroprusside was titrated to control MAP < 90 mm Hg, DO$_2$ increased rapidly during the initial 4 hours from 511 ± 56 to 643 ± 47 mL/min-m^2, and attained a maximum of ~700 mL/min-m^2 at 12 hours. On ICU admission these patients had elevated SVR and, coincident with Nipride infusion, there was a notable decrease in SVR.[43] While we have not made this part of our standard protocol, we are currently working on the logic and are testing it in isolated patients who present when we can intensively monitor them. The basic question is what level of PCWP to maintain after Nipride is started. We have noted that PCWP decreases significantly after Nipride is started in some patients. Maintaining PCWP at the pre-Nipride levels in these patients requires a lot of volume loading. An alternative strategy may be to use colloid and decrease the PCWP threshold at this time, because most of these patients would have already received large volumes of isotonic crystalloid.

Our observation that patients with persistently high SVR benefit from afterload reduction is consistent with recent observations from the Wake Forest group. In ongoing studies, they have shown that after preload optimization (described earlier), further improvement in myocardial performance can be achieved by the using inotropic agents and/or afterload reduction to optimize stroke work index (SWI) and ventricular-arterial coupling (VAC).[44] In their most recent work, they have validated that early optimized SWI and VAC by this approach is highly predictive for improved survival.[45] These data indicate that vasoactive agents should be used more frequently in the "nonresponders."

The Epidemic of Abdominal Compartment Syndrome (ACS)

With aggressive application of "damage control" surgery and early triage to the ICU to optimize resuscitation, patients who would have previously exsanguinated in the operating room were now surviving. However, with ongoing experience it became obvious that an epidemic of ACS was occurring. In the mid-1990s, reports from a number of well-known trauma centers documented that up to 36% of patients undergoing "damage control" surgery developed ACS.[46] In the late 1990s, a new entity called "secondary" ACS emerged.[47] This occurs in patients without intra-abdominal injuries who require massive resuscitation for injuries in which hemorrhage control is difficult or delayed (eg, pelvic fractures, mangled extremities). Recognition of this epidemic prompted our group to perform a series database studies in which we sought to clarify the epidemiology of ACS. We did this with the purpose of designing alternative strategies to avoid it.[48-51] In the initial study, 14% of patients developed ACS. Half were primary ACS (ie, associated with intra abdominal injuries).[49] These patients had undergone damage-control surgery and developed the "bloody vicious cycle" of hypothermia, acidosis, and coagulopathy. The other half developed secondary ACS patients. These patients arrived in the emergency department (ED) in shock; however, the severity of shock was not initially appreciated in the ED, excessive volumes of crystalloid were being administered, and/or the sources of bleeding were not immediately controllable. We found that ACS was associated with a high rate of MOF (55% in primary vs 53% in secondary vs 12% in non-ACS patients; p < 0.05) and death (63% in primary vs 53% in secondary vs 17 % in non-ACS patients, p < 0.05). Additionally, ACS was an independent risk factor for MOF (odds ratio = 9.2, 95% CI: 3.8-22.8) and death (odds ratio = 8.4, 95% CI: 3.0-20.6).

ACS is an Early Predictable ICU Event

We found that ACS was an early event occurring at a mean of 13 hours after arriving in the ED. We designed prediction models.[49] The first was based on clinical data that was readily available within 3 hours of admission (ED model) and the second was done with data available at 6 hours (ICU model). The independent predictors in the ED model for primary ACS were (1) crystalloid infusion = 3 L and (2) time to OR arrival = 75 min. The area under the curve (AUC) of the receiver operating characteristic (ROC) curve for this model was 0.92. The independent predictors in the ED model for secondary ACS were (1) crystalloid infusion = 3 L, (2) no urgent surgery, and (3) PRBC transfusion = 3 units. The AUC of the ROC curve for this model was 0.91. The independent predictors in the ICU model for primary ACS were (1) temperature = 34°C, (2) $PrCO_2$ – $PaCO_2$ = 16 mm Hg, (3) [Hb] = 8 g/dl, and (4) BD = 12 mEq/l, and AUC of the ROC curve was 0.97. The independent predictors in the ICU model for secondary ACS were (1) crystalloid infusion = 7.5L, (2) $PrCO_2$ – $PaCO_2$ = 16 mm Hg, and (3) urine output < 150 ml/h, and the AUC of the ROC curve was 0.98. Although these models need to be validated, the AUCs are surprisingly high, especially for the ICU model. This means that the clinical trajectory of primary and secondary ACS is fairly well set by the time these patients are admitted to the ICU.

Patients with Impending ACS Do Not Respond to Pre-load-Directed Interventions

Patients with impending ACS arrive in the ICU ~6 hours after hospital admission with high IAP (mean 19 mm Hg). They did not respond to preload-directed interventions, and, in fact, these interventions precipitated full-blown ACS.[51] The typical scenario is that major trauma patients present in the ICU with decreased CI, normal PCWP, and increased IAP. Conventional wisdom is that increased IAP artifactually increases PCWP to greater than normal. As a result, volume loading with crystalloid is recommended. Intravascular effects of crystalloid infusion include decreased colloid oncotic pressure and increased hydrostatic pressure. The latter increases PCWP, and in most patients CI increases. Increased preload also causes bowel edema, which increases IAP, causes venous obstruction and worsens bowel edema. The clinician does not recognize that this is happening. Preloading continues because CI continues to increase. At some point, however, increased bowel edema causes IAP to increase to a point that heart function can no longer be improved, and, if this happens early, the patient becomes a "nonresponder." Not recognizing that this has occurred, preloading continues, but now the only effect is progressive bowel edema, and worsening IAP and venous obstruction. IAP increases to a recognized pathologic pressure range and is associated with decreased CI, decreased urine output, and decreased systemic oxygenation. The full-blown ACS emerges. We termed this "futile crystalloid loading" (Fig. 19-3).

Decreasing DO₂ Goal Reduced Incidence of ACS

In September 2000, Velmahos et al published their above described PRT.[24] Based on these data plus our ongoing recognition of the "nonresponder," we decreased our DO_2 goal from ≥ 600 to 500 mL/min-m² in January 2001. After 17 months, we performed follow-up database analysis to determine the impact of this change in DO_2 goal. We compared 85 patients resuscitated to DO_2 ≥ 600 over 17 months prior to the change

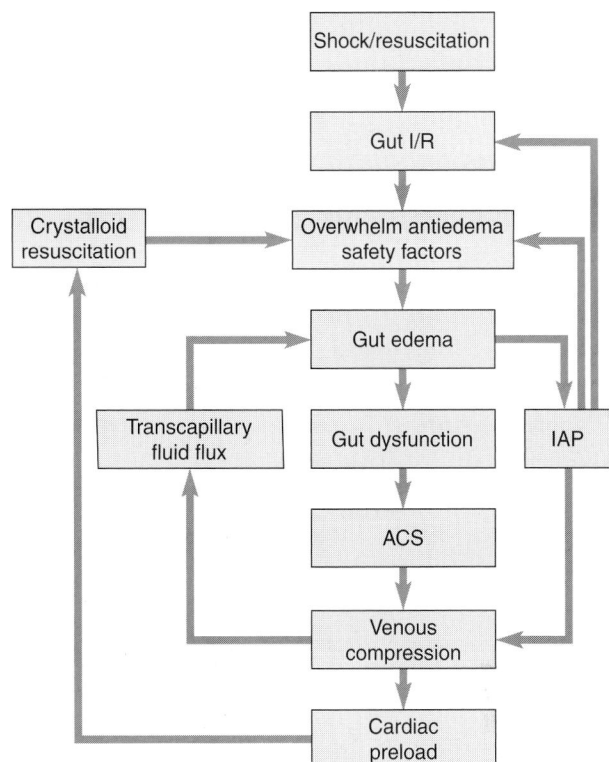

Figure 19-3 *I/R , ischemia/reperfusion; IAP, intra-abdominal pressure; ACS, abdominal compartment syndrome.*

to 71 patients resuscitated to a DO_2 ≥ 500 after the change.[50] The groups were comparable on ICU admission. The CI and SvO_2 response (Figs. 19-4A, 19-4B) to the ICU protocol and clearance of metabolic acidosis (Figs. 19-5A, 19-5B) were surprisingly similar. The DO_2 ≥ 600 cohort received significantly more crystalloid by protocol (Fig. 19-6A) and there was a trend for more PRBC transfusion (Fig. 19-6B). Of note, the DO_2 ≥ 600 cohort had greater incidence of IAP > 20 mm Hg (42%* vs 20%; * p < 0.05), ACS (16%* vs 8%), MOF (22%* vs 9%) and death (27%* vs 11%). Although this was not a PRT, these were prospectively collected data derived from a data-driven computerized decision support protocol. From these data, we conclude that supranormal DO_2 resuscitation in "nonresponders" is harmful.

Base Deficit as an Endpoint

Davis and colleagues showed ED BD to have strong association with blood loss, crystalloid fluid infusion, need for operative intervention, and mortality after trauma.[52-56] As a result, BD has become a standard method of assessing the severity of shock. In our experience, serial BD determinations can be used as an index of adequacy of resuscitation (Fig. 19-5B). Determination of BD requires discrete sample analysis that is typically done using a blood gas analyzer in a clinical laboratory. It is important to remember that sodium bicarbonate administration to correct acidosis improves BD but does not reverse shock.

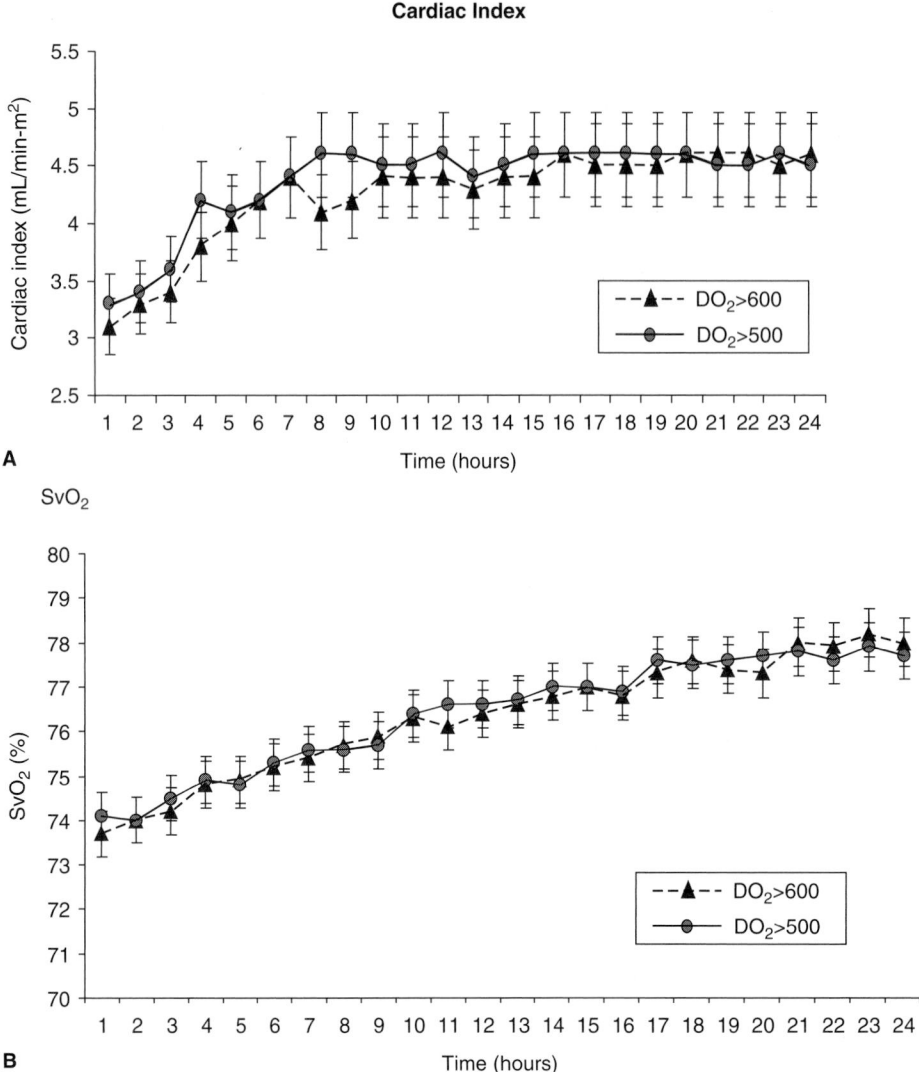

Figure 19-4 *SvO₂, mixed venous Hb O₂ saturation; DO₂, oxygen delivery.*

Lactate as an Endpoint

Lactate concentration is another variable that is commonly used to assess the severity of shock.[57,58] In the setting of traumatic shock, increased lactate concentration is assumed to be the result of anaerobic glycolysis, but increased lactate concentration can result from other causes. In our resuscitation experience, serial lactate concentration measurements have time course similar to serial BD determinations (Fig. 19-5A). Lactate is also an intermittent measurement done in the clinical laboratory. Increased lactate concentration that persists after 12 hours of ongoing resuscitation is probably indicative of defective mitochondrial function in peripheral tissues due to prolonged hypoperfusion, hypoxemia, and acidemia, and these patients are at high risk to develop late MOF.[59] Conceptually, this is similar to resuscitating patients with advanced septic shock. Early volume loading has been shown to be beneficial, but aggressive resuscitation in the later stages does not improve outcome

and a persistent increased lactate concentration is highly predictive of demise. An alternative metabolic explanation is that high lactate concentration occurs following severe insults because excessive mobilized substrates cannot be processed metabolically (ie, via the Krebs cycle).[60,61] As a result, there is a buildup of intracellular pyruvate that is converted to lactate which then exits the cell for transport back to the liver to be converted into glucose (ie, the Cori cycle). Thus, increased lactate concentration at the end of resuscitation simply reflects a more severe stress response.

Regional Gastric Mucosal PCO₂ (PrCO₂)

Disproportionate splanchnic vasoconstriction occurs with traumatic shock and does not normalize despite adequate systemic resuscitation. PrCO₂ measured by gastric tonometry increases in this situation and has been promoted to be a monitor of gut perfusion. Regional PCO₂ increases due to insufficient clearance of

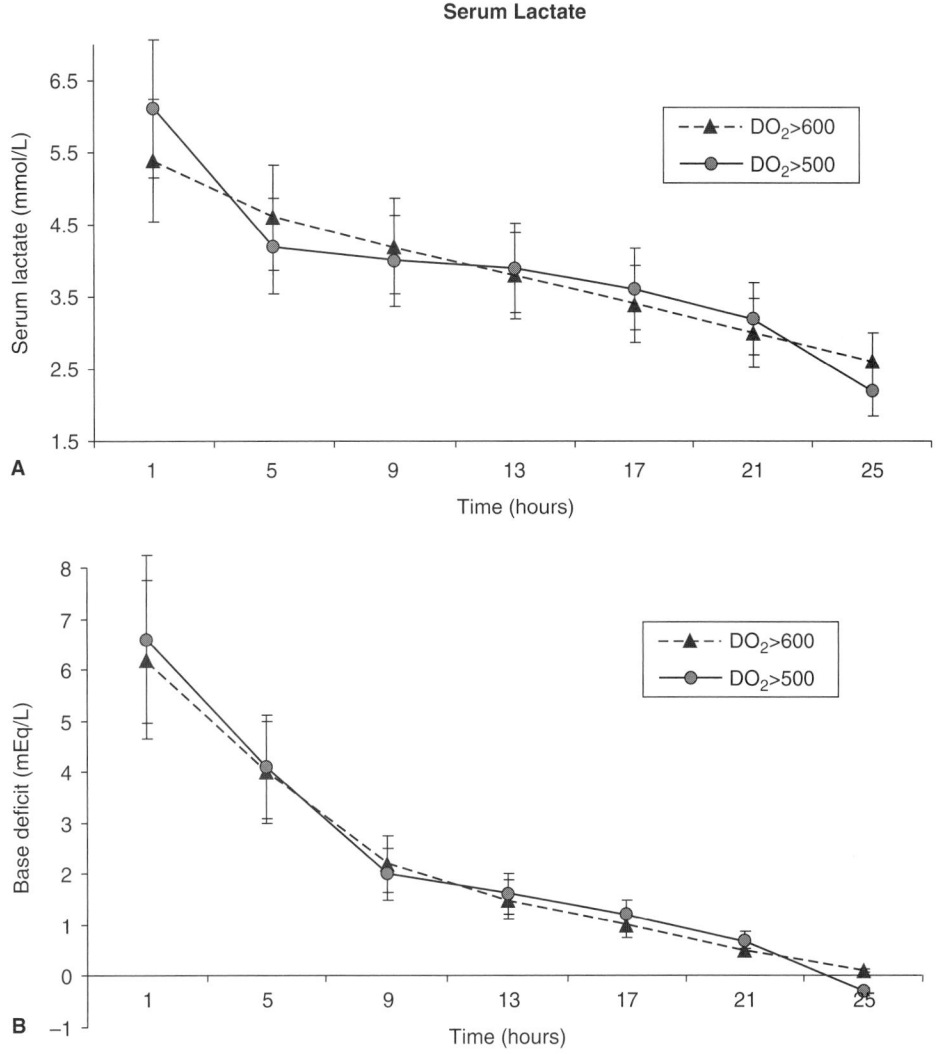

Figure 19-5 *DO₂, oxygen delivery.*

CO_2 produced by normal aerobic metabolism or due to buffering of acid production during anaerobic metabolism. Because gut ischemia reperfusion is believed to play a central role in MOF, this monitor is enticing. It has been considered as a valid alternative to the PAC and DO_2 to guide shock resuscitation.[62-66] In our experience, $PrCO_2$ is remarkably insensitive to our resuscitation process. Initially, it will be very elevated (ie, > 60 mmHg) in patients with severe systemic hypotension and decreases with resuscitation. However, it then begins to increase with ongoing resuscitation in the more severely injured as a result of increasing IAP characteristic of impending ACS.[51] As part of the protocol, we monitored $PrCO_2$ continuously and urinary bladder pressure (UBP) at 4-hour intervals. As $PrCO_2$ increases, we increase the frequency of UBP measurements to 1-hour intervals to not miss rapidly increases in IAP. With impending ACS (IAP >20 mm Hg), the abdomen is on the steep portion of its compliance curve where a modest increase in intra-abdominal contents can result in a sharp rise in IAP.

Fundamental Changes in Pre-ICU Care are Needed

A basic problem with this patient cohort is that virtually all require hemorrhage control interventions prior to ICU admission and the clinical course of the most severely injured is already set on ICU admission. The ICU resuscitation protocol does not help these patients; in fact, it harms them. The only recourse for these severely injured patients is to radically change pre-ICU care. Although standard of care ATLS (ie, large volume isotonic crystalloid infusion followed by PRBC transfusion to normal BP) is directed reversing shock, this does not limit reperfusion-induced inflammation and injury. The opposite occurs; it is worsened. Alternative types of fluids (eg, hypertonic saline) should be considered and are currently being tested. Additionally, standard of care ATLS also promotes coagulopathy. A good example is patients who have severe bleeding from pelvic fractures. Traditionally, these patients have been resuscitated to normal BP and observed for recurrent episodes of hypotension or ongoing transfusion requirement before

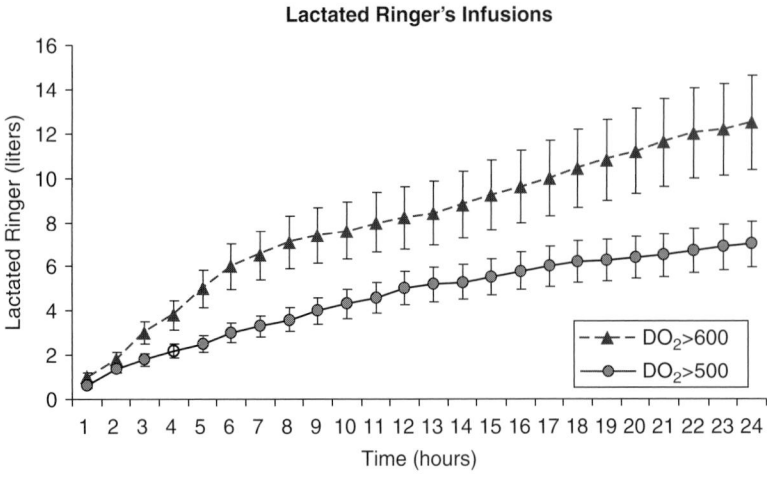

Figure 19-6 *A. Lactated Ringer infusions. B. Packed red blood cell transfusions. DO₂, oxygen delivery.*

angioembolization would be employed. Our new Pelvic Fracture Protocol (Fig. 19-7), prioritizes hemorrhage control and prevention of coagulopathy. Hemodynamically unstable patients undergo initial AP pelvic x-rays. If an unstable pelvic fracture is identified a pelvic binder is placed, the Orthopedic Service is consulted, and blood transfusions are started. Our Massive Transfusion Protocol is invoked as soon as the Trauma Surgeon recognizes that a massive transfusion will be required. Our blood bank has fresh thawed plasma immediately available. PRBC and fresh-thawed plasma are given in a ratio of 1:1[67] a trauma ultrasound exam is done and if positive the patient is triaged to the OR unless shock resolves with modest volume loading. If the trauma ultrasound is negative but patient is still in obvious shock, a peritoneal aspirate (PA) is done via a standard diagnostic peritoneal lavage catheter. If the PA is grossly positive the patient goes to the OR. Stabilized patients rapidly undergo for whole body CT scanning. If a vascular blush on pelvic CT scan the patient is triaged to interventional radiology for angioembolization. Unless there is a concern for a significant CHI, normalizing BP is strongly discouraged until hemorrhage control is complete.

Less Invasive Monitors Are Needed in the ED

Although our resuscitation protocol is a reliable process, it is restricted to the ICU where a PAC can be placed. Other less invasive monitors are needed, especially in the ED. Shoemaker and colleagues have demonstrated that transcutaneous PO_2 and PCO_2 monitoring is accurate and useful in shock resuscitation.[68-73] Additionally, they have demonstrated utility of transthoracic electrical bioimpedance (TEB) to monitor CO and to detect myocardial dysfunction in the ED. Using newer TEB technology they have successfully direct ED trauma resuscitation.[74]

Whereas placement of a PAC is difficult in the ED, the same fiber optic oximetry technology in a central venous catheter (CVC) to monitor central venous (superior vena cava) Hb O_2 saturation ($ScvO_2$) is now available, and placement a CVC in the ED is frequent if not standard practice.[75] Although $ScvO_2$ is not the same as mixed venous Hb O_2 saturation measured by a PAC, the principle that these variables reflect the balance between DO_2 and VO_2 is familiar to most clinicians. This technology is known to provide an accurate, stable measurement and a recent PRT in which $ScvO_2$ was used as the endpoint in ED resuscitation of

Pelvic Fracture Protocol

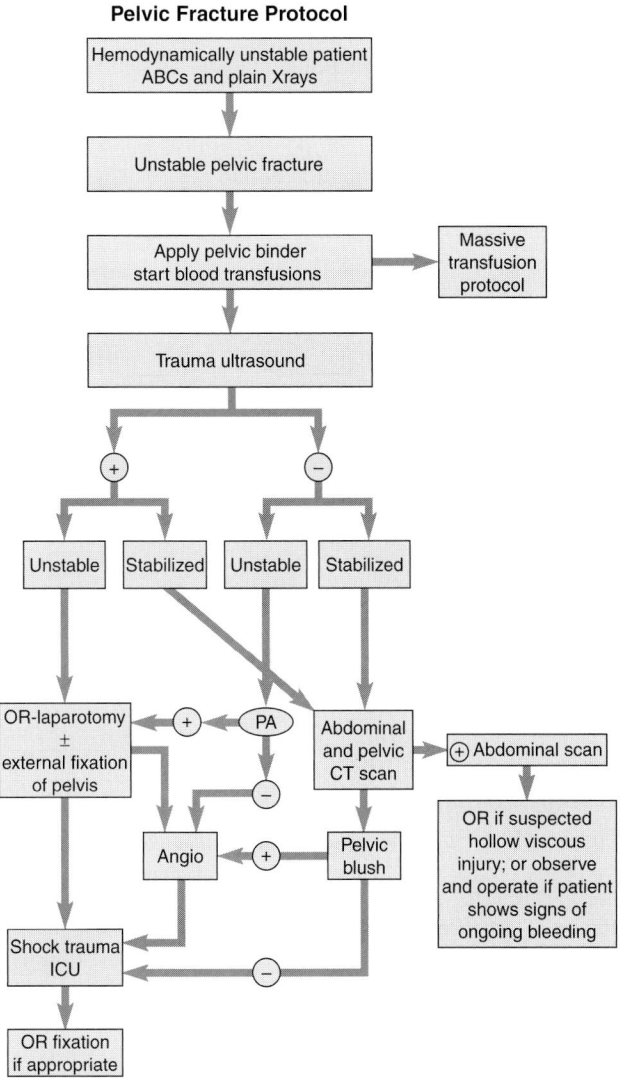

Figure 19-7 *Pelvic fracture protocol. ABCs, airway, breathing, and circulation; OR, operating room; PA, peritoneal aspirate.*

septic shock demonstrated improved survival compared to routine care.[76] Use of CVP, [Hb], SBP and ScvO$_2$ to monitor hemodynamic performance and to guide traditional intervention has the potential to improve resuscitation of the major trauma victim with earlier and less aggressive intervention.

Other monitor systems are available or in development that are minimally invasive, and provide measurements that are directed at use in the ED for early recognition of shock. For example, near infrared spectrometry (NIRS) quantitatively monitors Hb O$_2$ saturation in skeletal muscle and subcutaneous tissue (StO$_2$) and these can function as an index of tissue perfusion. In a recent study, we used NIRS to monitor StO$_2$ in the deltoid region during shock resuscitation and found that StO$_2$ closely correlated with DO$_2$.[77] NIRS also has the potential to simultaneously monitor the aa$_3$ redox

state, which reflects mitochondrial oxygen consumption.[59] Another monitor technology, fiber optic PO$_2$, PCO$_2$, and pH sensors could provide endpoints for resuscitation.[78] We have studied placement of extremely small probes with PO$_2$, PCO$_2$, and pH sensors directly in skeletal muscle and successfully monitored resuscitation responses.[79] Skeletal muscle pH (pHt) seems to be an index of overall resuscitation, PtO$_2$ a direct monitor of oxygenation, and PtCO$_2$ a sensitive monitor of perfusion.[80] Another monitor system that is available and was tested early in its development as a monitor of sepsis, shock, and resuscitation is the tissue electrode PO$_2$ sensor. Increased skeletal muscle interstitial PO$_2$ (PtO$_2$) has been shown to distinguish sepsis from cardiogenic shock.[81] Another technology related to fiber optic sensors and GI tract tonometry is sublingual PCO$_2$ measurement using a new hand-held fiber optic sensor system. This system is intended for use in early diagnosis of shock in the ED.[82]

CURRENT ALGORITHMS

From 2001 to 2005, we participated in the NIGMS sponsored Glue Grant entitled "Inflammation and the Host Response to Injury."[83] Our group was assigned to develop a Standard Operating Procedure (SOP) to guide shock resuscitation. The first section of the SOP provides a concise summary of the rationale of monitoring, interventions, and endpoints used in the protocol. The second section contains annotated algorithms to guide resuscitation in the ED and ICU. Figure 19-8 depicts initial resuscitation in the ED. In brief summary, patients who arrive in shock will be managed by ATLS and have an arterial blood gas (ABG) obtained. Patients with signs of significant shock (documented systolic blood pressure < 90 mm Hg or BD ≥ 6 mEq/L) will have a CVC placed. Patients will then be resuscitated until stable or until [Hb] ≥ 10 g/dl and CVP ≥ 10 mm Hg. Figure 19-9 depicts resuscitation in the ICU. The key ICU admission decision is whether to continue with the CVC protocol or to place a PAC to guide more intensive interventions. If a PAC is placed, then the goal should be to obtain CI ≥ 3.8 mL/min-m^2. Unrecognized myocardial dysfunction is the primary problem in patients not responding to volume loading. The transfusion trigger during acute resuscitation is [Hb] < 10 g/dl, then decreasing to < 7 g/dl once the patient stabilizes. We advised that aggressive preload-directed interventions (eg, "Starling curve") be used cautiously in nonresponding patients. We acknowledged that very little data existed on the optimal use of specific inotrope and vasoactive agents in refractory traumatic shock. We recommended specific agents based on known physiologic effects in less critically ill patients and recommended titration to the desired physiologic end points.

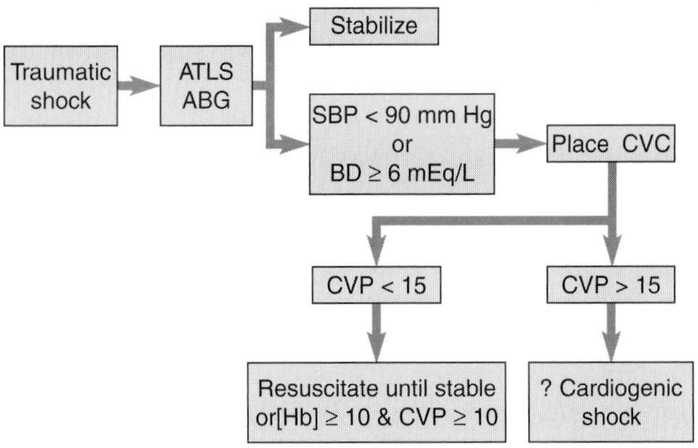

Initial CVC Resuscitation

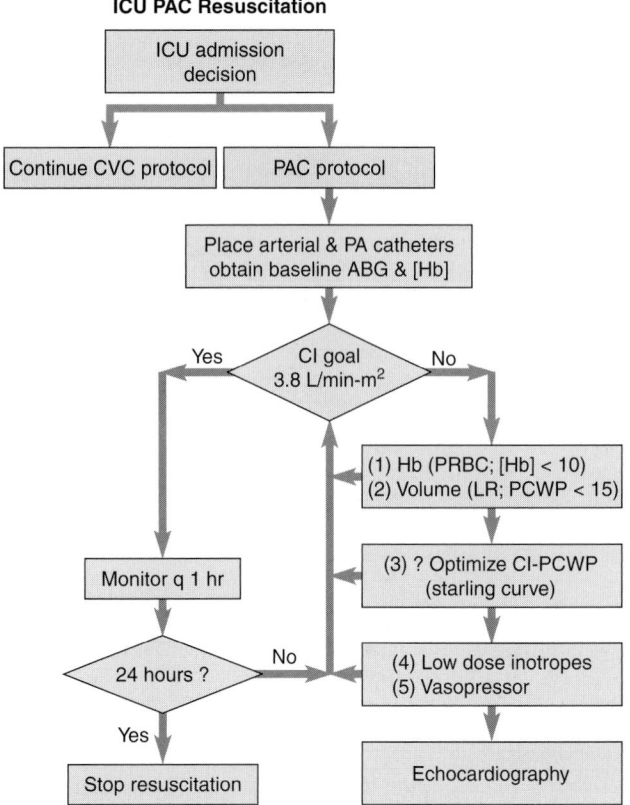

Figure 19-8   *Initial CVC resuscitation. ATLS, advanced trauma life support; ABG, arterial blood gas; SBP, systolic blood pressure; BD, base deficit; CVC, central venous catheter; CVP, central venous pressure; [Hb], hemoglobin concentration.*

CONCLUSION

Supranormal DO_2 ($\geq$ 600 mL O_2/min-m^2) is the only resuscitation endpoint that has been tested in PRTs and the results are inconclusive. Our experience indicates that a supranormal DO_2 should not be aggressively pursued. Responders generate this without difficulty, but the nonresponders are harmed by this approach. DO_2 is a useful endpoint because it integrates three important variables (ie, SaO_2, [Hb] and CI), but the key variable in detecting nonresponders is CI. The goal should be early identification of the nonresponders in the ED. Our prediction models suggest this is feasible. Alternative pre-ICU intervention strategies and monitoring technologies are needed. Early hemorrhage control and prevention of coagulopathy are of paramount importance. These patients should initially be resuscitated by the CVC protocol. Permissive hypotension should be encouraged as long as there is low suspicion for CHI until hemorrhage control is complete. When these patients arrive in the ICU they should be closely scrutinized for evidence of ongoing shock. Those that are not responding to volume preloading to CVP = 10 mm Hg should have a PAC placed to guide resuscitation. Aggressive preload interventions should be minimized in the nonresponders. Inotrope and vasodilator agents should be titrated for

Figure 19-9   *ICU PAC resuscitation. CVC; central venous catheter; PAC, pulmonary artery catheter; ABG, arterial blood gas; [Hb], Hemoglobin concentration; CI, cardiac index; LR, lactated ringers.*

known physiologic effects. The standardized process is more important than the specific endpoint. Our computerized decision support tool keeps the clinician focused on the key variables. It has permitted novel prospective data collection that describes what interventions were done, why, and how patients responded. Ongoing analysis of this data has permitted us to refine the process and identify patients who do not respond well to it. The next challenge will be to develop a similar process for pre- ICU resuscitation that will use less invasive monitors with different endpoints.

ACKNOWLEDGMENT

Supported by NIGMS P50 GM38529 and U54 GM62119.

REFERENCES

1. Bickell WH, Wall MJ Jr., Pepe PE, Martin RR, Ginger VF, Allen MK, Mattox KL. Immediate versus delayed fluid resuscitation for hypotensive patients with penetrating torso injuries. *N Engl J Med* 1994;331: 1105-1109.
2. Dutton RP, Mackenzie CF, Scalea TM. Hypotensive resuscitation during active hemorrhage: impact on in-hospital mortality. *J Trauma* 2002;52:1141-1146.
3. Dubick MA, Atkins JL. Small-volume fluid resuscitation for the far-forward combat environment: current concepts. *J Trauma* 2003;54:S43-45.
4. Holcomb JB: Fluid resuscitation in modern combat casualty care: lessons learned from Somalia. *J Trauma* 2003;54:S46-51.
5. Hebert PC, Wells G, Blajchman MA, et al: A multicenter, randomized, controlled clinical trial of transfusion

requirements in critical care. *N Engl J Med* 1999;340:409-417.

6. Moore FA, Chang M, Cryer HG, et al. Symposium: Monitoring in the SICU: Current controversies in the use of pulmonary artery catheters. *Contemp Surg* 1998;53:213-228.

7. Shoemaker WC, Montgomery ES, Kaplan E, et al. Physiologic patterns in surviving and nonsurviving shock patients. Use of sequential cardiorespiratory variables in defining criteria for therapeutic goals and early warning of death. *Arch Surg* 1973;106(5):630-636.

8. Shoemaker WC, Hopkins JA. Clinical aspects of resuscitation with and without an algorithm: relative importance of various decisions. *Crit Care Med* 1983;11(8):630-639.

9. Shoemaker WC, Fleming AW. Resuscitation of the trauma patient: restoration of hemodynamic functions using clinical algorithms. *Ann Emerg Med* 1986;15(12):1437-1444.

10. Shoemaker WC. Relation of oxygen transport patterns to the pathophysiology and therapy of shock states. *Intensive Care Med* 1987;13(4):230-243.

11. Shoemaker WC, Patil R, Appel PL, et al. Hemodynamic and oxygen transport patterns for outcome prediction, therapeutic goals, and clinical algorithms to improve outcome. Feasibility of artificial intelligence to customize algorithms. *Chest* 1992;102(5 suppl 2):617S-625S.

12. Shoemaker WC, Appel PL, Kram HB. Hemodynamic and oxygen transport responses in survivors and nonsurvivors of high-risk surgery. *Crit Care Med* 1993;21(7):977-990.

13. Bishop MH, Shoemaker WC, Appel PL, et al. Relationship between supranormal circulatory values, time delays, and outcome in severely traumatized patients. *Crit Care Med* 1993;21(1):56-63.

14. Shoemaker WC, Appel PL, Kram HB, et al. Prospective trial of supranormal values of survivors as therapeutic goals in high-risk surgical patients. *Chest* 1988;94(6):1176-1186.

15. Bishop MH, Shoemaker WC, Appel PL, et al. Prospective, randomized trial of survivor values of cardiac index, oxygen delivery, and oxygen consumption as resuscitation endpoints in severe trauma. *J Trauma* 1995;38(5):780-787.

16. Moore EE, Thomas G. Orr Memorial Lecture. Staged laparotomy for the hypothermia, acidosis, and coagulopathy syndrome. *Am J Surg* 1996;172(5):405-410.

17. Moore FA, Haenel JB, Moore EE, and Whitehill TA. Incommensurate oxygen consumption in response to maximal oxygen availability predicts post injury multiple organ failure. *J Trauma* 1992;33:58-67.

18. Moore FA and Moore EE. Evolving concepts in the pathogenesis of post injury multiple organ failure. Chapter in *Horizons in Trauma Surgery. Surg Clin. N Amer* 1995;75:257-277.

19. Gattinoni L, Brazzi L, Pelosi P, et al. A trial of goal-oriented hemodynamic therapy in critically ill patients. *NEJM* 1995;333(16):1025-1032.

20. Durham RM, Neunaber K, Mazuski JE, et al. The use of oxygen consumption and delivery as endpoints for resuscitation in critically ill patients. *J Trauma* 1996;41(1):32-39.

21. Hayes MA, Timmins AC, Yau EH, et al. Elevation of systemic oxygen delivery in the treatment of critically ill patients. *N Engl J Med* 1994;330(24):1717-1722.

22. Hayes MA, Yau EH, Timmins AC, et al. Response of critically ill patients to treatment aimed at achieving supranormal oxygen delivery and consumption. Relationship to outcome. *Chest* 1993;103(3):886-895.

23 Yu M, Takanishi D, Myers SA, et al. Frequency of mortality and myocardial infarction during maximizing oxygen delivery: a prospective, randomized trial. *Crit Care Med* 1995;23(6):1025-1032.

24. Velmahos GC, Demetriades D, Shoemaker WC, et al. Endpoints of resuscitation of critically injured patients: normal or supranormal? A prospective randomized trial. *Ann Surg* 2000;232(3):409-414.

25. Barone JE, Lowenfels AB. Maximization of oxygen delivery: a plea for moderation. *J Trauma* 1992;33(5):651-653.

26. Barone JE. Maximization of oxygen delivery: a plea for moderation, Part II. *J Trauma* 1994;37(3):337-338.

27. Heyland DK, Cook DJ, King D, et al. Maximizing oxygen delivery in critically ill patients: a methodologic appraisal of the evidence. *Crit Care Med* 1996;24(3):517-524.

28. Matuschak GM. Supranormal oxygen delivery in critical illness. *New Horiz* 1997;5(3):233-238.

29. Russell JA. Adding fuel to the fire—The supranormal oxygen delivery trials controversy. *Crit Care Med* 1998;26(6):981-983.

30. McKinley BA, Moore FA, Sailors RM, et al. Computerized decision support for mechanical ventilation of trauma induced ARDS: Results of a randomized clinical trial. *J Trauma* 2001;50(3):415-424.

31. Connors AF, Speroff T, Dawson NV, et al. The effectiveness of right heart catheterization in the initial care of critically ill patients. *JAMA* 1996;276(11):889-897.

32. The National Heart, Lung, Blood Institute Acute Respiratory Distress (ARDS) Clinical Trials Network. Pulmonary-Artery versus Central Venous Catheter to guide Treatment of Acute Lung Injury. *N Eng J Med* 2006;354:2213-2224.

33. Sauaia A, Moore FA, Moore EE, et al. Early predictors of post injury multiple organ failure. *Arch Surg* 1994;129(1):39-45.

34. Sauaia A, Moore FA, Moore EE, et al. Multiple organ failure can be predicted as early as 12 hours post injury. *J Trauma* 1998;45:291.

35. McKinley BA, Sailors RM, Glorsky SL, et al. Computer directed resuscitation of major torso trauma. *Shock* 2001;15(suppl):46.

36. Morris AH. Algorithm based decision making. In: Tobin MJ, ed. *Principles and Practice of Intensive Care Monitoring.* New York: McGraw-Hill, 1997:1355-1381.

37. Clemmer TP, Spuhler VJ. Developing and gaining acceptance for patient care protocols. *New Horizons* 1998;6(1):12-19.

38. McKinley BA, Marvin RG, Cocanour CS, et al. Blunt trauma resuscitation: the old can respond. *Arch Surg* 2002;48(4):637-642.

39. Scalea TM, Simon HM, Duncan AO, et al. Geriatric blunt multiple trauma: improved survival with early invasive monitoring. *J Trauma* 1990;30(2):129-134.

40. McKinley BA, Kozar RA, Cocanour CS, et al. Trauma resuscitation: Female hearts respond better. *Arch Surg* 2002;137(5):578-584.

41. Marr AB, McKinley BA, Sailors RM, et al. 'Starling curve' generation during shock resuscitation: Can it be done? *Shock* 2003;19(suppl):27.

42. Miller PR, Meredith JW and Chang MC. Randomized, prospective comparison of increased preload versus inotropes in the resuscitation of trauma patients: effects on cardiopulmonary function and visceral Perfusion. *J Trauma* 1998;44(1): 107-113.

43. McKinley BA, Marvin RG, Cocanour CS, et al. Nitroprusside in resuscitation of major torso trauma. *J Trauma* 2000;49(6):1089-1095.

44. Chang MC, Martin RS, Scherer, et al. Improving ventricular-arterial coupling during resuscitation from shock: effects on cardiovascular function and systemic perfusion. *J Trauma* 2002;53(4):679-685.

45. Martin RS, Norris PR, Kilgo PD, et al. Validation of stroke work and ventricular arterial coupling as markers of cardiovascular Performance during Resuscitation. *J Trauma* 2006; 60(5):930-935.

46. Balogh Z, McKinley BA, Cox CS, et al. Abdominal compartment syndrome: The cause or effect multiple organ failure? *Shock* 2003;20:483-492.

47. Maxwell RA, Fabian TC, Croce MA, Davis KA. Secondary abdominal compartment syndrome: an underappreciated manifestation of severe hemorrhagic shock. *J Trauma* 1999;47:995-999.

48. Balogh Z, McKinley BA, Cocanour CS, et al. Secondary abdominal compartment syndrome is an elusive early complication of traumatic shock resuscitation. *Am J Surg* 2002;184(6):538-543.

49. Balogh Z, McKinley BA, Holcomb JB, et al. Both primary and secondary abdominal compartment syndrome can be predicted early and are harbingers of bad outcome. *J Trauma* 2003;54:848-861.

50. Balogh Z, McKinley BA, Cocanour CS, et al. Supranormal trauma resuscitation causes more cases of abdominal compartment syndrome. *Arch Surg* 2003;138:637-643.

51. Balogh Z, McKinley BA, Cocanour CS, Kozar RA, Cox CS, Moore FA. Patients with impending abdominal compartment syndrome do not respond to early volume loading. *Am J Surg* 2003;186(6): 602-608.

52. Davis JW, Mackersie RC, Holbrook TL, et al. Base deficit as an indicator of significant abdominal injury. *Ann Emerg Med* 1991;20(8):842-844.

53. Davis JW, Shackford SR, Holbrook TL. Base deficit as a sensitive indicator of compensated shock and tissue oxygen utilization. *Surg Gynecol Obstet* 1991;173(6): 473-476.

54. Davis JW. The relationship of base deficit to lactate in porcine hemorrhagic shock and resuscitation. *J Trauma* 1994;36(2):168-172.

55. Davis JW, Parks SN, Kaups KL, et al. Admission base deficit predicts transfusion requirements and risk of complications. *J Trauma* 1996;41(5): 769-774.

56. Davis JW, Kaups KL, Parks SN. Base deficit is superior to pH in evaluating clearance of acidosis after traumatic shock. *J Trauma* 1998;44(1):114-118.

57. Broder G, Weil MH. Excess lactate: an index of reversibility of shock in human patients. *Science* 1964;143:1457.

58. Cady LD, Weil MH, Afifi AA, et al. Quantitation of severity of critical illness with special reference to blood lactate. *Crit Care Med* 1973;1(2):75-80.

59. Cairns CB, Moore FA, Haenel JB, et al. Evidence for early supply independent mitochondrial dysfunction in patients developing multiple organ failure after trauma. *J Trauma* 1997;42(3):532-536.

60. Gore DC, Jahoor F, Hibbert JM, et al. Lactic acidosis during sepsis is related to increased pyruvate production, not deficits in tissue oxygen availability. *Ann Surg* 1996;224(1):97-102.

61. James JH, Luchette FA, McCarter FD, et al. Lactate is an unreliable indicator of tissue hypoxia in injury or sepsis. *Lancet* 1999;354(9177):505-508.

62. Gutierrez G, Bismar H, Dantzker DR, et al. Comparison of gastric intramucosal pH with measures of oxygen transport and consumption in critically ill patients. *Crit Care Med* 1992;20(4):451-457.

63. Gutierrez G, Palizas F, Doglio G, et al. Gastric intramucosal pH as a therapeutic index of tissue oxygenation in critically ill patients. *Lancet* 1992;339(8787): 195-199.

64. Fiddian-Green RG, Haglund U, Gutierrez G, et al. Goals for the resuscitation of shock. *Crit Care Med* 1993;21(2 suppl):S25-31.

65. Chang MC, Cheatham ML, Nelson LD, et al. Gastric tonometry supplements information provided by systemic indicators of oxygen transport. *J Trauma* 1994;37(3):488-494.

66. Ivatury RR, Simon RJ, Islam S, et al. A prospective randomized study of end points of resuscitation after major trauma: global oxygen transport indices versus organ-specific gastric mucosal pH. *J Am Coll Surg* 1996;183(2):145-154.

67. Gonzalez EA, Moore FA, Holcomb JB, et al. Fresh frozen plasma should be given earlier to patients requiring massive transfusion. *J Trauma*, 2007;62:112-119.

68. Rooth G, Hedstrand U, Tyden H, et al. The validity of the transcutaneous oxygen tension method in adults. *Crit Care Med* 1976;4(3):162-165.

69. Al-Siaidy W, Hill DW. The importance of an elevated skin temperature in transcutaneous oxygen tension measurement. *Birth Defects Orig Artic Ser* 1979;15(4):149-165.

70. Lofgren O. Transcutaneous oxygen measurement in adult intensive care. *Acta Anaesthesiol Scand* 1979;23(6):534-544.

71. Tremper KK, Mentelos RA, Shoemaker WC. Effect of hypercarbia and shock on transcutaneous carbon dioxide at different electrode temperatures. *Crit Care Med* 1980;8(11):608-612.

72. Tremper KK, Shoemaker WC. Transcutaneous oxygen monitoring of critically ill adults, with and without low flow shock. *Crit Care Med* 1981;9(10): 706-709.

73. Waxman K, Sadler R, Eisner ME, et al. Transcutaneous oxygen monitoring of emergency department patients. *Am J Surg* 1983;146(1):35-38.

74. Velmahos GC, Wo CC, Demetriades D, et al. Early continuous noninvasive haemodynamic monitoring after severe blunt trauma. *Injury* 1999;30(3):209-214.

75. Rivers EP, Ander DS, Powell D. Central venous oxygen saturation monitoring in the critically ill patient. *Curr Opin Crit Care* 2001;7(3):204-211.

76. Rivers E, Nguyen B, Havstad S, et al. Early goal-directed therapy in the treatment of severe sepsis and septic shock. *N Engl J Med* 2001;345(19):1368-1377.

77. McKinley BA, Marvin RG, Cocanour CS, et al. Tissue hemoglobin oxygen saturation during resuscitation of traumatic shock monitored using NIR spectrometry. *J Trauma* 2000;48(4):637-642.

78. McKinley BA, Ware DN, Marvin RG, et al. Skeletal muscle pH, PCO_2 and PO_2 during resuscitation of severe hemorrhagic shock. *J Trauma* 1998;45(3):271-279.

79. McKinley BA, Butler BD. Comparison of skeletal muscle PO_2, PCO_2 and pH with gastric tonometric PCO_2 and pH in hemorrhagic shock. *Crit Care Med* 1999;27(9):1869-1877.

80. McKinley BA, Ware DN, Marvin RG, et al. Skeletal muscle pH, $P(CO_2)$, and $P(O_2)$ during resuscitation of severe hemorrhagic shock. *J Trauma* 1998;45(3): 633-636.

81. Boekstegers P, Weidenhofer S, Kapsner T, et al. Skeletal muscle partial pressure of oxygen in patients with sepsis. *Crit Care Med* 1994;22(4):640-650.

82. Weil MH, Nakagawa Y, Tang W, et al. Sublingual capnometry: A new noninvasive measurement for diagnosis and quantitation of severity of circulatory shock. *Crit Care Med* 1999;27:1225-1229.

83. Moore FA, McKinley BA, Moore EE, et al. Inflammation and the host response to injury, a large-scale collaborative project: Patient-oriented research core—Standard Operating Procedures for clinical care: Guidelines for resuscitation of the trauma patients. *J Trauma* 2006;61:82-89.

Part **II**
CRITICAL CARE

Chapter 20

POSTOPERATIVE PITFALLS

K. Inaba, MD, and D. Demetriades, MD

INTRODUCTION

The postoperative period is a difficult transition phase in the overall management of a patient requiring emergency surgery. Although the acute surgical problem may be corrected or temporized, the underlying disease process, operative tissue trauma and anesthetic can result in severe metabolic disturbances, intercompartmental fluid shifts and an up-regulated inflammatory system with secondary effects spanning all organ systems. Due to the urgent nature of the disease processes requiring emergency surgery, the normal preoperative history taking, evaluation, and medical optimization have often been abbreviated, which may also negatively impact the postoperative care.

In addition to these physiological derangements, as for all patients undergoing surgery, the postoperative period involves tremendous change. Intraoperatively, the patient is under continuous real time monitoring by both the surgical and anesthesia teams. From this carefully controlled situation, the patient must emerge from anesthesia, undergo a change to portable monitoring and be transported. In the post anesthetic recovery area, the patient will be placed into the care of nursing staff with a limited knowledge of the surgical procedure that the patient has undergone, with in most situations, a less than 1:1 patient monitoring ratio. With increasingly stringent work-hour regulations, the surgical team and the anesthesia team that performed the procedure may be due to leave the hospital. Consequently, a new team of surgeons, anesthetists, and intensivists is left to manage a patient that they have limited knowledge of. All of this places patients undergoing emergency surgery at very high risk of complications. A large prospective outcome study of patients requiring postanesthetic care documented postoperative complications in 23.7%, with emergent surgery being a major risk factor.[1] Although many of these complications may be due to minor self-limited problems such as nausea or vomiting, significant life-threatening complications can occur.

It is critical that surgeons performing emergency surgery be aware of the postoperative pitfalls that may lead to these complications. Once the patient has been transferred to the recovery room or intensive care unit, the surgical team must carefully follow the patient through the postoperative phase in order to ensure that normal homeostasis is achieved. During this time, these potential postoperative pitfalls need to be aggressively avoided. If the surgical team is postcall and due to leave, it is important that all relevant details about the patient's history, prior physiological state, procedure performed, and patient's performance be passed on to the oncoming surgical team, critical care team and nursing staff providing the ongoing postoperative care for the patient. This will provide optimal continuity of care and decrease the likelihood of the patient suffering a postoperative complication. The following chapter has been designed to illustrate common postoperative pitfalls in order to maximize avoidance and the early detection of these complications.

MYOCARDIAL ISCHEMIA

As our population ages, so does the proportion of older patients with concurrent cardiopulmonary disease who present to the hospital requiring emergency surgery. For these patients undergoing emergency surgery, the postoperative period is a critical time and unrecognized myocardial ischemia is a major potential pitfall. When the entire perioperative period is surveyed, myocardial ischemia is most prevalent postoperatively and occurs most frequently in the first 24-72 hours after operation.[2] Perioperative ischemia is not only associated with adverse cardiac events during the admission, but there is an increased risk of adverse cardiac events persisting for at least the subsequent 2 years.[3-5] Perioperative cardiovascular events are not uncommon, occurring in up to 5% of patients undergoing major emergency noncardiac operations.[6] An emergent operation remains one of the highest-risk situations for an adverse cardiac event during surgical intervention.

In patients undergoing elective operative procedures, the preoperative medical, surgical, and medication history is a critical part of the patient's risk stratification. In patients undergoing emergency surgery, a complete history may not be possible. If this could not be elicited preoperatively, every effort should be made perioperatively by another team member to obtain any collateral history from family, friends, or medical charts that would alert the team to the presence of an increased risk for a perioperative cardiac event. A medication history, targeted specifically at those agents used for rate control, cardiac remodeling, hypertension, diuresis, and anticoagulation can also provide valuable information regarding the preoperative physiological condition and subsequent risk of perioperative ischemia in these patients.

Monitoring for adverse cardiac events through the postoperative period is critical for early diagnosis (Table 20-1). Perioperative ST segment monitoring should be routinely carried on into the postoperative period. Unfortunately, although classic symptoms such as chest pain, dyspnea, arrhythmias, and congestive heart failure may occur, the majority of patients who experience postoperative myocardial ischemia are asymptomatic. This may be due to residual anesthetic effect or distracting incisional pain.[3,4,7] Reliance on classical symptoms for diagnosis is a potential pitfall. Because of this, ECG changes and cardiac biomarkers such as Troponin I have been studied in the postoperative monitoring of patients at risk for cardiac ischemia. In those patients with known or suspected coronary artery disease undergoing emergency surgery, a recovery room and daily electrocardiogram for the first two postoperative days may be cost-effective.[8] Cardiac Troponin has been evaluated for the diagnosis of myocardial injury in the perioperative period of noncardiac surgery and has been found to be a sensitive biomarker, utilizing traditional acute myocardial infarction cut-off values.[9,10] Cardiac troponin evaluation is warranted for those patients who are symptomatic or demonstrate ECG changes. Its role, however, as a routine screening biomarker in patients with suspected or known coronary artery disease undergoing emergency surgery is not known. Although routine perioperative pulmonary artery (PA) catheter monitoring has not been demonstrated to result in improved clinical outcomes, invasive monitoring may benefit specific patients undergoing emergency surgery. Those patients with congestive heart failure and either systolic or diastolic dysfunction, coronary artery disease with significant intraoperative hemodynamic abnormalities, cardiomyopathy, or valvular disease undergoing emergency surgery may, on an individual basis, benefit from PA catheterization. In this patient population, this may help with optimal fluid administration and, if required, the management of inotropic or vasopressive support.

Perioperative myocardial infarction is associated with a high mortality rate.[3,4,11] As there are treatment options even in the acute postoperative period, early diagnosis remains critical.

Although the treatment principles for those postoperative patients that have cardiac ischemia remain the same (reperfusion, antithrombotics, decreased O_2 demand, prevention of left ventricular remodeling), the acute postoperative state will limit therapeutic options. As in all patients, adequate pain management is highly desirable in order to minimize postoperative catecholamine surges and the resultant tachycardia. Tachycardia both intraoperatively and postoperatively can put significant stress on the myocardium by increasing myocardial oxygen demand. Maintenance of normothermia may reduce the incidence of adverse cardiac events.[12] This can be accomplished with passive ambient temperature maintenance, the use of blankets, warmed IV fluids, and forced air heating. Thrombolytics, antiplatelet agents, and anticoagulants in general will be contraindicated in the immediate postoperative period. Urgent catheterization and possible angioplasty should be considered. Beta-blockade and, in patients with associated heart failure, nitrates may be beneficial. A multidisciplinary approach to the evaluation and treatment of patients with myocardial ischemia including early cardiology consultation in the postoperative phase is essential to ensure optimal care.

POSTOPERATIVE HYPERTENSION

Normally, uncontrolled preoperative hypertension is a contraindication to elective surgery. Uncontrolled hypertension with a diastolic blood pressure > 110 mm Hg has been shown to be associated with significant operative risks due to large fluctuations in systemic vascular resistance both during induction and maintenance anesthesia. This pressure lability has been associated with an increased incidence of myocardial ischemia, dysrhythmias, renal dysfunction, and pulmonary edema.[13,14] For those patients that do present with preoperative hypertension requiring emergency surgery, perioperative control is essential and in most cases can be accomplished. These patients are at high risk of postoperative myocardial ischemia and dysrhythmias and will need to be carefully monitored throughout the perioperative period.

New and unexpected *postoperative* hypertension, can occur in patients presenting with normal blood

Table 20-1   Methods for Reducing Postoperative Cardiac Complications
Preoperative hypertension control.
Perioperative beta-blockade.
Optimize intraoperative anesthesia.
Minimize perioperative fluid shifts.
Maintain normothermia.
Adequate postoperative pain control.
Close postoperative monitoring +/− ECG/Troponin.

pressures or even hypotension. These patients may have had pharmacologically controlled hypertension or may never have had hypertension in the preoperative period.[15] For patients undergoing emergency surgery, preoperative hypertension may be masked by a hyperinflammatory state, large fluid shifts, vascular redistribution or relative volume depletion. In the general surgical population, postoperative hypertension is seen in approximately 3% of patients, the majority occurring early, within the first 30 minutes. Half of these patients will have had no evidence of preoperative hypertension. The etiology is not known; however, it is likely to be multifactorial with contributions from the autonomic nervous system and the renin angiotensin system. The most common treatable inciting cause is anxiety and pain with the dissipation of the anesthetic. This is an especially important pitfall in the paralyzed or head injured patient. This can be treated effectively with sedation and analgesia. Bladder and gastric distention is also known to cause hypertension[16] and hypothermia may contribute by decreasing the reuptake of circulating catecholamines.

A postoperative hypertensive emergency is rare; the vast majority of these episodes are self-limited. Neglecting the common causes of postoperative hypertension and moving directly to pharmacological control is a pitfall to be avoided. Although it is rare that pharmacological management is required, once the common causes have been corrected, the drug chosen should be short acting and titratable to effect. Especially in patients with an abnormal fluid balance in a hyperinflammatory milieu, as the body continues to regulate itself to a state of homeostasis, overshoot, with resultant hypotension may occur. Although the evidence to support the use of perioperative beta blockade in noncardiac surgery is unclear, pending the completion of a large multinational randomized controlled trial (Peri Operative Ischemic Evaluation—POISE),[17] initiating therapy with short-acting intravenous beta blockade may be reasonable.

CONGESTIVE HEART FAILURE

In critically ill patients undergoing emergency surgery, a potent hyperinflammatory state is induced. Major fluid shifts within body compartments as a result of redistributed vascular beds, inflammatory mediator induced capillary leak and massive fluid resuscitation may result in acute pulmonary edema. Attributing postoperative pulmonary edema to "fluid overload" is a pitfall that may be exacerbated by the blind administration of diuretics. Excess pulmonary fluid requires an aggressive search for potential treatable underlying causes such as myocardial ischemia and left-sided failure, electrical conduction abnormalities, and renal failure.

True congestive heart failure is a well-known postoperative complication occurring in the early postoperative period.[18,19] This is most commonly seen in those patients with preoperative congestive heart failure, previous myocardial infarction and valvular disease. In general, oxygen, fluid normalization (including restriction, diuresis, or dialysis), supportive ventilation, and pain control will apply to all patients. With left ventricular systolic dysfunction, phosphodiesterase inhibitors, vasodilators such as nitroglycerin to decrease afterload and hypertension especially if there is associated myocardial infarction and nitroprusside with aortic or mitral regurgitation may be indicated.

RESPIRATORY FAILURE

For the patient undergoing emergency surgery, the postoperative period has the potential for severe life-threatening pulmonary complications. The first potential pitfall is premature extubation. Successful extubation requires a patient to be mentally capable of driving their respiratory system and protecting their airway. If this cannot be accomplished or the patient is scheduled to undergo a second look procedure shortly or is hemodynamically fragile and in need of ongoing resuscitation that may be complicated by respiratory failure, extubation should be delayed. The patient can be transferred directly to the ICU for the postoperative recovery phase, can have their ventilatory support weaned and then, when ready, can undergo extubation in a controlled manner.

Postextubation, careful monitoring of both the airway and pulmonary gas exchange is required. The incidence of respiratory failure varies depending on the definition used, the patient population studied and the underlying disease process requiring the general anesthetic. It is, however, most common in those patients that are older with underlying pulmonary pathology, primarily obstructive disease and congestive heart failure. Those that present with a higher ASA classification have also been found to be at higher risk and a moderate association with smoking has also been shown.[20,21] When examining the procedure related risk, patients undergoing emergency surgery, particularly if intra-abdominal or prolonged greater than 3 hours, are at increased risk of respiratory failure when compared to patients undergoing elective surgery.

Although the etiology of postoperative respiratory failure is often a mixed problem, to facilitate the search for causes, the problem can be separated (Table 20-2) into those that are primarily hypoxemic in nature (inadequate oxygenation, where the PCO_2 may be normal or low) and those that are hypercapnic (inadequate ventilation, often associated with a hypoxemia). The former is often caused by problems such as contusion, pneumothorax, pulmonary edema, atelectasis, aspiration, pulmonary embolism, bronchospasm, and mucous plugging. The most common cause is a right to left shunt secondary to atelectasis. Even without a visible

Table 20-2   Common Causes of Postoperative Respiratory Complications
Hypoxic
Pulmonary contusion
Pneumothorax
Pulmonary edema
Atelectasis
Aspiration
Pulmonary embolism
Mucus plugging
Hypercarbic
Decreased efferent drive
Head injury
Cervical spine injury
Oversedation
Mechanical impairment
Chest wall injury
Abdominal compartment syndrome

region of atelectasis on x-ray, diffuse airway collapse can cause a significant right to left shunt. In general, the causes of hypercapnic failure are decreased CNS drive or mechanical respiratory impairment. The mechanical impairment that may be seen in emergency surgical patients include diverse problems such as associated chest wall injury, abdominal compartment syndrome, and severe ARDS. General anesthesia will have an effect on the respiratory system of all patients in the postoperative phase. Most lung volumes including the forced vital capacity and functional residual capacity are decreased. This is especially pronounced after abdominal operations. Diaphragmatic function may be impaired from pain and residual neuromuscular blockade. The volatile anesthetic itself can directly affect the ventilatory compensation to both hypoxemia and hypercarbia. In addition, excess sedatives or narcotics for pain management may cause a significant decrease in ventilatory drive. Conversely, inadequate pain control may also result in a hypercarbic response from hypoventilation. Hypercapnic failure often has an associated VQ mismatch as well. For example, with inadequate analgesia, the splinting will be associated with atelectasis adding a hypoxemic component to the respiratory failure.

Patients with respiratory failure may present slowly with symptoms of increased work of breathing, tachypnea, accessory muscle use, a dysynchronous breathing pattern, evidence of a catecholamine surge (tachycardia, dysrhythmias, blood pressure changes) or may demonstrate a progressive decrease in level of consciousness ranging from agitation to frank coma. In fact, a common pitfall in the postoperative period is the treatment of agitation and confusion secondary to hypoxia with further sedation leading to a downward spiral that will end in intubation and mechanical ventilation.

As a general approach to the postoperative patient in respiratory distress, investigations include arterial blood gas sampling, hemoglobin, electrolyte, and creatinine measurement. Pulse oximetry should be utilized and if an inadequate waveform is visualized, the sensor should be resituated. Causes of misreadings include poor peripheral perfusion, dark skin pigment, intravascular dyes, nail polish, acrylic nails, motion artifact, carboxy-hemoglobin, and methemoglobin. A chest x-ray should be obtained.

For patients who have undergone emergency surgery, the use of lung expanding treatments such as chest physiotherapy, incentive spirometry, intermittent positive pressure breathing, and continuous positive airway pressure may help prevent postoperative pulmonary complications.[20] In most cases, supplemental oxygen to drive the partial pressure gradient between the alveoli and blood will benefit the patient. Although high-concentration, high-flow oxygen may actually exacerbate hypoventilation due to the lack of hypoxemic drive in some patients, oxygen therapy should be instituted and titrated to oximetry saturation while the cause of the hypoxemia and hypercarbia is investigated. The oxygen can be delivered by nasal cannula, an entrainment facemask, or reservoir facemask. The magnitude of the response depends on the degree of shunt fraction; the smaller the shunt, the more pronounced is the response to supplemental oxygen. If there is inadequate response with 100% FiO_2, mechanical ventilation and addition of positive end expiratory pressure will increase the functional residual capacity (FRC) and reduce closing volume (CV). The increase in FRC in relation to CV will reduce the shunt fraction. Noninvasive positive pressure ventilatory strategies may also improve oxygenation provided the patient is able to participate, can protect their airway, and does not have facial trauma. This can allow the administration of functional PEEP. Noninvasive ventilation can also address hypoventilation with bilevel positive airway pressure. This may act as a bridge to avoiding orotracheal intubation.

One of the commonest causes of hypoventilation in the postoperative period remains iatrogenic medications such as narcotics. This is treatable with antagonists. Naloxone should be titrated to effect rather than being used as a fixed bolus dose to prevent overshoot and a pain response with its associated catecholamine surge. In addition, Naloxone has a short half-life relative to most narcotics so that its effects may wear off resulting in the original respiratory depression if not carefully monitored. Nonnarcotic neuromuscular blockers may also contribute to postoperative respiratory depression. Failed reversal of the neuromuscular blockade may be potentiated by renal failure, increased serum magnesium and hypothermia.

Finally, although rare, acute airway obstruction in the post anesthetic period may occur, most commonly due to pharyngeal obstruction, laryngeal spasm, vocal cord paralysis, or direct airway injury and swelling. Patients at increased risk include those with obstructive sleep apnea and those that had a difficult intubation. Acutely, the patient should be given oxygen, have their sedation held and if required, anterior displacement of the mandible. Airway control and positive pressure ventilation may be required. The temporary use of a laryngeal mask airway may be helpful.

ABDOMINAL COMPARTMENT SYNDROME

In the postoperative period, patients undergoing emergency surgery are at high risk of developing abdominal compartment syndrome (ACS). Unrecognized ACS may lead to severe physiological derangements that if not recognized and treated promptly may result in organ failure and even death. The key to avoiding this pitfall is the early identification of those patients who are at risk (Table 20-3). For the acute care surgeon, the majority of the critically ill patient load remains at high risk of developing this complication. This includes patients undergoing major emergency intra-abdominal surgery, significant extra-abdominal surgery or even no surgery with a heightened systemic inflammatory response requiring massive fluid resuscitation.

In patients undergoing emergency abdominal operations, especially those with an infectious or inflammatory component to their underlying disease process, the hyperinflammatory state along with aggressive fluid resuscitation will lead to visceral and retroperitoneal fluid sequestration and edema. Specific surgical disease processes such as bowel obstruction or the reduction of hernias with loss of domain are at especially high risk for ACS due to the physical space constraints of the abdominal cavity. In injured patients, traumatic hemorrhage may also result in a hyperinflammatory state with visceral edema which can be worsened by intra-abdominal hematoma or bleeding. In damage control situations, the physical presence of intracavitary packs can also contribute to increased intra-abdominal pressures. Even patients undergoing emergency nonabdominal surgery (thoracotomy, burns, extremity vascular or crush) or no operation at all, but a major physiological insult with massive resuscitation in a hyperinflammatory milieu may develop intra-abdominal hypertension and progress to ACS.

Unrecognized, IAH may go on to cause end organ complications and ACS. Several critical organ systems may be involved resulting in renal failure, respiratory failure, cardiac failure, increased ICP, and gut ischemia. The renal system is affected early on with an increase in intra-abdominal pressure. This is a direct result of decreased renal blood flow from both direct compression of both the renal veins and cortical arterioles as well as the added effect of decreased cardiac output. This will result in decreasing urine output, which is only minimally responsive to a volume challenge. Ureteral compression itself is not an etiological factor as stenting has been demonstrated to be ineffective protection against the renal failure secondary to elevated intra-abdominal pressures. The pulmonary effects of ACS are also seen early with the elevation of intra-abdominal pressure. As the compliance of the respiratory system decreases, both the peak and plateau pressures will increase. Both hypercarbia and hypoxemia can result. In the nonventilated patient progressive tachypnea with low tidal volumes will progress to respiratory distress and eventual failure. Finally, the cardiovascular response to the decreased venous return will result in tachycardia and hypotension. Invasive monitoring will demonstrate significantly decreased cardiac output with increased CVP, SVR, PAP, and PAWP. The decreased cardiac output is a direct result of decreased preload and increased afterload. This is seen on a background of relatively normal or even increased PAWP. This decreased cardiac output will in turn exacerbate the renal dysfunction and may cause GI tract ischemia.

Ideally, this process will be anticipated and prevented. With increasing awareness of the clinical situations that put patients at risk for IAH and eventually ACS, prophylactic steps can be taken. For the acute care surgeon, practically, these patients can be subdivided into those that have undergone abdominal operation and those that have not. For those undergoing laparotomy, intraoperative visceral edema, bleeding, a requirement for damage control packing, or any difficulty in closure without elevated airway pressures signals the possibility of IAH if the abdomen were to be inappropriately closed. It is important to remember that the intra-abdominal pressure will increase even further postoperatively as the neuromuscular blockade is removed. In these clinical situations, early consideration needs to be given to the use of a temporary abdominal closure. Although it is tempting to simply close the skin, this may not be sufficient as a compartment syndrome can still occur with skin closure alone. If ACS is a concern, temporary closure utilizing a perforated x-ray cassette drape to protect the bowel, sponges, and perforated drains sandwiched with a clear adhesive dressing or any variation of this setup can be utilized.

For the other group of patients, those in whom the abdomen is already closed or did not undergo abdominal surgery, the diagnosis can be challenging. Although clinical examination of the abdomen may reveal a distended and firm abdomen, relying on this alone is a

Table 20-3 Risk Factors for Abdominal Compartment Syndrome
Major intra-abdominal surgical procedure
Blunt or penetrating intra-abdominal trauma
Ruptured abdominal aortic aneurysm
Severe pancreatitis
Major intra-abdominal infection
Thermal injury
Massive fluid resuscitation or transfusion

potential pitfall. Objective measurement is possible for the documentation of intra-abdominal pressure. At our institution, a protocol of routine intra-abdominal pressure monitoring every 8 hours for the first 48 hours after operation for critically ill patients in the ICU has been implemented. Surrogate pressures transmitted through either the bladder or the stomach can be used.

In those patients that have a closed abdomen or did not have an abdominal operation, bladder pressure measurements can aid in the diagnostic process. With IAH or ACS, there are few medical treatments that have been found to be effective. If detected in the burn patient population, paracentesis may have a role;[22] however, this has not been definitively demonstrated. For all other patients, sedatives and paralytics may allow temporization. The definitive treatment however remains abdominal decompression and temporary abdominal closure. Although the exact indication for surgical decompression as intra-abdominal pressure escalates is not known, ACS, where there is organ dysfunction, remains an absolute indication for abdominal decompression. For early intra-abdominal hypertension without organ dysfunction however, the exact indication for decompression remains elusive and warrants further focused investigation.

EXTREMITY COMPARTMENT SYNDROME

Missed extremity compartment syndrome (ECS) is a devastating pitfall that can eventually lead to limb loss and even death (Table 20-4). Elevated compartment pressures can be caused by hematoma from a fracture or trauma, edema secondary to crush injury, or after arterial or venous vascular injury. Iatrogenic causes include intracompartmental extravasation of IV fluid or contrast from a power injector and external compression from a cast. The acute care surgeon must maintain a high index of suspicion when managing any of these injury patterns. Repeat clinical examination of high risk patients remains critical to diagnosis. In the evaluable patient, the 5 Ps (pain, pulselessness, pallor, parasthesias, poikilothermia) are unreliable and late signs of a

Table 20-4 Pitfalls in the Identification of Extremity Compartment Syndrome
Failure to recognize the "at risk" limb, especially without signs of external trauma
Failure to repeat frequent clinical examination
Reliance on the classical "Ps"
Delayed compartment pressure measurement
Treatment of persistent extremity pain with escalating analgesia
Casts or splints covering toes
The unevaluable patient (sedation, head or cord injury, children)

nonviable limb. Reliance on the 5 Ps is a pitfall. Any pain out of proportion to the injury either at rest or with passive stretch warrants close evaluation and objective compartment pressure monitoring. More challenging is the unevaluable patient or child. In these patients, a swollen compartment on physical exam warrants pressure monitoring. Objective pressure monitoring can be done with either a commercially available transduction system or with an arterial line. The actual pressure threshold for which definitive treatment (fasciotomy) is warranted is not known. There is evidence to support the use of a compartment perfusion pressure.[23] In a prospective study, McQueen monitored pressures in patients with tibial fractures utilizing anterior compartment pressure monitoring. Utilizing a diastolic blood pressure–compartment pressure threshold of less than 30 mm Hg detected all compartment syndrome patients requiring surgical intervention. In this study, utilizing an isolated threshold of 40 mm Hg would have resulted in a 23% nontherapeutic fasciotomy rate with a mean follow-up of 15 months.

Definitive treatment remains release of external causes such as casts when present and surgical fasciotomy. After extremity revascularization, perioperative mannitol may reduce the incidence of ECS. Close clinical follow-up in the postoperative period is essential. For those patients requiring surgical intervention, a final pitfall is a missed compartment, especially the anterior compartment. In the operating room, care must be taken to decompress all compartments at risk.

POSTOPERATIVE BLEEDING

In the patient undergoing emergency surgery, postoperative bleeding is a major concern. Laboratory values such as hemoglobin or hematocrit may be confirmatory; however, during an acute bleed, these may not accurately reflect blood loss and reliance on this is a clinical pitfall to be avoided. Examination of the patient may demonstrate abdominal tenderness or distention with evidence of intra-abdominal hypertension. The abdomen however can sequester liters of blood which, especially in a sedated critically ill patient, may be asymptomatic. If drains were left in place intraoperatively they may not discharge blood if they become clotted, kinked or are away from a walled-off area of hemorrhage. Any patient in whom bleeding is a concern will require baseline hemoglobin, hematocrit, and coagulation parameters to be checked. Concurrently, aggressive fluid resuscitation, the correction of any detected coagulation defects, and replacement of packed red blood cells should be considered. With evidence of active ongoing bleeding, surgical reexploration is often required. If the patient is a trauma patient with a known solid organ injury such as a complex liver injury, proceeding directly to angiography may be preferable. In the multitrauma patient, identification of the source of bleeding may pose a major challenge and assuming that it is localized to a known injury is a diagnostic pitfall. All areas of potential hemorrhage including the thorax, intraperitoneal space, retroperitoneum, pelvis, long bones, and soft tissues must be considered. Once the bleeding has been localized, therapeutic pitfalls include a delay in returning to the operating room or angiography to address surgical bleeding. This may increase the patient's exposure to blood products, induce coagulopathy, and magnify the inflammatory response. In the operating room, underutilization of packing and damage control principles to allow physiologic normalization should also be avoided.

In the critically ill patient requiring emergency surgery, especially if there is massive resuscitation and transfusion, a coagulopathy may result. This acquired postoperative coagulopathy may be the primary problem or may be a major contributing problem to the bleeding. Failure to recognize this is a major potential pitfall. The etiology of this coagulopathy is multifactorial. Preinjury anticoagulant or antiplatelet agent use including over the counter medications may not have been obtained during the urgent preoperative history. Intraoperatively, platelet and coagulation factor loss from hemorrhage, dilution from volume replacement, disseminated and local consumption, temperature derangements, and acidosis may all contribute to the coagulopathy that occurs in patients undergoing emergency surgery.

As a global approach to the management of all patients with coagulopathy, early identification and surgical or endovascular hemostasis is critical. If there is known pharmacological use of anticoagulants preoperatively or if there is an abnormality detected on the screening coagulation assays, the defect should be aggressively corrected with fresh frozen plasma or platelets. Especially in the trauma population, upward of a quarter of patients may present with a screening laboratory abnormality in their coagulation parameters.[24]

Because it is common, preventable, and has a detrimental effect on coagulation, aggressive prevention of further thermal energy loss should be instituted in all patients. Patient core temperatures should be monitored closely throughout all phases of resuscitation, diagnosis, operation, and critical care. Wet clothing should be removed and heat loss prevented with the use of blankets and head coverings as possible. Ambient room temperatures should be kept high, all fluids and inhaled gases should be warmed, and, if required, external forced air warming systems may be utilized. The coagulation process relies on a variety of temperature-dependent enzymatic reactions that are slowed by hypothermia. Clinically, for the surgeon in the operating room, the magnitude of this effect is difficult to quantitate as blood samples sent to the laboratory are routinely warmed to 37 degree Celsius for testing, which will not accurately reflect the actual *in vivo* coagulation parameters of the hypothermic trauma patient. Experimental data shows that even with normal factor levels, temperatures of 33 degree Celsius can result in a functional factor deficiency of greater than 50%. Platelet adhesion is also impaired by hypothermia. In fact, at milder levels of hypothermia, the depression in core body temperature will have a greater effect on platelet function than on the enzymatic clotting cascade.

Laboratory result–guided treatment requires the measurement of PT (INR), aPTT, platelet count, and fibrinogen and uses these results to detect component deficits, initiate replacement, and monitor response. In general, an INR > 1.5, aPTT > 1.5 X normal, platelet count < 100,000/mL (assuming normal function) and a fibrinogen level < 100 mg/dL are all clear indications for plasma, platelet, or cryoprecipitate replacement in the bleeding patient. Unfortunately, lab results, which can take up to an hour to obtain, may lag behind the patient's clinical status and not accurately reflect the minute-to-minute coagulation parameters of the acutely bleeding patient. In rapid bleeds, empiric replacement may be required.

Empiric replacement therapy applies to situations where there is massive or rapid ongoing hemorrhage. At some institutions, this has been protocolized so that for every X units of packed red blood cells, X units of plasma and platelets are infused concurrently without waiting for laboratory results. No class 1 data to support these protocols exists. Not surprisingly, institutional protocols and individual practices vary widely. This lack of a standardized approach stems from our inability to quickly measure the rapidly changing coagulation profile in the bleeding patient being actively resuscitated. Practically, however, in situations where laboratory results cannot keep up with the rapidly changing clinical situation, empiric replacement is warranted.

For trauma patients, several case series and a large multinational randomized placebo controlled double-blinded trial have been published documenting the results of the investigational use of recombinant activated factor VII (rFVIIa – NovoSeven). Although these results have been promising, the cost to benefit ratio is unknown. At this time, rFVIIa is being used on an off label basis at many centers around the world. A multicenter randomized placebo controlled double-blinded trial with survival as a primary endpoint has been initiated by the manufacturer and is currently under way at the time of this writing.

STEROID INSUFFICIENCY

In critically ill septic patients undergoing emergency surgery, there are many possible etiologies for the shock state. Failure to recognize adrenal insufficiency as a treatable cause of persistent hypotension is a potential pitfall. This must be considered in any critically ill or injured patient with persistent hypotension not responding to standard treatment. Glucocorticoids play an important hemodynamic role in the physiologic stress response. They exert direct effects on vasomotor tone and interact indirectly with the regulatory vasodilators and catecholamines that act on both the venous and arterial systems. They are also important in the maintenance of fluid balance. In septic shock, multiple possible causes for adrenal insufficiency have been reported. These include direct damage to the hypothalamic-pituitary-adrenal axis from trauma, necrosis, hemorrhage, and inflammation. A multitude of drugs used in this patient population from antibiotics to sedatives such as etomidate used in rapid sequence intubation to suppressive exogenous glucocorticoid treatment can all cause a relative deficiency. In addition to this deficiency, there may be a tissue resistance to the activity of circulating glucocorticoid in this patient population.

The traditional clinical presentation of steroid deficiency (mental status changes, hypoglycemia, hyponatremia, hyperkalemia, neutropenia, and eosinophilia) may not be readily separable from the clinical presentation of the critically ill patient after surgical intervention. In those patients who remain refractory to traditional fluid resuscitation, empiric treatment with low-dose hydrocortisone should be initiated.[25] Concurrent plasma cortisol response to cosyntropin stimulation should be tested. Treatment should be stopped in responders and continued for 7 days in nonresponders.

HEPARIN INDUCED THROMBOCYTOPENIA

A final consideration in the bleeding patient postoperatively is heparin induced thrombocytopenia (HIT). Any intraoperative exposure to heparin may result in this antibody mediated prothrombotic activation of platelets.[26,27] Although most commonly occurring with unfractionated heparin in up to 1% of exposed patients, this can occur with low molecular weight heparin as well. HIT can be classified into immune-mediated and non–immune mediated etiologies. Non–immune mediated HIT is more common, occurring in 20%-30% of exposed patients and is rarely clinically significant. Immune-mediated HIT however is rare, occurring in 1%-3% of exposed patients, and can be severe. The immune-mediated process is triggered by the recognition of heparin and platelet factor 4 complexes by IgG antibodies resulting in both platelet activation, the generation of thrombin, and clearance of the antibody coated platelets by the reticuloendothelial system.

Clinically, thrombocytopenia is one of the clinical hallmarks of HIT. A 50% drop from the preoperative levels or a drop to an absolute value less than 150,000/mL is suggestive and should trigger laboratory testing. Although most likely to be seen between days 3-5 after exposure to heparin, it is possible to see this acutely in the postoperative period in the emergency surgery patient that may have been in hospital, for example, with acute cholecystitis prior to being taken to the operating room. Any patient that has received heparin within the 6 months prior to an emergency operation may also manifest rapid onset heparin induced thrombocytopenia, occurring within 24 hours of exposure. In addition to the thrombocytopenia, the patient may present with an acute arterial or venous thrombosis. These prothrombotic complications are responsible for the morbidity associated with HIT. This may range from skin necrosis or erythema to peripheral limb ischemia or gangrene. Laboratory confirmation of the clinical symptomatology can be performed by either heparin/PF4 solid phase ELISA, or platelet activation based assays (platelet activation assay, serotonin release assay, platelet aggregation assay).

As the use of heparin is ubiquitous, a careful search for exposure to either unfractionated heparin or low molecular weight heparin and documentation of this exposure is required. Although rare, HIT can be triggered by even minimal exposure to heparin from intravenous or intra-arterial flushes or heparin coated catheters. The primary treatment for HIT is halting the exposure to heparin, including low molecular weight heparins due to cross reactivity. In general, platelet administration is contraindicated as it may worsen the thrombotic complications. Anticoagulation is necessary to prevent subsequent thrombosis and can be accomplished by factor Xa inhibition with Danaproid or thrombin inhibition with either Lepirudin or Argatroban. A multimodality approach to this problem with early hematology consultation is essential for the long-term treatment of this condition.

MALIGNANT HYPERTHERMIA

Malignant hyperthermia (MH) is a genetic disorder that results in massive cytoplasmic calcium release. This results in local muscle cell damage with a hypermetabolic response, increased oxygen demand, carbon dioxide and heat production. Serum hyperkalemia, myoglobinemia-induced renal failure, cardiac arrhythmias, and disseminated intravascular coagulopathy may result. It is triggered by depolarizing muscle relaxants such as succinylcholine and inhalational anesthetics. The incidence of MH varies from 1 in 6000 to 1 in 40 000, depending on when the study was published, likely due to the variability in preoperative testing as well as differences in the anesthetic agents used (28-30). Although traditionally thought of as an intraoperative event, its presentation may be delayed into the postoperative period and is a potential pitfall if not given consideration as this is a treatable problem. In fact, institution of early treatment has allowed this once highly lethal condition to become fatal in less than 5% of cases.

Our understanding of the genetic basis of MH has grown rapidly over the last decade with linkage of MH to the Ryanodine type 1 receptor (RYR1) gene. Although a genetic screening evaluation is not yet available, preoperative in vitro caffeine halothane muscle contracture testing and a detailed history of prior anesthetics (although a history of an uneventful anesthetic does not preclude the disease) and family history will allow the diagnosis to be made preoperatively in some patients.

In patients undergoing emergency surgery, a complete history may not be available and preoperative testing is not feasible. In these patients, succinylcholine is often used for rapid sequence intubation with maintenance using inhalational vapors. Therefore, in the postoperative phase, MH needs to be considered in patients demonstrating hypermetabolism, muscle rigidity, increasing end tidal CO_2 or electrical conduction disorders. Although there is no definitive gold standard laboratory test to diagnose MH, in this postoperative patient with an escalating hypermetabolic state unresponsive to fluid resuscitation and increased ventilation, strong consideration should be given to MH and treatment initiated.

If occurring in the acute postoperative state, all volatile triggering anesthetics should be stopped and hyperventilation with anesthetic free oxygen should be initiated. Maintenance anesthesia should be changed to intravenous techniques and the procedure should be abbreviated. Dantrolene 1-2 mg/Kg IV preferably through a central line is given. Dantrolene will cause weakness and will preclude extubation. Electrolyte abnormalities and conduction dysrhythmias should be treated and aggressive diuresis promoted to prevent rhabdomyolysis. These patients will require intensive monitoring postoperatively and family counseling for anesthetic preparation prior to further surgical interventions.

RETAINED FOREIGN BODY

Retained foreign bodies remain an ongoing concern. Although the true incidence is not known, it is estimated that this occurs in 1 in 1000 to 1 in 3000 procedures.[31,32] An emergency surgical procedure was of the three independent risk factors including unplanned changes in procedure and higher BMI that were identified for the occurrence of a retained foreign body in the 2003 study by Gawande. Emergency surgical interventions are often highly unplanned and may be carried out late at night by a tired team. There may not have been time for a preoperative instrument count and in emergency trauma surgery, sponges may even be left behind intentionally as part of a damage control procedure. In both trauma and nontrauma surgery with an open abdomen, the patient may have a prolonged course with multiple reoperations and washouts

with different teams, all of which may increase the chance of a retained foreign body. In attempting to avoid this pitfall, the American College of Surgeons has recommended consistent application and adherence to standardized counting procedures, performance of a methodical wound exploration prior to closure of the surgical site, use of radiographic detectable items only, maintenance of an optimal operating room environment allowing focused performance of operative tasks, implement of radiographic studies as indicated to ensure that there is no retained foreign bodies and suspension of these measures as required in life-threatening situations.[33]

Although it is possible for the retained sponges and instruments to cause an acute foreign body reaction with local systemic signs, obstruction, or fistulization to a contiguous structure, these symptoms are nonspecific and are not expected to occur immediately after an operation. Therefore, it is important that in avoiding this pitfall a high index of suspicion be maintained for retained foreign bodies. In any situation where an emergent surgical procedure is performed and there is inadequate time for a sponge count or the count is found to be incorrect, radiographic evaluation should be completed. Furthermore, if an open abdomen, damage control procedure, or a second-look laparotomy is required, prior to the final definitive closure, a radiographic survey of the chest or abdominal cavity to ensure that there are no retained foreign bodies should be performed.

MISSED INJURIES

For the acute care surgeon, missed injuries intraoperatively in trauma constitute a major potential pitfall. In multisystem trauma, missed injuries are not uncommon. This is especially true in patients that are unevaluable with traumatic brain injury and those patients who proceed directly to emergency surgery. It is critical that all trauma patients undergo a tertiary survey with a complete head to toe examination and radiographic survey as warranted. This has been documented to decrease the incidence of missed injuries.[34] For trauma patients requiring operative intervention, there are numerous potential pitfalls. In penetrating trauma, the path of each projectile needs to be carefully followed to determine the areas at risk of injury. Common areas where injuries are missed intraoperatively include the diaphragm, ureters, retroperitoneal colon, and duodenum. In penetrating injuries, all hematomas require exploration. With shotgun wounds, the multiple small pellet holes are difficult to track and careful examination of the hollow viscus structures is required in order to avoid missed injuries. In blunt trauma, complete examination of all structures is required to exclude injury including the duodenum, diaphragm, and lesser sac.

For penetrating cardiac trauma, emergent wall repair is often required in order to salvage the patient. After sternal closure and stabilization, early postoperative examination of the heart sounds and transthoracic echocardiography is required in order to exclude a missed valvular or septal injury as the incidence of this complication is approximately 20%.[35]

Missed injuries are a pitfall that continues to occur, even with experienced trauma surgeons. For patients undergoing operation, careful and complete intraoperative evaluation is required. Postoperatively and for patients not requiring surgery, a comprehensive tertiary survey and review of radiographic studies is essential to decrease the incidence of this complication.

ALCOHOL WITHDRAWAL

Alcohol is a widely abused substance across all socioeconomic levels around the world. With direct toxic effects on virtually all organ systems, the paradox lies in the potentially life-threatening effects that may result from the abrupt cessation of its use. Alcohol withdrawal is seen commonly in the surgical patient, especially in those sustaining trauma.[36-38] The early preoperative detection of alcohol abuse would allow for effective prophylaxis;[36-38] however, even in the elective surgical patient this is commonly missed. In acutely ill patients about to undergo emergency surgery, this history can be even more difficult to elicit. Awareness of the prevalence of this problem, the clinical manifestations and its treatment is critical to avoidance of this postoperative pitfall. Acute alcohol withdrawal often manifests within 6 to 24 hours of the last ingestion. This is a diagnosis that must be considered in all patients of all ages. An up-regulated autonomic response results in nausea, vomiting, hyperthermia, tremors, anxiety and agitation. Patients may present with seizure activity. This may progress to delirium tremens with hallucinations, confusion, and altered level of consciousness in addition to the autonomic abnormalities. Cardiopulmonary collapse and death may occur if not detected and treated. The differential diagnosis includes hypoxia, sepsis, fluid, and electrolyte abnormalities.

Postoperatively, if a history was not available, this should be elicited either from the patient, family, or friends. If the patient is intubated or is otherwise unable to provide a history, at the earliest exhibition of symptoms, treatment should be initiated. Although a variety of laboratory markers are being investigated, at this time, none are available for clinical use. Treatment is pharmacological. In the surgical patient, the severity of the symptoms and the amount of medication required is considerably greater than the nonsurgical patient, likely due to differences in the set point autonomic state, effects of the anesthetic, and pain. The mainstay of treatment remains benzodiazepines.[39] Adjunctive medications such as Clonidine and Haloperidol are also in common use; however, both can decrease the seizure threshold, result in QT-interval prolongation and Clonidine may decrease cerebral blood flow and therefore both should not be used as single agents. These medications should be titrated to effect. In patients undergoing withdrawal, it is important to monitor for the other effects of alcohol that may effect the postoperative course including malnutrition, chronic liver disease (coagulation, metabolism, healing), myocardial damage (arrhythmias, cardiomyopathy, hypertension), neurological problems, and a host of associated GI problems, some of which may have necessitated the acute surgical intervention.

REFERENCES

1. Hines R, Barash PG, Watrous G, et al. Complications occurring in the postanesthesia care unit: a survey. *Anesth Analg* 1992;74(4):503-509.
2. Mangano DT, Browner WS, Hollenberg M, et al. Association of perioperative myocardial ischemia with cardiac morbidity and mortality in men undergoing noncardiac surgery: The Study of Perioperative Ischemia Research Group. *N Engl J Med* 1990;323(26):1781-1788.
3. Mangano DT, Hollenberg M, Fegert G, et al. Perioperative myocardial ischemia in patients undergoing noncardiac surgery—I: Incidence and severity during the 4 day perioperative period. The Study of Perioperative Ischemia (SPI) Research Group. *J Am Coll Cardiol* 1991;17(4):843-850.
4. Mangano DT, Wong MG, London MJ, et al. Perioperative myocardial ischemia in patients undergoing noncardiac surgery—II: Incidence and severity during the 1st week after surgery: The Study of Perioperative Ischemia (SPI) Research Group. *J Am Coll Cardiol* 1991;17(4):851-857.
5. Mangano DT, Layug EL, Wallace A, et al. Effect of atenolol on mortality and cardiovascular morbidity after noncardiac surgery. Multicenter Study of Perioperative Ischemia Research Group. *N Engl J Med* 1996;335(23):1713-1720.
6. Eagle KA, Berger PB, Calkins H, et al. ACC/AHA guideline update for perioperative cardiovascular evaluation for noncardiac surgery: executive summary: a report of the American College of Cardiology/American Heart Association Task Force on Practice Guidelines (Committee to update the 1996 Guidelines on perioperative cardiovascular evaluation for noncardiac surgery). *J Am Coll Cardiol* 2002;39(3):542-553.
7. Charlson ME, MacKenzie CR, Ales KL, et al. The postoperative electrocardiogram and creatine kinase: implications for diagnosis of myocardial infarction after non-cardiac surgery. *J Clin Epidemiol* 1989;42(1):25-34.
8. Charlson ME, MacKenzie CR, Ales K, et al. Surveillance for postoperative myocardial infarction after noncardiac operations. *Surg Gynecol Obstet* 1988;167(5):407-414.

9. Kemp M, Donovan J, Higham H, et al. Biochemical markers of myocardial injury. *Br J Anaesth* 2004;93(1):63-73.

10. Adams JE III, Sicard GA, Allen BT, et al. Diagnosis of perioperative myocardial infarction with measurement of cardiac troponin I. *N Engl J Med* 1994;330(10):670-674.

11. Mangano DT, Browner WS, Hollenberg M, et al. Long-term cardiac prognosis following noncardiac surgery. The Study of Perioperative Ischemia Research Group. *JAMA* 1992;268(2):252-253.

12. Frank SM, Fleisher LA, Breslow MJ, et al. Perioperative maintenance of normothermia reduces the incidence of morbid cardiac events. A randomized clinical trial. *JAMA* 1997;227(14):1127-1134.

13. Charlson ME, MacKenzie CR, Gold JP, et al. Preoperative characteristics predicting intraoperative hypotension and hypertension among hypertensives and diabetics undergoing noncardiac surgery. *Ann Surg* 1990;212(1):66-81.

14. Browner WS, Li J, Mangano DT. In-hospital and long-term mortality in male veterans following noncardiac surgery: The Study of Perioperative Ischemia Research Group. *JAMA* 1992;268(2):228-232.

15. Gal TJ, Cooperman LH. Hypertension in the immediate postoperative period. *Br J Anaesth* 1975;47(1):70-74.

16. Albert SN, Penlivanian Z, McClure K Urinary bladder distention: a cause of hypertension during anesthesia. *Anesth Analg* 1971;50(5):794-797.

17. Deveraux PJ, Yusuf S, Yang H, et al. Are the recommendations to use perioperative beta-blocker therapy in patients undergoing noncardiac surgery based on reliable evidence. *CMAJ* 2004;171(3):245-247.

18. Cooperman LH, Price HL. Pulmonary edema in the operative and postoperative period: a review of 40 cases. *Ann Surg* 1970;172(5):883-891.

19. Goldman L, Caldera DL, Nussbaum SR, et al. Multifactorial index of cardiac risk in noncardiac surgical procedures. *N Engl J Med* 1977;297(16):845-850.

20. Qaseem A, Snow V, Fitterman N, et al. Risk assessment for and strategies to reduce perioperative pulmonary complications for patients undergoing noncardiothoracic surgery: a guideline from the American College of Physicians. *Ann Intern Med* 2006;144(8):575-580.

21. Taylor S, Kirton OC, Staff I, et al. Postoperative day one: a high risk period for respiratory events. *Am J Surg* 2005;190(5):752-756.

22. Latenser BA, Kowal-Vern A, Kimball D, et al. A pilot study comparing percutaneous decompression with decompressive laparotomy for acute abdominal compartment syndrome in thermal injury. *J Burn Care Rehabil* 2002;23(3):190-195.

23. McQueen MM, Court-Brown CM. Compartment monitoring in tibial fractures. The pressure threshold for decompression. *J Bone Joint Surg Br* 1996;78(1):99-104.

24. MacLeod JB, Lynn M, McKenney, et al. Early coagulopathy predicts mortality in trauma. *J Trauma* 2003;55(1):39-44.

25. Gonzalez H, Nardi O, Annane D. Relative adrenal failure in the ICU: an identifiable problem requiring treatment. *Crit Care Clin* 2006;22(1):105-118, vii.

26. Davoren A, Aster RH. Heparin-induced thrombocytopenia and thrombosis. *Am J Hematol* 2006;81(1):36-44.

27. de Maistre E, Gruel Y, Lasne D. Diagnosis and management of heparin-induced thrombocytopenia. *Can J Anaesth* 2006;53(6 suppl):S123-S134.

28. Hopkins PM. Malignant hyperthermia: advances in clinical management and diagnosis. *Br J Anaesth* 2000;85(1):118-128.

29. Heggie JE. Malignant hyperthermia: considerations for the general surgeon. *Can J Surg* 2002;45(5):369-372.

30. Krause T, Gerbershagen M, Fiege M, et al. Dantrolene—a review of its pharmacology, therapeutic use and new developments. *Anaesthesia* 2004;59(4):363-373.

31. Bani-Hani KE, Gharaibeh KA, Yaghan RJ Retained surgical sponges (gossypiboma). *Asian J Surg* 2005;28(2):109-115.

32. Gawande AA, Studdert DM, Orav EJ, et al. Risk factors for retained instruments and sponges after surgery. *N Engl J Med* 2003;348(3):229-235.

33. Gibbs VC, McGrath MH, Russell TR. The prevention of retained foreign bodies after surgery. *Bull Am Coll Surg* 2005;90(10):15-16.

34. Biffl WL, Harrington DT, Cioffi WG. Implementation of a tertiary trauma survey decreases missed injuries. *J Trauma* 2003;54(1):38-43; discussion 43-44.

35. Demetriades D, Charalambides C, Sareli P, et al. Late sequelae of penetrating cardiac injuries. *Br J Surg* 1990;77(7):813-814.

36. Spies CD, Rommelspacher H. Alcohol withdrawal in the surgical patient: prevention and treatment. *Anesth Analg* 1999;88:946-954.

37. Spies CD, Neuner B, Neumann T, et al. Intercurrent complications in chronic alcoholic men admitted to the intensive care unit following trauma. *Intensive Care Med* 1996;22(4):286-293.

38. Spies CD, Nordmann A, Brummer G, et al. Intensive care unit stay is prolonged in chronic alcoholic men following tumor resection of the upper digestive tract. *Acta Anaesthesiol Scand* 1996;40(6):649-656.

39. Mayo-Smith MF. Pharmacological management of alcohol withdrawal: a meta-analysis and evidence-based practice guideline: American Society of Addiction Medicine working group on pharmacological management of alcohol withdrawal. *JAMA*, 1997;278(2):144-151.

Chapter 21

GENERAL EVALUATION AND RESUSCITATION

Jason W. Smith, MD, Scott B. Armen, MD, and Larry C. Martin, MD

INTRODUCTION

The initial assessment of the patient who presents with an acute surgical emergency confronts the physician with a complex problem. This is true if the patient is a victim of trauma or has life-threatening abdominal pathology. In either case, the priorities are the same and the decisions must be made expeditiously. Patient stability must be assured while diagnostic studies are undertaken and plans made for definitive therapy instituted. This begins with the assessment of the airway, breathing, and circulation with ongoing resuscitation. Each life-threatening emergency must be dealt with as it is identified. Often obtaining any history has to be delayed until the patient is stable.

PRIMARY EVALUATION

AIRWAY

Airway assessment should be straightforward. The awake, talking patient can be assumed to have a patent stable airway. However, the potential for airway obstruction must also be determined so that intubation can be accomplished prior to any airway compromise. Obstruction may result from soft tissue or tongue edema, blood, foreign bodies, teeth, or vomit. Facial fractures may cause obstruction due to anatomical changes, soft tissue swelling, or bleeding. These problems may not be obvious initially, but any chance of problems should be addressed before they become emergent and more difficult. This is particularly important in facial burns and inhalation where airway edema may develop quickly during resuscitation with resulting obstruction. The combative patient may be assumed to have a closed head injury or be intoxicated but in reality have hypoxemia as a cause of their agitation. In general, patients that are unconscious and have a Glasgow Coma Scale (GCS) score of 8 or less and cannot protect their airway should be intubated.

Rapid sequence intubation (RSI) (Table 21-1) by the orotracheal route is preferred if someone with experience with the agents used and technique is available. This involves the use of a short acting depolarizing agent, succinylcholine, which provides short-term paralysis. This is often used with etomidate for anesthetic and amnestic properties as well as minimal impact on cardiovascular function with hypotension even in hypovolemic patients.[1] The paralytic and anesthetic effects last less than 10 minutes. Caution should be used with succinylcholine in patients with neuromuscular disease, paralysis, prolonged immobilization, and burns after 48 hours due to the possibility of life-threatening hyperkalemia.[2,3]

Despite the success of RSI via the oral route occasionally, this cannot be accomplished. Nasotracheal intubation is a good alternative if the patient is breathing spontaneously and there are no contraindications such as midface fractures. This can be done with minimal or no sedation. If oral- or nasotracheal intubation cannot be accomplished then the clinician must be prepared to perform a cricothyroidotomy emergently.

If there is concern that a cervical spinal cord injury may be present, then immobilization should be maintained at all times. In the unconscious patient with obvious head or facial injuries this is particularly important, but oral intubation can be done safely with careful support of the cervical spine in the neutral position using a two-person technique, one for spine control and one for intubation. Obtaining airway control should take precedence over spine x-rays, which should never delay intubation in the emergent circumstance and they are usually inadequate for cervical spine "clearance."

BREATHING

Once the airway has been evaluated, the adequacy of ventilation should be addressed. Symmetrical chest wall motion, equal breath sounds on auscultation, and depth of tidal volume should be determined. Pulse

Table 21-1   Rapid sequence intubation
Preparation: Universal precautions and assemble equipment
Cervical spine stabilization: Remove anterior collar and hold in-line traction
Preoxygenation: 100% O_2 for 3 minutes if possible
Pretreatment: Consider atropine or lidocaine and cricoid pressure
Anesthesia: Etomidate (0.3 mg/kg), or thiopental (2-4 mg/kg), or propofol (2 mg/kg)
Paralysis: Succinylcholine (1-2 mg/kg) or rocuronium (1 mg/kg)
Oral intubation with neck immobilized in traction
Confirm tube position and bilateral breath sounds
End-tidal CO_2 confirmation of tracheal intubation
Firmly secure the endotracheal tube and note the position
Replace cervical collar for neck immobilization

oximetry may be helpful in determining the oxygen saturation quickly and noninvasively. The causes of inadequate ventilation may be related to trauma such as a tension pneumothorax, open pneumothorax, massive hemothorax, flail chest with pulmonary contusion, or rib fractures with significant pain. Also, the patient with increased ventilation requirements due to a metabolic acidosis or onset of respiratory insufficiency will require emergent intervention. Correction of the underlying cause, if possible, is optimal, such as placing a chest tube, or pain control, but often ventilatory support is needed before the underlying pathology can be corrected.

A hemothorax or pneumothorax may be the result of penetrating or blunt injury. It may also result from the improper placement of central venous catheters for volume infusion. These may result in massive tension hemo- or pneumothoraces with the pressure in the chest caused lung collapse and mediastinal shift with decreased venous return to the heart. In the unstable patient, needle decompression with a 14-gauge IV catheter inserted in the 2nd intercostal space in the midclavicular line can be done. This should be followed by insertion of a tube thoracostomy as definitive treatment for evacuation of air and blood. This should be done with a large (36 or 40 French) chest tube inserted in the 4th or 5th intercostal space (nipple level) between the mid and anterior axillary lines. The tube should be directed posteriorly and to the apex of the hemithorax which should evacuate both blood and air in the supine patient. The use of trocars for chest tube insertion should be avoided.

An open pneumothorax with a wound that is two-thirds the diameter of the trachea may also compromise breathing. During inspiration air moves through the open chest wound which decreases the amount that comes through the trachea into the lungs with resultant hypoxemia. This air entering the pleural space may also cause shifting of the mediastinum and interfere with venous return to the heart causing hypotension. The initial treatment is placement of a three-sided occlusive dressing over the wound to prevent air from entering the pleural space during inhalation but allowing escape of trapped air from the chest during exhalation. A tube thoracostomy should be inserted for definitive management and closure or occlusion of the open chest wound is necessary to prevent an air leak from the chest wall. Once connected to a collection system (Pleur-Evac), the amount of blood and presence of an air leak with bubbles in the water seal chamber should be documented.

A massive hemothorax is defined as greater than 1500 cc of blood on initial insertion of a tube thoracostomy.[4] This is an indication of a very significant thoracic injury and a thoracotomy is indicated for hemorrhage control. A thoracotomy is also indicated if there is continued bleeding from the thorax greater than 100-200 cc/hr. The presence of an air leak may signify a parenchymal lung injury, bronchial, or tracheal injury. This results in respiratory compromise and large loss of tidal volume with positive pressure ventilation and hypercapnia. Bronchoscopy can be utilized to determine the site of injury.[5]

A flail chest, defined as fracture of three or more consecutive ribs in more than one place or fractures associated with costochondral separation at the sternum, may also compromise breathing. This results in paradoxical movement of the chest wall such that the flail segment moves inward while the chest wall moves outward during inspiration and is due to the negative inspiratory force during inspiration.[6] Disruption of the chest wall anatomy from eight or more fractures results in the inability to take an adequate tidal volume. However, the underlying pulmonary contusion and tremendous pain associated with the fractures causes most of the respiratory problems. Pain control is vital and use of regional anesthetic techniques, such as epidural analgesia, can be useful without the sedative effects of systemic agents. The resulting hypoxemia from the pulmonary contusion may require mechanical ventilatory support and may not be evident initially as the physiologic changes tend to progress over the first 48 to 72 hours after injury and patients should be monitored closely for this time period.

Shock as a result of blood or intravascular volume loss may cause significant respiratory derangement as a compensatory mechanism. Tachypnea may be evident early as patients attempt to increase minute ventilation due to the effects of a severe metabolic acidosis. This may result from trauma, gastrointestinal bleeding, or a response to sepsis. Often mechanical ventilation is necessary while volume infusion of crystalloid or blood is undertaken.

CIRCULATION

Adequacy of circulation and tissue perfusion is of utmost importance. Hypovolemia is the most common cause of circulatory failure in the patient with a surgical emergency. Obviously, the trauma patient usually will be hemorrhaging, but so will the patient with an acute massive gastrointestinal bleed. After trauma, the likelihood of cardiac tamponade, tension pneumothorax, or blunt cardiac injury should be addressed also. Patients with acute abdominal problems may have substantial volume losses due to vomiting or diarrhea. In addition, the effects of ongoing severe infection with sequestration of fluid can have profound effects whether from a perforated viscus or a necrotizing soft tissue infection. Placement of adequate venous access, usually at least two large-bore catheters in upper extremity veins and volume infusion should be instituted with warm crystalloid solution. External hemorrhage should be controlled with direct pressure on the bleeding site until definitive control is attained. This is more effective than large dressings and tape. Scalp lacerations can cause extensive hemorrhage and rapid closure with staples or a running suture will stop the bleeding in the majority of cases.

The assessment of circulation involves physiologic parameters that are easily measured in the emergent situation. These include heart rate, blood pressure, urine output, and level of consciousness. The nature and strength of the pulse should be determined. Tachycardia with a rate greater than 120 in adults is a sign of hypovolemia in the trauma patient. This may be affected by pacemakers, beta-blocking, or calcium channel blocking drugs as well so the absence of tachycardia does not mean a patient is not in shock. In general, a strong femoral pulse means that a patient has a blood pressure of at least 70-80 mm Hg and those with a carotid pulse a blood pressure of 60-70 mm Hg.

Blood pressure may not reflect to degree of shock and can be normal until a patient has lost greater than 35% of their blood volume. Furthermore, accuracy is questionable when there is a mismatch in cuff size and patient size. The use of automated blood pressure cuff devices further complicates obtaining a representative value. A manual blood pressure can be obtained quickly and should be used in the initial determination. Particular attention should be given to the pulse pressure, which may more accurately reflect intravascular volume status. The pulse pressure will decrease with 15%-20% or blood volume loss, which is before an actual fall in systolic pressure would be noted.

In the trauma patient, the possibility of cardiac tamponade or tension pneumothorax must also be considered. Each of these will result in hypotension but will also have distended neck veins or elevated central venous pressure which would not be found with hemorrhagic shock. If cardiac tamponade is suspected, an ultrasound (FAST) can be performed to identify fluid in the pericardial space. If this is indeterminate either needle pericardiocentesis or a pericardial window can be done which would be followed by thoracotomy if positive. Needle pericardiocentesis is often described but rarely performed because the use of ultrasound has become prevalent and the technique is rarely used in a trauma situation. A tension pneumothorax should be suspected with absent breath sounds on chest examination and tracheal deviation toward the opposite hemithorax. Needle or tube thoracostomy decompression of the chest will alleviate the tension and restore cardiac venous return.

DISABILITY

The neurologic status should be assessed after the life-threatening conditions are treated. This baseline examination should include papillary size and reaction, Glasgow Coma Scale (GCS) determination, and the presence of any focal motor or sensory findings.

The GCS includes is assessed for three areas: (1) best motor response, (2) eye opening, and (3) verbal response. The lowest score is a 3 and the highest 15. Those patients with a GCS of 8 or less are considered unconscious. For those patients that cannot give a verbal response due to intubation the best score would be 11. The utility of the GCS is that it can be repeated during the assessment of the patient and afterward to detect changes in neurologic condition and is highly reproducible by multiple examiners over time.

Pupillary size and reaction as well as any asymmetry in the neurologic assessment may indicate the possibility of an intracranial mass lesion that require emergent surgical intervention. Furthermore, evidence of motor or sensory deficit may indicate the presence of a spinal cord injury. The need for computed tomography should be determined as well based on this examination and the history.

EXPOSURE AND ENVIRONMENT

Prior to patient arrival, the area for evaluation should be warmed to prevent hypothermia. Patients must be completely examined and all clothes quickly removed. This is often done by cutting the clothes off in an emergent situation. Warm fluids should be used for resuscitation and warm blankets placed over the patient once the examination is concluded. Hypothermia is more difficult to correct than to prevent and body temperature should be monitored closely.

HISTORY AND COMPLETE EXAMINATION

Once the primary evaluation is complete and the life-threatening conditions treated, a history and complete examination should be done. The history may come from family members or prehospital personnel may provide much or the relevant information. Essential information includes allergies to medications, previous illnesses, medical conditions and operations, current medications, and the nature of the current illness or injury.

A detailed examination should be performed when possible. This is often described as the secondary survey for trauma patients when a "head to toe" evaluation of all injuries is done. Naso- or orogastric tubes and urinary catheters should be inserted routinely in most patients with emergent surgical problems. Also, the necessary diagnostic studies required such as computed tomography should be arranged. While the secondary evaluation is ongoing, monitoring of the patient's condition should be done to include vital signs, urine output, arterial oxygen saturation, and end tidal CO_2 for patients on mechanical ventilation. During this time the patient is reassessed for any change in condition that may warrant expeditious surgical intervention.

RADIOGRAPHS AND DIAGNOSTIC STUDIES

Chest radiographs should be done in most if not all patients with acute surgical emergencies and in all blunt trauma patients. Also, in the blunt trauma patient, a pelvic film should be performed, as this may be a site of ongoing hemorrhage. These films can be done while the initial assessment is in progress and may identify serious conditions that need immediate therapy. Evaluation of the cervical spine with plain x-rays has be supplanted by CT scan of the neck in most cases.[7]

Ultrasound or focused abdominal sonogram for trauma (FAST) can be used to determine the presence of intra-abdominal blood or fluid and is a fast, noninvasive method to determine if the abdomen is a site of significant bleeding. It does not interfere with ongoing resuscitation and does not require patient transport to the radiology department. However, use of ultrasound is operator dependent and someone familiar with the interpretation of the images must be available. In cases where the FAST is not an option, Diagnostic Peritoneal Lavage (DPL) is a very sensitive method for determining intra-abdominal hemorrhage. This, too, can be performed while there is ongoing activity and without patient transport but is an invasive procedure with approximately a 2% complication rate.[8] Other radiologic studies are usually done after the patient has been stabilized and can be transported to the radiology department. This would include computed tomography of the head, neck, chest, abdomen, and pelvis as indicated.

RESUSCITATION

Resuscitation of the emergency surgery/trauma patient encompasses much more than selecting the appropriate fluid to administer. These patients present an extreme challenge to the clinician due to an underlying derangement in the basic physiologic processes of life. Emergency surgery patients are often hypothermic, acidotic, coagulopathic and in various stages of shock and only by correcting these derangements by appropriate and rapid resuscitation will patients survive.

THE LETHAL TRIAD: HYPOTHERMIA, ACIDOSIS, AND COAGULOPATHY[9]

Hypothermia is defined as a core body temperature of less than 35°C and is usually caused by prolonged exposure to the elements usually during colder, winter months. While exposure to the elements can certainly become a factor in trauma patients, most emergency surgery patients become hypothermic due to iatrogenic causes. Large body surface areas are often exposed for long periods of time in the operating room leading to increased heat loss. Room temperature IV fluid administration can lower the body's core temperature. Skeletal muscle hypoperfusion can lead to hypothermia and negate the shivering response which is an important internal mechanism for heat production. Decreased body temperature can slow cardiac conduction decreasing heart rate and cardiac output. Peripheral vasoconstriction results in a shunting of blood to the central circulation which can worsen acidosis due to skeletal muscle ischemia. Acid-base and electrolyte derangements hypovolemia develop due to a "cold" diuresis and extracellular fluid shifts.

Correction of hypothermia is a priority in emergency surgery patients and can usually be accomplished by passive techniques. Covering the patient with warm blankets and keeping the environment warm allows endogenous heat production to correct the hypothermia. All fluids and blood products given to emergency surgery patients should be warmed to 40°C. Breathing warm humidified oxygen via face mask or ET tube is effective in many cases. Active rewarming techniques such as warm body cavity lavage or extracorporeal blood warming are not indicated and should be reserved for patients in sever hypothermia due to exposure or cold water immersion.

The most important question regarding ongoing bleeding in an emergency surgery patient is: Is there a surgically correctable cause for the bleeding? Ongoing blood loss from a surgically correctible cause cannot be dealt with by resuscitation, rewarming, and fluid and blood product administration. Alternately, bleeding from multiple sites implies an ongoing coagulation defect that further surgery cannot help. Emergency surgery patients are often coagulopathic due to multiple reasons and correction of the ongoing acquired coagulation disorder is required.

In a normal coagulation cascade, tissue injury leads to exposed collagen, endothelial damage, and release of various intracellular products (ie, adenosine diphosphate, ADP). This results in platelet aggregation and adherence to the injured area. Then a complex interaction between platelet phospholipase A_2 and the injured cellular membrane leads to the activation of the arachidonic acid pathway. This results in the production of thromboxane A_2, which causes vasoconstriction of the microcirculation and leads to further platelet aggregation. Thrombin deposition begins to occur at the platelet plug from the activated coagulation cascade. This is primary hemostasis. Secondary hemostasis continues this process as the exposed collagen and platelet factor 3 activate the intrinsic pathway of coagulation. Tissue thromboplastin then activates the extrinsic pathway. The net effect is the activation of factor X and conversion of prothrombin to thrombin and thus fibrinogen to fibrin. Fibrin stabilizes the entire clot and completes secondary hemostasis. Tissue plasminogen activator, TPA, then converts plasminogen to plasmin which in the presence of factors C and S causes fibrin degradation. This balancing mechanism controls bleeding but does not allow for "runaway" hemostasis.

Several acquired coagulation defects are seen in emergency surgery patients and must be corrected if resuscitation is going to succeed. Consumptive coagulopathy is a broad term that identifies an acquired coagulopathy due to resuscitation of blood loss using products devoid of coagulation factors. The endogenous coagulation proteins are used in the normal coagulation process. However, as bleeding continues, no other products are available leading to a significant bleeding diathesis. Fresh frozen plasma and platelet transfusions are often required after significant red blood cell transfusion. Calcium can be chelated by the citrate in blood products requiring the administration of exogenous calcium. Activated factor VII has recently been shown to be of benefit in a select subgroup of patients.

Another significant defect found in emergency surgery patients is thrombocytopenia. This is often due to platelet consumption; however, chronic medical conditions such as renal failure and HIV infection can lead to this as well. Clinical bleeding due to thrombocytopenia rarely occurs below platelet counts of 20,000 and transfusions should be aimed at maintaining a count higher than this during initial resuscitation of the emergency surgery patient. It is important to remember that many emergency surgery patients will have been taking aspirin, NSAIDS, or Plavix prior to surgery. Without adequate time to stop administration of these products, significant platelet dysfunction can occur with normal platelet counts. In this case, it will often be necessary to transfuse platelets in spite of a normal platelet count in order to correct a bleeding diathesis.

Correction of acidosis in the emergency surgery patient is at the core of all successful resuscitations. Acidosis in the emergency surgery patient can come from multiple sources. Nongap metabolic acidosis can occur after resuscitation with hypertonic resuscitation fluids such as normal saline and 3% saline. Renal failure can lead to acidosis secondary to accumulation of organic acids and renal tubular acidosis. Respiratory acidosis can occur as the systemic inflammatory mediators lead to hypercarbia and progressive respiratory failure. However, the most common cause of acidosis in the emergency surgery patient is a lactic acidosis due to poor tissue perfusion and reliance on anaerobic metabolism for energy. Regardless of the cause of the acidosis, it must be corrected because endogenous proteins have a very narrow pH range of activity. Outside of this range, physiologic function slows and then ceases leading the eventual cellular death. In severe lactic acidosis, sodium bicarbonate may be used to temporarily increase the circulating pH; however, it is not without drawbacks and usually is reserved for patients with a pH below 7.2. Eventually, correction of the acidosis requires the restoration of tissue oxygenation and correction of the patient's shock state.

SHOCK

Shock represents a syndrome of derangement in the supply to or utilization of oxygen by the peripheral tissues. This can represent a failure of the pumping mechanism (cardiogenic shock), a failure of the delivery substrate (hemorrhagic/hypovolemic shock) or a failure in the delivery system itself (septic/neurogenic shock). Regardless of the inciting event, the end result is a decrease in adenosine triphosphate production by oxidative metabolism and the near total reliance on anaerobic metabolism for the production of energy. This reliance on anaerobic metabolism leads to excess organic acid production, cellular ischemia, tissue hypoxia, and eventual organ dysfunction.

Classification of shock is based on the etiology of the inciting event (Table 21-2). It must be emphasized that the emergency surgery patient may be affected by any combination of causes, making the diagnosis and treatment more difficult. Hypovolemic shock is a condition that causes decreased preload secondary to plasma volume loss. Hemorrhagic shock is a subtype of hypovolemic shock due to blood loss; however, any condition that causes a decrease in plasma volume (vomiting, diarrhea) or extravascular fluid sequestration (bowel obstruction, increased vascular permeability) can lead to this condition. Table 21-3 shows the classification of degrees of hypovolemic shock with each degree increasing in severity. Treatment of hypovolemic/hemorrhagic shock is replacement of circulating blood volume. Initiation of vasopressor agents is contraindicated as it will worsen tissue ischemia and acidosis, leading to a worsening in the overall condition/outcome.

Cardiogenic shock indicates a failure in the pump of the vascular system, the heart. This can come from

Table 21-2 Etiology and Manifestations of Shock

Etiology	Skin	Urine Output	Cardiac Output	PAOP	SVR	SvO$_2$
Hypovolemic	Cool, pale	Decreased	Decreased	Decreased	Increased	Decrease
Cardiogenic	Cool, pale	Decreased	Decreased	Increased	Increased	Decreased
Septic: early	Warm, pink	Normal	Increased	Normal	Normal or Decreased	Normal to Increased
Septic: late	Cool, pale	Decreased	Decreased	Decreased	Decreased	Decreased
Neurogenic	Warm, pink	Decreased	Decreased	Decreased	Decreased	Decreased
Anaphylactic	Cool, pale	Decreased	Decreased	Decreased	Increased	Decreased

various sources such as tamponade, arrhythmia, valvular lesions, and so on. However, the most classic example is that of myocardial infarction. Whatever the cause, the underlying pathophysiology is a decrease in cardiac output resulting from contractile dysfunction of the myocardium. Clinical presentation depends on the degree of myocardium affected and can include tachycardia, jugular venous distension, oliguria, pulmonary edema, and hypotension. Treatment of cardiac failure depends on the recognition and treatment of the underlying cause. Preload, afterload, and cardiac output should be optimized using invasive monitoring if necessary, and intra-aortic balloon pump augmentation may be needed.

Neurogenic shock results from a loss of sympathetic tone causing a pooling of blood in the capacitance vessels of the venous system. This causes a relative decrease in the plasma volume available for circulation leading to the same downward spiral as hypovolemic shock. The classic situation where this occurs is after a high spinal cord injury (T4 level or higher); however, oliguria/hypotension after spinal anesthesia is related to the same mechanism. Treatment entails initial volume resuscitation with early institution of vasopressor agents to normalize vascular tone.

Anaphylactic shock results from exposure of a sensitized individual to an antigen that results in the massive release of histamine and other vasoactive substances from mast cells and basophils. Clinical manifestations of anaphylaxis typically occurs within minutes of exposure and consist of angioedema, urticaria, flushing, laryngeal edema, bronchospasm, and, eventually, hypotension and vascular collapse. Treatment of anaphylactic shock consists of removal

Table 21-3 Classification of Hemorrhagic Shock

	Class I	Class II	Class III	Class IV
Blood loss (%)	< 15	15-30	30-40	> 40
Heart rate	Normal	Mild tachycardia (100-120 bpm)	Significant tachycardia (120-140 bpm)	Severe Tachycardia (> 140 bpm)
Systolic blood pressure	Normal	Normal	Decreased	Decreased
Pulse pressure	Normal	Decreased	Decreased	Decreased
Capillary refill	Normal	Delayed	Delayed	Delayed
Urinary output	Normal (> 30 ml/h)	Slight decrease (20-30 ml/h)	Significant decreased (5-15 ml/h)	Oliguria
Mental status	Normal	Anxiety	Confusion	Lethargy
Fluid replacement	Crystalloid	Crystalloid	Crystalloid and PRBCs	Crystalloid and PRBCs

of the offending antigen, endotracheal intubation to secure the patients airway, epinephrine, glucocorticoids and supportive therapy until the anaphylactic response subsides.

Sepsis and septic shock are variations of the same pathophysiologic response. Both describe a syndrome of increased vascular permeability, cardiac dysfunction, and hemodynamic collapse due to an overproduction of endogenous inflammatory mediators in response to an infectious focus. If organ failure results it is deemed septic shock. Any of the previously mentioned shock syndromes can precipitate a systemic inflammatory response syndrome (SIRS) giving a similar clinical picture as sepsis. It is these entities that are most often encountered in the emergency surgery patient.

TREATMENT OF SHOCK

Interventions to correct the shock state rely upon the normalization of tissue oxygen delivery and utilization. Figure 21-1 shows the concept of oxygen supply dependency. As oxygen delivery exceed demand oxygen consumption will "plateau" and further increase will not affect consumption. Supply dependency occurs in this critical section where supply does not meet demand, an increase in oxygen delivery can make a significant impact on tissue oxygenation. The method of doing this varies considerably between the different shock syndromes; however, a single standard response to the initial resuscitation of the emergency general surgery patient can be elucidated. The calculation of systemic oxygen delivery (DO_2) is:

$$DO_2 = CaO_2 \times CO$$

where CaO_2 is the arterial oxygen content as blood leaves the heart, and CO is cardiac output. Arterial oxygen content can further be defined as

$$CaO_2 = \text{oxygen bound by hemoglobin (98\%)}$$
$$+ \text{oxygen dissolved in blood (2\%)}$$

or

$$CaO_2 = (1.34 \times Hgb \times SaO_2) + (0.0031 \times PaO_2)$$

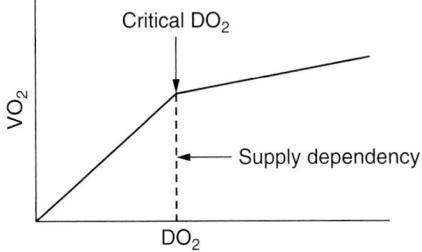

Figure 21-1 *Oxygen supply dependency.*

where Hgb is hemoglobin concentration of the blood, SaO_2 is the saturation of hemoglobin with oxygen, and PaO_2 is the alveolar oxygen tension. The factor 1.34 comes from the fact that 1.34 ml of oxygen can be carried by each gram of human hemoglobin. Cardiac output is defined as the product of heart rate (HR) and stroke volume (SV). Therefore, the overall equation for DO_2 is:

$$DO_2 = (HR \times SV) \times [(1.34 \times Hgb \times SaO_2)$$
$$+ (0.0031 \times PaO_2)]$$

Several clinical interventions can be made using this equation as guidance to increase oxygen delivery. First, heart rate should be controlled between a rate of 50 and 150 beats per minute. Below 50 beats per minute cardiac output can be significantly affected and above 150 beats per minute left ventricular filling is decreased to the point that cardiac output can be compromised. Second, PaO_2 and SaO_2 should be optimized by the application of oxygen support, ventilatory support and positive end-expiratory pressure (PEEP). These two interventions can be made quickly and easily in most patients and can augment oxygen delivery significantly. One of the most important determinants of tissue oxygen delivery is the arterial hemoglobin concentration. While oxygen delivery from the left ventricle is linearly related to the hemoglobin concentration, capillary flow may be impaired at extremely high hematocrits. Theoretically, the optimal hemoglobin concentration to maximize tissue oxygen delivery seems to be in the range of between 10 and 13 g/dL and transfusion to achieve these goals has shown to increase tissue oxygen delivery. However, it has been difficult to demonstrate this benefit in clinical practice and some studies document a lack of improvement in tissue oxygenation after RBC transfusion, despite increases in oxygen delivery. Dietrich et al observed no improvement in oxygen consumption among patients with shock who had hemoglobin levels increased from 8.3 g/dL to 10.5 g/dL by transfusion of RBCs. Similarly, in another study of septic patients, blood transfusion did not improve tissue oxygen uptake, despite an increase in oxygen delivery.

Once these factors have been optimized the last remaining variable to increase is stroke volume (SV). Stroke volume of the left ventricle is determined by three important physiologic concepts: preload, afterload, and contractility of the myocardium. By optimizing each of these variables, stroke volume can be increased, thus increasing cardiac output, which increases oxygen delivery to the peripheral tissues.

Preload is broadly defined as the stretch on a skeletal or cardiac muscle prior to contraction (Fig. 21-2). By increasing the stretch on the muscle, more actin and myosin interact giving a stronger muscle contraction. If preload is increased too much, less interaction occurs and contraction strength decreases. This is

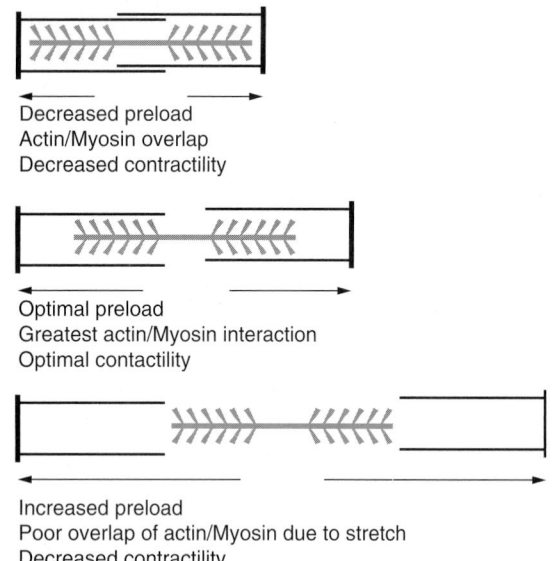

Decreased preload
Actin/Myosin overlap
Decreased contractility

Optimal preload
Greatest actin/Myosin interaction
Optimal contactility

Increased preload
Poor overlap of actin/Myosin due to stretch
Decreased contractility

Figure 21-2 *Actin/myosin interaction and preload.*

demonstrated by the Frank-Starling curve. In the heart, preload is defined as left ventricular end diastolic volume (LVEDV) and represents the blood available to the heart to pump. Optimizing preload can be done with intravenous fluids, volume expanders, or blood products in hypovolemic shock or by diuretics in cardiogenic shock; however, increasing/decreasing preload to maximize contractile force is a key component in the treatment of all forms of shock.

Optimization of afterload is another key concept and is the second step in the augmentation of stroke volume. Afterload is conceptually the force the heart must overcome to expel a given stoke volume. An elevated afterload, as evidenced by hypertension or elevated systemic vascular resistance, should be decreased in order to increase the stroke volume of the left ventricle. Vasodilators such as nitroprusside, nicardipine, and ACE inhibitors are typical agents used to reduce afterload. Mechanical augmentation of afterload can be accomplished with the placement of an intra-aortic balloon pump, which can also augment coronary artery filling.

Increasing myocardial contractility is the final step in the augmentation of stroke volume. Preload and afterload should be optimized before contractility is augmented. It does no good to cause a heart to pump harder, when there is no substrate to pump (preload) or when it is pumping against a brick wall (afterload). Augmentation of contractility often increased myocardial oxygen consumption due to increased cardiac work. In the case of the ischemic heart this can worsen cardiogenic failure long term and should not be undertaken lightly. Beta-agonists such as dobutamine and epinephrine and isoproterenol are pharmacologic agents used to increase cardiac contractility.

Critically ill patients frequently demonstrate evidence of inadequate tissue perfusion manifested by

anaerobic metabolism and lactic acidosis. As stated earlier, the primary resuscitation goal in such patients is to restore tissue perfusion and oxygenation and maintain end organ function through volume resuscitation. The optimal resuscitation fluid, however, remains a subject of debate. Crystalloids may be classified as hypotonic, isotonic, or hypertonic. For purposes of resuscitation, only isotonic and hypertonic fluids are of use as hypotonic fluids (such as D5W and 0.45 normal saline) do not remain intravascular long enough to affect a significant physiologic response. Isotonic fluids (such as lactated ringer solution and normal saline) are the foundation of crystalloid resuscitation. Hypertonic fluids (such as 3%, 6%, or 7.5% normal saline) are largely experimental and not commonly used in everyday resuscitation; however, several studies have recently shown some benefits to initial resuscitation with hypertonic fluids.[10-12] Crystalloids have the advantage of being inexpensive and readily available, resuscitate both the intravascular and interstitial space, and promote urinary output. Disadvantages to the use of crystalloid infusions include edema formation and the need for large resuscitation volumes as only one-third of transfused fluids will remain intravascular.

Colloids may be divided into protein and nonprotein colloids. In the United States, the only available protein colloid is serum albumin (5% and 25%). Albumin has the advantage of remaining intravascular longer than the crystalloids; therefore, less resuscitation volume is required. Albumin is expensive (55 times that of an equivalent volume of crystalloid) and does not restore the interstitial space. The nonprotein colloids include the starches (6% hetastarch, 10% pentastarch) and the dextrans (dextran-40 in 0.9 NS, dextran-70 in D5W). They have been found to be equivalent to albumin as a resuscitation fluid. Their primary drawbacks are their expense (10 times that of isotonic crystalloid), a dose-related coagulopathy (greatest with hetastarch), and occasional anaphylaxis (greatest with the dextrans). There have also been reports that these starch molecules may adversely affect renal function by causing tubular injury.[13]

Theoretically, colloid resuscitation represents a viable alternative to crystalloid resuscitation in the clinical setting. The real question is whether (1) colloids improve patient morbidity and mortality and (2) whether their use is worth the added expense. Several meta-analyses of prospective, randomized clinical trials evaluating the use of crystalloids versus colloids in critical care resuscitation were performed in the 1990s, and all demonstrated a survival advantage to patients resuscitated with crystalloids.[14-17] These studies consistently concluded that there is no advantage to colloid resuscitation and that crystalloids are the resuscitation fluid of choice. In 2001, Wilkes et al[18] performed a meta-analysis evaluating 55 studies including 3504 randomized patients (27 studies with 1504 surgical/trauma patients). Although no statistically significant increase in mortality was seen, the analysis indicated an increase in relative risk of death of more than 10% for surgical and trauma patients. In 2003, Rizoli et al published a review of some of the larger meta-analyses and concluded that "even when all limitations and nuances of interpretation are considered, one piece of evidence that comes out is that trauma patients should probably continue to be resuscitated with crystalloids."[19]

In 2004, the SAFE trial was published.[20] This was a very large (~7000 patients) multicenter, randomized, double-blind trial comparing 4% albumin (n = 3497) to normal saline (n = 3500) for intravascular-fluid resuscitation. This study found no difference in mortality, ICU or hospital days, days of mechanical ventilation, or days of renal-replacement therapy. Subgroup analysis noted that the relative risk of death among trauma patients in the albumin group was 1.36 compared to the saline group. The group concluded that albumin and saline should be considered clinically equivalent treatments for volume resuscitation in a heterogeneous population of patients in the ICU. While the SAFE Study authors purport that this study demonstrates that albumin can be utilized as a resuscitation fluid, the lack of a survival benefit of albumin and the significant economic burden associated with its use suggests that albumin should be reserved for specific, limited indications. In fact a Cochrane Database Review on the subject concluded that "As colloids are not associated with an improvement in survival, and as they are more expensive than crystalloids, it is hard to see how their continued use in these patients can be justified outside the context of randomized controlled trials."[21,22]

BLOOD PRODUCTS

Blood product use in resuscitation for emergency surgery patients has changed greatly over the last 25 years. In a study published in 1977 by Czer and Shoemaker, the optimal hematocrit was thought to be 32%.[23] New evidence suggests that a lower transfusion trigger might be more appropriate. In a multicenter, randomized, controlled clinical trial of two different transfusion approaches for packed red blood cells in medical and surgical ICU patients, Hebert et al[24] reported that a restrictive strategy of RBC transfusion was at least as effective as a more liberal policy. Also, recent data questioning the safety and efficacy of RBC transfusion raises concern in view of the high blood use in the emergency surgery/trauma population.[25-27] One of the greatest problems associated with transfusion of RBCs is the fact that transfused RBCs are also not the same as endogenous RBCs. The CRIT study showed that blood transfused to critically ill patients in a large tertiary care center was on average 21 days old and was an independent predictor of mortality.[28] Storage of RBCs decreases 2,3-diphosphoglycerate levels, interfering with the ability of RBCs to unload oxygen. Studies have demonstrated that packed RBCs contain potent proinflammatory mediators that may have an impact on the inflammatory response. In a study of patients suffering from septic shock, those receiving RBC units stored for > 15 days developed more evidence of ischemia when compared with those receiving blood stored for < 15 days. Another demonstrated that transfusion of fresh RBCs increased systemic oxygen uptake, whereas transfusion of RBCs stored for 28 days failed to improve tissue oxygenation. These findings may in part explain the clinical observations of RBC transfusions being independently associated with various types of infections. In the face of mounting evidence, a more cautious approach to blood transfusion should be adopted in emergency surgery patients.[29-39]

Correction of acidosis, hypothermia, coagulopathy can stop what has been described as the "bloody vicious cycle" and will lead to successful resuscitations and the end point of resuscitation in emergency surgery patients is patient survival. No single number, guideline, or hemodynamic parameter can be the end-all-be-all guide to resuscitation. In the end, the clinician must examine the patient, collect all the data and come to a gestalt regarding the care of that specific patient.

REFERENCES

1. Choi, YF, Wong TW, Lau CC. Midazolam is more likely to cause hypotension than Etomidate in emergency department rapid sequence intubation. *Emerg Med J* 2004;21(6):700.
2. Hansen D. Suxamethonium-induced cardiac arrest and death following 5 days of immobilization. *Eur J Anaesthesiol* 1998;15(2):240.
3. Schow, AJ, Lubarsky DA, Olson RP, et al. Can succinylcholine be used safely in hyperkalemic patients? *Anesth Analg* 2002;95(1):119.
4. American College of Surgeons Committee on Trauma. Advanced Trauma Life Support, 116, 1998.
5. Flynn AE, Thomas AN, Schecter WP. Acute tracheobronchial injury. *J Trauma* 1989;29:1326.
6. Cappello M, Legrand A, De Troyer A. Determinants of rib motion in flail chest. *Am J Respir Crit Care Med* 1999;159:886.
7. Schenarts PJ, Diaz J, Kaiser C, et al. Prospective comparison of admission computed tomographic scan and plain films of the upper cervical spine in trauma patients with altered mental status. *J Trauma* 2001;51:663.
8. Fischer RP, Beverlin BC, Engrav LH, et al. Diagnostic peritoneal lavage: 14 years and 2586 patients later. *Am J Surg* 1978;136:701.

9. Shapiro MB, Jenkins DH, Schwab CW, et al. Damage control: collective review. *J Trauma* 2000;49:969.

10. Homma, H, Deitch, EA, Feketeova A. Small volume resuscitation with hypertonic saline is more effective in ameliorating trauma-hemorrhagic shock-induced lung injury, neutrophil activation and red blood cell dysfunction than pancreatic protease inhibition. *J Trauma* 2002;59(2):266.

11. Kramer, GC. Hypertonic resuscitation: Physiologic mechanisms and recommendations for trauma care. *J Trauma* 2003;54(5) Supplement:S89.

12. Shackford SR, Bourguignon PR, Wald SL. Hypertonic saline resuscitation of patients with head injury: A prospective, randomized clinical trial. *J Trauma* 1998;44(1):50.

13. Gore DC, Dalton JM, Gehr Todd WB. Colloid infusions reduce glomerular filtration in resuscitated burn victims. *J Trauma* 1996;40(3):356.

14. Velanovich V. Crystalloid versus colloid fluid resuscitation: A meta-analysis of mortality. *Surgery* 1989;105:65.

15. Schierhout G, Roberts L. Fluid resuscitation with colloid or crystalloid solutions in critically ill patients: A systematic review of randomized trials. *BMJ* 1998; 316:961.

16. Cochrane Injuries Group Albumin Reviewers. Human albumin administration in critically ill patients: Systematic review of randomized controlled trials. *BMJ* 1998;317:235.

17. Choi PTL, Yip G, Quinonez LG, et al. Crystalloids vs. colloids in fluid resuscitation: A systematic review. *Crit Care Med* 1999;27:200.

18. Wilkes MM, Navickis RJ. Patient survival after human albumin administration: A meta-analysis of randomized, controlled trials. *Ann Intern Med* 2001;135:149.

19. Rizoli SB. Crystalloids and colloids in trauma resuscitation: A brief overview of the current debate. *J Trauma* 2003;54:S82.

20. The SAFE Study Investigators. A comparison of albumin and saline for fluid resuscitation in the intensive care unit. *N Engl J Med* 2004;350:2247.

21. Bunn F, Alderson P, Hawkins V. Colloid solutions for fluid resuscitation. *Cochrane Database Syst Rev* 2003;

22. Roberts I, Bunn F, Chinnock P, Ker K, Schierhout G. Colloids versus crystalloids for fluid resuscitation in critically ill patients. *Cochrane Database Syst Rev* 2004

23. Czer LS, Shoemaker WC. Optimal hematocrit value in critically ill postoperative patients. *Surg Gynecol Obstet* 1978;147:363.

24. Hebert PC, Wells G, Blajchman MA, et al. A multicenter, randomized, controlled clinical trail of transfusion requirements in critical care. *N Engl J Med* 1999;340:409.

25. Offner PJ, Moore EE, Biffl WL, Johnson JL, Silliman C. Increased rate of infection associated with transfusion of old blood after severe injury. *Arch Surg* 2002;137:711.

26. Taylor RW, Manganaro L, O'Brien J, Trottier SJ, Parkar N, Veremakis C. Impact of allogenic packed red blood cell transfusion on nosocomial infection rates in the critically ill patient. *Crit Care Med* 2002;30:2249.

27. Claridge JA, Sawyer RG, Schulman AM, McLemore EC, Young JS. Blood transfusions correlate with infections in trauma patients in a dose-dependent manner. *Am Surg* 2002;68:566.

28. Corwin HL, Gettinger M, Pearl RG, et al. The CRIT Study: Anemia and blood transfusion in the critically ill—current clinical practice in the United States. *Crit Care Med* 2004;32(1):39.

29. Simon TL, Alverson DC, AuBuchon J, et al. Practice parameter for the use of red blood cell transfusions: Developed by the Red Blood Cell Administration Practice Guideline Development Task Force of the College of American Pathologists. *Arch Pathol Lab Med* 1998;122:130.

30. Vincent JL, Baron JF, Reinhart K, et al. Anemia and blood transfusion in critically ill patients. *JAMA* 2002;288:1499.

31. Shapiro MJ, Gettinger A, Corwin HL. Anemia and blood transfusion in trauma patients admitted to the intensive care unit. *J Trauma* 2003;55(2):269.

32. Levy MM, Abraham E, Zilberberg M, A descriptive evaluation of transfusion practices in patients receiving mechanical ventilation. *Chest* 2005;127(3):928.

33. Fransen E, Maessen J, Dentener M, Senden N, Buurman W. Impact of blood transfusions on inflammatory mediator release in patients undergoing cardiac surgery. *Chest* 1999;116:1233.

34. Marik PE, Sibbald WJ. Effect of stored-blood transfusion on oxygen delivery in patients with sepsis. *JAMA* 1993;269:3024.

35. Dietrich KA, Conrad SA, Hebert CA, Levy GL, Romero MD. Cardiovascular and metabolic response to red blood cell transfusion in critically ill volume-resuscitated nonsurgical patients. *Crit Care Med* 1990;18:940.

36. Lorente JA, Landin L, De Pablo R, Renes E, Rodriguez-Diaz R, Liste D. Effects of blood transfusion on oxygen transport variables in severe sepsis. *Crit Care Med* 1993;21:1312.

37. Fitzgerald RD, Martin CM, Dietz GE, Doig GS, Potter RF, Sibbald WJ. Transfusing red blood cells stored in citrate phosphate dextrose adenine-1 for 28 days fails to improve tissue oxygenation in rats. *Crit Care Med* 1997;25:726.

38. Purdy FR, Tweeddale MG, Merrick PM. Association of mortality with age of blood transfused in septic ICU patients. *Can J Anaesth* 1977;44:1256.

39. Zallen G, Offner PJ, Moore EE, et al. Age of transfused blood is an independent risk factor for postinjury multiple organ failure. *Am J Surg* 1999;178:570.

Chapter 22

NUTRITION AND VENOUS ACCESS

James H. Holmes, IV, MD

INTRODUCTION

Many of the foremost advances in medical nutrition have been made by surgeons—ranging from the development of total parenteral nutrition (TPN) by Dudrick to the clear demonstration of improved outcomes with early, aggressive total enteral nutrition (TEN) in the critically ill by the Moores, Kudsk, and others. This seems only logical as decades of data clearly indicate that surgical and medical complications increase in direct proportion to the degree of malnutrition. Hence, surgeons, and in particular "acute care" surgeons, will be expected to remain at the forefront of developments in medical nutrition, thus necessitating a current and ever-evolving understanding of nutritional support. As "Acute Care Surgery" is not fully defined from a clinical perspective at this time, some assumptions have to be made regarding the particular patient population to be encountered. It will be assumed that the "acute care surgery" patient is equivalent to the well-defined surgical critical care and trauma patient populations from a physiologic, metabolic, and nutritional standpoint. Consideration of nutritional support in the elective surgery patient population, although potentially applicable, is beyond the scope of this chapter. Thus, further discussion will be limited to the acutely ill surgical patient suffering critical physiologic and metabolic stress. An evidence-based algorithm for nutritional support in acute care surgery patients is provided in Fig. 22-1.

IDENTIFYING PREMORBID MALNUTRITION AND ESTIMATING INITIAL NUTRITIONAL REQUIREMENTS

There is no universally accepted, evidence-based definition of malnutrition; however, it is appropriate to classify malnourished acute care surgery patients as having protein energy malnutrition (PEM). Numerous biochemical markers, clinical tests, and screening instruments have been promulgated as means to assess the patient at risk for PEM, but no single modality has

proven vastly superior to another. Nonetheless, the most consistently reliable clinical method of diagnosing premorbid PEM is eliciting a history of recent unintentional weight loss, specifically an unintentional weight loss ≥ 10% of usual body weight in the preceding 6 months.[1] Although many acute care surgery patients will require some form of nutritional supplementation, identification of those who are premorbidly malnourished may allow for more rapid intervention and potentially the greatest improvement in outcomes.

As with defining malnutrition, there is no universally accepted, evidence-based methodology for estimating nutritional requirements. For years, indirect calorimetry has been considered the "gold standard" for not only the initial assessment of nutritional requirements, but also for monitoring on-going responses to nutritional support and interventions. However, recent data have called this practice into question. First, the American Society of Parenteral and Enteral Nutrition (ASPEN) guidelines recommend weight-based initial estimates for nutritional support, with acute care surgery patients typically receiving 30 kcal/kg according to the guidelines.[2] Furthermore, the most widely used and generally accepted instrument for assessing initial nutritional requirements is the Harris-Benedict equation (Fig. 22-2), which is based on gender, height, weight, and age for estimating resting or basal energy expenditure (REE). In metabolically stressed patients, the Harris-Benedict equation is typically modified by multiplying the REE by a conversion factor that takes into account patient activity and the severity of illness. A conversion factor of 1.5 would be warranted in acute care surgery patients. Finally, a recent prospective, observational study comparing the estimated nutritional requirements as determined by indirect calorimetry, the ASPEN guidelines, and the modified Harris-Benedict equation clearly refutes the superiority of indirect calorimetry.[3] In fact, the weight-based ASPEN guidelines of 30 kcal/kg and the modified Harris-Benedict equation with a conversion factor of 1.5 estimated nutritional requirements as accurately as indirect calorimetry; the three methods were clinically equivalent. Thus, from an evidence-based perspective,

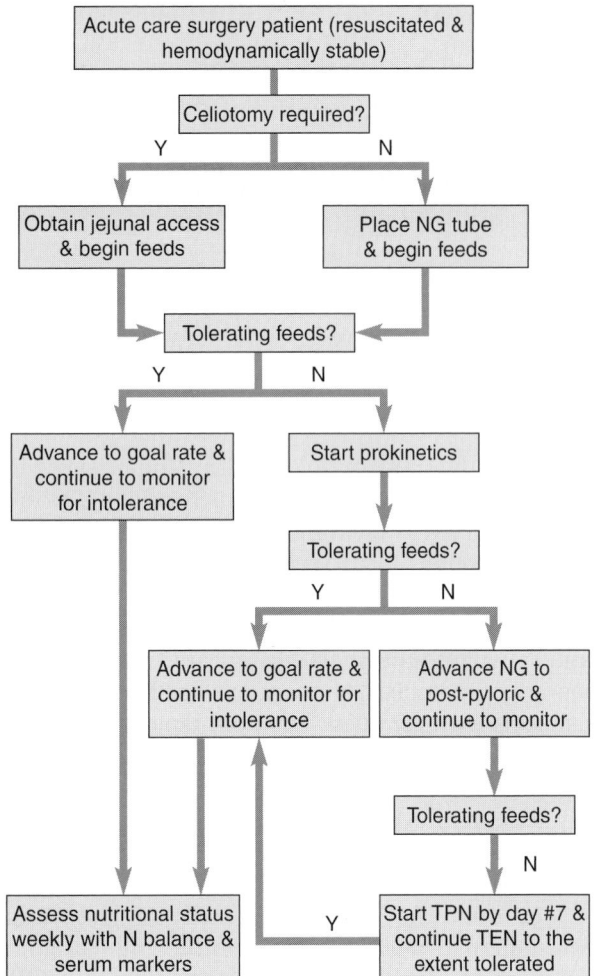

Figure 22-1 *Evidence-based algorithm for nutritional support in acute care surgery patients.*

the use of either 30 kcal/kg, the modified Harris-Benedict equation with a conversion factor of 1.5, or indirect calorimetry is an appropriate method for estimating initial nutritional requirements. It is our practice to use the ASPEN guidelines of ~30 kcal/kg.

NUTRITIONAL COMPOSITION

Once energy requirements are estimated, the composition of the nutritional support to be administered has to be determined, keeping in mind certain metabolic limitations. The Recommended Daily Allowance (RDA) for protein intake in the healthy, well-nourished

REE (male) = 66.5 + 13.8 (weight in kg) + 5 (height in cm) –
6.8 (age in years
REE (female) = 655 + 9.6 (weight in kg) + 1.85 (height in cm) –
4.7 (age in years)
Modified REE for acute care surgery patient = 1.5 (REE)

Figure 22-2 *Harris-Benedict equation.*

individual is 0.8 g/kg/day, with each gram of protein providing 4 kcal in energy. It is well-established that protein requirements increase to 1.5-2 g/kg/day in acutely ill/stressed patients without renal dysfunction. In those patients with renal dysfunction who are acutely ill/stressed, the protein requirements are 1-1.5 g/kg/day depending on dialysis status. The maximal rate of glucose oxidation in man is 4-5 mg/kg/min (~7 g/kg/day), and overall total carbohydrate administration should not exceed these levels. The balance of nonprotein caloric requirements is met with fats. If enteral nutrition is being administered, this component is predetermined in the particular formula employed for nutritional support. The only way to adjust fat intake is to change formulas. However, with total parenteral nutrition, a maximal dose of 2.5 g/kg/day of lipid should never be exceeded. Enterally, fat provides 9.1 kcal/g, while parenterally it provides 10 kcal/g with the added energy coming from emulsifiers and glycerol. In normal, healthy individuals a nonprotein calorie:nitrogen ratio of 150:1 should be maintained to prevent catabolism; however, in the catabolic acute care surgery patient this ratio decreases to 80-100:1.

ENTERAL NUTRITION

Total enteral nutrition (TEN) has become the nutritional support modality of choice over the past two decades. During this evolution, there have been significant advances in the composition of TEN formulas to the extent that manufacturers promulgate almost disease-specific diets. Germane to the acute care surgery patient, these specialized formulas are referred to as "enhanced" TEN or immune enhancing diets (IED). IEDs contain variable but increased concentrations of arginine and glutamine in addition to standard amino acids, omega-3 fatty acids (fish oils) as opposed to omega-6 (vegetable oils), and nucleotides when compared to standard TEN formulas. The caloric densities of IEDs and standard TEN formulas are similar at 1-1.5 kcal/cc. The evidence supporting the claims of improved outcomes with IEDs compared to standard formulations is lacking at this time. Currently, IEDs offer no outcome benefits over standard TEN for the acute care surgery patient, and there may be potential adverse consequences in the septic patient.[4,5]

To deliver TEN, one must have secure, reliable access to the GI tract. This can be obtained via numerous methods: nasogastric/enteric, gastrostomy, or jejunostomy. No method of GI access has been shown to be superior and depends more on the individual patient and the surgeon's preference. It is quite clear that the outcomes, benefits, and complications are equivalent whether TEN is delivered into the stomach, duodenum, or jejunum, assuming appropriate motility and tolerance at a given anatomic site.[6,7,8] One caveat may apply to specific techniques for surgical jejunal access. It appears that needle catheter jejunostomy may be the method of choice for surgically accessing the jejunum in trauma patients, while a standard Witzel jejunostomy is acceptable in all other acute care surgery patients.[9]

Once GI access is established and nutritional requirements estimated, the timing of TEN administration has to be decided. Many authors and most medical societies issuing consensus statements pertaining to nutritional support espouse a policy of withholding TEN until resolution of shock via adequate resuscitation and discontinuation of any pressors (the exception being in the burn patient population). This philosophy is predicated on the theoretical concern of increasing GI perfusion and oxygen demand in the face of a limited supply, thus potentially precipitating GI ischemia/necrosis. This is controversial as no clear data support this practice or the converse of feeding acute care surgery patients during active resuscitation. In fact, the definition of "early" TEN is without consensus in the literature and ranges between 4 and 72 hours following admission. Nonetheless, aggregate analysis of the published data relating to the timing of TEN initiation demonstrates the following: there is no outcome advantage to initiating TEN within 24 hours of admission as compared to 72 hours following admission.[10,11]

Complications associated with TEN include diarrhea, aspiration, technical misadventures in tube placement/migration, GI perforation, and intestinal necrosis. Most of these can be averted via close monitoring of feeding tolerance and tube placement, but unfortunately there is virtually no evidence-based data to help guide monitoring and allow early detection of intolerance or even stratify patients at high-risk of feeding intolerance.

PARENTERAL NUTRITION

The successful development of total parenteral nutrition (TPN) was a monumental advancement in clinical nutrition, as well as medicine as a whole. It changed nutritional practices forever and has undoubtedly saved numerous lives. Nonetheless, TPN has significant limitations. The delivery of substrates via TPN has to be closely monitored as overfeeding can easily occur, and the aforementioned maximum doses of glucose (7 g/kg/day) and lipids (2.5 g/kg/day) must be strictly maintained. In fact, the weight of the evidence suggests that if TPN is to be used in acute care surgery patients, then intravenous lipids probably should not be used as an energy source at all. They are associated with increased overall morbidity in the form of infectious complications, increased ICU and hospital

lengths of stay, and increased ventilator days.[12-14] This can be explained by the immunosuppressive properties of intravenous lipids.[14,15]

TPN requires central venous access, which in itself carries attendant infectious, thrombotic, and procedural/mechanical complications. It appears that subclavian central venous catheters (CVC) are superior to peripherally inserted central catheters (PICC) for delivery of TPN in hospitalized patients from the infectious and cost-benefit perspectives.[16] Regardless of the type or location of the catheter used, a dedicated single-lumen CVC or dedicated lumen in a multilumen CVC should be used for TPN delivery, which will decrease complications.[2]

In addition to catheter-related complications, TPN is associated with some significant metabolic complications. Acutely, TPN can precipitate hyperglycemia, hyperglycemic hyperosmolar nonketotic syndrome, hepatic steatosis, hypertriglyceridemia, fat overload syndrome, and acid-base/electrolyte aberrations. The majority of these can be avoided with close monitoring of the TPN prescription and metabolic indices. However, chronically, TPN will eventually induce parenteral nutrition associated cholestasis (PNAC), which is ultimately fatal. The mechanisms underlying PNAC remain unclear, and the only known way to prevent or arrest PNAC is to liberate the patient from TPN.

TEN VERSUS TPN

Collectively, the evidence absolutely supports the notion that enteral nutrition is superior to parenteral nutrition ... PERIOD! Although either nutritional route has no appreciable effect on mortality, a thorough review of the current literature demonstrates a consistent reduction in morbidity with TEN compared to TPN. This remains constant irrespective of the patient population studied. In the acute care surgery patient population, all published studies have universally demonstrated reduced septic morbidity with TEN,[17-23] whereas a few have shown reduced cost of care parameters in addition.[22,23]

The *sole* absolute contraindication to TEN is insufficient small bowel surface area for nutrient absorption (ie, "short gut"). This is the only patient group who would benefit from TPN over TEN *a priori*; all other patients should be given TEN as their initial nutritional intervention. In patients with gastroparesis or ileus who are not fully tolerating TEN, prokinetics (erythromycin or metoclopramide) usually can overcome this GI dysmotility,[24] allowing full tolerance of TEN without resorting to TPN supplementation. In the rare instance where a patient is intolerant of TEN while receiving maximal prokinetics at 7 days following admission, TPN should be added to complete the goal nutritional prescription.[2]

MONITORING NUTRITIONAL INTERVENTIONS

Once nutritional support is implemented and the patient is tolerating goal TEN, or alternatively TPN, a monitoring strategy to assess the efficacy of nutritional replacement is of paramount importance. Although conclusive evidence is lacking, it appears that nitrogen balance provides the best assessment of ongoing nutritional support in the catabolic acute care surgery patient.[25] To augment the accuracy of nutritional monitoring, numerous biochemical tests have been proposed. The most common serum assays of visceral proteins used in nutritional monitoring are: C-reactive protein (CRP), albumin, prealbumin/transthyretin, transferrin, and retinol-binding protein (RBP).[26-28] CRP trends are typically followed as a gauge of the magnitude of the acute phase response (APR), with decreasing CRP levels corresponding with reprioritization of the APR and a shift toward anabolism. Prealbumin/transthyretin and RBP levels vary inversely with CRP levels and, given their short half-lives of ~2d and ~12h, respectively, are good acute markers of adequate nutritional support and correlate well with anabolism. The long half-lives of albumin and transferrin, ~20 and 8 days, respectively, render them obsolete for modern nutritional support monitoring. In addition to the aforementioned labs, serum electrolytes, liver function tests, and triglycerides need to be monitored on a regular basis if the patient is receiving TPN.

The monitoring of TEN tolerance is even more problematic, as there is no direct way to accurately monitor GI motility. Furthermore, there is no scientific evidence to guide current practices of attempts at indirect monitoring of TEN tolerance, namely, checking gastric residuals. In fact, recent data clearly refute the concept that gastric residuals are an accurate marker of impending aspiration of gastric contents and demonstrate that what constitutes a "high" residual is completely arbitrary.[29] One evidence-based practice that has been shown to reduce episodes of aspiration of gastric contents is elevating the head of the bed $\geq 30°$,[30] which is now part of many ICU "ventilator bundles." Until more sophisticated monitoring devices for GI motility are developed, clinical acumen and gestalt will drive TEN tolerance monitoring.

VENOUS ACCESS

In the era of evidence-based medicine, many aspects of venous access with central venous catheters (CVC) are beyond the individual surgeon's control. For instance, many hospitals are employing "central line sets" that include the hospital-designated intravascular device kit with prepping solution and occlusive dressing, full sterile attire and drapes, and full barrier precautions. CVC can only be placed using the "central line sets," which are successful in reducing catheter-related bloodstream infections (CRBSI) and evidence-based in their design.[31] However, the type of CVC used, location of placement, and technique are in the hands of the surgeon, and there is sufficient scientific evidence to provide guidance. With respect to choosing the actual CVC, antimicrobial-impregnated CVC are clearly associated with reduced rates of CRBSI when compared to standard catheters.[32,33] There are two antimicrobial-impregnated CVC commercially available in the United States, and they are not equivalent. One is impregnated intra- and extraluminally with minocycline and rifampin, while the other is impregnated extraluminally with chlorhexidine and silver sulfadiazine. The rifampin-minocycline impregnated CVC is significantly more efficacious at reducing CVC colonization and CRBSI when compared to the chlorhexidine-silver sulfadiazine impregnated CVC.[33] Furthermore, cost analysis clearly shows that the rifampin-minocycline CVC performs better financially saving ~$9600/CRBSI averted, which translated to a cost savings of $81/patient.[34]

Historically, CVC location was typically driven by a surgeon's perceptions with respect to the relative cleanliness of a given anatomic location. It has been believed and espoused that the area of highest CRBSI rates was the femoral vein (FV), followed by the internal jugular vein (IJ) and then the subclavian vein (SCV). Recent prospective, observational data questions this belief. In 657 ICU patients with 831 CVCs and 4735 catheter days, there was no difference in CRBSI rates between the FV, IJ, or SCV sites.[35] However, in a prospective randomized study comparing SCV with FV, the FV site was associated with a significantly higher rate of CRBSI than the SCV.[36] Hence, the question remains unanswered. Practically speaking, a CVC should be placed at the safest location in a given patient. For now, this will be based on the judgment of the operating surgeon without the benefit of evidence-based guidelines.

Aside from CRBSI, the majority of other complications associated with CVCs are periprocedural and related to technique. In efforts to reduce technical complications with CVC placement, ultrasound techniques have been developed to elucidate the anatomy more clearly to allow more accurate venous access. In fact, the SOAP-3 Trial clearly demonstrated how ultrasound guidance for CVC placement was superior to landmark based techniques.[37]

Finally, there is no evidence that routine, scheduled CVC changes or exchanges over a wire reduce CRBSI rates or improve outcomes at all. In fact, the converse holds in that routine CVC changes/exchanges actually increases the risk of infectious complications and technical misadventures.[38]

REFERENCES

1. Alberda C, Graf A, and McCargar L. Malnutrition: Etiology, consequences, and assessment of a patient at risk. *Best Practice & Research Clinical Gastroenterology* 2006;20:419-439.

2. ASPEN Board of Directors and the Clinical Guidelines Task Force. Guidelines for the use of parenteral and enteral nutrition in adult and pediatric patients. *J Parenter Enteral Nutr* 2002;26(Suppl):1SA-138SA.

3. Davis KA, Kinn T, Esposito TJ, et al. Nutritional gains versus financial gain: The role of metabolic carts in the surgical ICU. *J Trauma* 2006;61:1436-1440.

4. Heyland DK, Novak F, Drover JW, et al. Should immunonutrition become routine in critically ill patients? A systematic review of the evidence. *JAMA* 2001;286:944-953.

5. Anonymous. Consensus recommendations from the US summit on immune-enhancing enteral therapy. *J Parenter Enteral Nutr* 2001;25:S61-S63.

6. Kortbeek JB, Haigh PI, Doig C. Duodenal versus gastric feeding in ventilated blunt trauma patients: a randomized controlled trial. *J Trauma* 1999;46:992-998.

7. Ho KM, Dobb GJ, Webb SAR. A comparison of early gastric and postpyloric feeding in critically ill patients: a meta-analysis. *Intensive Care Med* 2006;32:639-649.

8. Marik PE, Zaloga GP. Gastric versus post-pyloric feeding: a systematic review. *Crit Care* 2003;7(3):R46-R51.

9. Holmes JH IV, Brundage SI, Yuen P, et al. Complications of surgical feeding jejunostomy in trauma patients. *J Trauma* 1999;47(6):1009-1012.

10. Jacobs DG, Jacobs DO, Kudsk KA, et al. Practice management guidelines for nutritional support of the trauma patient. *J Trauma* 2004;57:660-679.

11. Marik PE, Zaloga GP. Early enteral nutrition in acutely ill patients: a systematic review. *Crit Care Med* 2001;29(12):2264-2270.

12. Heyland DK, Montalvo M, MacDonald S, et al. Total parenteral nutrition in the surgical patient: a meta-analysis. *Canadian Journal of Surgery* 2001;44(2):102-111.

13. Heyland DK, MacDonald S, Keefe L, et al. Total parenteral nutrition in the critically ill patient: a meta-analysis. *JAMA* 1998;280(23):2013-2019.

14. Battistella FD, Widergren JT, Anderson JT, et al. A prospective, randomized trial of intravenous fat emulsion administration in trauma victims requiring total parenteral nutrition. *J Trauma* 1997;43:52-60.

15. Waitzberg DL, Lotierzo PH, Logullo AF, et al. Parenteral lipids emulsions and phagocytic systems. *British Journal of Nutrition* 2002;87(S1):S49-S57.

16. Cowl CT, Weinstock JV, Al-Jurf A, et al. Complications and cost associated with parenteral nutrition delivered to hospitalized patients through either subclavian or peripherally-inserted central catheters. *Clinical Nutrition* 2000;19(4):237-243.

17. Moore FA, Moore EE, Jones TN, McCroskey BL, Peterson VM. TEN versus TPN following major abdominal trauma—reduced septic morbidity. *J Trauma* 1989;29:916-923.

18. Kudsk KA, Croce MA, Fabian TC, et al. Enteral versus parenteral feeding: effects on septic morbidity following blunt and penetrating trauma. *Ann Surg* 1992;215: 503-513.

19. Moore FA, Feliciano DV, Andrassy RJ, et al. Early enteral feeding, compared with parenteral, reduces postoperative septic complications: the results of a meta-analysis. *Ann Surg* 1992;216:172-183.

20. Peter JV, Moran JL, Philips-Hughes J. A metaanalysis of treatment outcomes of early enteral versus early parenteral nutrition in hospitalized patients *Crit Care Med* 2005;33:213-220.

21. Simpson F, Dog GS. Parenteral vs. enteral nutrtion in the critically ill patient: a meta-analysis of trials using the intention totreat principle. *Intensive Care Med* 2005;31:12-23.

22. Gramlich L, Kichian K, Pinilla J, et al. Does enteral nutrition compared to parenteral nutrition result in better outcomes in critically ill adult patients? A systematic review of the literature. *Nutrition* 2004;20: 843-848.

23. Radrizzani D, Bertolini G, Facchini R, et al. Early enteral immunonutrition vs. parenteral nutrition in critically ill patients without severe sepsis: a randomized clinical trial. *Intensive Care Med* 2006;32(8):1191-1198.

24. Booth CM, Heyland DK, Paterson WG. Gastrointestinal promotility drugs in the critical care setting: A sytematic review of the evidence. *Crit Care Med* 2002;30:1429-1435,.

25. Manning EM, Shenkin A. Nutritional assessment in the critically ill. *Crit Care Clin* 1995;11:603-634.

26. Winkler MF, Gerrior SA, Pomp A, Albina JE. Use of retinol-binding protein and prealbumin as indicators of the response to nutrition therapy. *J Am Diet Assoc* 1989;89:684-687.

27. Spiekerman AM. Proteins used in nutritional assessment. *Clin Lab Med* 1993;13:353-369.

28. Raguso CA, Dupertuis YM, Pichard C. The role of visceral proteins in the nutritional assessment of intensive care unit patients. *Curr Opin Clin Nutr Metab Care* 2003;6:211-216.

29. McClave SA, Lukan JK, Stefater JA, et al. Poor validity of residual volumes as a marker for risk of aspiration in critically ill patients. *Crit Care Med* 2005;33:324-330.

30. Torres A, Serra-Batlles J, Ros E, et al. Pulmonary aspiration of gastric contents in patients receiving mechanical ventilation: the effect of body position. *Ann Intern Med* 1992;116:540-543.

31. O'Grady NP, Alexander M, Dellinger EP, et al. Guidelines for the prevention of intravascular catheter-related infections. *Infection Control and Hospital Epidemiology* 2002;23(12):759-769.

32. Veenstra DL, Saint S, Saha S, et al. Efficacy of antiseptic impregnated central venous catheters in preventing catheter-related bloodstream infection: a meta-analysis. *JAMA* 1999;281(3):261-267.

33. Darouiche RO, Raad II, Heard SO, et al. A comparison of two antimicrobial-impregnated central venous catheters. *NEJM* 1999;340(1):1-8.

34. Shorr AF, Humphreys CW, Helman DL. New choices for central venous catheters: Potential financial implications. *Chest* 2003;124:275-284.

35. Deshpande KS, Hatem C, Ulrich HL. The incidence of infectious complications of central venous catheters at the subclavian, internal jugular, and femoral sites in an intensive care unit population. *Crit Care Med* 2005;33:13-20.

36. Merrer J, DeJonghe B, Golliot F, et al. Complications of femoral and subclavian venous catheterization in critically ill patients: a randomized controlled trial. *JAMA* 2001;286(6):700-707.

37. Milling TJ, Rose J, Briggs WM, et al. Randomized, controlled clinical trial of point-of-care limited ultrasonography assistance of central venous cannulation: The 3rd Sonography Outcomes Assessment Program (SOAP-3). *Crit Care Med* 2005;33:1764-1769.

38. Cook D, Randolph A, Kernerman P, et al. Central venous catheter replacement strategies: A systematic review of the literature. *Crit Care Med* 1997;25(8):1417-1424.

Chapter 23

ANTIBIOTIC SELECTION

Philip S. Barie, MD, MBA, and, Soumitra R. Eachempati, MD

INTRODUCTION

Infections remain the leading cause of morbidity and mortality of hospitalized patients. Antimicrobial therapy is a mainstay of treatment, but widespread overuse and misuse of antibiotics have led to an alarming increase in multiple-drug-resistant (MDR) pathogens. New agents may allow shorter courses of therapy and prophylaxis, which are desirable for cost control and control of microbial flora.

PHARMACOKINETIC PRINCIPLES

To provide effective therapy with no toxicity requires understanding the principles of drug absorption, distribution, and metabolism, known as *pharmacokinetics*.[1] The dose-response relationship is influenced by dose, dosing interval, and route of administration. Drug concentrations in plasma and tissue are influenced by absorption, distribution, and elimination, which in turn depend on drug metabolism and excretion. Plasma and tissue concentrations may or may not correlate, depending on tissue penetration. Relationships between local drug concentration and effect are defined by pharmacodynamic (PD) principles (see below).[2]

Basic concepts of pharmacokinetics (PK) include *bioavailability*, the percentage of drug dose that reaches the systemic circulation. Bioavailability is 100% after intravenous (IV) administration, but varies after oral administration, being affected by absorption, intestinal transit time, and the degree of hepatic first-pass metabolism. *Half-life* ($T_{1/2}$) is the time required for the drug concentration to reduce by one-half, reflecting both clearance and *volume of distribution* (V_D).[1] Half-life is useful to estimate when a steady-state drug concentration will be achieved, for interpretation of drug concentration data. The proportionality constant V_D is useful for estimating the plasma drug concentration achievable from a given dose. A derived parameter of no particular physiologic significance that is independent of a drug's clearance or $T_{1/2}$, V_D can vary substantially due to pathophysiology. Reduced V_D causes a higher plasma drug concentration for a given dose, whereas fluid overload and hypoalbuminemia (with decreased drug binding) increase V_D, making dosing more complex.

Clearance refers to the volume of liquid from which drug is eliminated completely per unit of time, whether by tissue distribution, metabolism, or elimination; it is important for determining the dose of drug necessary to maintain a steady-state concentration. Drug elimination may be by metabolism, excretion, or dialysis. Most drugs are metabolized by the liver to polar compounds for eventual renal excretion, which may occur by filtration or either active or passive transport. The degree of filtration is determined by molecular size and charge and by the number of functional nephrons. In general, if ≥ 40% of administered drug or its active metabolites is eliminated unchanged in the urine, decreased renal function will require a dosage adjustment.

PHARMACODYNAMIC PRINCIPLES

Pharmacodynamics (PD), the relationship of a drug to its intended effect, are complex for antibiotic therapy, because drug-patient, drug-microbe, and microbe-patient interactions must be accounted for.[2] In contrast to most pharmacotherapy, the key drug interaction is not with the host, but with the microbe. Microbial physiology, inoculum size, microbial growth phase, mechanisms of resistance, microenvironmental factors such as pH at the local site of infection, and the host's response are important factors. Because of microbial resistance, mere administration of drug may not be microbicidal. Factors that may induce resistance are drug-inactivating enzymes, altered cell surface receptor target molecules, and decreased bacterial permeability to antimicrobial penetration. Crucial to the microbe-patient interaction is the patient's immune system, as are drug-patient factors that may influence PK.

Antibiotic PD are determined by laboratory analysis. *In vitro* analyses include the *minimal inhibitory concentration* (MIC), the lowest serum drug concentration that inhibits bacterial growth (MIC_{90} refers to 90% inhibition). However, some antibiotics may suppress bacterial growth at subinhibitory concentrations (*postantibiotic effect*, PAE). Appreciable PAE can be observed with aminoglycosides and fluoroquinolones for gram-negative bacteria, and with some β-lactam drugs (notably carbapenems) against *Staphylococcus aureus*. However, MIC testing may not detect resistant bacterial subpopulations within the inoculum (a particular problem with "heteroresistance" of gram-positive bacteria, particularly *S aureus*).[3,4] Moreover, *in vitro* results may be irrelevant to the patient if bacteria are inhibited *in vitro* only by drug concentrations that cannot be achieved clinically.

Sophisticated analytic strategies utilize both PK and PD, for example, by determination of the peak serum concentration: MIC ratio, the duration of time that plasma concentration remains above the MIC, and the area of the plasma concentration-time curve above the MIC (the "area under the curve," or AUC).[5] Through such analyses, certain drugs (eg, aminoglycosides) have been characterized as having concentration-dependent killing, whereby a higher peak concentration increases the efficacy of bacterial killing (up to a point).[6,7] Most β-lactam agents exhibit concentration-independent bactericidal properties; rather, efficacy is determined by the length of time that the drug concentration remains above the MIC.[8] For β-lactam antibiotics with short $T_{1/2}$, it may be efficacious to administer the agents by continuous infusion.[9,10] Some agents (eg, fluoroquinolones) exhibit both properties; bacterial killing increases as drug concentration increases up to a saturation point, after which the effect becomes concentration independent.

EMPIRIC ANTIBIOTIC THERAPY

Empiric antibiotic therapy must be administered carefully. Injudicious therapy could result in nontreatment of established infection, or unnecessary therapy when the patient has only inflammation or bacterial colonization; either may be deleterious. Inappropriate therapy (eg, delay, therapy misdirected against usual pathogens, failure to treat MDR pathogens) leads unequivocally to increased mortality.[11-14]

A number of strategies have been promulgated to optimize the administration of antibiotics, including reliance on physician prescribing patterns, computerized decision support,[15] antibiotic administration by protocol (eg, a predetermined agent or schedule),[16-20] and formulary restriction programs (Table 23-1). Owing to the increasing prevalence of MDR pathogens causing serious infections, it is crucial for initial empiric antibiotic therapy to be targeted appropriately

Table 23-1 Descriptive Strategies for the Administration of Antibiotic Therapy

Monotherapy
Combination Therapy
Heterogeneity
Protocolized Therapy
Synergistic Therapy
Computerized Decision Support
Cycling
Deescalation
Formulary Restriction

at the likely pathogens, administered in sufficient dosage so that bacterial killing is assured insofar as possible, narrowed in spectrum (called *de-escalation*)[21] as soon as possible based on microbiology data and clinical response, and continued for only as long as necessary. Appropriate antibiotic prescribing is essential not only for optimal patient care, but also for infection control and maintenance of the microbial ecology of the unit.[22,23]

Several questions must be asked whenever empiric therapy is considered. Are antibiotics indicated at all? The answer may ultimately be no, but the decision to treat the unstable patient must often be made before definitive information is available. The decision to start antibiotics empirically considers the likelihood of infection, its likely source, and whether delay will be detrimental. Outcome from serious infections is improved if antibiotics are started promptly. By contrast, only about 50% of fever episodes in hospitalized patients are caused by infection[24] (Table 23-2). Many causes of the systemic inflammatory response syndrome (SIRS) are not due to infection (eg, aspiration pneumonitis, burns, trauma, pancreatitis), although they may be complicated later by infection.[25] Multiple organ dysfunction syndrome (MODS) may progress

Table 23-2 Nosocomial Infections in the Intensive Care Unit

COMMON
Pneumonia
Catheter-related infection
Intraabdominal (in surgical units)
Urinary tract
Skin/soft tissue
    Decubitus ulcer
    Surgical site infection

UNCOMMON
Sinusitis
Empyema
Endocarditis
Endophthalmitis
Parotitis
Suppurative phlebitis

Table 23-3   Rank Order of Key Pathogens in ICU Infections (By Incidence)

	Blood stream infection	Urinary tract infection	Pneumonia
Gram-positive	1: Coag-neg staphylococci 2: *Enterococcus* 3: *S. aureus*	1: *Enterococcus* 2: Coag-neg staphylococci 3: *S. aureus*	1: *S. aureus*
Gram-negative	1: *Enterobacter* 2: *P. aeruginosa* 3: *K. pneumoniae* 4: *E. coli*	1: *E. coli* 2: *P. aeruginosa* 3: *K. pneumoniae* 4: *Enterobacter*	1: *P. aeruginosa* 2: *Enterobacter* 3: *K. pneumoniae* 4: *E. coli*

even after an infectious precipitant has been controlled, due to a dysregulated host response.[26]

Must antibiotics be started immediately? If the presumed infection is not destabilizing, the overall status of the patient is considered, including age, debility, renal and hepatic function, and immunosuppression. Culture yields are highest before antibiotics are administered, which for certain types of specimens (eg, blood, cerebrospinal fluid) can be crucial. However, for many infections (eg, bacteremia, intra-abdominal infection, pneumonia), early appropriate therapy improves outcome.[14,27,28]

Which organisms are the likely pathogens, and are they likely to be MDR? The clinical setting must be considered (eg, nosocomial vs health care [eg, nursing home] vs community-acquired infection, recent antimicrobial therapy), as must the patient's environment (eg, recent hospitalization or antibiotic treatment, the presence of MDR pathogens in the unit, and any recent positive cultures).

Will a single antibiotic suffice? The likely diagnosis and the probable pathogens are crucial determinants (Tables 23-3 and 23-4). If a nosocomial gram-positive pathogen is suspected (eg, wound or surgical site infection, catheter-related infection, prosthetic device infection, pneumonia), and methicillin-resistant *S. aureus* (MRSA) is endemic, then empiric vancomycin (or linezolid) is appropriate. Some authorities recommend dual-agent therapy for serious *Pseudomonas* infections (ie, an antipseudomonal β-lactam drug plus

an aminoglycoside), but evidence of efficacy is scant.[29] It is important to use at least two antibiotics for empiric therapy of any infection that may be caused by either a gram-positive or -negative infection (eg, nosocomial pneumonia)[30] (Figs. 23-1 and 23-2).

CHOICE OF ANTIBIOTIC

The choice of which antibiotic(s) to prescribe is based on several interrelated factors (Table 23-5). Paramount is activity against identified or likely (for empiric therapy) pathogens, presuming infecting and colonizing organisms can be distinguished, and that narrow-spectrum coverage is always desired. Estimation of likely pathogens depends on the disease process believed responsible; whether the infection is community, health care, or hospital acquired; whether MDR organisms are present; and proximity to other infected patients. Knowledge of antimicrobial resistance patterns is essential, especially in one's own institution and unit. Also important are patient-specific factors, including age, debility, immunosuppression, intrinsic organ function, prior allergy or another adverse reaction, and recent antibiotic therapy. Institutional factors of importance include guidelines that may specify a particular therapy, formulary availability of specific agents, and antibiotic control programs. Numerous agents are available for therapy (Table 23-6).[31,32] Agents may be chosen based on spectrum, whether broad or targeted (eg, antipseudomonal, antianaerobic), in addition to these factors.

ANTIFUNGAL PROPHYLAXIS AND THERAPY

The incidence of invasive fungal infections has doubled in the past decade, with the greatest increase in critically ill surgical patients. Several conditions (both patient dependent and disease specific) are predictors for invasive fungal complications during critical illness, including intensive care unit length of stay, the degree or morbidity, alterations of immune response, and the number of medical devices placed. Neutropenia, diabetes mellitus, new-onset hemodialysis, total parenteral nutrition, broad-spectrum antibiotic administration, bladder catheterization, azotemia, diarrhea,

Table 23-4   Flora in Different Types of Intra-abdominal Infection

Primary (Monomicrobial)	Secondary (Polymicrobial)	Tertiary (Polymicrobial)
E. coli	*B. fragilis* group	*S. epidermidis*
Klebsiella spp.	Other anaerobes	Enterococci
S. pneumoniae	*E. coli*	*P. aeruginosa*
Enterococci	*Klebsiella* spp.	*Candida* spp.
Anaerobes rare	Other enterics Enterococci	

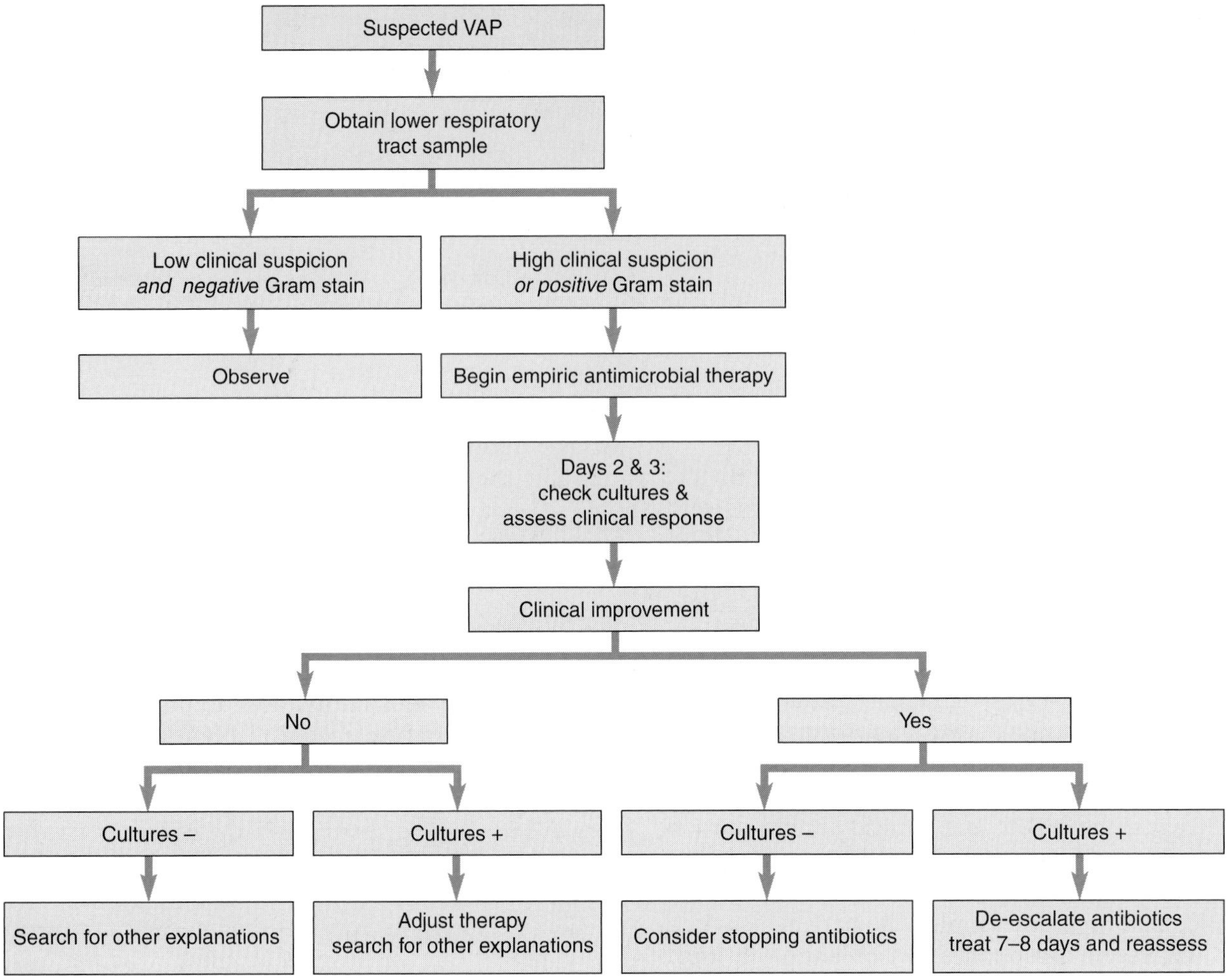

```
                        ┌─────────────────────┐
                        │   Suspected VAP     │
                        └──────────┬──────────┘
                                   ↓
                        ┌─────────────────────┐
                        │ Obtain lower         │
                        │ respiratory          │
                        │ tract sample         │
                        └──────────┬──────────┘
              ┌────────────────────┴────────────────────┐
              ↓                                          ↓
   ┌──────────────────────┐              ┌──────────────────────┐
   │ Low clinical suspicion│              │ High clinical suspicion│
   │ and negative Gram stain│             │ or positive Gram stain │
   └──────────┬───────────┘              └──────────┬───────────┘
              ↓                                      ↓
   ┌──────────────────────┐              ┌──────────────────────┐
   │      Observe          │              │ Begin empiric        │
   └──────────────────────┘              │ antimicrobial therapy │
                                         └──────────┬───────────┘
```

Days 2 & 3: check cultures & assess clinical response

Clinical improvement

No

Yes

| Cultures − | Cultures + | Cultures − | Cultures + |

Search for other explanations

Adjust therapy search for other explanations

Consider stopping antibiotics

De-escalate antibiotics treat 7–8 days and reassess

Figure 23-1 *Ventilator-associated pneumonia management algorithm. VAP; ventilator-associated pneumonia. Adapted from American Thoracic Society. Guidelines for the management of adults with hospital-acquired, ventilator-associated, and healthcare-associated pneumonia.* Am J Resp Crit Care Med *2005;171:388-416.*

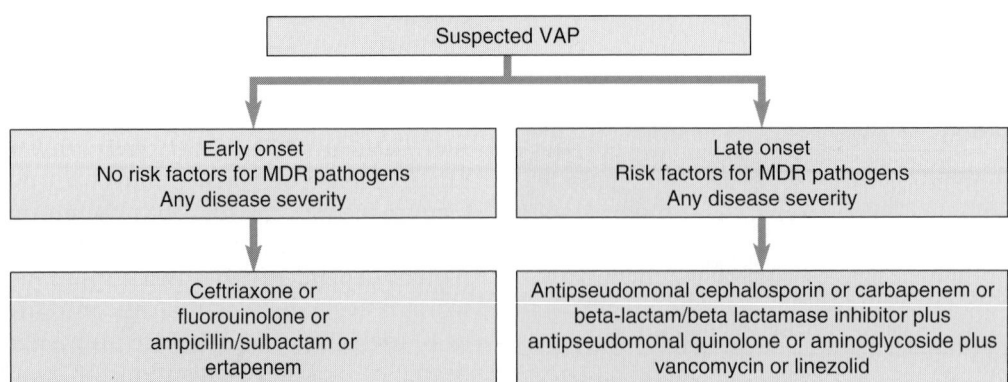

Suspected VAP

Early onset
No risk factors for MDR pathogens
Any disease severity

Late onset
Risk factors for MDR pathogens
Any disease severity

Ceftriaxone or
fluorouinolone or
ampicillin/sulbactam or
ertapenem

Antipseudomonal cephalosporin or carbapenem or
beta-lactam/beta lactamase inhibitor plus
antipseudomonal quinolone or aminoglycoside plus
vancomycin or linezolid

Figure 23-2 *Algorithm for selection of initial antimicrobial therapy in suspected ventilator-associated pneumonia. Early onset: Pneumonia within the first five days after onset of mechanical ventilation; VAP, ventilator-associated pneumonia; MDR, multi-drug-resistant. Adapted from American Thoracic Society. Guidelines for the management of adults with hospital-acquired, ventilator-associated, and healthcare-associated pneumonia.* Am J Resp Crit Care Med *2005;171:388-416.*

Table 23-5   Factors Influencing Antibiotic Choice
Activity against known/suspected pathogens
Disease believed responsible
Distinguish infection from colonization
Narrow-spectrum coverage most desirable
Antimicrobial resistance patterns

Patient-specific factors
   Severity of illness?
   Age?
   Immunosuppression
   Organ dysfunction
   Allergy

Institutional guidelines/restrictions

and corticosteroid therapy are also associated with invasive fungal infection.[33,34]

The recovery of *Candida* spp. from multiple sites of colonization (without symptoms) has been linked to a high likelihood of invasive candidiasis. Risk factors for the development of *Candida* colonization include prior use of antibiotics or a bacterial infection prior to ICU admission, a prolonged stay in the ICU, and multiple gastrointestinal operations. The source of most of the outbreaks of systemic candidiasis in the context of colonization is frequently the gastrointestinal tract.

Table 23-6   Antibacterial Agents for Empiric Use
Antipseudomonal Piperacillin-tazobactam Cefepime, ceftazidime Imipenem, meropenem ? Ciprofloxacin, levofloxacin (depending on local   susceptibility patterns) Aminoglycoside
Targeted-spectrum *Gram-positive* Glycopeptide Lipopeptide (not for known/suspected pneumonia) Oxazolidinone *Gram-negative* Third-generation cephalosporin (not ceftriaxone) Monobactam *Anti-anaerobic* Metronidazole
Broad-spectrum Piperacillin-tazobactam Carbapenems Fluoroquinolones Tigecycline (plus an antipseudoomonal agent
Anti-anaerobic Metronidazole Carbapenems Beta-lactam/beta-lactamase combination agents Tigecycline

Some data suggest a that prophylactic antifungal therapy for colonized, non-neutropenic critically ill surgical patients can decrease the risk of invasive candidiasis,[35] whereas other data suggest that antifungal prophylaxis with fluconazole leads to resistance in previously susceptible fungi.[36]

Numerous new antifungal agents have been introduced in the past 10 years, including less-toxic lipid-complexed formulations of amphotericin B, improved triazoles (eg, voriconazole, posaconazole), and echinocandins (eg, caspofungin, micafungin, anidulafungin), and other agents that target the fungal cell wall. The safety profile of azole and echinocandin agents, combined with decreasing cost owing to marketplace competition, have resulted in markedly decreased usage of amphotericin B in any form. Independent of the species, infection by fluconazole-resistant *Candida* doubles the mortality rate; considering that fluconazole-resistant strains of *Candida* (eg, *C. glabrata, C. krusei*) are causing an increasing percentage of invasive fungal infections, empiric antifungal therapy should begin with an agent other than fluconazole. Table 23-7 presents a list of selected antifungal agents and susceptibility to *Candida* spp.[37]

DURATION OF THERAPY

The endpoint of therapy is largely undefined, in part because quality data are few.[26,38,39] If *bona fide* evidence of infection is evident, then treatment is continued as indicated clinically. Often, however, cultures are negative and the decision must be arbitrary. A clinical response to therapy in the absence of positive cultures may be a coincidence or a result of false-negative cultures (which is unlikely with good specimen collection technique and modern microbiology laboratories; false-positive cultures are a larger clinical problem). Unnecessary antibiotic therapy in the absence of infection clearly increases the risk of MDR infection; therefore, continuing empiric antibiotic therapy with negative cultures beyond 48-72 hours is unjustifiable, with two possible exceptions: Suspected fungal infection (the organisms are fastidious), and a need for deep cultures from an inaccessible area (additional time may be necessary to arrange image-guided aspiration). The morbidity of antibiotic therapy includes allergic reactions; development of nosocomial superinfections, including fungal infections, enterococcal infections, and *Clostridium difficile*–related disease;[40-42] organ toxicity; promotion of antibiotic resistance; reduced yield from subsequent cultures; and induced vitamin K deficiency with coagulopathy or accentuation of warfarin effect.

Many infections can be treated with therapy lasting five days or less. Every decision to start antibiotics must be accompanied by a decision regarding the duration of therapy.[26] A reason to continue therapy beyond the predetermined endpoint must be compelling. Bacterial killing is rapid in response to effective

Table 23-7   Usual Susceptibilities of *Candida* Species to Selected Antifungal Agents

Candida species	Fluconazole	Itraconazole	Voriconazole	Amphotericin B	Caspofungin
C. albicans	S	S	S	S	S
C. tropicalis	S	S	S	S	S
C. parapsilosis	S	S	S	S	S to I (?R)
C, glabrata	S-DD to R	S-DD to R	S to I	S to I	S
C. krusei	R	S-DD to R	S to I	S to I	S
C. lusitaniae	S	S	S	S to R	S

Modified from Reference 37
S = Susceptible
S-DD = Susceptible-dose dependent (increased MIC may be overcome by higher dosing—eg, 12 mg/kg/day fluconazole)
I = Intermediate
R = Resistant

agents, but the host response may not subside immediately. Therefore, the clinical response of the patient should not be the sole determinant for continuation of therapy. If a patient still has SIRS at the predetermined end of therapy, it is more useful to stop therapy and obtain a new cultures to look for persistent or new infection, resistant pathogens, and noninfectious causes of SIRS.

Infections that require 24 hours of therapy or less (sometimes just a single dose) include uncomplicated acute appendicitis or cholecystitis, uncomplicated bacterial cystitis (with some agents), and intestinal infarction without perforation. There is seldom justification to continue antibacterial therapy for more than 7-10 days. Examples of bacterial infections that require more than 14 days of therapy include tuberculosis of any site, endocarditis, osteomyelitis, and selected cases of brain abscess, liver abscess, lung abscess, postoperative meningitis, and endophthalmitis.

DEVELOPMENT OF BACTERIAL RESISTANCE

Although antibiotic selection pressure is the major factor in the development of bacterial resistance and MDR pathogens, other risk factors have been identified

Table 23-8   Factors Contributing to Antibiotic Resistance

Increased severity of illness

Severely immunocompromise

Invasive devices and procedures

Resistant organisms in the community

Ineffective infection control and compliance

Inappropriate antibiotic usage

Greater antibiotic usage

(Table 23-8). Hospitalized patients are more severely ill than ever before, and may be immunosuppressed owing to illness (eg, cancer, trauma) or therapy (eg, antineoplastic therapy, transplant immunosuppression, glucocorticoid therapy). Invasive procedures (even in this era of minimal-access surgery) breach natural epithelial barriers to bacterial invasion of the host, and increase the risk of infection. Ineffective infection control practice is a major issue in health care facilities; hand washing is the single most effective deterrent of infection that has been described.

In general, bacteria develop resistance to antibiotics via four different mechanisms.[43-46] Cell wall permeability is decreased by changes in porin channels (especially important for gram-negative bacteria with complex cell walls, affecting aminoglycosides, β-lactam drugs, chloramphenicol, sulfonamides, tetracyclines, and possibly quinolones). Production of antibiotic-inactivating enzymes by either plasmid- or chromosomally mediated mechanisms affects aminoglycosides, β-lactam drugs, chloramphenicol, and macrolides. Altered binding targets in the cell wall affect β-lactam drugs and vancomycin, whereas alteration of target enzymes can inhibit β-lactam drugs, sulfonamides, quinolones, and rifampin. Drugs that bind to the bacterial ribosome (ie, aminoglycosides, chloramphenicol, macrolides, lincosamides, streptogramins, and tetracyclines) are susceptible to alteration of the ribosomal receptor. Antibiotics may be extruded actively via efflux pumps, affecting macrolides, lincosamides, oxazolidinolones, streptogramins, quinolones, and tetracyclines.

Cephalosporin resistance among gram-negative bacilli may result from induction of chromosomal β[GR4]-lactamases after antibiotic exposure, particularly third-generation cephalosporin use.[47] More than 500 mutations have now been described in virtually clinically relevant species of gram-negative bacteria. The carbapenems generally retain useful microbicidal activity against extended-spectrum β-lactamase (ESBL)-producing strains.[48] Increasingly, *Pseudomonas aeruginosa* produces metalloproteinases that inactivate carbapenems.

Quinolone resistance, which is increasing rapidly,[49] is chromosomally mediated for the most part, primarily by changes in target binding sites (DNA gyrase or topoisomerase IV). Changes in permeability or efflux may sometimes cause resistance to quinolones as well. Quinolone resistance is relatively easy to induce if a less-than-maximally effective drug or dose is chosen for initial therapy. Resistance to one quinolone may also increase the MIC for the other quinolones against the organism, so if used, a highly active agent given in adequate dosage is essential.

ANTIBIOTIC SPECTRUM OF ACTIVITY

Susceptibility testing of specific organisms is necessary for management of serious infections (including all nosocomial infections). Recommended agents for specific organisms are guidelines only, because *in vitro* susceptibilities may not correlate with clinical efficacy.

CELL-WALL-ACTIVE AGENTS: β-LACTAM ANTIBIOTICS

The β-lactam antibiotic group consists of penicillins, cephalosporins, monobactams, and carbapenems. Within this group, several agents have been combined with β-lactamase inhibitors to broaden the spectrum and increase the efficacy of the drugs. Several subgroups of antibiotics are recognized within the group, notably several "generations" of cephalosporins and penicillinase-resistant penicillins.

PENICILLINS

With the exception of carboxy- and ureidopenicillins, penicillins retain little or no activity against most gram-negative bacilli. Penicillin is useful against most strains of *Streptococcus*, except for penicilin-resistant *S. pneumoniae* (PRSP, up to 40% of isolates). Penicillins also have activity against *Enterococcus faecalis* (but not *E. faecium*), *Corynebacterium diphtheriae*, and *Listeria monocytogenes*. Gram-negative bacteria that are susceptible to penicillins include *Neisseria meninigitidis* (highly resistant strains exist), some strains of *Proteus mirabilis*, and *Pasturella multocida*. Penicillins are also effective against all *Clostridium* spp. other than *C. difficile*.

The penicillinase-resistant semisynthetic penicillins include methicillin, nafcillin, oxacillin, cloxacillin, and dicloxacillin. The primary use of these agents is as therapy for sensitive strains of staphylococci. Hospitalized patients should not be treated empirically with these agents, because 60% of strains of *S. aureus* (MRSA), 90% of strains of *S. epidermidis* (MRSE), and virtually all enterococcal strains are resistant.[50] However, these drugs are the treatment of choice for infections caused by susceptible isolates of *S. aureus*.

The aminopenicillins include ampicillin and amoxicillin. Ampicillin is effective against *E. faecalis*, including some vancomycin-resistant strains (VRE), but only rarely against *E. faecium*. Useful activity remains against *N. meningitidis*, *Moraxella catarrhalis*, community-acquired strains of *E. coli* and *Klebsiella* spp., *Salmonella* and *Shigella* spp., and *Proteus* spp. Ampicillin remains reasonably effective against community-acquired strains of *Hemophilus influenzae*, but *H. influenzae* is an increasingly important nosocomial pathogen.

The carboxypenicillins (ticarcillin and carbenicillin) and ureidopenicillins (azlocillin, mezlocillin, and piperacillin; sometimes referred to as acylampicillins) have enhanced activity against gram-negative bacteria and some activity against *P. aeruginosa*. Ureidopenicillins have greater intrinsic activity against *Pseudomonas*, but with the advent of β-lactamase inhibitor combination drugs, none are used widely any more. Combination with a β-lactamase inhibitor (sulbactam, tazobactam, clavulanic acid) enhances the effectiveness of the parent β-lactam agent (piperacillin > ticarcillin > ampicillin), and to a lesser extent the inhibitor (tazobactam > sulbactam ~ clavulanic acid). The spectrum of activity varies within the class, and the treating clinician needs to be familiar with each of the drugs. All of these drugs are effective against streptococci, and methicillin-sensitive strains of *S. aureus*, and widely effective against anaerobes (except for *C. difficile*). Piperacillin-tazobactam has the widest spectrum of activity against gram-negative bacteria, and the most potency among β-lactam drugs against *P. aeruginosa*. Although ampicillin-sulbactam is unreliable against *E. coli* and *Klebsiella* (resistance rate ~ 50%), it has useful activity against *Acinetobacter* spp. because of sulbactam.[51]

CEPHALOSPORINS

More than twenty cephalosporins comprise the class; the characteristics of the drugs thus vary widely, but are similar within four broad "generations." "First-generation" agents retain useful activity against gram-positive organisms, whereas "second-generation" agents generally lose that activity in favor of antianaerobic activity. "Third-generation" agents have enhanced activity against gram-negative bacilli (some have specific anti-pseudomonal activity), but most are ineffective against gram-positive cocci and none against anaerobes. Cefepime, the "fourth-generation" cephalosporin available in the United States, has enhanced anti-pseudomonal activity and has regained activity against most gram-positive cocci, but not methicillin-resistant *S. aureus* (MRSA). None of the cephalosporins are useful against enterococci. The heterogeneity of spectrum, especially among third-generation agents, requires broad familiarity with all of these drugs.

First-Generation Cephalosporins

First-generation cephalosporins (cefadroxil, cefazolin, cephalexin, cephalothin, cephapirin, and cephradine) are useful to treat community-acquired gram-negative infections caused by *E. coli* and *Klebsiella* spp., but not nosocomial pathogens. Parenteral first-generation cephalosporins still have a major role in surgical prophylaxis. Oral first-generation cephalosporins are used mostly for outpatient therapy of skin and soft tissue and urinary tract infections. First-generation agents are the most active cephalosporins against staphylococci (not MRSA) and streptococci.

Second-Generation Cephalosporins

Second-generation cephalosporins are useful to the abdominal surgeon, but they are in short supply. These agents include cefaclor, cefamandole, cefmetazole, cefonicid, cefotetan, cefoxitin (technically a cephamycin), and cefuroxime. These drugs retain activity against aerobic and anaerobic streptococci, but lose some activity against methicillin-sensitive staphylococci. Activity against gram-negative bacilli is intermediate between that of the first-and third-generation agents. In general, there is activity against the *Enterobacteriaceae* except for *Enterobacter*, but no activity against *Acinetobacter*, *Pseudomonas*, or *Stenotrophomonas*. Cefmetazole, cefotetan, and cefoxitin have some activity against anaerobic gram-negative bacilli, including *Bacteroides fragilis*, but not to the extent of beta-lactamase combination drugs, carbapenems, or metronidazole.

Third-Generation Cephalosporins

Third-generation cephalosporins include cefoperazone, cefotaxime, cefpodoxime, cefprozil, ceftazidime, ceftibuten, ceftizoxime, ceftriaxone, and lorcarbicef. They possess a modestly extended spectrum of activity against gram-negative bacilli, but not against gram-positive bacteria (except for ceftriaxone) or anaerobic bacteria. Third-generation cephalosporins, particularly ceftazidime, have been associated with the induction of ESBLs among many of the *Enterobacteriaceae*.[52] Activity is reliable only against non-ESBL producing species of *Enterobacteriaceae* including *Enterobacter*, *Citrobacter*, *Providencia*, and *Morganella*. Activity is no longer reliable for empiric use against nonfermenting gram-negative bacilli (eg, *Acinetobacter* spp., *P. aeruginosa*, *S. maltophilia*).

Fourth-Generation Cephalosporins

The gram-negative spectrum of cefepime is more broad than that of the third-generation cephalosporins (the antipseudomonal activity exceeds that of ceftazidime), whereas the anti-gram-positive activity is comparable to that of a first-generation cephalosporin. The excellent safety profile of the cephalosporins is retained, and the potential for induction of ESBL production appears to be less. In common with all cephalosporins, there is no activity against either enterococci or enteric anaerobic flora. Similar to the carbapenems, cefepime appears to be intrinsically more resistant to hydrolysis by β-lactamases, but cefepime has variable activity against ESBL-producing bacteria.[53]

MONOBACTAMS

The single available agent of this class, aztreonam, has a spectrum of activity against gram-negative bacilli that is similar to the third-generation cephalosporins, with no activity against either gram-positive organisms or anaerobes. Aztreonam is not a potent inducer of β-lactamases. Resistance to aztreonam is widespread, but the drug may be useful for directed therapy against known susceptible strains, and may be used safely for penicillin-allergic patients because the incidence of cross-reactivity is low.

CARBAPENEMS

Carbapenems have a five carbon-ring attached to the beta-lactam nucleus. The alkyl groups are oriented in a transconfiguration rather than the cis-configuration characteristic of other β-lactam agents, making these drugs resistant to beta-lactamases. Three drugs, imipenem-cilastatin, meropenem, and ertapenem, are available for clinical use in the United States. Imipenem-cilastatin and meropenem have the widest antibacterial spectrum of any antibiotics, with excellent activity against aerobic and anaerobic streptococci, methicillin-sensitive staphylococci, and virtually all gram-negative bacilli except *Legionella*, *P. cepacia*, and *S. maltophilia*.[54] Activity against the *Enterobacteriaceae* exceeds that of all antibiotics with the possible exceptions of piperacillin-tazobactam and cefepime, and activity of meropenem against *P. aeruginosa* is approached only by that of amikacin. All carbapenems are superlative antianaerobic agents, thus there is no reason to combine a carbapenem with metronidazole except, for example, to treat concurrent *C. difficile* colitis in a patient with a life-threatening infection that mandates continuance of the carbapenem.

Meropenem may have less potential for neurotoxicity than imipenem-cilastatin, 55 which is contraindicated in patients with active central nervous system disease or injury (excepting the spinal cord), because of the rare (~0.5%) appearance of myoclonus or generalized seizures in patients who have received doses > 3 g/day (with normal renal function) or who have not had dosage reductions in the setting of renal insufficiency. With both drugs, widespread disruption of the host microbial flora may lead to superinfections (eg, fungi, *C. difficile*, *Stenotrophomonas*, or resistant enterococci).

Ertapenem is not useful against *Pseudomonas* spp., *Acinetobacter* spp., Enterobacter spp., or MRSA, but its long half-life and substantial PAE permit once-daily dosing.[56] Ertapenem is highly active against ESBL-producing *Enterobacteriaceae*, and has less potential for neurotoxicity than imipenem-cilastatin.

CELL WALL ACTIVE AGENTS: LIPOGLYCOPEPTIDES

Vancomycin, a soluble lipoglycopeptide, is rapidly bactericidal, but only on dividing organisms. A PAE persists for about 2 hours. Unfortunately, tissue penetration of vancomycin is poor for almost all tissues, which can limit its effectiveness. Both *S. aureus* and *S. epidermidis* are susceptible to vancomycin, although MICs for S. *aureus* are increasing, requiring higher doses for effect.[52] *Streptococcus pyogenes*, group B streptococci, *S. pneumoniae* (including PRSP), and *C. difficile* are also susceptible. Most strains of *E. faecalis* are inhibited (but not killed) by attainable concentrations, but *E. faecium* is increasingly resistant to vancomycin (VRE).

It is important for the public health that widespread inappropriate usage of vancomycin should be curtailed (Table 23-9). *Bona fide* indications include serious infections caused by MRSA/MRSE, gram-positive infections in patients with serious penicillin allergy, and oral therapy (or by enema in patients with ileus) for *C. difficile*–related colitis in patients who have failed or are intolerant of metronidazole. Parenteral vancomycin (a dose of 15 mg/kg is now recommended) must be infused over at least 1 hour.

CELL WALL ACTIVE AGENTS: CYCLIC LIPOPEPTIDES

Daptomycin has potent, rapid bactericidal activity against most gram-positive organisms. The mechanism of action is novel, causing rapid membrane depolarization, potassium ion efflux, arrest of DNA, RNA, and protein synthesis, and cell death. Daptomycin exhibits concentration-dependent killing, has a long half-life (8 hours), and demonstrates a prolonged PAE, up to 6.8 hours.[58]

A dose regimen of 4 mg/kg once daily is recommended for complicated skin/skin structure infections (cSSSI) (6 mg/kg/day for bacteremia). Daptomycin is excreted renally, therefore, the dosing interval should be increased to 48 hours when creatinine clearance < 30 mL/min. No antagonistic drug interactions have been observed.

Daptomycin is active against many aerobic and anaerobic gram-positive bacteria, including MDR strains such as MRSA, MRSE, and VRE. Furthermore, daptomycin is also effective against a variety of anaerobes, including *Peptostreptococcus* spp., *C. perfringens*, and *C. difficile*. Resistance to daptomycin remains rare.

Importantly, daptomycin must not be used for the treatment of pneumonia or empiric therapy when pneumonia is in the differential diagnosis, even when caused by a susceptible organism, because daptomycin penetrates lung tissue poorly and is also inactivated by pulmonary surfactant.[59]

PROTEIN SYNTHESIS INHIBITORS

Several classes of antibiotics, although dissimilar structurally and having widely divergent spectra of activity, exert their antibacterial effects via binding to bacterial ribosomes, thereby inhibiting protein synthesis. This classification is valuable mechanistically, linking several classes of antibiotics conceptually that have few clinically useful members.

AMINOGLYCOSIDES

Once disdained as toxic and superceded by newer antibiotics, it is ironic that a resurgence of aminoglycoside use has occurred as resistance to these newer antibiotics (especially third-generation cephalosporins and quinolones) has developed. Aminoglycosides bind to the bacterial 30S ribosomal subunit, inhibiting protein synthesis. With the exception of slightly better activity against gram-positive cocci possessed by gentamicin, the spectrum of activity for the various agents is nearly identical. Differences among the agents are based upon toxicity and local resistance patterns. Gentamicin, tobramycin, and amikacin are still used frequently. Netilmicin is comparable in toxicity, but seldom used. Kanamycin is now used only topically, owing to marked toxicity. Streptomycin, also quite toxic, is used rarely in antimycobacterial regimens.

Nevertheless, the potential toxicity is real, and aminoglycosides are now seldom first-line therapy, except in a synergistic combination to treat a serious *Pseudomonas* infection, enterococcal endocarditis, or an infection caused by a MDR gram-negative bacillus. As second-line therapy, these drugs are highly efficacious against the *Enterobacteriaceae*, but there is less activity against *Acinetobacter*, and limited activity against *P. cepacia*, *Aeromonas* spp., and *S. maltophilia*.

Aminoglycosides kill bacteria most effectively with a concentration peak: MIC > 12, therefore a loading dose is necessary and serum drug concentration

Table 23-9 Situations in which the use of vancomycin is discouraged
Routine surgical prophylaxis in the absence of life-threatening allergy to beta-lactam antibiotics
Empiric therapy of febrile neutropenia in the absence of evidence for a gram-positive infection
Continued empiric use when microbiologic data suggest a reasonable alternative
Systemic or local (ie, catheter flush) prophylaxis of indwelling vascular catheters
Selective decontamination of the digestive tract
Eradication of colonization of methicillin-resistant staphylococci
Primary treatment of antibiotic-associated colitis due to *Clostridium difficile*
Routine prophylaxis for patients on hemodialysis or continuous ambulatory peritoneal dialysis
Use for topical irrigation or application

monitoring is often performed.[7] Synergistic therapy with a β-lactam agent is theoretically effective because damage to the bacterial cell wall caused by the β-lactam drug enhances intracellular penetration of the aminoglycoside, but evidence of improved clinical outcomes is lacking.[29] Serious infections require 5 mg/kg/day of gentamicin or tobramycin after a 2 mg/kg loading dose, or 15 mg/kg day of amikacin after a loading dose of 7.5 mg/kg. Clearance and V_D are variable and unpredictable in critically ill patients, and higher doses are sometimes necessary (eg, burn patients). High doses (eg, gentamicin 7 mg/kg/day, amikacin 20 mg/kg/day) administered as a single daily dose can obviate these problems in selected patients.[6] Marked dosage reductions are necessary in renal failure, but the drugs are dialyzed and a maintenance dose should be given after each hemodialysis treatment.

TETRACYCLINES

Tetracyclines bind irreversibly to the 30S ribosomal subunit, but unlike aminoglycosides, they are bacteriostatic agents. Widespread resistance limits their utility in the hospital setting (with two exceptions, doxycycline and tigecycline), but they are still prescribed as oral agents. Tetracyclines are active against anaerobes; *Actinomyces* can be treated successfully. Doxycycline is active against B. *fragilis*, but seldom used for the purpose. Many spirochetes are susceptible, including *Borrelia burgdorferi*, as are rickettsiae, *Chlamydophila* spp., mycoplasmas, and to some extent protozoa (*Entamoeba histolytica, Plasmodium* spp.). All tetracyclines are contraindicated in pregnancy and for children under the age of 8 years, owing to dental toxicity.

Tigecycline is a novel glycylcycline derived from minocycline.[60] With the major exceptions of *Pseudomonas* spp and *P. mirabilis*, the spectrum of activity is broad, including many MDR gram-positive and –negative bacteria. Tigecycline is able to overcome typical bacterial resistance to tetracyclines because of modification at position 9 of its core structure, which enables binding to the 30S ribosomal unit with greater affinity. Tigecycline is active against aerobic and anaerobi streptococci, staphylococci, MRSA, MRSE, and enterococci including VRE. Activity against gram-negative bacilli is directed against *Enterobacteriaceae* including ESBL-producing strains, *P. multocida, A. hydrophila, S. maltophila, E. aerogenes*, and *Acinetobacter* spp. Antianaerobic activity is excellent.

OXAZOLIDINONES

Oxazolidinones bind to the ribosomal 50S subunit, preventing complexing with the 30S subunit.[61] Assembly of a functional initiation complex for protein synthesis is blocked, preventing translation of mRNA. This mode of action differs from that of extant protein synthesis inhibitors such as chloramphenicol, macrolides, lincosamides, and tetracyclines, which permit mRNA translation but then inhibit peptide elongation. This difference is important in two respects. Linezolid, the first marketed oxazolidinone, is particularly effective in preventing the synthesis of staphylococcal and streptococcal virulence factors (eg, coagulase, hemolysins, protein A). Second, linezolid's target binding site does not overlap with those of existing protein synthesis inhibitors; consequently, it is unaffected by the rRNA methylases that modify the 23S rRNA so as to block binding of macrolides, clindamycin, and group B streptogramins. Preventing the initiation of protein synthesis is no more inherently lethal than prevention of peptide elongation, therefore linezolid is bacteriostatic similar to chloramphenicol, clindamycin, macrolides, and tetracyclines. The ribosomes of *E. coli* are as susceptible to linezolid as those of gram-positive cocci but, with minor exceptions, gram-negative bacteria are oxazolidinone-resistant, because oxazolidinones are excreted by efflux pumps.

Linezolid is equally active against MSSA and MRSA, vancomycin-susceptible enterococci and VRE, and against susceptible and PRSP pneumococci. Most gram-negative bacteria are resistant, but *Bacteroides* spp are susceptible. Linezolid exhibits excellent tissue penetration, and requires no dosage reduction in renal insufficiency. Some retrospective data suggest that linezolid may be superior to vancomycin for hospital-acquired pneumonia[62] and cSSSI,[63] but prospective confirmation is required if linezolid is to supplant vancomycin as first-line therapy for serious infections caused by gram-positive cocci.

THE MACROLIDE-LINCOSAMIDE-STREPTOGRAMIN (MLS) FAMILY
Clindamycin
The only lincosamide antibiotic in active clinical use is clindamycin, which also binds to the 50S ribosome. Clindamycin has good antianaerobic activity (although *B. fragilis* resistance is increasing), and reasonably good activity against susceptible gram-positive cocci (not MRSA or VRE). Clindamycin is used occasionally for anaerobic infections, and is preferred over vancomycin for prophylaxis of clean surgical cases in penicillin-allergic patients. Because clindamycin inhibits production of exotoxins *in vitro*, it has been advocated in preference to penicillin as first-line therapy of invasive *S. pyogenes* infections. Use of clindamycin has been associated with the development of antibiotic-associated colitis caused by *C. difficile*.

Macrolides and Ketolides
Azithromycin, clarithromycin, dirithromycin, and erythromycin (the available macrolide antibiotics) and telithromycin (the first ketolide), are characterized by a macrocyclic lactone ring. Clarithromycin was developed against atypical mycobacteria in immunosuppressed patients, for which it is undeniably effective, and it is extremely active against *Helicobacter pylori*. Most macrolide usage is among outpatients, for upper

respiratory tract infections and sometimes for uncomplicated skin infections. Activity is excellent against aerobic streptococci, but azithromycin and clarithromycin are better against MSSA. There is no appreciable activity against MRSA or MRSE. Azithromycin is available orally and parenterally for therapy of severe community-acquired pneumonia caused by atypical organisms, including *L. pneumophilia*.

Most macrolides inhibit the function of the cytochromes P_{450}. Patients on theophylline should be monitored carefully when clarithromycin or erythromycin are used concurrently, but not azithromycin. Interactions between erythromycin or clarithromycin and other drugs that prolong the QTc interval, such as fluoroquinolones, may precipitate ventricular dysrhythmias such as torsades de pointes.

DRUGS THAT DISRUPT NUCLEIC ACIDS
Quinolones

Quinolones inhibit bacterial DNA synthesis by inhibiting DNA gyrase, which folds DNA into a superhelix in preparation for replication. The fluoroquinolones exhibit a broad spectrum of activity, excellent oral absorption and bioavailability, and are generally well tolerated. These are potent agents with an unfortunate propensity to develop resistance rapidly. Agents with both parenteral and oral formulations include ciprofloxacin, levofloxacin, and moxifloxacin (which has some antianaerobic activity).

Quinolones are most active against enteric gram-negative bacteria, particularly the *Enterobacteriaceae* and *Hemophilus* spp. There is activity against *P. aeruginosa*, *S. maltophilia*, and gram-negative cocci. Activity against gram-positive cocci is variable, being least for ciprofloxacin and best for the so-called respiratory quinolones (eg, moxifloxacin). Ciprofloxacin is most active against *P. aeruginosa*. However, rampant overuse of fluoroquinolones is rapidly causing resistance that may limit severely the future usefulness of these agents.[48,64] Fluoroquinolone use has been associated with the emergence of resistant *P. aeruginosa*[48] and MRSA.[65]

Rifampin

The rifamycins, of which rifampin is used most often, inhibit DNA-dependent RNA polymerase at the β-subunit, which prevents chain initiation. Rifampin penetrates well almost all body tissues, with a unique ability to penetrate living neutrophils and kill phagocytized intracellular bacteria. Rifampin is available both orally and parenterally, and is active against a wide range of pathogens. Oral bioavailability approaches 100% with the usual dose of 600 mg once daily, but the rapid development of resistance relegates this agent to combination therapy in virtually all circumstances.

Rifampin is active against staphylococci (including MRSA), and also active against other gram-positive and gram-negative cocci, including gonococci and meningococci. Among gram-negative bacilli, it is active against *H. influenzae*, but there is little activity against the *Enterobacteriaceae*. It is the most active known agent against *L. pneumophilia*, more so than the macrolides (which are the drugs of choice). It is as active as vancomycin in vitro against *C. difficile*, useful against *M. tuberculosis*, and also useful against *C. pneumoniae*.

In addition to antituberculosis chemotherapy, rifampin is used for meningococcal meningitis prophylaxis of close contacts, synergistic therapy of MSSA endocarditis (this is controversial, because of questions about antagonism and a propensity to develop resistance), the staphylococcal carrier state (including MRSA), chronic staphylococcal arthritis or osteomyelitis, synergistic therapy of Legionnaire's disease, and staphylococcal prosthetic device infections. Synergistic therapy with rifampin and vancomycin is controversial for MRSA endocarditis; no data support synergistic therapy for other MRSA infections.

Rifampin is a potent inducer of hepatic microsomal enzymes. Reduced oral bioavailability and decreased serum half-life occur for a number of drugs, including barbiturates, benzodiazepines, calcium channel blockers, chloramphenicol, cyclosporine, digitalis, estrogens, fluconazole, haloperidol, histamine H_2-antagonists, metoprolol, phenytoin, prednisone, propranolol, quinidine, theophylline, and warfarin.

CYTOTOXIC ANTIBIOTICS
Metronidazole

Metronidazole is active against nearly all anaerobic pathogens, and against many protozoa that are human parasites. Metronidazole has potent bactericidal activity, including activity against *B. fragilis*, *Prevotella* sp., *Clostridium* spp. (including *C. difficile*), and anaerobic cocci, although it is ineffective in actinomycosis. Resistance remains rare and is of negligible clinical significance. Also sensitive are *Campylobacter fetus*, *Gardnerella vaginalis*, *H. pylori*, *Giardia lamblia*, *Trichomonas vaginalis*, and *E. histolytica*.

Metronidazole causes DNA damage after intracellular reduction of the nitro group of the drug. Acting as a preferential electron acceptor, it is reduced by low-redox potential electron transport proteins, decreasing the intracellular concentration of the unchanged drug and maintaining a transmembrane gradient that favors uptake of additional drug.

The drug penetrates nearly all tissues, including neural tissue, well, making it effective for deep-seated infections even against bacteria that are not multiplying rapidly. Absorption after oral or rectal administration is rapid and nearly complete. The $T_{1/2}$ of metronidazole is 8 hours, owing to an active hydroxy metabolite. Increasingly, intravenous metronidazole is administered every 8-12 hours in recognition of the active metabolite, but once-daily dosing is possible.[66] No dosage reduction is required for renal insufficiency, but the drug is dialyzed effectively and administration should be timed to follow dialysis if twice-daily dosing is used. Pharmacokinetics in patients with hepatic insufficiency suggests a dosage reduction of 50% with marked impairment.

Trimethoprim-Sulfamethoxazole (TMP-SMX)

Sulfonamides exert bacteriostatic activity by interfering with bacterial folic acid synthesis, a necessary step in DNA synthesis. Resistance is widespread, and use is limited. The addition of sulfamethoxazole to trimethoprim, that prevents the conversion of dihydrofolic acid to tetrahydrofolic acid by the action of dihydrofolate reductase (downstream from the action of sulfonamides), accentuates the bactericidal activity of trimethoprim.

The combination of TMP-SMX is active against *S. aureus, S. pyogenes, S. pneumoniae, E. coli, P. mirabilis, Salmonella* and *Shigella* spp., *Yersinia enterocolitica, S. maltophilia, L. monocytogenes,* and *Pneumocystis carinii.* Used for urinary tract infections, acute exacerbations of chronic bronchitis, and *Pneumocystis* infections, TMP-SMX is the treatment of choice for infections caused by *S. maltophilia* and outpatient treatment of skin infections caused by community-acquired MRSA (CA-MRSA).

A fixed-dose combination of TMP-SMX of 1:5 is available for parenteral administration. The standard oral formulation is 80:400 mg, but lesser and greater strength tablets are available. Oral absorption is rapid and bioavailability is nearly 100%. Tissue penetration is excellent. Ten mL of the parenteral formulation contains 160:800 mg drug. Full doses (150-300 mg TMP in 3-4 divided doses) may be given if creatinine clearance is > 30 mL/min, but the drug is not recommended when the creatinine clearance is < 15 mL/min.

ANTIBIOTIC TOXICITIES

BETA-LACTAM ALLERGY

Allergic reaction, although less common than generally believed, is the most common toxicity of β-lactam antibiotics. The incidence is approximately 7-40/1,000 treatment courses of penicillin.[67] Reactions of four distinct types are recognized, but some reactions are not easily classified. Immediate hypersensitivity reactions occur via interaction with preformed β-lactam-specific IgE antibodies bound to mast cells or circulating basophils. Cytotoxic antibody reactions occur when β-lactam-specific IgG (usually) or IgM antibodies bind to antigen-fixed red blood cells or renal interstitial cells, resulting in complement-dependent cell lysis. Complement-independent toxicity (eg, leukopenia, thrombocytopenia, hemolytic anemia, interstitial nephritis) may result from binding to neutrophil or macrophage cell membranes. Immune complex (Arthus) reactions occur when circulating antigen-antibody (IgG, IgM) complexes fix complement and lodge in various tissue sites, causing serum sicknesslike reactions and possibly drug fever. The onset of these reactions is usually 7-14 days after therapy has begun, even if drug has already been stopped. In cell-mediated hypersensitivity, β-lactam antigen-specific T-cell receptors bind the antigen, causing cytokine release and lymphocyte proliferation. Contact dermatitis is the usual manifestation. Certain reactions do not fall under these classifications, including pruritus, maculopapular reactions, erythema multiforme, erythema nodosum, photosensitivity, and exfoliative dermatitis.

The immunochemistry of penicillin reactions is well defined. Penicillin binds tissue proteins to produce multivalent hapten-protein complexes necessary for induction of immunity. The most common hapten form of penicillin *in vivo* is the penicilloyl derivative, which is called the *major determinant*. Accelerated (1- to 72-hour) and late reactions are usually in response to the major determinant. Small quantities of other *minor determinants* may be formed by metabolic activity, and induce a variable response. Anaphylactic reactions are usually in response to a minor determinant.

Parenteral therapy causes more clinical allergic reactions as a dose-dependent function. Most serious reactions occur in patients with no history of penicillin allergy, simply because a history of penicillin allergy is sought commonly, and reported by 5-20% of patients (far in excess of the true incidence). Patients with a prior reaction have a four- to six fold increased risk of another reaction compared to the general population. However, this risk decreases with time, from 80-90% skin test reactivity at 2 months to 20% reactivity at 10 years. The risk of cross-reactivity between penicillins and carbapenems and cephalosporins is 5-10%, being highest for first-generation cephalosporins.[68] There is negligible cross-reactivity to monobactams.

"RED MAN" SYNDROME

Tingling and flushing of the face, neck, or thorax may occur with parenteral vancomycin therapy, but is less common than fever, rigors, or local phlebitis. Although a hypersensitivity reaction, it is not an allergic phenomenon owing to the clear association with too-rapid infusion of the drug (which can also cause hypotension). The cause is believed to be histamine release due to local hyperosmolality. A maculopapular rash due to hypersensitivity occurs in about 5% of patients.

NEPHROTOXICITY

There is little difference among aminoglycosides in terms of potential nephrotoxicity. Aminoglycosides do not provoke inflammation, thus there are no allergic components to any manifestation of aminoglycoside toxicity. The mechanisms of clinical toxicity relate both to ischemia and toxicity to the renal proximal tubular cell (PTC).[69] Aminoglycosides cause afferent arteriolar vasoconstriction, thus ischemia is prominent. Aminoglycoside binding to the brush border membrane of PTC leads to enzymuria, excretion of calcium and magnesium, and internalization by pinocytosis. The consequence is perturbation of the phosphatidyl inositol "middle messenger" system, with membrane damage and increased excretion of membrane phospholipids. Subsequently, there is rapid perinuclear localization of drug, with disturbed protein synthesis and mitochondrial respiration. Ultimately, the injury is manifested by necrosis of the PTC, reduction of the glomerular filtration rate (GFR), and decreased creatinine clearance. Postulated mechanisms of reduced GFR include release of vasoconstrictive hormones, transepithelial back-leak of toxins, obstruction by necrotic cellular debris, or a change in glomerular fenestrae and the ultrafiltration coefficient. Injury is usually reversible. Most patients develop a nonoliguric decrease in creatinine clearance; progression to dialysis dependence is rare. Aminoglycoside nephrotoxicity is accentuated by frequent dosing, older age, sodium and volume depletion, acidemia, hypokalemia, hypomagnesemia, coexistent liver disease, and other nephrotoxins. The risk of injury is ameliorated by single-daily-dose therapy. If renal function deteriorates, it is advisable to discontinue therapy unless treatment is for a life-threatening (ie, *Pseudomonas*) infection.

Vancomycin nephrotoxicity is less common than previously believed. Multiple courses of therapy, administration of very high doses (dosage reductions are necessary in renal insufficiency), and concurrent administration of aminoglycosides are known risk factors for toxicity.

OTOTOXICITY

Aminoglycosides cause cochlear or vestibular toxicity that is usually irreversible, and may develop after the cessation of therapy.[70] Repeated exposures create cumulative risk. Most patients develop either cochlear toxicity or a vestibular lesion; rarely are both organs injured. Cochlear toxicity can be a subtle diagnosis to make, because baseline audiograms are virtually never available, and formal screening programs are seldom undertaken. Few patients complain of hearing loss, yet when sought, the incidence of cochlear toxicity may be more than 60%. Clinical hearing loss may occur in 5-15% of patients.

The outer hair cells of the basal turn of the cochlea, which detect high-frequency sound, are most susceptible to aminoglycosides. Amikacin and netilmicin are less ototoxic than gentamicin and streptomycin, and tobramycin is intermediate in toxicity. Risk factors include treatment duration, high serum drug concentrations, a large cumulative dose, concomitant ototoxic drug therapy (especially vancomycin or furosemide), hypovolemia, and renal or liver disease. There is no correlation with nephrotoxicity.

The target of vestibular toxicity is the type I hair cell of the summit of the ampullar cristae. The true incidence of vestibular toxicity is unknown (estimate, ~5%). Patients can suffer considerable injury before the onset of symptoms, owing to the compensatory contribution of visual and proprioceptive cues (symptoms may therefore be worse at night). Complaints of nausea, vomiting, and vertigo are most common, and patients may exhibit nystagmus.

Ototoxicity caused directly by vancomycin is accepted as fact, but poorly documented in the literature. Hearing loss attributed to vancomycin is better described as neurotoxicity, manifesting as auditory nerve damage, tinnitus, and loss of acuity for high-frequency tones. Synergistic injury is possible with co-administration of other ototoxic drugs, especially aminoglycosides and furosemide.

QUINOLONE TOXICITY

Quinolones are generally well tolerated. For the most part, adverse effects increase with higher doses and prolonged therapy. Gastrointestinal side effects are common (up to 13%), but mild; *C. difficile*–related disease has been reported.

Adverse central nervous system effects are also common (up to 7%). Headache and dizziness predominate, followed by insomnia and mood alteration. Hallucinations, delirium, and seizures are rare. Allergic and skin reactions occur in up to 2% of patients. Phototoxicity after exposure to ultraviolet A light (sunlight is sufficient exposure) occurs in some patients. Anaphylactoid reactions are rare. Arthropathy and tendinitis, reversible bone marrow depression, leukopenia, and hemolytic anemia have been reported. Rare but important is prolongation of the electrocardiogram QTc interval, which may precipitate the dangerous ventricular dysrhythmia torsades de pointes.[71]

AVOIDING TOXICITY: ADJUSTMENT OF ANTIBIOTIC THERAPY

HEPATIC INSUFFICIENCY

The liver metabolizes and eliminates drugs that are too lipophilic for renal excretion. The cytochromes P_{450} (a gene superfamily consisting of more than 300 different enzymes) oxidize lipophilic compounds to water-soluble products. Other enzymes convert drugs or metabolites by conjugating them with sugars, amino acids, sulfate, or acetate to facilitate biliary or renal excretion, whereas enzymes such as esterases and hydrolases act by other distinct mechanisms. Many of these functions are disrupted when liver function is impaired, especially oxidative metabolism.

Drug dosing in hepatic insufficiency is complicated by insensitivity of clinical assessments to quantify liver function, and changing metabolism as the degree of impairment fluctuates (eg, resolving cholestasis).

Changes in renal function with progressive hepatic impairment add considerable complexity. Renal blood flow is decreased in cirrhosis, and GFR is decreased in cirrhosis with ascites. Adverse drug reactions are more frequent with cirrhosis than other forms of liver disease.

The effect of liver disease on drug disposition is difficult to predict in individual patients; none of the usual tests of liver function can be used to guide dosage.[72] Generally, a dosage reduction of up to 25% of the usual dose is considered if hepatic metabolism is 40% or less and renal function is normal (Table 23-10). Greater dosage reductions (up to 50%) are advisable if the drug is administered chronically, there is a narrow therapeutic index, protein binding is significantly reduced, or the drug is excreted renally and renal function is severely impaired.

RENAL INSUFFICIENCY

Renal drug elimination depends on the GFR, tubular secretion, and reabsorption, any of which may be altered with renal dysfunction. Renal failure may

affect hepatic as well as renal drug metabolic pathways. Drugs whose hepatic metabolism is likely to be disrupted in renal failure include aztreonam, cefmetazole, cefonicid, cefotaxime, ceftizoxime, erythromycin and imipenem-cilastatin (Tables 23-11 and 23-12).

Different types of renal disease, or acute versus chronic renal failure, may result in different drug

Table 23-10 Antimicrobials Requiring Dosage Reduction in Hepatic Disease

Aztreonam
Cefoperazone
Chloramphenicol
Clindamycin
Erythromycin
Isoniazid
Metronidazole
Nafcillin
Quinupristin/dalfopristin
Rifampin
Tigecycline

Table 23-11 Antibiotic Therapy Considerations in Renal inSufficiency

■ Formula for estimation of creatinine clearance [CCr]:

$$CCr\ [mL/min] = \frac{140\text{-age} \times (1.00\ [\text{male}]\ 0.85\ [\text{female}]) \times \text{weight}\ [Kg]}{\text{Serum Cr concentration}\ [mg/dL] \times 72}$$

Dosage Reductions for Selected Antimicrobials in Renal Insufficiency

Drug (Usual Dose)	Dose for CCr 10-50 mL/min	Dose for CCr < 10 mL/min	Dialyzed?*
Aminoglycosides	Individualize	Individualize	Yes
Ampicillin (1-2 g q4h)	0.5-1 g q6h	0.5-1 g q12h	Yes
Aztreonam (1 g q8h)	0.5 g q8h	0.5 g q12h	HD only
Cefamandole (1-2 g q6h)	1-2 g q8-12h	1-2 g q8-24h	HD/CRRT
Cefazolin (1 g q8h)	1 g q12-24h	1 g q48h	HD only
Cefepime (2 g q12h)	1 g q12h	1 g q24h	Yes
Cefotaxime (1 g q 6h)	1 g q8-12h	1 g q24h	HD only
Cefotetan (1 g q12h)	1 g q24h	0.5-1g q24h	No
Cefoxitin (1-2 g q6h)	1-2 g q8-12h	1-2 g q24h	HD/CRRT
Ceftazidime (1 g q8h)	1 g q24h	1 g q48h	Yes
Ceftizoxime (1 g q8h)	1 g q12-24h	1 g q48h	HD only
Ciprofloxacin (0.4 g q8-12h)	0.4 g q8h	0.4 g q16h	No
Imipenem/cilastatin (0.5 g q6h)	0.25-0.5 g q6-8h	0.25-0.5 g q12h	HD only
Levofloxacin (0.5-0.75 g q12h)	0.5g q24h	0.5 g q248h	CRRT only
Piperacillin (2-4 g q4h)	2-4 g q6h	2-3 g q8h	HD/CRRT
Vancomycin (1 g q12h)	Individualize	Individualize	High-flux HD only

*Dialysis by hemodialysis (HD), peritoneal dialysis (PD), or continuous renal replacement therapy (CRRT)

Table 23-12 Dosing of Selected Antibiotics in Dialysis Patients	
Hemodialysis (Supplement after Dialysis)	
■ Parenteral Antibiotics	
■ Amikacin	2.5-3.75 mg/kg
■ Ampicillin	1 g
■ Azlocillin	3 g
■ Aztreonam	0.125 g
■ Cefamandole	0.5-1 g
■ Cefepime	0.5 g
■ Cefoxitin	1 g
■ Ceftazidime	1 g
■ Ceftizoxime	1-3 g
■ Cefuroxime	0.75 g
■ Chloramphenicol	1 g
■ Gentamicin	1.0-1.7 mg/kg
■ Imipenem/cilastatin	0.25-0.5 g
■ Meropenem	0.5 g
■ Mezlocillin	2-3 g
■ Netilmicin	2 mg/kg
■ Piperacillin	2 g
■ Piperacillin/tazobactam	2.25 g
■ Ticarcillin	3 g
■ Ticarcillin/clavulanic acid	3.1 g
■ Tobramycin	1.0-1.7 mg/kg
■ Trimethoprim/	5 mg/kg trimethoprim sulfamethoxazole
■ Vancomycin	0.5 g if using polysulfone dialysis membrane, otherwise no supplement

clearance rates among patients with the same GFR. Renal failure can change V_D due to fluid overload or hypoproteinemia. Antimicrobials known to have increased V_D in renal failure are aminoglycosides, azlocillin, cefazolin, cefoxitin, cefuroxime, cloxacillin and dicloxacillin, erythromycin, trimethoprim, and vancomycin. Chloramphenicol and methicillin are examples of agents with decreased V_D in renal failure.

Accurate estimates of renal function are important in patients with mild-to-moderate renal dysfunction, because the clearance of many drugs by dialysis actually makes management easier. Factors influencing drug clearance by hemofiltration include molecular size, aqueous solubility, plasma protein binding, equilibration kinetics between plasma and tissue, and the apparent V_D.[72,73] New high-flux polysulfone membranes can clear molecules up to 5 kD (the molecular weight of vancomycin is 1.486 kD) efficiently. The need to dose patients during or after a renal replacement therapy treatment must be borne in mind; during continuous renal replacement therapy, the estimated creatinine clearance is ~15 mL/min in addition to the patient's intrinsic clearance (73,74). Cefaclor, cefoperazone, ceftriaxone, chloramphenicol, clindamycin, cloxacillin and dicloxacillin, doxycycline, erythromycin, linezolid, methicillin/nafcillin/oxacillin, metronidazole, rifampin, and tigecycline do not require dosage reductions in renal failure.

REFERENCES

1. Fry DE. The importance of antibiotic pharmacokinetics in critical illness. *Am J Surg* 1996;172(Suppl): 20S-25S.

2. DiPiro JT, Edmiston CE, Bohnen JMA. Pharmacodynamics of antimicrobial therapy in surgery. *Am J Surg* 1996;171:615-622.

3. Naimi TS, LeDell KH, Como-Sabetti K, et al. Comparison of community- and health care-associated methicillin-resistant *Staphylococcus aureus* infection. *JAMA* 2004; 290:2976-2984.

4. Anstead GM, Owens AD. Recent advances in the treatment of infections due to resistant *Staphylococcus aureus*. *Curr Opin Infect Dis* 2004;17:549-555.

5. Schentag JJ, Gilliland KK, Paladino JA. What have we learned from pharmacokinetic and pharmacodynamic theories? *Clin Infect Dis* 2001; 32:S39-S46.

6. Nicolau DP, Freeman CD, Belliveau PP, et al. Experience with a once-daily aminoglycoside program administered to 2,184 adult patients. *Antimicrob Agents Chemother* 1995;39:650-655.

7. Kashuba AD, Bertino JS Jr, Nafziger AN. Dosing of aminoglycosides to rapidly attain pharmacodynamic goals and hasten therapeutic response by using individualized pharmacokinetic monitoring of patients with pneumonia caused by gram-negative organisms. *Antimicrob Agents Chemother* 1998;42:1842-1844.

8. Thomas JK, Forrest A, Bhavnani SM, et al. Pharmacodynamic evaluation of factors associated with the development of bacterial resistance in acutely ill patients during therapy. *Antimicrob Agents Chemother* 1998;42:521-527.

9. Benko AS, Cappelletty DM, Kruse JA, et al. Continuous infusion versus intermittent administration of ceftazidime in critically ill patients with suspected Gram-negative infections. *Antimicrob Agents Chemother* 1996; 40:691-695.

10. Lau WK, Mercer D, Itani KM, et al. Randomized, open-label, comparative study of piperacillin-tazobactam administered by continuous infusion versus intermittent infusion for treatment of hospitalized patients with complicated intra-abdominal infection. *Antimicrob Agents Chemother* 2006;50:3556-3561.

11. Kollef MH, Ward S, Sherman G, et al. Inadequate treatment of nosocomial infections is associated with certain empiric antibiotic choices. *Crit Care Med* 2000;28:3456-3464.

12. Alvarez-Lerma F. Modification of empiric antibiotic treatment in patients with pneumonia acquired in the intensive care unit: ICU-Acquired Pneumonia Study Group. *Intensive Care Med* 1996; 22:387-394.

13. Iregui M, Ward S, Sherman G, et al. Clinical importance of delays in the initiation of appropriate antibiotic treatment for ventilator-associated pneumonia. *Chest* 2002;122:262-268.

14. Garnacho-Montero J, Garcia-Garmendia JL, Barrero-Almodovar A, et al. Impact of adequate empirical

antibiotic therapy on the outcome of patients admitted to the intensive care unit with sepsis. *Crit Care Med* 2003; 31:2742-2751.

15. Evans RS, Pestotnik SL, Classen DC, et al. A computer-assisted management program for antibiotics and other antiinfective agents. *N Engl J Med* 1998; 338: 232-238.

16. Kollef MH, Vlasnik J, Sharpless L, et al. Scheduled rotation of antibiotic classes: A strategy to decrease the incidence of ventilator-associated pneumonia due to antibiotic-resistant gram-negative bacteria. *Am J Respir Crit Care Med* 1997;156:1040-1048.

17. Gruson D, Hilbert G, Vargas F, et al. Strategy of antibiotic rotation: Long term effect on incidence and susceptibilities of gram-negative bacilli responsible for ventilator-associated pneumonia. *Crit Care Med* 2003;31:1908-1914.

18. Raymond DP, Pelletier SJ, Crabtree TD, et al. Impact of a rotating empiric antibiotic schedule on infectious mortality in an intensive care unit. *Crit Care Med* 2001;29:1101-1108.

19. van Loon HJ, Vriens MR, Fluit AC, et al. Antibiotic rotation and development of gram-negative antibiotic resistance. *Am J Respirir Crit Care Med* 2005;171: 480-487.

20. Kollef MH. Is antibiotic cycling the answer to preventing the mergence of bacterial resistance in the intensive care unit? *Clin Infect Dis* 2006;43:S82-S88

21. Niederman MS: Appropriate use of antimicrobial agents: Challenges and strategies for improvement. *Crit Care Med* 2003; 31:608–616.

22. Kollef MH, Micek ST. Strategies to prevent antimicrobial resistance in the intensive care unit. *Crit Care Med* 2005;33:1845-1853.

23. LeDell K, Muto CA, Jarvis WR, et al. SHEA guideline for preventing nosocomial transmission of multidrug-resistant strains of *Staphylococcus aureus* and *Enterococcus*. *Infect Control Hosp Epidemiol* 2003; 24:639-641.

24. Talmor M, Hydo L, Barie PS. Relationship of systemic inflammatory response syndrome (SIRS) to organ dysfunction, length of stay, and mortality in critical surgical illness: Effect of intensive care unit resuscitation. *Arch Surg* 1999;134:81-87.

25. Barie PS, Hydo LJ. Epidemiology of multiple organ dysfunction syndrome in critical surgical illness. *Surg Infect* 2000;1:173-186.

26. Barie PS, Hydo LJ, Eachempati SR. Characteristics and consequences of fever complicating critical surgical illness. *Surg Infect* 2004;5:145-159.

27. Mosdell DM, Morris DM, Voltura A, et al. Antibiotic treatment for surgical peritonitis. *Ann Surg* 1991;214:543-549.

28. Montravers P, Gauzit R, Muller C, et al. Emergence of antibiotic-resistant bacteria in cases of peritonitis after intraabdominal surgery affects the efficacy of empirical antimicrobial therapy. *Clin Infect Dis* 1996;23:486-494.

29. Paul M, Benuri-Silbiger I, Soares-Weiser K, et al. Beta-lactam monotherapy versus beta-lactam-aminoglycoside combination therapy for sepsis in immunocompetent patients: systematic review and meta-analysis of randomized trials. *BMJ* 2004; 328(7441):668-672.

30. American Thoracic Society. Guidelines for the management of adults with hospital-acquired, ventilator-associated, and healthcare-associated pneumonia. *Am J Resp Crit Care Med* 2005; 171:388-416.

31. Bosso JA.The antimicrobial armamentarium: Evaluating current and future treatment options. *Pharmacotherapy* 2005;25:55S-62S.

32. Padmanabhan RA, Larosa SP, Tomecki KJ. What's new in antibiotics? *Dermatol Clin* 2005;23:301-312.

33. Eggimann P, Pittet D. Postoperative fungal infections. *Surg Infect* 2006;7 Suppl 2:S53-S56.

34. Pittet D, Monod M, Suter PM, et al. Candida colonization and subsequent infections in critically ill surgical patients. *Ann Surg* 1994;220:751-758.

35. Lipsett PA. Surgical critical care: fungal infections in surgical patients. *Crit Care Med* 2006;34(9 Suppl): S215-S224.

36. Gleason TG, May AK, Caparelli D, et al. Emerging evidence of selection of fluconazole-tolerant fungi in surgical intensive care units. *Arch Surg* 1997;132: 1197-1201.

37. Pappas PG, Rex JH, Sobel JD, et al. Infectious Diseases Society of America. Guidelines for treatment of candidiasis. *Clin Infect Dis* 2004;38:161-189.

38. Dellinger EP. Duration of antibiotic treatment in surgical infections of the abdomen. Undesired effects of antibiotics and future studies. *Eur J Surg* 1996;576(Suppl):29-31.

39. Chastre J, Wolff M, Fagon JY, et al. Comparison of 15 vs. 8 days of antibiotic therapy for ventilator-associated pneumonia in adults: a randomized trial. *JAMA* 2003; 290:2588-2598.

40. Bartlett JG, Perl TM. The new *Clostridium difficile*—What does it mean? *N Engl J Med* 2005;343:2503-2505.

41. Loo V, Poirier L, Miller MA, et al. A predominantly clonal multi-institutional outbreak of *Clostridium difficile*-associated diarrhea with high morbidity and mortality. *N Engl J Med* 2005;353:2442-2449.

42. McDonald LC, Kilgore GE, Thompson A, et al. An epidemic, toxin gene-variant strain of *Clostridium difficile*. *N Engl J Med* 2005;353:2433-2441.

43. Livermore DM. Bacterial resistance: origins, epidemiology, and impact. *Clin Infect Dis* 2003; 36:S11-S23.

44. Gold HS, Moellering RC. Antimicrobial drug resistance. *N Engl J Med* 1996;335:1445-1453.

45. Naiemi NA, Duim B, Savelkoul PH, et al. Widespread transfer of resistance genes between bacterial species in an intensive care unit: implications for hospital epidemiology. *J Clin Microbiol* 2005;43:4862-4864.

46. Clark NM, Hershberger E, Zervosc MJ, et al. Antimicrobial resistance among gram-positive organisms in the intensive care unit. *Curr Opin Crit Care* 2003; 9:403-412.

47. Brahmi N, Blel Y, Kouraichi N, et al. Impact of ceftazidime restriction on gram-negative bacterial resistance in an intensive care unit. *J Infect Chemother* 2006;12:190-194.

48. Livermore DM, Woodford N. The beta-lactamase threat in Enterobacteriaceae, *Pseudomonas* and *Acinetobacter*. *Trends Microbiol* 2006;14:413-420.

49. Neuhauser MM, Weinstein RA, Rydman R, et al. Antibiotic resistance among Gram-negative bacilli in

US intensive care units: Implications for fluoro-quinolone use. *JAMA* 2003; 289:885-888.

50. National Nosocomial Infections Surveillance System. National Nosocomial Infections Surveillance (NNIS) System Report, data summary from January 1992 through June 2004, issued October 2004. *Am J Infect Control* 2004;32:470-485.

51. Ferrara AM. Potentially multidrug-resistant non-fermentative gram-negative pathogens causing nosocomial pneumonia. *Int J Antimicrob Agents* 2006;27:183-195.

52. McGowan JE Jr. Resistance in nonfermenting gram-negative bacteria: multidrug resistance to the maximum. *Am J Med* 2006;119(6 Suppl 1):S29-S36.

53. Labombardi VJ, Rojtman A, Tran K. Use of cefepime for the treatment of infections caused by extended spectrum beta-lactamase-producing *Klebsiella pneumoniae* and Escherichia coli. *Diagn Microbiol Infect Dis* 2006;56:313-315.

54. Rodloff AC, Goldstein EJ, Torres A. Two decades of imipenem therapy. *J Antimicrob Chemother* 2006;58:916-929.

55. Edwards SJ, Emmas CE, Campbell HE. Systematic review comparing meropenem with imipenem plus cilastatin in the treatment of severe infections. *Curr Med Res Opin* 2005;21:785-94.

56. Zhanel GG, Johanson C, Embil JM, et al. Ertapenem: review of a new carbapenem. *Expert Rev Anti Infect Ther* 2005;31:23-39.

57. Jones RN. Microbiological features of vancomycin in the 21st century: minimum inhibitory concentration creep, bactericidal/static activity, and applied break-points to predict clinical outcomes or detect resistant strains. *Clin Infect Dis* 2005;42:S13-S24.

58. Lee SY, Fan HW, Kuti JL, Nicolau DP. Update on daptomycin: the first approved lipopeptide antibiotic. *Expert Opin Pharmacother* 2006;7:1381-1397.

59. Silverman JA, Mortin LI, Vanpraagh AD, et al. Inhibition of daptomycin by pulmonary surfactant: in vitro modeling and clinical impact. *J Infect Dis* 2005;191:2149-2152.

60. Stein GE, Craig WA. Tigecycline: a critical analysis. *Clin Infect Dis* 2006;43:518-524.

61. Wilcox MH. Update on linezolid: the first oxazolidi-none antibiotic. *Expert Opin Pharmacother* 2005;6:2315-2326.

62. Kollef MH, Rello J, Cammarata S, et al. Clinical cure and survival in gram-positive ventilator-associated pneumonia: retrospective analysis of two double-blind studies comparing linezolid with vancomycin. *Intensive Care Med* 2004;30:388-394.

63. Peppard WJ, Weigelt JA. Role of linezolid in the treatment of complicated skin and soft tissue infections. *Expert Rev Anti Infect Ther* 2006;4:357-366.

64. Nseir S, Di Pompeo C, Soubrier S, et al. First-generation fluoroquinolone use and subsequent emergence of multiple drug-resistant bacteria in the intensive care unit. *Crit Care Med* 2005;33:283-289.

65. Charbonneau P, Parienti JJ, Thibon P, et al. Fluoroquinolone use and methicillin-resistant Staphylococcus aureus isolation rates in hospitalized patients: a quasi experimental study. *Clin Infect Dis* 2006;42:778-784.

66. Sprandel KA, Drusano GL, Hecht DW, et al. Population pharmacokinetic modeling and Monte Carlo simulation of varying doses of intravenous metronidazole. *Diagn Microbiol Infect Dis* 2006;55:303-309.

67. Demoly P, Romano A. Update on beta-lactam allergy diagnosis. *Curr Allergy Asthma Rep* 2005;5:9-14.

68. Madaan A, Li JT. Cephalosporin allergy. *Immunol Allergy Clin North Am* 2004;24:463-476.

69. De Broe ME, Giuliano RA, Verpooten GA. Aminoglycoside nephrotoxicity: mechanism and prevention. *Adv Exp Med Biol* 1989;252:233-245.

70. Bates DE. Aminoglycoside ototoxicity. *Drugs Today* 2003;39:277-278.

71. Owens RC Jr, Ambrose PG. Antimicrobial safety: focus on fluoroquinolones. *Clin Infect Dis* 2005;41 Suppl 2:S144-S155.

72. Roberts JA, Lipman J. Antibacterial dosing in intensive care: pharmacokinetics, degree of disease and pharmacodynamics of sepsis. *Clin Pharmacokinet* 2006;45:755-773.

73. Pinder M, Bellomo R, Lipman J. Pharmacological principles of antibiotic prescription in the critically ill. *Anaesth Intensive Care* 2002;30:134-144.

74. Trotman RL, Williamson JC, Shoemaker DM, et al. Antibiotic dosing in critically ill adult patients receiving continuous renal replacement therapy. *Clin Infect Dis* 2005;41:1159-1166.

Chapter 24

PROPHYLAXIS

Patricia A. O'Neill, MD, Lisa S. Dresner, MD, and Robert Schulze, MD

INTRODUCTION

Management of the acute surgical patient presents multiple challenges. In addition to the primary injury or disease process, the nature, circumstances, and treatment of the primary problem puts the patient at risk for the development of secondary complications, which are themselves associated with significant morbidity and mortality.

In general, the acute surgical patient is older, has comorbid conditions, and is frequently dehydrated at the time of presentation. The severely injured trauma patient is often younger in age with less likelihood of comorbidities, but critical injuries predispose the trauma patient to acute hemorrhage, shock, and inflammatory response syndromes. Regardless of age or type of primary illness most acute surgical patients experience some degree of hypoperfusion and require varying levels of resuscitation throughout the perioperative period. Many patients are critically ill and need ventilator support with prolonged periods of bedrest and ICU stays postoperatively. The combination of hypoperfusion, resuscitation, and the need for anesthesia and surgery markedly increases the risk for secondary complications. The more serious of these complications include infection and sepsis, organ failure, venous thromboembolic (VTE) complications, and secondary gastrointestinal bleeding. Each of these complications is associated with increased morbidity and mortality, lengths of stay, and hospital costs. It is essential that the acute care surgeon become familiar with these complications and make every effort to minimize their occurrence in order to assure the best outcome for the patient.

Prophylaxis is defined as the "preventative or protective treatment against disease."[1] At present, it is not possible to completely prevent complications in this patient population but there are prophylactic measures that can be instituted to help minimize their incidence. In a very broad and general sense, prophylaxis in the perioperative setting should include the delivery of standard, evidence-based clinical care with strict attention to detail. This includes timely and appropriate management of the patient's presenting illness along with the timely reestablishment of adequate tissue perfusion through rapid and effective resuscitation. Judicial wound management, prevention of ventilator-associated pneumonia and uncompromised attention to sterile technique for vascular access all fall into this category. These basic principles of perioperative management are an essential part of minimizing complications in the acute surgical patient and should thus be followed as the first step in surgical prophylaxis.

The more common concept of prophylaxis in the perioperative setting, however, usually refers to three specific interventions for prevention; antibiotic prophylaxis, VTE prophylaxis, and gastric protection. The principles of antibiotic prophylaxis have been addressed in detail in the preceding chapter. The present chapter will now address the principles of VTE and gastrointestinal (GI) prophylaxis. Significant emphasis will be placed on measures to reduce thromboembolic complications such as deep vein thrombosis (DVT) and pulmonary embolism (PE) because they pose the greater risk to both short- and long-term morbidity and mortality. We will review the incidence, risk assessment, and current recommendations for DVT and PE prophylaxis. We will also review the incidence of secondary gastrointestinal hemorrhage in the acutely ill patient population; its pathophysiology, risk factors, and recommendations for gastric mucosal protection.

VENOUS THROMBOEMBOLISM

The pathophysiology of venous thrombosis has been fairly well-defined since Virchow first described the interrelationship between the three factors that contribute to venous thrombosis; venous stasis, vascular endothelial damage, and increased blood coagulability.[2] Despite this insight, deep vein thrombosis and pulmonary embolism continue to be a major cause of death and morbidity among hospitalized patients. In the long term, DVT may lead to postthrombotic venous insufficiency, which will negatively impact the patient's quality of life and increase long-term health costs. A review of several long-term studies, demonstrated that the incidence of postthrombotic syndrome was as high as 35% to 69% in patients studied 3 years after treatment for DVT and as high as 49% to 100% in patients studied 5 to 10 years after treatment.[3]

In the short term, the greater concern is that a deep vein thrombosis may lead to a fatal pulmonary embolism. PE is responsible for the hospitalization of more than 100,000 patients per year and contributes to death in another 100,000.[4,5] In one community-wide study conducted by 16 acute-care hospitals in Worchester, Massachusetts, PE was confirmed in 23 of 100,000 hospitalized residents per year and had an in-hospital case fatality rate of 12%.[6] More disconcerting is the fact that venous thromboembolic disease is often clinically silent. Relying on the presence of clinical signs and symptoms to prevent clinically important thromboembolic events is insensitive and unreliable.[7] Studies have shown that in patients proven at autopsy to have died from PE, the diagnosis of PE was never suspected by the treating physicians in 70% to 80% of the patients prior to death.[8,9] Moreover, the first manifestation of VTE is often sudden death or near-sudden death from PE. In one study, patients with a proven diagnosis of PE succumbed to the PE within 30 minutes of the acute event making meaningful intervention for those patients impossible.[10] Routine serial screening of all patients for the presence asymptomatic DVT by Doppler ultrasonography (DUS) has been proposed as an option to prevent fatal PE by some clinicians. However, in general, the routine use of surveillance studies for all patients has been found to be logistically difficult, not cost effective, and does not completely prevent fatal PE.[11,12,13,14,15] For these reasons, it is generally recommended that serial screening for asymptomatic DVT be reserved for patients in whom adequate prophylactic measures cannot be achieved or for patients in clinical research trials where objective documentation of DVT occurrence is essential to the safety or outcome of the study. At present, aggressive prophylaxis against VTE remains the best and most cost-effective strategy to reduce the acute and chronic sequelae of DVT and PE.

INCIDENCE

The true incidence of thromboembolic complications in the "acute surgical" population has not been specifically studied. The best that can be done is to extrapolate this incidence by review of previous studies performed in a mix of general surgical and multitrauma patients. It should be pointed out that elective general surgical patients and acute trauma patients are quite different in terms of their risk for and incidence of VTE complications. Trauma patients are generally at a much higher risk for VTE. The incidence of VTE for the emergent surgical patient will fall somewhere between these two spectrums depending on individual factors such as age, primary illness, and comorbid factors.

INCIDENCE IN GENERAL SURGICAL PATIENTS

Clagett and Reisch reviewed the overall incidence of thromboembolic complications in general surgical patients by pooling data and performing a meta-analysis of all trials of DVT prophylaxis published in the English language[16] (Table 24-1). The bulk of these studies were conducted in patients undergoing elective gastrointestinal surgery but some also included patients undergoing gynecologic, thoracic, urologic, and vascular operations. In their review, the overall incidence of DVT in surgery patients not given prophylaxis when assessed by fibrinogen uptake test (FUT) was 25%. In the studies in which a positive FUT was subsequently confirmed by venography the incidence was somewhat lower at 19%, suggesting that FUT studies may be somewhat oversensitive. The subset of surgical patients presenting with malignant disease had the highest incidence of DVT with a rate of 29%.

In this pooled data, the overall incidence of clinically recognized PE (fatal and nonfatal) was 1.6% and the rate of fatal PE was 0.8%.[16] It should be noted, however, that the incidence of PE among the control patients in these studies may have been lower than what might occur in surgical patients not given prophylaxis because the control patients in these trials underwent serial surveillance with FUT studies. Because patients were given anticoagulant therapy if serial FUT studies were positive, the incidence of PE in subjects with otherwise clinically silent DVT would likely have been higher if serial screening for DVT was not performed.

INCIDENCE IN TRAUMA PATIENTS

The literature on the incidence of thromboembolic complications in the trauma patient is more difficult to interpret as trauma patients are inherently dissimilar to each other and, trauma patients often have injuries that themselves pose additional risks for venous thrombosis. However, despite these dissimilarities, trauma patients have been shown consistently to have an extremely high rate of VTE after injury.[3,12,13,14,15]

In 1994, Geerts and colleagues sought to determine the incidence of DVT and PE in multi-injured trauma patients in a cohort of 716 patients admitted to their trauma unit.[17] In this hallmark study, prophylaxis against thromboembolism was not used. Instead patients were routinely screened by serial impedance plethysmography and lower extremity venography. Of the initial cohort of 716 patients, adequate venogram studies could be achieved in only 349 patients. Of these 349 patients, 201 (58%) developed deep-vein thrombosis of which 63 (18%) had proximal vein thrombosis. In addition, only 3 of the 201 patients with DVT (1.5%) had clinical findings suggestive of thrombosis before the diagnosis was made by venography.

Table 24-1 Venous Thromboembolism in General Surgery Patients Not Given Prophylaxis

End Point	No. of Trials	No. of Patients (with DVT / without DVT)	Incidence (%)	95% Confidence Limit
DVT (FUT)	54	1,084/4,310	25	24-26
Confirmed DVT (FUT, venogram)	20	288/1,507	19	7-21
DVT (FUT) (malignant disease)	16	159/546	29	25-33
DVT (FUT) (Europe)	37	824/2,775	30	28-31
DVT (FUT) (North America)	14	178/1,111	16	14-18
Proximal DVT	16	83/1,206	7	6-8
All PE	32	82/5,091	1.6	1.3-1.9
Fatal PE	33	48/5,547	0.9	0.7-1.1

Modified with permission from reference 16.
DVT = deep vein thrombosis, FUT = fibrinogen uptake test, PE = pulmonary embolism.

During the surveillance period, pulmonary embolism was suspected in 39 patients but conclusively ruled out in 22. Of the remaining 17 patients suspected of having PE, pulmonary embolism was confirmed in only 7 patients (0.98%). Three of which were diagnosed at autopsy. All of the remaining 10 patients suspected of having a PE had an equivocal ventilation perfusion scan. In 8 of them, DVT was present on venography and since DVT warranted treatment, subsequent pulmonary angiograms were not performed. The other 2 patients refused angiography. Thus, although the confirmed rate of PE in Geerts' study is reported as 0.98%, the true incidence of PE was likely underestimated. If these additional 10 patients were further studied and confirmed to have PE, the incidence of PE in that study could have been as high as 4.9% (17/349). Also of importance is the fact that none of the 3 patients with fatal pulmonary embolism in his study had any clinical features of VTE before their sudden deaths on days 15, 16, and 18. This further demonstrates the difficulty in clinically diagnosing DVT in this patient population and shows that serial surveillance studies for DVT will not completely prevent fatal PEs.

RISK FACTORS

There are several risk factors that have been shown to contribute to VTE. Some factors pose a greater risk than others but, more importantly, the effect of these risk factors is cumulative. The more risk factors present in any individual patient the greater the likelihood for that patient to develop thromboembolic complications.[18] In general, the risk factors for VTE can be categorized into one of the three etiologic factors described in Virchow's triad; an increase in blood coagulability, stasis of blood flow, or direct vascular endothelial damage.

Both congenital and acquired hypercoagulable states predispose to venous thrombosis. Congenital abnormalities include activated protein C resistance, antithrombin III deficiency, heparin cofactor II, and protein C and protein S deficiencies. The acquired hemostatic abnormalities include the development of lupus anticoagulant and anticardiolipin antibodies as well as myeloproliferative disorders and hyperviscosity syndromes. Patients with disorders of plasminogen, plasminogen activation, or abnormalities in the fibrinolytic system will also be at risk for venous thrombosis. It is not the general practice to screen all surgical and trauma patients for coagulation dyscrasias. However, any patient who presents with a prior history of VTE or develops new onset VTE should undergo full screening for any of these abnormalities of coagulation.

Other predisposing risk factors for thromboembolism are listed in Table 24-2 and include advanced age (clinically significant at 40 years and continues to increase with age), obesity, prior VTE, malignancy, prolonged bedrest, major surgery, congestive heart failure, varicose veins, fractures of lower extremities, estrogen treatment, stroke, multiple trauma, childbirth, and myocardial infarction.[19] In 2003 Anderson and Spencer stratified these factors into strong, moderate, and weak risks for VTE after studying 1231 consecutive patients treated for acute DVT and/or PE and calculating the odds ratio for each risk factor[19] (Table 24-3). The strongest risk factors for venous thrombotic complications included fractures to the hip or leg, hip or knee replacement, major surgery (defined as abdominal or thoracic operations that require general anesthesia lasting ≥ 30 minutes), major trauma, and spinal cord injury. Risk factors

Table 24-2 Risk Factors in Patients Treated for Acute DVT or PE	
Risk Factors	Patients (%)[a]
Age > 40 years	88.5
Obesity	37.8
History of VTE	26.0
Cancer	22.3
Bed rest > 5 days	12.0
Major surgery	11.2
Congestive heart failure	8.2
Varicose veins	5.8
Fracture (hip or leg)	3.7
Estrogen treatment	2.0
Stroke	1.8
Multiple trauma	1.1
Childbirth	1.1
Myocardial Infarction	0.7
1 or more risks	96.3
2 or more risks	76.0
3 or more risks	39.0

[a]N = 1231 consecutive patients.
Reproduced with permission from reference 19.

Table 24-3   Strong, Moderate, and Weak Risk Factors for VTE
Strong Risk Factors (odds ratio > 10)
Fracture (hip or leg)
Hip or knee replacement
Major general surgery
Spinal cord injury
Moderate Risk Factors (odds ration 2 to 9)
Arthroscopic knee surgery
Central venous catheters
Chemotherapy
Congestive heart failure or respiratory failure
Hormone replacement therapy
Malignancy
Oral contraceptive therapy
Paralytic stroke
Pregnancy / postpartum
Previous VTE
Thrombophilia
Weak Risk Factors (odds ratio < 2)
Bed rest > 3 days
Immobility due to sitting (eg, prolonged car or air travel)
Increasing age
Laproscopic surgery
Obesity
Pregnancy/antepartum
Varicose veins

Reproduced with permission from reference 19.

were categorized as moderate risk if odds ratios were calculated to be between 2-9 and weak risks if odds ratios were < 2.

Major surgery and trauma patients are at particular risk for thromboembolic complications for a number of reasons. Many are immobilized for prolonged periods of time. The administration and duration of general anesthesia increases the incidence of DVT. Studies suggest that the acute venous dilatation from general anesthesia leads to exposure of the endothelial surface which then serves as a nidus for platelet and leukocyte aggregation setting the stage for clot formation.[20] A similar mechanism may explain the high incidence of VTE in spinal injury patients since acute spinal injury also results in pronounced peripheral vasodilatation from the sudden loss of sympathetic tone. Trauma patients may have direct injuries to veins in association with bony fractures or from direct vessel puncture from penetrating trauma. The use of large bore venous access devices is also associated with thrombosis from direct venous injury.[21] Unfortunately, large bore central and femoral venous catheters may be unavoidable in the early management of the acute surgical patient.

OPTIONS FOR VTE PROPHYLAXIS

Once one appreciates the multiple risk factors for DVT and PE in the acute surgical patient, it is hard to argue against the need for an aggressive approach to prophylaxis. There are several prophylactic options available. Generally, these measures can be divided into two different categories; mechanical and pharmacologic. Like many forms of treatment, the different measures of VTE prophylaxis have different levels of efficacy and cost and some measures may be contraindicated in certain patient populations such as the use of anticoagulants in patients with head injury. Thus, to provide both safe and effective VTE prophylaxis it is essential to understand the available options and contraindications for prophylaxis and to be able to assess the degree of risk in each individual patient so that the best method of prophylaxis can be tailored for that specific patient.

MECHANICAL DEVICES

Mechanical methods for VTE prophylaxis can be further divided to include (1) simple physical measures such as early ambulation, leg elevation > 20 degrees, and leg exercises and (2) the use of mechanical devices such as elastic stocking (ES), sequential compression devices (SCDs), and venous foot pumps (VFP). In one study, the use of leg elevation and exercise coupled with early ambulation decreased the incidence of DVT by 50% (from 30% to 15%) in surgical patients ≥ 60 years of age.[22] Unfortunately, many acute surgical patients are not able to perform leg exercises or early ambulation because of the severity of their illness or injuries, but these simple techniques are both therapeutic and cost effective and should be used for any patient who is physically capable of performing them.

The application of ES, SCDs, and VFP to the lower extremities reduces venous stasis, improves venous valvular function, and, in the case of SCDs, stimulates activity of tissue plasminogen activator.[23] Unfortunately, there is limited data on the effectiveness of mechanical prophylaxis since these methods have been studied much less thoroughly than anticoagulant-based options. In addition, most studies performed to evaluate mechanical methods of prophylaxis were not blinded and thus further limit the quality of the available data for evaluation. Still, despite these limitations there is evidence to suggest that all three mechanical methods reduce the risk of DVT in patients when compared to no prophylaxis.[3,24] Similarly, there is little quality data comparing one mechanical device to another. In practice, the mechanical device chosen for prophylaxis is often determined by institutional or patient factors such as cost, patient comfort and compliance, and whether certain devices are contraindicated or not physically feasible.

It is the general consensus that mechanical methods of prophylaxis do have benefit but that they are not as efficacious as anticoagulation regimens for the prevention of DVT.[3,24] The main advantage of mechanical prophylaxis is that they provide some protection against DVT without increasing bleeding risk. Thus, they are considered an acceptable (although suboptimal) alternative in patients who are felt to be at too high a risk for bleeding with anticoagulation prophylaxis. These devices can also be used in combination with anticoagulation prophylaxis in patients at very high risk for VTE to provide added benefit.

When mechanical devices are used, extra care must be taken to assure compliance with their use. Studies have shown that when used outside of research protocols the overall compliance with the use of these devices is poor unless actively monitored.[25] There are few contraindications to the use of mechanical devices. However, it is generally recommended that SCDs be used with caution in patients with acute CHF or arterial insufficiency because the extrinsic compression will increase venous return in the former and interfere with arterial perfusion in the later. In addition, some patients have developed compartment syndromes of the lower extremity particularly patients undergoing surgical procedures in lithotomy position.[26]

UNFRACTIONATED HEPARIN

Unfractionated heparin (UH) is a heterogenous mixture of glycosaminoglycans with molecular weights that range from 4 to 30 kDaltons. Its main anticoagulation effect is mediated by the activation of antithrombin. Antithrombin inhibits thrombin, factor Xa, and other activated clotting factors. Under normal circumstances, these reactions are slow. In the presence of heparin, however, the rate of inhibition of these clotting factors is accelerated about 1000-fold.[27] Unfractionated heparin has other less significant anticoagulation effects, which include inhibition of platelets and antithrombin-independent mechanisms. Heparin has a short half-life in plasma ($t_{1/2}$ = 1.5 hours) and binds extensively to plasma proteins.

Low dose unfractionated heparin (LDUH) has been the most widely studied of all the methods of prophylaxis. The usual recommended dose for prophylaxis is 5000 units given subcutaneously 1 to 2 hours before surgery and then twice a day (BID) or three times a day (TID) until the patient is ambulating or discharged from the hospital. Its effectiveness in preventing DVT has been well established in multiple randomized clinical trials. A meta-analysis of 46 randomized clinical trials in general surgical patients comparing LDUH to no prophylaxis or placebo showed that the rate of DVT with LDUH was significantly reduced from 22% to 9% (odds ratio [OR], 0.3) (Collins et al).[28] The rate of symptomatic PE was reduced from 2.0 to 1.3% (OR, 0.5) and fatal PE from 0.8% to 0.3% (OR, 0.4).

Prophylaxis with LDUH was however associated with a small increase in the rate of bleeding events (from 3.8 to 5.9%; OR, 1.6) but most of these were considered to be minor in nature.[28] Similar findings were found in another meta-analysis in which the rate of wound hematomas was increased with LDUH (6.3% vs 4.1% in controls; OR, 1.6) but the rate of major bleeding events were not.[16] Both of these meta-analyses also concluded that the administration of LDUH threes times a day (q 8 hours) was more efficacious than twice a day (q 12 hours) and that this increased dosing was not associated with increased bleeding events. However, it should also be cautioned that these conclusions were based on indirect comparisons and there are no studies at present that have directly compared these two dose regimens.

Although heparin is considered safe, a small population of patients receiving unfractionated heparin may develop heparin induced thrombocytopenia (HIT). Type II (immune mediated) heparin induced thrombocytopenia will occur in about 1% to 5% of patients receiving heparin.[29] Of these patients, approximately 30% will develop limb or life-threatening venous or arterial thrombosis. Thus, all patients receiving heparin should have their platelet counts monitored at least every other day and heparin should be immediately stopped if there is any suspicion for the development of the HIT syndrome.

LOW-MOLECULAR-WEIGHT HEPARIN

Low-molecular-weight heparin is created by the fragmentation of the parent heparin molecule yielding chains of glycosaminoglycans with a molecular weight in the range of 5000 to 6000 Daltons. These shorter chains retain their anticoagulant activity by interacting with antithrombin but have less activity against thrombin and platelets when compared to unfractionated heparin. The shorter chains also have increased bioavailability, a longer half-life, and a lower risk of heparin-induced thrombocytopenia when compared to UH. The incidence of HIT in patients receiving LMWHs is reported to be in the range of 0% to 0.9%.[29] These properties make the anticoagulant response of LMWH more predictable than UH and, in theory, should simultaneously reduce the risk for bleeding. The increased bioavailability and longer half-life of LMWHs also allows for once a day dosing for prophylaxis.

There are currently three isoforms of LMWH available in the United States: dalteparin, enoxaparin, and tinzaparin. It is important to know that each isoform exhibits different pharmacokinetic patterns and has a different potency when normalized to the same injected dose (1000 IU antifactor Xa). For example, when normalized, the actual amount of plasma anti-Xa activity generated by enoxaparin is 2.28 times greater than that of dalteparin.[30] These differences in isoforms likely account for the differences in clinical effect and bleeding risk of LMWHs reported in clinical trials.

The use of LMWHs in general surgery patients has been evaluated extensively in recent years. One meta-analysis found that LMWH reduced the risk of both asymptomatic DVT and symptomatic VTE in general surgery patients by > 70% when compared to no prophylaxis.[31]

Other studies have compared the use of LMWH to LDUH. In their most recent analysis of the current literature on the use of LMWHs, the 7th ACCP Conference Group reviewed more than nine meta-analyses and systematic reviews comparing LMWH to LDUH. Unfortunately after their review, the consensus panel determined that when prophylaxis with LMWH in general surgical patients was directly compared to LDUH, no single study thus far showed a difference in the rates of symptomatic VTE. Some trials did show that LMWH was associated with fewer asymptomatic DVTs when compared to LDUH however the clinical significance of these findings in not yet clear.[24]

Similar to the studies of LDUH, studies performed to evaluate different dosing regimens of LMWHs in high-risk surgery patients demonstrated that higher doses of LMWHs provided greater protection against DVT than lower doses of LMWH.[25] Thus, both LDUH and LMWH appear to be more effective when given at the higher dosing regimens.

In regards to bleeding, some studies reported significantly fewer wound hematomas and other bleeding complications with LMWH than with LDUH while other studies demonstrated the opposite effect.[24] The differences in reported bleeding complications between studies may be attributed, in part, to the differences in the isoform of LMWH (eg, different anti-Xa activities) or different dosing regimens between studies. Two meta-analyses found similar efficacy for LDUH and LMWH but described differences in bleeding rates that were dependent on the dose of LMWH used. Lower doses of LMWH were associated with less bleeding than with LDUH ((3.8% vs 5.4%) respectively, OR, 0.7),

whereas higher doses resulted in more bleeding events (7.9% vs 5.3%, OR, 1.5).[24] Thus at present, based on the current available data, it is generally agreed that for prophylaxis in general surgical patients, the standard doses of LDUH and LMWHs have similar efficacy and bleeding rates. Additional studies are needed to determine the safety and efficacy of higher dosing regimens and the different isoforms of LMWH.

There are some clinical advantages of LMWH over LDUH, which include its once-a-day dosing regimen and its lower risk for heparin-induced thrombocytopenia. However, LMWHs are also significantly more costly than LDUH and, as mentioned, may be a higher bleeding risk if higher dosing regimens are used.

Unlike in the general surgical patient, there is evidence to suggest that LDUH is not as effective in preventing VTE in the high-risk multitrauma patient.[30,31] A recent meta-analysis of studies of prophylaxis performed in multi-injured trauma patients demonstrated that LDUH was no more effective than no prophylaxis in this high-risk patient population (OR, 0.97; CI, 0.35 to 2.64).[32] In one double-blind randomized clinical trial, LMWH was shown to be superior to LDUH in 344 major trauma patients.[11] The overall rate of major bleeding in that study was < 2% with no reported difference in bleeding rates between the two treatment groups. However, it should be pointed out that that study excluded all patients with intracranial bleeding or uncontrolled bleeding at other sites of injury. In addition, anticoagulant prophylaxis was not administered for up to 36 hours after injury making definitive conclusions about bleeding risks in the early postinjury period impossible.

At present, LMWH is considered to be the most effective form of prophylaxis against VTE in high-risk multitrauma patients. However, due to its high cost and the fact that potential risks for bleeding with LMWH in trauma patients has not been conclusively determined, the use of LMWH has not uniformly replaced LDUH in clinical practice. Many institutional protocols for VTE prophylaxis still provide the option for LMWH or LDUH. Until additional studies are performed to clarify this safety issue, the surgeon will need to follow his own judgment or institutional policy in choosing LMWH over LDUH prophylaxis in trauma patients.

PROPHYLACTIC VENA CAVAL FILTERS

Traditionally, vena caval filters (VCFs) have been used to prevent pulmonary embolism in patients with a known DVT in whom anticoagulation therapy has either failed or is contraindicated. Its effectiveness to prevent PE is well established. There are now many trauma centers who advocate the use of VCFs as a form of prophylaxis against PE in high-risk trauma patients since studies have shown that the use of standard prophylactic methods can not always be accomplished. In addition, when standard mechanisms of prophylaxis are given there is still a significant failure rate in protecting against VTE in high-risk trauma patients.[14,15] Studies have also shown that 35% of high-risk trauma patients cannot have SCDs applied and 14% cannot receive anticoagulation because of their injuries.[11,33] Other studies have shown that DVT and PE have occurred in up to 10% of multitrauma patients when given adequate prophylaxis.[15] For these reasons, many trauma surgeons (including the present authors) are presently placing VCFs in high-risk trauma patients regardless of their ability to use other methods of prophylaxis. These high risk groups are usually defined as patients with (1) spinal cord injury and deficits, (2) pelvic fracture and/or long bone fractures requiring immobilization, or (3) significant head injury with prolonged immobilization.

We should note, however, that there are no randomized prospective studies in the literature evaluating the prophylactic use of VCFs in trauma patients with and without the use of other methods of prophylaxis. But there is data to show that the use of prophylactic VCF filters is effective, safe, and durable. In two long-term follow-up studies in trauma patients in which vena caval filters were placed for prophylaxis against PE, no patient in either study developed a PE during or after hospitalization. The complication rates related to filter placement in both studies were very low and there were no specific long-term complications identified specific to the presence of the filters. Patients with vena caval filters should still receive other forms of prophylaxis if able. In the long-term study by Patton and colleagues, approximately 35% of the patients with VCFs had postphlebitic complications when studied several years after filter placement.[33] This study confirms the effectiveness of filters to prevent acute and long-term PE but also reiterates that vena caval filters themselves do nothing to prevent DVT formation and its subsequent long-term sequelae.

Filters are also not completely infallible. Recurrent PE has been reported in 3% of trauma patients. In addition, rare cases of filter migration and vascular injury at the time of insertion have been reported as well as untoward mechanical complications during procedures for placement of central venous catheters such as trapping of guide-wires within the indwelling filter.

RISK STRATIFICATION AND RECOMMENDATIONS FOR PROPHYLAXIS

There are two general approaches to determining prophylaxis strategies. One approach is to assess the specific VTE risk in individual patients by determining all of a patient's predisposing risk factors including the risks imposed by their current illness, surgery, and other invasive procedures. The prophylactic regimen is then prescribed based on the patient's cumulative risk estimate. The risk estimate will fall somewhere along a continuous point scale. Risk assessment models have

been created to assist with these calculations.[34] However, these models are generally cumbersome to use, have not yet been validated, and have poor physician compliance when applied to the clinical setting.

A more common approach is to use a simplified version of this model. This strategy assigns a weighted point scale for each risk factor present in the individual patient and the assigned points are then calculated into a risk score. Unlike the previous models where prophylactic measures are recommended based on a continuous point scale, the cumulative score calculated in this model is used instead to assign patients into low-, moderate-, and high-risk groups. Prophylactic regimens are then recommended based on the group (category of risk) that the patient falls into. This method simplifies the process, is associated with better compliance among clinicians, and provides an easier way to statistically evaluate the effectiveness of the prophylaxis recommendations for future reassessment.

Using this approach, Geerts and colleagues developed a classification system for general surgical patients in 2001.[35] This model assigned surgical patients into one of four VTE risk levels based on the type of operation (minor or major), age (< 40 years, 40 to 60 years, and > 60 years), and the presence of additional risk factors (malignancy, prior DVT). These classifications were derived using prospective study data. With that data, the authors were also able to provide both an estimate of VTE risk as well as recommendations for prophylaxis for each group. The four categories of patients, their relative VTE risk and recommendations for prophylaxis are outlined in Table 24-4. These recommendations formed the foundation for most prophylactic strategies subsequently developed for use in surgical patients.

In 2004, these original recommendations for prophylaxis for general surgical patients were reassessed at the 7th ACCP Conference on Antithrombotic and Thrombolytic Therapy. After reviewing additional studies published in the literature, the members of the 7th AACP Conference modified these recommendations and placed a stronger emphasis on pharmacologic prophylaxis in the moderate- and high-risk patients. More specifically, the previous recommendations offered the option of using *either* anticoagulation *or* sequential compression devices in moderate- and high-risk general surgical patients. The most current recommendation for prophylaxis in moderate- and high-risk surgical groups is to use LDUH (5000 units bid) or LMWH (≤ 3400 units once daily) (Fig. 24-1).

Unfortunately, the recommendations for the multitrauma patient are not so clearly defined. The 7th AACP Consensus Group did provide recommendations for VTE prophylaxis for the multitrauma patient. However, due to the still unresolved questions regarding the potential for bleeding in trauma patients and the limited ability to stratify trauma

Table 24-4   Stratification of VTE Risk in Surgical Patients without Prophylaxis

Level of Risk	% DVT		% PE		Successful Prevention Strategies
	Calf	Proximal	Clinical	Fatal	

Low Risk
  Minor surgery in patients < 40 yrs
  With no additional risk factors
	2	0.4	0.2	<0.01	No specific prophylaxis; Early and aggressive mobilization

Moderate Risk
  Minor surgery in patients with
  Additional risk factors
	10-20	2-4	1-2	0.1-0.4	LDUH (q12h), LMWH (<3,400 U daily), ES, or SCD[a]

Surgery in patients aged 40-60 yr With no additional risk factors					

High Risk
  Surgery in patients >60 yr, or age
  With additional risk factors
	20-40	4-8	2-4	0.4-1.0	LDUH (q8h), LMWH (>3,400 U daily), or SCD[*]

Highest Risk
  Surgery in patients with multiple
  Factors
  Hip or knee arthroplasty, HFS
  Major trauma, SCI
	40-80	10-20	4-10	0.2- 5	LMWH (>3,400 U daily)[a] fondaparinux, oral VKAs (INR 2-3), or SCD/ES + LDUH/LMWH

Modified with permission from reference 35.

[*] Note: These recommendations for moderate and high risk patients were later modified by the 7th ACCP Conference on Antithrombotic and Thrombolytic Therapy (see Fig. 23-1).

LDUH = low dose unfractionated heparin, LMWH = low molecular weight heparin, SCD = sequential compression devices, VKA = vitamin K antagonists, INR = international normalized ratio, ES = elastic stockings, HFS = hip fracture surgery, SCI = spinal cord injury.

patients into low-, moderate-, and high-risk groups these recommendations are not very precise. The recommendations given for prophylaxis in trauma patients are by the 7th ACCP Consensus Group are listed in Table 24-5.

A somewhat more definitive strategy for VTE prevention in multitrauma patients was first developed by Greenfield and coauthors in 1997.[14] The authors, a group of experienced trauma, vascular, and orthopedic surgeons, created an assessment tool known as the risk assessment profile for thromboembolism (RAPT) score. The purpose of the RAPT score (also referred to as the RAP score) was to help identify trauma patients at high risk for VTE. It was devised using risk factors known to be associated with VTE in trauma patients. The risk factors were weighted by the panel based on their own

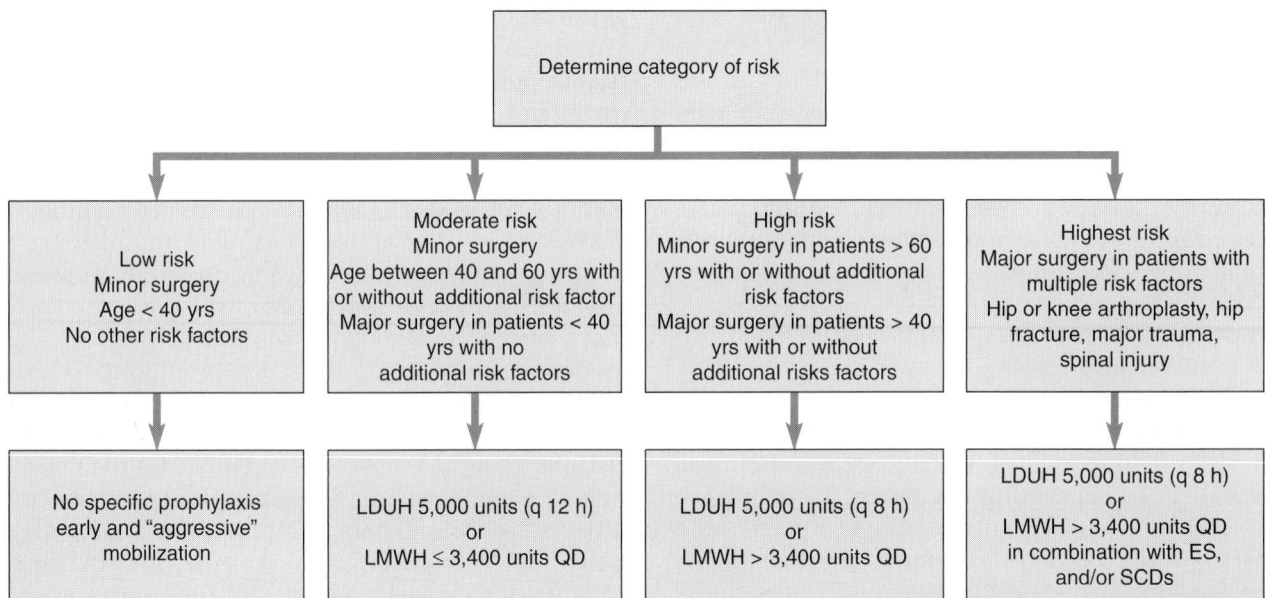

Figure 24-1   *Algorithm showing most current recommendations for venothromboembolism prophylaxis in general surgical patients according to risk classification.*

Table 24-5   Recommendations for VTE Prophylaxis in Multitrauma Patients by the 7th ACCP Consensus Group

1. All trauma patients with at least one risk factor should receive VTE prophylaxis.

2. In the absence of a major contraindication, it is recommended that clinicians administer LMWH prophylaxis as soon as it is considered safe to start.

3. Mechanical prophylaxis with SCDs, or possibly ESs alone, should be used if LMWH prophylaxis is delayed or contraindicated because of bleeding risk.

4. Doppler Ultrasound screening should be performed in patients at high risk for DVT who have received suboptimal or no prophylaxis.

experience and that cited in the literature (Table 24-6). A RAPT score of 5 or more, which required a minimum of two risk factors, was used to define the high-risk group.

The authors then evaluated the ability of the score to successfully define the high risk group in a small prospective series of trauma patients. A RAPT score was calculated for each patient at the time of admission. The patients with a RAPT score ≥ 5 were given some form of prophylaxis then followed for VTE complications. Patients with RAPT < 5 were not given prophylaxis

Table 24-6   Risk Factors and Points Allotted to Calculate the Risk Assessment Profile (RAP) Score

	Points
Underlying Condition	
Obesity	2
Malignancy	2
Abnormal coagulation	2
History of thromboembolism	3
Iatrogenic Factors	
Femoral venous line	2
Transfusion, >4 units	2
Operation, >2 h	2
Major venous repair	3
Injury-related factors	
Chest AIS, >2	2
Abdomen AIS, >2	2
Head AIS, >2	2
Spinal fractures	3
Glascow Coma Score, <8	3
Severe lower extremity fracture	4
Pelvic fracture	4
Spinal cord injury	4
Age (y)	
≥ 40, < 60	2
≥ 60, < 75	3
≥ 75	4

Borrowed with permission from reference 14.
Low risk = RAPT score < 5, high risk = RAPT score ≥ 5.

and were not followed for VTE in this study. The authors identified 53 patients with a RAPT score ≥ 5. Of these, 23 patients (43%) developed DVT despite some form of prophylaxis. In 17 cases, the DVT was in a proximal vein (65%) and in nine cases in a distal vein (35%). Twenty-two percent (22%) of patients had thrombus in both proximal and distal veins. Thus, the RAPT score of ≥ 5 was successful in defining the trauma patients at high risk for VTE. However, there was no correlation between the magnitude of the RAPT score and the likelihood to development of DVT. Thus, the score was successful in identifying patients at high risk to develop VTE, but it could not further stratify patients within the high-risk group or, predict the likelihood of VTE complications for that patient.

In the year 2000, Gearhart and colleagues attempted to validate the RAPT score and prophylaxis regimen in a prospective study of 184 trauma patients.[15] These authors also successfully demonstrated the ability of the RAPT to separate trauma patients into low-risk (RAPT score < 5) and high-risk (RAPT score ≥ 5) groups.[15] In Gearhart's study the high-risk group received both pharmacologic and mechanical prophylaxis where feasible. All but two high-risk patients received anticoagulation therapy. When anticoagulation was given, either unfractionated heparin (5000 units subcutaneously every 12 hours) or enoxaparin (30 mg subcutaneously every 12 hours) was prescribed based on the choice of the treating trauma surgeon. Compression devices included below-the-knee sequential compression devices or arteriovenous foot pumps for those patients that could not wear SCDs. Surveillance Doppler duplex scans were performed during the first 7 days of admission and then each week during hospitalization on all study participants. Low-risk patients did not receive any prophylaxis but did undergo serial duplex scanning. There were 160 participants who completed all phases of the study; 58 patients (36.3%) were categorized as low risk by the RAPT score and 102 patients (63.8%) were categorized as high risk.

Of significance, none of the low-risk patients in Gearhart's study developed a DVT. However, 11 of the high-risk patients (10.8%) still developed DVT despite combined pharmacologic and mechanical prophylaxis. Seven of the 11 patients who developed DVT (64%) were asymptomatic and were diagnosed by serial duplex scan. Thus, Gearhart's study reconfirmed that the RAP score is an effective tool to separate trauma patients into low-risk and high-risk groups. The greatest benefit of the RAPT score appears to be its ability to direct the clinician in identifying the low-risk patient in whom DVT prophylaxis can be withheld. Withholding prophylaxis in this low-risk group has been shown to calculate into a significant cost savings for the institution without increasing VTE complications.[15]

Although still not perfect, the authors believe that the RAPT score and the prophylaxis strategy followed by Greenfield, Gearhart, and their colleagues (Fig. 24-2) provides the most practical and evidence-based algorithm for DVT prophylaxis in trauma patients at the present time. However, because 10% of high-risk trauma patients still developed DVT despite combined pharmacologic and mechanical prophylaxis, an aggressive VTE prophylaxis strategy may need to include the use of surveillance duplex scanning or the insertion of a prophylactic VCF in this high-risk group. VCF placement has the advantage of eliminating the need for serial duplex scanning while simultaneously reducing the risk for fatal PE.

In summary, VTE prophylaxis in the general surgical patient is presently well-defined and when followed has been shown to reduce the rate of DVT and PE with reasonable success. The multitrauma patient, however, is a different entity. The calculation of a RAPT score will help the surgeon determine which trauma patients are at low risk for VTE and do not need prophylaxis. Aggressive prophylaxis strategies should be followed for high-risk patients and should include combination therapies if not otherwise contraindicated. Of the pharmacologic agents available, the LMWHs are probably more efficacious but unresolved questions regarding its bleeding risk in trauma patients have prevented the uniform replacement of LDUH by LMWH in current prophylaxis recommendations. Most important, it is clear that current options for VTE prophylaxis are still suboptimal for preventing DVT and PE in the high risk trauma patient and alternative prophylaxis regimens and strategies need to be studied. It is likely that there are other factors not yet identified that contribute to the high risk of VTE in the trauma patient and are resistant to present modes of prophylaxis.

GASTROINTESTINAL BLEEDING

It is well known that critical illness can be complicated by upper gastrointestinal hemorrhage. Because many acute surgical patients are often critically ill or injured it is important to review the pathophysiology, risk factors, and potential prophylactic methods available to prevent upper GI bleeding for this patient population.

Curling first described acute duodenal ulcers in patients after burn injury as early as 1842. Harvey Cushing later described the association between CNS injury and gastoduodenal ulcers in 1932. Subsequently, numerous terms have been used to describe the stress related gastric mucosal damage (SRMD) seen in critically ill and injured patients over the years. These include "stress gastritis," "stress ulcerations," and "erosive gastritis."

Bleeding from SRMD may range from occult (guiac positive gastric aspirate or stool) to clinically significant bleeding. Clinically significant bleeding is generally defined as overt bleeding (coffee grounds or blood in nasogastric tube) accompanied by one of the following: a spontaneous drop in blood pressure > 20 mm Hg,

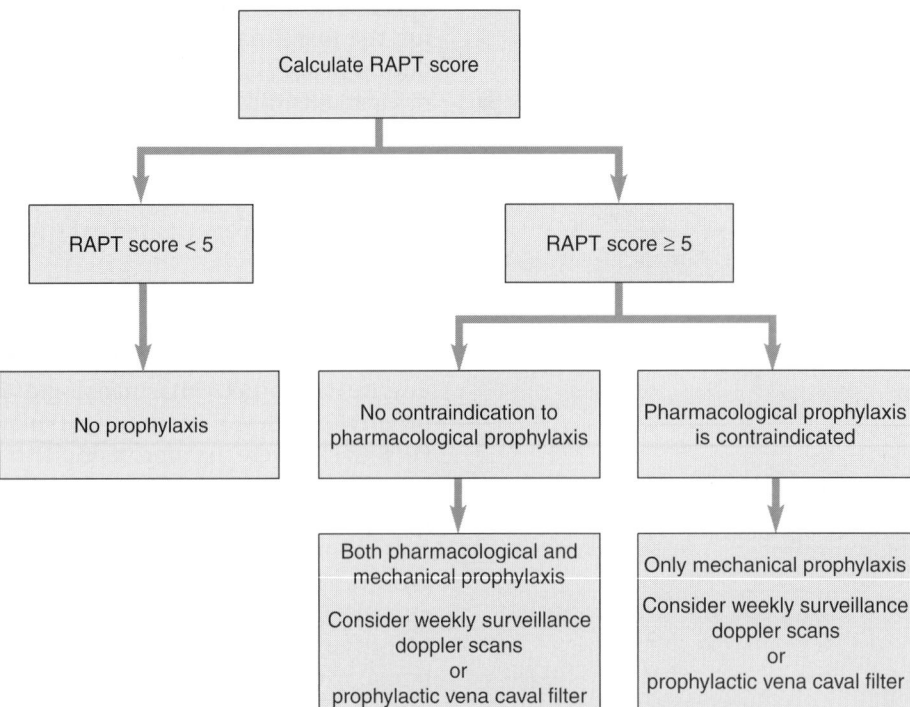

Figure 24-2 *Algorithm to determine venothromboemolism prophylaxis in multitrauma patients based on the RAPT score and ability to use anticoagulants. Modified with permission from reference 14.*

a decrease in hemoglobin of 2 g/dL or, the failure to increase hemoglobin after transfusion.[36] Similarly, endoscopic findings of SRMD may range from sporadic subepithelial petechia to superficial discrete erosions in the gastric mucosa. Microscopic findings demonstrate disruption of the epithelium, coagulation necrosis and intramucosal hemorrhage. Perforation is uncommon in SRMD and when bleeding is present it is usually diffuse and from the superficial gastric vessels. The diffuse nature of this bleeding makes it poorly responsive to usual endoscopic therapies.

INCIDENCE

Nearly all patients with acute critical illness develop some degree of SRMD and will therefore be at risk for complications of mucosal bleeding. The actual incidence of bleeding complications however depends on how one defines bleeding. Approximately 75%-100% of all critically ill patients will show some degree of erosive gastritis as early as 24 hours after admission to the Intensive Care Unit (ICU). In 1994, Maier demonstrated that 99% of critically injured patients had guiac positive nasogastic aspirates when tested.[37] The incidence of clinically significant bleeding, however, is lower. Clinically significant gastric bleeding has been shown to occur in 1.5% of all critically ill patients but was as high as 4% in the ICU patients who were mechanically ventilated for more than 48 hours.[38] In one study, clinically significant UGI hemorrhage was associated with significantly longer ICU stays and a fourfold increase in mortality.[39] Thus, although the incidence of clinically significant gastric bleeding is not that high, the increase in morbidity and mortality associated with it when it does occur supports prophylactic strategies to try to prevent it occurrence. Some form of GI prophylaxis is now recommended in the management of critically ill patients by both the Institute for healthcare improvement[40] and the "surviving sepsis campaign."[41]

PATHOPHYSIOLOGY

Although "stress gastritis" was once thought to result from excessive gastric acid production during states of high physiologic stress, this is no longer the case. There is good evidence that SRMD is actually caused by the hypoperfusion of the upper GI tract during these high-stress states. Under normal circumstances healthy gastric mucosa will maintain its integrity despite constant exposure to very low gastric pH. But, even with a neutralized stomach, systemic or splanchnic ischemia and reperfusion have resulted in mucosal injury and ulceration. Low-grade mucosal ischemia is known to occur in sepsis and multiple system organ failure as a result of changes in blood volume the redistribution of blood flow away from the splanchnic bed. In one human study, Spirt demonstrated that septic patients had a 50%-60% decrease in upper GI blood flow when compared to controls.[36] Thus, aggressive resuscitation

and timely correction of underlying disease processes are important factors in limiting the development and severity of SRMD in critical patients.

Although gastric acid secretion is no longer felt to be the primary cause of SRMD in critical patients, gastric acid probably does contribute, at least in part, to the development of SRMD. The macroscopic ulcerations seen in SRMD are usually found in the gastric fundus where acid is produced and not in the antrum or duodenal bulb as is typically seen in peptic ulcer disease. It is felt that episodes of mucosal ischemia or underperfusion lead to a disruption in the normal cellular defense mechanisms of the gastric mucosa, which then leaves the mucosa more susceptible to acid erosion.

Although *Helicobacter pylori* (*H. pylori*) is known to be a causative agent in the pathogenesis of chronic gastritis and peptic ulcer disease, it may play only a limited role in pathogenesis of SRMD.[37] In one study, less than half of all patients with clinically occult gastric bleeding were seropositive for *H. pylori*. By contrast, nearly all of the patients who developed clinically significant gastric hemorrhage in that study were *H. pylori* positive.[42] This data suggests that patients with *H. pylori* associated gastritis may be at increased risk for mucosal injury when subjected to an acute stress. It also suggests that ICU patients with existing *H. pylori* infection will have a higher degree of mucosal injury if it occurs and thus a greater likelihood to develop clinically significant bleeding.

RISK FACTORS

Risk factors for developing clinically significant bleeding from SRMD include the patient's underlying disease process and the therapeutic interventions required during the patient's management (Table 24-7). In 1994 Cook and colleagues[38] followed more than

Table 24-7   Risk Factors Associated with Stress-Related Mucosal Damage in Critically Ill Patients
Risk factors
Coagulopathy
Mechanical ventilation > 48 hours
Respiratory failure
Burns
Major trauma
Extraabdominal sepsis
Peritonitis
Jaundice
Established liver failure
Established renal failure
Hypotension

2200 patients (most were cardiovascular surgery patients) admitted to the intensive care unit. Patients with a history of peptic ulcer disease, head trauma, and multitrauma were excluded from study but all other patients were observed without giving any form of gastric prophylaxis. Cook's study identified two independent risk factors for subsequent development of clinically significant bleeding; the need for more than 48 hours of mechanical ventilation (odds ratio 15.6) and the presence of coagulopathy (odds ratio 4.3). Among patients with both risk factors, 4% developed clinically significant bleeding, whereas only 0.1% of patients with neither risk factor developed bleeding. Other risk factors for bleeding identified include extra-abdominal sepsis, peritonitis, jaundice, preexisting liver and renal failure, burns, hypotension, and major trauma.[43]

Of note, the incidence of stress gastritis in critically ill and injured patients has decreased dramatically in the past decade as clinicians achieved a better understanding of its pathophysiology. Its prevalence is currently thought to be in the range of 1.5%-6% of critically ill patients.[44] The decline is attributed to improvements in resuscitation and monitoring, a better understanding of the hemodynamic support of the critically ill patient, and the liberal use of agents to raise intraluminal gastric pH.

Thus, an effective strategy to prevent stress-related bleeding in the ICU actually requires a three prong approach; rapid and effective resuscitation, preventing or minimizing episodes of gastric mucosal ischemia, and protecting the gastric mucosa from gastric acid injury by either increasing mucosal barriers or by decreasing gastric acid production. There is good evidence that pharmaceutical agents that either help to protect the mucosal barrier from the effects of gastric acid or those that reduce the production of gastric acid help to reduce the incidence of UGI bleeding. Pharmaceutical agents that help to protect the mucosal barrier include antacids and sucralfate and agents that reduce acid production include H_2 receptor antagonists (H_2RAs) and proton pump inhibitors (PPIs).

OPTIONS FOR PROPHYLAXIS

Antacids

Antacids work by either buffering or neutralizing gastric acid and by inactivating the proteolytic activity of pepsin. With frequent dosing and diligent monitoring, antacids can achieve a reliable increase in gastric ph > 3.5. Antacids are effective in decreasing the rate of stress-related bleeding when compared to placebo. However, in one study, mortality was higher in patients receiving frequent antacid dosing via the nasogastric tube. This data suggests that the increase in gastric volume from frequent nasogastric dosing may increase the rate of aspiration with resulting complications. Of note, antacids contain aluminum and magnesium and thus should be used with caution in patients with renal dysfunction as they may result in toxicity.[45]

Sucralfate

Sucralfate is an aluminum hydroxide-sucrose compound. When taken orally, it coats the gastric mucosa and forms a protective layer between the mucosa and the acid in the gastric lumen. Sucralfate also appears to trigger prostaglandin E_2 release, which provides an additional cytoprotective effect. Sucralfate has been shown to be better than placebo at protecting the gastric mucosa and was equal in efficacy to administered antacids. One meta-analysis comparing sucralfate to H_2RAs found sucralfate to be at least as effective as these agents. Because sucralfate is not systemically absorbed but coats the gastric mucosa, it may decrease the absorption of orally administered H_2RAs if these agents are given simultaneously. Like antacids, sulcralfate contains aluminum hydroxide and also been associated with toxicity in patients with renal failure.[45,46,47]

Histamine 2 Receptor Antagonists

The use of H_2RAs is currently the standard of care for the prevention of stress ulcer bleeding in the ICU. There are a number of studies and metaanalysis[44,48] suggesting that H_2RA administration is associated with a lower rate of clinically important bleeding when compared to antacids and sucralfate. Of note, cimetidine is the least potent of all the H_2 receptor blockers but it is the only H_2RA with FDA approval for the prevention of UGI bleeding. However, the use of cimetidine is associated with several potential side effects including thrombocytopenia, CNS manifestations, and interactions with the cytochome p450 metabolizing enzymes. Interference with the cytochrome p450 system by the H_2RAs increases the potential for multiple drug interactions with their use and as such, its use in the ICU may be problematic. In addition, prolonged administration of H_2RAs over time may result in drug tolerance and thus limit their effectiveness.

Cimetadine can be administered by either continuous IV infusion or intermittent IV bolus. Although continuous infusion is better at maintaining a gastric ph > 4, there are no studies to date that compare the safety, efficacy, prevention, or healing rates between the two methods of administration. Because it is thought that some of the drug-related side effects are associated with high serum concentrations, clinicians often prefer continuous infusions over intermittent bolus administration to avoid the spikes in serum concentration. Oral administration is an option for patients with functioning GI tracts.[44]

Proton Pump Inhibitors

Proton pump inhibitors are the most potent antisecretory agents available. They block the final pathway for acid secretion by irreversibly inhibiting the proton pump H^+K^+ ATPase found on the secretory surface of the gastric parietal cells. PPIs elevate and maintain gastric ph > 6. Whereas H_2 receptor blockers are the most widely used agents in stress ulcer prophylaxis, PPIs have replaced H_2 receptor blockers in the treatment of many other acid related conditions. Few clinical trials as yet have investigated the use of PPIs in the prophylaxis of stress ulceration in critically ill patients.[46] PPIs are more expensive than the H_2RA agents but PPIs have the advantage that they achieve a more rapid and sustained increase in gastric pH and they are not associated with tachyphylaxis.[9] PPIs are generally well tolerated and appear to be more effective than H_2 receptor blockers in the treatment of patients with peptic ulcer disease, gastroesophageal reflux, and Zollinger-Ellison syndrome. PPIs have few side effects and few drug interactions. In the past, the lack of an intravenous formulation and difficulties with oral administration had limited the use of PPIs in critically ill surgical patients. However, Pantoprazole is now available in intravenous form here in the United States. The IV form is equipotent to the oral form in suppressing acid secretions and does not require dose adjustment in patients with organ failure. Inhibition of acid secretion is dose dependent and 80 mg/day seems to suppress acid secretion by 90%.[46]

Enteral feeding is also used as a preventative strategy for SRMD although its efficacy has not been well studied. Early enteral nutrition appears to be effective in preventing gastric ulcerations in severely burned patients. Because enteral feedings are known to increase GI mucosal blood flow it is believed that its administration acts more to prevent mucosal ischemia rather than by neutralizing gastric pH.[44]

It has been suggested by some that the absence of improvement in survival with SRMD prophylaxis may be due to an increased rate of nosocomial pneumonia in ventilated patients. In a meta-analysis comparing ranitidine to sucralfate, the incidence of nosocomial pneumonia was increased in patients treated with ranitidine when compared to sucralfate.[45,46] In a more recent, well-powered, prospective randomized trial comparing treatments for GI prophylaxis and assessing the subsequent nosocomial pneumonia rate, the study found that ranitidine was somewhat more effective than sucralfate in preventing clinically significant GI hemorrhage (1.7% vs 3.8%) but was not associated with an increased risk of nosocomial pneumonia.[45] In practice, the risk of ventilator associated pneumonia can be reduced through the adoption of a number of fundamental measures including elevation of the head 30 degrees, oral care, and good hand washing practices.[40]

In summary, stress-related mucosal damage is an erosive gastritis that occurs rapidly after severe physiologic insults such as major trauma, surgery, sepsis and burns. It is present in 75%-100% of patients studied 24 hours after admission to an intensive care unit. Clinically important bleeding is less common, but appears to occur in about 3.5%-4% of patients who are mechanically ventilated for longer than 48 hours. Best prevention of SRMD is by improving mucosal perfusion with aggressive treatment of underlying disease. Removal of mucosal irritants such as gastric acid is important to prevent progression of disease once it occurs. Although it is clear that prophylactic strategies reduce the incidence of significant bleeding, its actual impact on survival is small. At present, there is no consensus regarding optimal GI prophylaxis and no single strategy of stress ulcer prophylaxis is preferred when mortality is used as the outcome.[48]

In general, however, H_2RAs and PPIs appear to provide better protection than antacids and sucralfate. There is also limited, but good data, to show that in high-risk patients PPIs perform better than H_2 receptor blockers. PPIs achieve the highest suppression of gastric acid secretion and have a lower incidence of adverse effects and drug interactions. The high cost and limited availability of intravenous forms of PPIs, however, have limited its use in patients with nonfunctional GI tracts. One commonly used and cost-effective strategy is to use H_2RAs as the first line of GI prophylaxis in ICU patients but switch to the intravenous PPI if the patient develops an episode of clinically significant bleeding.

REFERENCES

1. The English Institute of America. *The Living Webster Encyclopedic Dictionary of the English Language.* 1st ed. Winnipeg: North American Educational Guild, Ltd.; 1971.
2. Virchow R. Neuer Jall von todlicher emboli der lungenarteric. *Arch Pathol Anat* 1956;10:225-228.
3. Nicolaides AN, Bergqvist D, Hull R, et al. Prevention of venous thromboembolism. International Consensus Statement. *International Angiology* 1997;16(1):3-38.
4. Dalen JE, Alpert JS. Natural history of pulmonary embolism. *Prog Cardiovasc Dis* 1975;17:257-270.
5. Alpert JS, Dalen JE. Epidemiology and natural history of venous thromboembolism. *Prog Cardiovasc Dis* 1994;36:417-422.
6. Anderson FA, Wheeler HB, Goldberg RJ, et al. A population-based perspective of the hospital incidence of case fatality rates of deep vein thrombosis and pulmonary embolism. *Arch Intern Med* 1991;151;93:3-38.
7. Hirch J, Hull RD (eds.). Diagnosis of venous thrombosis, *Venous Thromboembolism: Natural History, Diagnosis, and Management.* Florida; FL: CRC Press; 1987:23.

8. Goldhaber SZ, Hennekens CH, Evans DA, et al. factors associated with correct antemortem diagnosis of major pulmonary embolism. *Am J Med* 1982;73:822-826.
9. Rubenstein I, Murray D, Hoffstein V. Fatal pulmonary embolism in hospitalized patients. *Arch Intern Med* 1988;148:1425-1426.
10. Hull RD, Hirsh J, Sackett DL, et al. Cost effectiveness of primary and secondary prevention of fatal pulmonary embolism in high-risk surgical patients. *Can Med Assoc J* 1982;127:990-95.
11. Geerts WH, Jay RM, Code KI, et al. A comparison of low-dose heparin with low molecular weight heparin as prophylaxis against venous thromboembolism after major trauma. *N Engl J Med* 1996;335:701-707.
12. Meyer CS, Blebea J, Davis K. Surveillance venous scans for deep vein thrombosis in multiple trauma patients. *Ann Vasc Surg* 1995;9:109-114.
13. Cipolle MD, Wojcik R, Seislove E, et al. The role of surveillance duplex scanning in preventing venous thrombosis in trauma patients. *J Trauma* 2002;52:453-462.
14. Greenfield LJ, Proctor MC, Rodriguez JL, et al. Posttrauma thromboembolism prophylaxis. *J Trauma* 1997;42(1):100-103.
15. Gearhart MM, Luchette FA, Proctor MC, et al. The risk assessment profile score identifies trauma patients at risk for deep vein thrombosis. *Surgery* 2000;128:631-640.
16. Clagett GP, Reisch JS. Prevention of venous thromboembolism in general surgical patients. Results of a meta-analysis. *Ann Surgery* 1988;208(2):227-240.
17. Geerts WH, Code KI, Richard MJ, et al. A prospective study of venous thromboembolism after major trauma. *N Eng J Med* 1994;331(24):1601-1606.
18. Salzman EW, Hirsh J. The epidemiology, pathogenesis, and natural history of venous thrombosis. In: Coleman RW, Hirsh J, Marder VJ, et al. (eds.) *Hemostasis and Thrombosis, Basic Principles and Clinical Practice.* 3rd ed. Philadelphia, PA: JB Lippincott; 1994:1275-1296.
19. Anderson FA Jr, Spencer FA. Risk Factors for venous thromboembolism. *Circulation* 2003;107:I-9-I-16.
20. Knaggs AL, Delis KT, Mason P, et al. Perioperative lower limb venous haemodynamics in patients under general anaesthesia. *Br J Anaesth* 2005;94:292-295.
21. Mian NZ, Bayly R, Schreck DM, et al. Incidence of deep vein thrombosis associated with femoral venous catheterization. *Acad Emerg Med* 1997;4:1118-1121.
22. Arcelus, JI, Caprini JA, Traverso CI, et al. Physical methods for the prevention of post-operative venous thromboembolism: graduated compression stockings, intermittent pneumatic compression, electrical stimulation. In: Samama M, Clerque F (eds.) *La Maldie Thrombembolique Perioperatoire.* Paris, France: Arnette; 1992:47-62.
23. Comerota AJ, Choulan V, Harada RN, et al. The fibrinolytic effects of intermittent pneumatic compression: Mechanism of enhanced fibrinolysis. *Ann Surgery* 1997;226(3):306-314.
24. Geerts WH, Graham FP, Heit JA, et al.: Prevention of venous thromboembolism: The seventh ACCP conference on antithrombotic and thrombolytic therapy. *Chest* 2004;126:338-400.
25. Comerota AJ, Katz ML, White JV. Why does prophylaxis with external pneumatic compression for deep vein thrombosis fail? *Am J Surg* 1992;164:265-268.
26. Lachman EA, Rook JL, Tunkel R, et al. Complications associated with intermittent pneumatic compression. *Arch Phys Med Rehab* 1992;73:482-485.
27. Hirsch J. Heparin. *N Engl J Med* 1991;324:1565-1574.
28. Collins R, Scrimgeour A, Yusuf S, et al. Reduction in fatal pulmonary embolism and venous thrombosis by perioperative administration of subcutaneous heparin. Overview of results in randomized trials in general, orthopedic, and urologic patients. *N Engl J Med* 1988;318:1162-1173.
29. Arepally GM, Ortel TL. Heparin-induced thrombocytopenia. *N Eng J Med* 2006;355:809-817.
30. Collignon F, Fryman A, Caplain H, et al. Comparison of the pharmacokinetic profiles of three low molecular heparins; dalteparin, enoxaparin and nadropin—administered subcutaneously in healthy volunteers (doses for prevention of thromboembolism). *Thromb Haemost* 1995;73:630-640.
31. Mismetti P, Laporte S, Darmon J, et al. Meta-analysis of low molecular heparin the prevention of venous thromboembolism in general surgery. *Br J Surg* 2001;88:913-930.
32. Velmahos G, Kern J, Chan L, et al. Prevention of venous thromboembolism after injury: an evidence-based report: Part I. Analysis of risk factors and evaluation of the role of vena caval filters. *J Trauma* 2000;49:132-139.
33. Shackford SR, Davis JW, Hollingsworth-Fridlund P, et al. Venous thromboembolism in patients with major trauma. *Am J Surg* 1990;159:365-369.
34. Patton JH, Fabian, TC, Croce MA, et al. Prophylactic Greenfield filters: Acute complications and long-term follow-up. *J Trauma* 1996;41(2):231-237.
35. Geerts WH, Heit JA, Clagett GP, et al. Prevention of venous thromboembolism. *Chest* 2001;119:132S-175S.
36. Spirt MJ. Stress-related mucosal disease: Risk factors and prophylactic therapy. *Clin Ther* 2004;26:197-213.
37. Maier RV, Mitchell D, Gentillo L. Optimal therapy for stress gastritis. *Ann Surgery* 1994;220(3):353-363.
38. Cook D, Fuller H, Guyatt G, et al. For the Canadian Critical Care Trials Group. Risk factors for gastrointestinal bleeding in critically ill patients. *N Engl J Med* 1994;330:377-381.
39. Cook D, Heyland D, Griffith L, et al. Risk factors for clinically important upper gastrointestinal bleeding in patients requiring mechanical ventilation. *Crit Care Med* 1999;27:2812-2817.
40. Institute for healthcare improvement: resources http://www.ihi.org/IHI/Topics/CriticalCare/Intensive-Care/Changes/IndividualChanges/PepticUlcerDiseaseprohylaxis. Accessed June 11, 2008.
41. Dellinger RP, et al. Surviving Sepsis Campaign: guidelines for management of severe sepsis and septic shock. *Crit Care Med* 2004;32(3):858-873.
42. Robertson MS, Clancy RL, Cade JF. Helicobacter pylori in intensive care: why we should be interested. *Intensive Care Medicine* 2004;28:1881-1888.
43. Hastings PR, Skillman JJ, Bushnell LS, et al. Antacid titration in the prevention of acute gastrointestinal bleeding: a controlled randomized study in

100 critically ill patients. *N Engl J Med* 1978;298: 1041-1045.

44. Stollman N, Metz DC. Pathophysiology and prophylaxis of stress ulcer in intensive care unit patients. *J Crit Care* 2005;20:35-45.

45. Cook DJ, Reeve BK, Guyatt GH, et al. Stress ulcer prophylaxis in critically ill patients: resolving discordant meta-analyses. *JAMA* 1996;275:308-314.

46. Brett S. Science review: The use of proton pump inhibitors for gastric acid suppression in critical illness. *Crit Care* 2004;9:45-50.

47. Cook D, Guyatt G, Marshall J, et al. For the Canadian Critical Care Trials Group. A comparison of sucralfate and ranitidine for the prevention of upper gastrointestinal bleeding in patients requiring mechanical ventilation. *N Engl J Med* 1998;338:791-527.

48. Kahn JM, Doctor JN, Rubenfeld GD. Stress ulcer prophylaxis in mechanically ventilated patients: integrating evidence and judgment using a decision analysis. *Intensive Care Med* 2006;32(8):1151-1158.

Chapter 25

ANALGESIA AND SEDATION

Bryan A. Cotton, MD, and Addison K. May, MD

INTRODUCTION

Recent guidelines from the Society of Critical Care Medicine have reinforced the importance of attaining the goals of pain control and relief of anxiety and agitation.[1] Achievement of these end points is often viewed by patients and families with equal or greater importance than surgical technique or outcome. The interrelated nature of pain, anxiety, sleep, and delirium is frequently under appreciated, poorly taught, often mismanaged, and the impact on patient outcomes incompletely understood.[2] Both analgesia and sedation are utilized to address each of these clinical parameters and we have chosen to organize our discussion in the context of each (pain, anxiety, agitation, delirium, sleep) rather than organizing the discussion in the context of generic management strategies of analgesia and sedation.

PAIN

SOURCES AND PATHOPHYSIOLOGY OF PAIN

Two-thirds of critically ill patients will experience pain of a moderate to severe nature as a result of invasive procedures, mechanical ventilation, physical therapy, dressing changes, or prolonged immobilization and the presence of pain exerts direct effects on outcome.[2,3] Unaddressed, pain stimuli alter pathophysiology by the stimulated release of numerous cytokines (IL-1, IL-6, TNF-α), the augmentation of the sympathetic nervous system's response to stress and injury, increased levels of corticotropin and antidiuretic hormone, and activation of components of the renin-angiotensin-aldosterone axis.[2] In addition, immunological dysfunction, hypercoagulability, and electrolyte disturbances have been connected to the perception of pain.[3,4]

ASSESSMENT AND RECOGNITION OF PAIN

The level of pain reported by the patient should be considered the "gold standard" for both initial evaluation as well as response to analgesia.[1] However, the ability to consistently and systematically achieve adequate pain control is enhanced by utilizing quantifiable pain scales, particularly in the ICU setting where verbal communication is frequently hindered.[1,2] These objective scales help to avoid the error of assuming "sedation equals analgesia."[2,3]

Pain Scales

For patients who can appropriately indicate pain, several one-dimensional reporting scales are available to evaluate the intensity of pain and the change in pain in response to intervention including the visual analog scale (VAS), the verbal rating scale (VRS), and the numeric rating scale (NRS) (Fig. 25-1).[1,2] The VAS is a well-validated tool that utilizes a single horizontal line along, with "no pain" on the left end and "worst pain imaginable" on the right end, whereas the NRS uses a numeric scale of 0 through 10 to help patients rate their pain ("no pain" to "worst imaginable"). The NRS has the advantage of allowing both verbal and nonverbal documentation while providing a quantifiable number for assessment and compliance monitoring.

Objective Findings

In the sedated, delirious, or intubated patient, physicians must often rely on objective clinical findings to guide care and analgesic administration. Tachycardia, hypertension, and tachypnea have traditionally been recognized as evidence of patient discomfort and pain. However, physiological signs have not shown reliable correlation with pain and may greatly underestimate its presence; less than one-third of pain events are associated with abnormal vital signs in postoperative patients.[5,6] Thus, the evaluation of both subjective "pain-related behaviors" (body movement, facial expressions) and objective parameters are often necessary.

PHARMACOLOGIC MANAGEMENT OF PAIN

OPIATES

Opiates are the most common agents used for analgesia in the surgical patient and remain the gold standard against which all others are measured (Table 25-1).[1,2]

Visual Analog Scale (VAS)

No pain   *Worst pain
                                                                        imaginable*

Verbal Descriptor Scale (VDS)

| *No pain* | *Mild pain* | *Moderate pain* | *Severe pain* | *Very severe pain* | *Worst pain imaginable* |

Numeric Rating Scale (NRS)

0   1   2   3   4   5   6   7   8   9   10

No pain   *Moderate
                           pain*   *Worst pain
                                                       imaginable*

Figure 25-1   *Visual pain scales.*

Opiates work through both central and peripheral opioid receptors, with the mu and kappa receptors having the most analgesic effects. The other receptors (sigmoid, delta, lambda) contribute to the majority of their adverse effects (respiratory depression, hypotension, urinary retention, ileus, and pruritus).[1,2] Respiratory depression may occur with all members of this class at higher dosing ranges and is more frequently observed when combined with benzodiazepines. Hypotension may occur after opiates as a result of reversal of endogenous catecholamine effects on vascular smooth muscle constriction. Thus, hypotension after opioid administration is more common in the patients with hypovolemia or in those already demonstrating cardiovascular collapse (morphine, codeine, and meperidine).[2]

Morphine: Morphine is the most commonly prescribed of the opioid analgesics as it is well known, inexpensive, and has an excellent analgesic effect. It has a long duration of action allowing intermittent dosing to achieve adequate pain control. Morphine does, however, have several active metabolites that require renal clearance, and its use in patients with renal failure increases the risk of toxicity and adverse event. In addition, morphine is associated with histamine release causing an associated pruritus.

Fentanyl: Fentanyl has a very rapid onset and a short duration, making intermittent dosing of fentanyl for continuous pain control problematic. It may be given to those with morphine allergies and does not cause histamine release. It does not have active metabolites requiring renal clearance and can be used safely in those with renal failure without dose adjustment.[1] Fentanyl has been shown to demonstrate tachyphylaxis in chronic exposure which may require significant increasing in dosing requirements or even change to other agents.[2,3] Additionally, fentanyl is extremely fat-soluble and demonstrates accumulation within repeated dosing.

Other opiates: Hydromorphone is similar to morphine in its duration and onset, but lacks active metabolites and the histamine release often seen with morphine. As such, it may be used in those with hemodynamic concerns and renal insufficiency. Meperidine has a significant side effect profile and should be avoided for the management of acute pain in the surgical patient.[1] Meperidine has active metabolites that often lead to confusion, delirium, and even seizures. It may not be given by constant infusion or frequent

Table 25-1	Opioids Employed in the Acute Care of Surgical Patients				
Opioid	Initial dosing	Half-life	Renal dosing	Hepatic dosing	Adverse events
Morphine	2-10 mg I.V. q 2-6h	3-7 hr	Reduce by 25-50% if CrCL < 50	Not defined	Histamine release
Fentanyl	25-100 mcg I.V. q 1-2h	1.5-6 hr	Reduce by 25-50% if CrCL < 50	Not defined	Significant accumulation in fat, tachyphylaxis, rigidity with higher doses
Hydromorphone	0.2-0.6 mg I.V. q 2-3 h	2-3 hr	Not defined	Not defined	Pancytopenia, agranulocytosis
Remifentanil	0.025 mcg/kg/min continuous infusion	3-10 min	Not defined	Not defined	Muscle rigidity
Oxycodone	5-10 mg PO q 4 hr	2-3 hr	Reduce by 25-50% if CrCL < 50	Decrease initial dosing	Constipation, pruritus
Hydrocodone	7.5 mg PO q 4-6 hr	2-4 hr	Avoid with severe impairment	Avoid with severe impairment	Headache, pruritus
Methadone	2.5-5 mg PO q 8 hr	12 hr-6 d	Reduce by 25-50% if CrCL < 10	Decrease initial dosing	QTc prolongation, ventricular arrhythmias
Codeine	15-30 mg q 4-6 hr	2-4 hr	Reduce by 25-50% if CrCL < 50	Avoid with severe impairment	Constipation, pruritus

intervals for this reason. Meperidine also interacts with many other medications, including MAO inhibitors and selective serotonin reuptake inhibitors.

NONSTEROIDAL ANTI-INFLAMMATORY DRUGS (NSAIDS)

NSAIDs provide analgesia through a nonselective, competitive inhibition of the cyclo-oxygenase (COX) enzyme, a critical component of the inflammatory cascade. Utilization of these medications may help reduce opioid requirements and is often adequate pain control for musculoskeletal pain (Table 25-2). Ibuprofen and ketorolac are the most commonly utilized oral and enteral forms of NSAIDs, respectively.[1-3] However, NSAIDs are associated with gastrointestinal (GI) bleeding, platelet inhibition, and renal insufficiency. The adverse renal effects are more common in those patients who are hypovolemic, elderly, or receiving the medications for an extended period.[1-3] Selective COX-2 inhibitors appear to be associated with less GI bleeding, but several have been withdrawn from the market by their manufacturers due to concern of increased risk of cardiovascular complications.[7] Although widely used as an over-the-counter analgesic, aspirin is also associated with GI bleeding and platelet dysfunction. Therefore, its use as an analgesic in the acute setting is fairly limited.

ACETAMINOPHEN
Acetaminophen is often utilized as a primary medication for mild to moderate pain and as an adjunct in more severe pain. When combined with an opioid, the two medications achieve an analgesic effect much greater than with the opioid alone. Overdose and subsequent hepatotoxicity may occur when combination agents are not recognized as containing acetaminophen. Daily administration of the total acetaminophen dose should be limited to less than 4 grams (Table 25-2). However, both alcohol abuse and malnutrition lower the threshold for hepatotoxicity. Care must be taken to limit dosing to less than 2 grams in these patients.[1,8]

ALPHA-2 RECEPTOR AGONISTS
Alpha-2 agonists (clonidine, dexmedetomidine) have been shown to be effective in primary and adjunctive control of pain and lack the side effect profile observed with opiates.[9] These agents are relatively lipid-soluble and absorbed and distributed fairly quickly. Several mechanisms for their nociceptive effects have been debated, including spinal level inhibition of noradrenergic descending pathways and a reduction in pain perception.[1-3,9]

KETAMINE
Ketamine is a phencyclidine derivative with superb analgesic properties at subanesthetic doses that may provide excellent periprocedure pain control without the development of respiratory depression, airway compromise, or hemodynamic deterioration.[1,2,10] However, its use may be associated with hallucinations, emergence "delirium," and aspiration; use should be limited to monitored settings.

Table 25-2	Nonopioid options for acute pain control (primary and adjuncts)				
	Initial dosing	Route of administration	Renal dosing	Hepatic dosing	Adverse events
Ibuprofen	600-800 mg q 6-8 hours	Oral	Avoid with renal insufficiency and hypovolemia; do not use with advanced renal disease	Not defined	Avoid in late pregnancy; gastroin testinal (GI) bleeding; perforation
Ketorolac	15-30 mg I.V., 30-60 mg I.M., or 10 mg P.O. every 6-8 hours	Intravenous, intramuscular, or oral	Avoid with renal insufficiency and hypovolemia; do not use with advanced renal disease	Not defined	For short-term use (< 5days); GI bleeding, perforation
Celecoxib	200 mg every 12 hours	Oral	Avoid use with severe impairment	Decrease dose by 50% with Child-Pugh B; avoid with Child-Pugh C	May increase risk of fatal cardiovascular thrombotic events (myocardial infarct, stroke)
Acetaminophen	325-650 mg every 4-6 hours	Oral	Adjust frequency with CrCL 10-50 to q 6; CrCL < 10 to q 8	Limit use to 500 mg per dose and no more than 2000 mg/d	Do not exceed total acetaminophen dose of > 4000 mg/d
Aspirin	325-650 mg every 4 hours	Oral	Adjust frequency with CrCL 10-50 to q 6; avoid with CrCL < 10	Not defined	Do not exceed total aspirin dose of > 4000 mg/d

DELIVERY OPTIONS

Oral and transdermal delivery: The duration of analgesia and tolerance of adverse effects with oral forms of opioids makes the enteral tract the preferred administration route. In patients requiring frequent dosing, sustained release options are available but should only be administered orally (not through nasogastric or nasoenteric routes). Fentanyl patches have shown adequacy in achieving pain control, but their use should be closely monitored and usually restricted to those with chronic pain issues.

Intravenous or epidural delivery: In patients requiring intravenous opioids, scheduled dosing (morphine, hydromorphone) or a continuous infusion (fentanyl, morphine) should be utilized to provide consistent analgesia. Although intermittent (as needed) regimens are often associated with inadequate pain control, excellent results (and superior patient satisfaction on pain scales) can be achieved through a patient-controlled analgesia (PCA) device.[2,3,11] Therefore, if the patient is capable of operating such a device, a PCA, utilizing morphine or hydromorphone, should be employed.[1] Neuraxial (epidural) anesthesia has been shown to achieve superior pain control following thoracoabdominal procedures or trauma (rib fractures) compared to PCA.[11] Epidural analgesia has also been shown to decrease nosocomial pneumonia rates and shorten duration of mechanical ventilation. Catheter placement, however, is associated with hypotension, dural puncture, spinal cord injury, and urinary retention.[12]

SPECIAL POPULATIONS

Acute abdomen: Recent studies have shown acute abdominal pain is one of the most poorly managed and undertreated pain conditions. In fact, over 70% of emergency room physicians withhold analgesic medications until surgeon evaluation of the abdomen. Additionally, two-thirds of surgeons believe administration of such medications will interfere with diagnostic accuracy of their examination.[13] However, investigations into the "masking" of an acute abdomen with judicious opiate administration have not supported these suspicions. In fact, randomized controlled trials have found opiate administration significantly reduced discomfort without impairing the ability to perform an adequate and accurate examination.[14,15]

Acute pain management in patients with opioid dependence: The analgesic properties of methadone and buprenorphine differ quite considerably from those utilized for acute pain. Additionally, tolerance and hyperalgesia associated with these agents likely diminishes any analgesic effect. Used alone, these agents usually prove grossly inadequate in providing acute analgesia. As well, cross-tolerance between these medications and other opioids may explain why this population often requires higher and more frequent doses of opiates.[16,17] Management should focus on delivering uninterrupted therapy (to address baseline opioid requirements) and aggressive pain management strategies (to achieve acute analgesia). Similar to the managing opioid naïve patients, strategies should employ nonpharmacologic and nonopioid interventions as well.[18] Although physicians are often concerned that opioid administration in treating acute pain will result in relapse to active drug use, there is no evidence to support this bias.[16-18]

ANXIETY

In the absence of adequate control of anxiety and agitation, achievement of other objectives and therapeutic end points is greatly impaired.[1,3,19] Anxious or agitated patients are more likely to remove feeding tubes, bladder catheters, and endotracheal tubes, resulting in loss of nutritional support, trauma, and potential airway complications. However, unresponsive, comatose patients are often the end result of "overshooting" sedation and this is equally detrimental. As such, the delicate balance of sedation and agitation is often difficult to achieve (even among the most experienced physicians) and even more difficult to teach to those in training.

SEDATION-AGITATION SCALES

In the absence of rational and agreed-on target levels, different members of the patient's health care team will demonstrate quite disparate treatment goals, increasing the risk of complications and decreasing recovery potential.[19] Scales such as the Riker Sedation-Agitation Scale (SAS) and Ramsay Scale have been developed to address this problem and are in wide use in many ICUs and hospitals. However, the Richmond Agitation-Sedation Scale (RASS) is the only scale demonstrated to be a valid and reliable tool for measuring the sedation-agitation levels over the patient's hospital course (Fig. 25-2).[20] The RASS utilizes the duration of eye contact following verbal stimulation as the primary method of assessment and means of titrating sedation. Similar to the Glasgow Coma Scale, the RASS separates verbal and physical stimulation to allow for better grading of arousal levels. It is for these reasons that our institution universally utilizes the RASS in all trauma and surgical patients.

DAILY AWAKENING AND INTERRUPTION OF SEDATION

Continuous sedative infusions result in delayed awakening that appears to increase ICU stays through prolonging time on mechanical ventilation. Several studies have noted a reduction in ICU length of stay and mechanical ventilator days with daily interruption of

+4	Combative	Combative, violent, immediate danger to staff
+3	Very agitated	Pulls or removes tube (s) or catheter (s); aggressive
+2	Agitated	Frequent nonpurposeful movement, fights ventilator
+1	Restless	Anxious, apprehensive, but movements are not aggressive or vigorous
0	Alert and calm	
−1	Drowsy	Not fully alert, but has sustained awakening to voice (eye opening and contact >10 seconds)
−2	Light sedation	Briefly awakens to voice (eye opening and contact <10 seconds)
−3	Moderate sedation	Movement or eye opening to voice (but no eye contact)
−4	Deep sedation	No response to voice, but movement or eye opening to physical stimulation
−5	Unarousable	No response to voice or physical stimulation

Figure 25-2 *Richmond Agitation and Severity Scale (RASS).*

sedation.[21,22] Daily awakening trials involve the interruption of sedating medications until the patient is awake and responsive to commands or until the patient becomes agitated. Not surprisingly, such trials have been met with resistance as some physicians question the feasibility of performing daily "awakening trials" in their ICUs and because of concerns of long-term psychological effects. However, these trials have actually been associated with a lower risk for posttraumatic stress disorder.[22]

PHARMACOLOGICAL MANAGEMENT OF ANXIETY

BENZODIAZEPINES

Benzodiazepines may be used to provide brief procedural sedation, anxiolysis, or a continuous sedated state. Although they lack any actual analgesic effect, their impact on reducing opioid requirements by attenuating anticipatory pain is well documented. In addition, some drugs in this class (most notably midazolam) carry potent antegrade amnestic effects. Elderly and those with hepatic or renal insufficiency are most likely to experience adverse events from these agents. Respiratory depression, slurred speech, nystagmus, and obtundation are but a few side effects of this class. Additionally, these agents may contribute to delirium, particularly in the elderly population and consideration of their use must be balanced by the potential to lead to prolonged delirium in this populations.

The most common agents used for sedation are midazolam and lorazepam. Lorazepam has a longer half-life and can be given by both intermittent and continuous administration to achieve continuous sedation; whereas midazolam's short half-life usually mandates continuous infusion to achieve continuous sedation. Midazolam has a significant propensity for tachyphylaxis requiring escalating dosages.

Intermittent administration: In patients with baseline anxiety or persistent benzodiazepine requirements, use of intermittent (but scheduled) enteral diazepam or lorazepam is preferred. An as-needed approach is preferable in the hospitalized patient requiring occasional dosing for illness-related stress and anxiety (Table 25-3).

Continuous infusions: In patients requiring frequent repeat dosing, utilization of a continuous infusion may be preferred to offer smoother titration and maintenance of RASS targets. Midazolam should be used for continuous infusion as it has a fairly rapid onset and much shorter half-life than other benzodiazepines. However, its active metabolites may result in prolonged sedation in those with renal insufficiency.

PROPOFOL

Propofol is an intravenous general anesthetic agent whose sedation properties can be achieved at lower doses. The rapid onset and short duration of action make this drug a preferred agent in many clinical settings, including those requiring frequent neurological assessments. It may be used as a continuous infusion, with initial achievement obtained through bolus administration. Propofol provides similar depth and quality of sedation to midazolam but demonstrates quicker extubation and recovery times.[23] Adverse

Table 25-3 Sedative Agents for Intermittent and Continuous Administration

	Initial dosing	Half-life	Renal dosing	Hepatic dosing	Adverse events/comments
Diazepam	2-5 mg IV q 4-6 hour	20-80 hour	No adjustment	Use with caution in hepatic impairment	Active metabolites that may produce quite prolonged sedation.
Lorazepam	0.5 mg-1.0 mg IV q 4-8 hour	6-8 hour	Avoid with renal failure	Avoid with hepatic failure	No active metabolites
Midazolam	1.0 mg/hr IV, titrate for desired RASS	2-3 hour	Decrease dose by 50% with CrCL < 10	Use with caution in hepatic failure	Hypotension, significant respiratory depression
Dexmedetomidine	0.2 mcg/kg/hr IV, titrate for desired RASS	1.5-2 hour	Decrease dose with CrCL < 50	Decrease dose with any Child-Pugh class	May load with 1.0 mcg/kg IV, but beware hypotension, bradycardia; do not exceed 24-hour infusion
Propofol	5 mcg/kg/min, titrate by 5-10 mcg/kg/min for desired RASS	3-12 hour	None	None	"Infusion syndrome" seen with doses > 80 mcg/kg/min; hypotension, apnea; fatty tissue distribution may prolong effect

Cardiac and respiratory monitoring are mandatory with all the above agents.

events are primarily related to duration of therapy (pancreatitis, hypertriglyceridemia, lactic acidosis); therefore, propofol use should be limited to 48 hours or less. Additionally, propofol has no analgesic properties and should be administered in conjunction with opiates.

ALPHA-2 AGONISTS

Selective alpha-2 adrenergic receptor agonists exhibit sedative, analgesic, and anxiolytics effects.[24] These agents maintain adequate sedation with less risk for producing hemodynamic instability or respiratory depression. Dexmedetomidine has the added benefit of analgesia (with fewer opiate requirements) and lacks the respiratory depression seen with propofol.[24] When employed in settings where other agents have been unsuccessful (but the patient is successfully controlled with dexmedetomidine), we transition these patients to clonidine. In our experience, enteral (0.1-0.3 mg TID) and or transdermal clonidine (0.1-0.3 mg patch) helps maintain light sedation and agitation control in those responsive to dexmedetomidine. Adverse events associated with its use include hypotension, hypertension, severe bradycardia, and other arrhythmias.

AGITATION

Agitation, a heightened state of arousal and nonpurposeful motor activity, represents the extreme of the arousal continuum. Its onset is usually quite abrupt, almost universally disruptive to patient care, and frightening to the patient and their family members.[3,25]

IMMEDIATE EVALUATION OF AGITATION

A rapid assessment should begin with ruling out any life-threatening situations. Many of these conditions (tension pneumothorax, occluded endotracheal tubes) can present with severe agitation and mental status changes and should be excluded first. Simultaneously, the patient should be protected from harming themselves through falls, self-extubation, and tube removal. Identifying and correcting less life-threatening issues should follow; ruling out ventilator dyssynchrony, bladder catheter occlusion, unaddressed pain, or pending bowel incontinence (especially in patients unable to communicate).[3,25] Once such diagnoses have been excluded, appropriate management of agitation can proceed.

PHARMACOLOGICAL MANAGEMENT OF AGITATION

HALOPERIDOL

Haloperidol is often utilized for the rapid control of the acutely and severely agitated patient. Initial dosing of 5 mg intravenously should be used and may be repeated every 10-15 minutes (usually with increasing dosages) until adequate control is achieved.[25] If intravenous access is lost or unobtainable, intramuscular use is also successful but likely to take longer to achieve results. Its side effect profile, however, has historically limited the enthusiasm for its use (Table 25-4). Concomitant use of benzodiazepines or benztropine

Table 25-4 Agents Utilized for Agitation and Delirium

	Initial dosing	Half-life	Renal dosing	Hepatic dosing	Adverse events/comments
Haloperidol	2-5 mg IM/IV*; double dose until effect achieved; use effective dose (?PO) scheduled q 6 h	21-24 hr	No adjustment	Caution with severe hepatic impairment	Neuroleptic malignant syndrome (NMS), akathisia, tardive dyskinesia, arrhythmias
Olanzapine	2.5-5 mg IM (or 5-10 mg PO/PT) q 2 hr prn; if effective, start 2.5-5 mg PO/PT qhs	21-50 hr	No adjustment	Caution with severe hepatic impairment	NMS, akathisia, tardive dyskinesia, severe hyperglycemia
Risperidone	0.5 mg-1 mg PO/PTq 6 hour prn, then use effective dose q 12 hr	20-36 hr	Half dose with CrCL < 50; half dose and use qd with CrCL < 10	Half dose and use qd with severe impairment	Available as dissolving tablet; NMS, akathisia, tardive dyskinesia
Quetiapine	25-50 mg PO/PT q 4-6 hr prn, then use effective dose q 12 hr	6-8 hr	No adjustment	Half dose and use qd with severe impairment	NMS, tardive dyskinesia, QTc prolongation, headache, severe hyperglycemia, hyperlipidemia
Ziprasidone	10-20 mg IM q 2-4 prn or 20 mg PO/PT q 4-6 hr prn, then use effective dose q 12 hour	6-8 hr	Avoid IM use	No adjustment	NMS, tardive dyskinesia, QTc prolongation, headache, akathisia

*Not FDA-approved for intravenous administration

decreases extra-pyramidal symptoms (EPS) in the acutely agitated patient.[26]

ATYPICAL ANTIPSYCHOTICS

Atypical antipsychotics have gained increased attention for use as alternative agents for management of acute agitation. In lower doses than that required for acute psychoses management, risperidone, ziprasidone, and olanzapine have been shown to be appropriate alternatives for treatment of acute agitation.[26,27] Their safety profiles include lower incidence of EPS and better patient tolerance. As well, once agitation is under control, these agents can be changed to the enteral route for continued use until agitation has resolved. However, these agents carry equal, if not higher, risk of arrhythmias. As such, they have failed to demonstrate a superior safety profile to haloperidol in managing the acutely agitated patient.[25-27]

SPECIAL POPULATIONS

AGITATION FOLLOWING HEAD INJURY

In the setting of severe traumatic brain injury (TBI), patients may develop paroxysmal episodes of hypertension, tachycardia, diaphoresis, tachypnea, and severe agitation.[28] Often dismissed as an exaggerated systemic inflammatory response, these episodes have been correlated with significant increases in plasma catecholamine levels and, unaddressed, are associated with an increased mortality rate. Beta-blockers have been shown to reduce episode frequency and severity and we have recently demonstrated a significant reduction in mortality when these patients are managed with beta-blockers.[29] We utilize intravenous agents (labetalol or propranolol) for acute episodes, with concurrent scheduled enteral agents (propranolol, beginning at 10 mg every 8 hours). Doses are titrated to control of agitation and attenuation of the hyperdynamic state.

ALCOHOL WITHDRAWAL SYNDROME

As with the anxiety-agitation continuum, alcohol withdrawal syndrome (AWS) presents along a wide, varied presentation, both in depth and intensity. It is often characterized by tachycardia, hypertension, confusion, altered level of consciousness, and, additionally, seizures. Undetected, this symptom complex will predictably disrupt delivery of appropriate care and management of the patient's primary presenting diagnosis. Prophylaxis and management strategies have traditionally centered on the attenuation of the withdrawal and prevention of seizure activity.

Medications can be administered using fixed-schedule or symptom-triggered regimens. With fixed schedule regimens, benzodiazepines are administered at specific intervals, with additional doses given based on severity of symptoms. Other therapies include using ethanol itself as a continuous infusion (5-10% ethanol infusion initiated at 0.5-0.8 mL/kg ideal body weight/hour).[30] Once symptoms develop, however, rapid control of acute agitation is best controlled by use of intravenous lorazepam (2-4 mg) or diazepam (5-10 mg), titrated to severity of symptoms.[30,31] As with other withdrawal states, clonidine (0.1-0.3 mg PO/PT every 8 hours) has been successfully employed to prevent, decrease severity, and shorten duration of AWS.[31]

DELIRIUM

Delirium is a global disturbance of consciousness characterized by fluctuating mental status, inattention, and disorganized thinking. Delirium has been historically dismissed as an expected complication of the hospitalized elderly patient, and its impact on outcomes thought to be negligible. However, recent studies have shown that delirium is significantly underdiagnosed, not limited to the elderly patient, and is associated with a threefold higher mortality.[32,33] Additionally, patients with delirium have higher hospital costs and experience significant cognitive impairment long after discharge.[32] We have recently demonstrated that delirium occurs in 80% of mechanically ventilated medical ICU patients and over 75% of mechanically ventilated patients in surgical ICUs.[33-35] Surprisingly, we noted that the trauma ICU population, which is much younger than that of either medical or surgical ICU patients and less likely to have comorbidities, has an almost 70% prevalence of delirium.

ASSESSMENT OF DELIRIUM

The Confusion Assessment Method for the ICU (CAM-ICU) tool is a valid and extremely reliable tool, taking an average of 60 seconds to perform. The CAM-ICU is comprised of four features: acute change or fluctuation in mental status (Feature 1), inattention (Feature 2), disorganized thinking (Feature 3), or an altered level of consciousness (Feature 4) (Fig. 25-3). In patients who are medically, traumatically, or pharmacologically comatose (RASS of –4 or –5), CAM-ICU is not assessed due to lack of any response to verbal stimulation. In patients with RASS scores of –3 or higher, CAM-ICU should be utilized. To be diagnosed as delirious, the patient should have an RASS score of –3 or higher, with an acute change or fluctuation in mental status (Feature 1), accompanied by inattention (Feature 2) and either disorganized thinking (Feature 3) or an altered level of consciousness (Feature 4).

RISK FACTORS FOR THE DEVELOPMENT OF DELIRIUM

Sleep deprivation, hypoxia, sensory impairment, as well as exposure to numerous medications (sedatives, analgesics, anticholinergics, antihistamines, antiarrhythmics, and steroids) have all been implicated as risk factors for delirium.[32-34] In a recent study of surgical and trauma patient, we identified only two risk factors for developing delirium.[35] Midazolam was

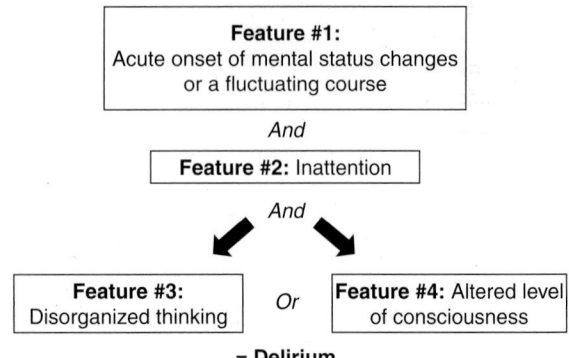

Step #1: Sedation assessment (RASS)

If RASS is –4 or –5, then **Stop** and **Reassess** patient at a later time. If RASS is above –4 (–3 through –4), **Proceed to step 2.**

Step #2: Delirium assessment (CAM-ICU)

Feature #1:
Acute onset of mental status changes or a fluctuating course

And

Feature #2: Inattention

And

Feature #3:
Disorganized thinking

Or

Feature #4: Altered level of consciousness

= **Delirium**

Figure 25-3   *CAM-ICU assessment to detect delirium.*

associated with a threefold-higher risk of developing delirium. This is consistent with data from our MICU study in which lorazepam was an independent risk factor.[32] In addition, fentanyl demonstrated an increased risk for development of delirium, whereas morphine appeared to have a protective effect. This "protective effect," however, needs to be considered in the context that fentanyl is often (inappropriately?) used as a sedative, while morphine is exclusively used as an analgesic.

PREVENTION OF DELIRIUM

Avoiding high-risk medications, preserving sleep hygiene, and treating symptoms with appropriately targeted medications (ie, opiates for pain, benzodiazepines for anxiety, antihistamines for pruritus, not for sleep) are the foundations on which one can hope to prevent delirium. Preserving or reestablishing the patient's senses (eyeglasses and hearing aids) and providing sufficient daytime cognitive stimulation (through staff and family interactions) may help to prevent development of delirium or at least shorten its duration and reduce symptom severity.

TREATMENT OF DELIRIUM
Initial Management

Initial treatment is aimed at reversing and/or treating any underlying medical conditions suspected of contributing to its development (Fig. 25-4). After evaluating potential metabolic or infectious sources, all efforts should be made to remove "deliriogenic" medications. These include benzodiazepines, antihistamines, anticholinergics (specifically diphenhydramine), and corticosteroids. Instituting daily interruption of sedatives and analgesics, and using these agents within a strict protocol, has both been shown to improve patients' outcomes.[36] Next, interventions focusing on environmental control, cognitive reorientation, and "normalization"

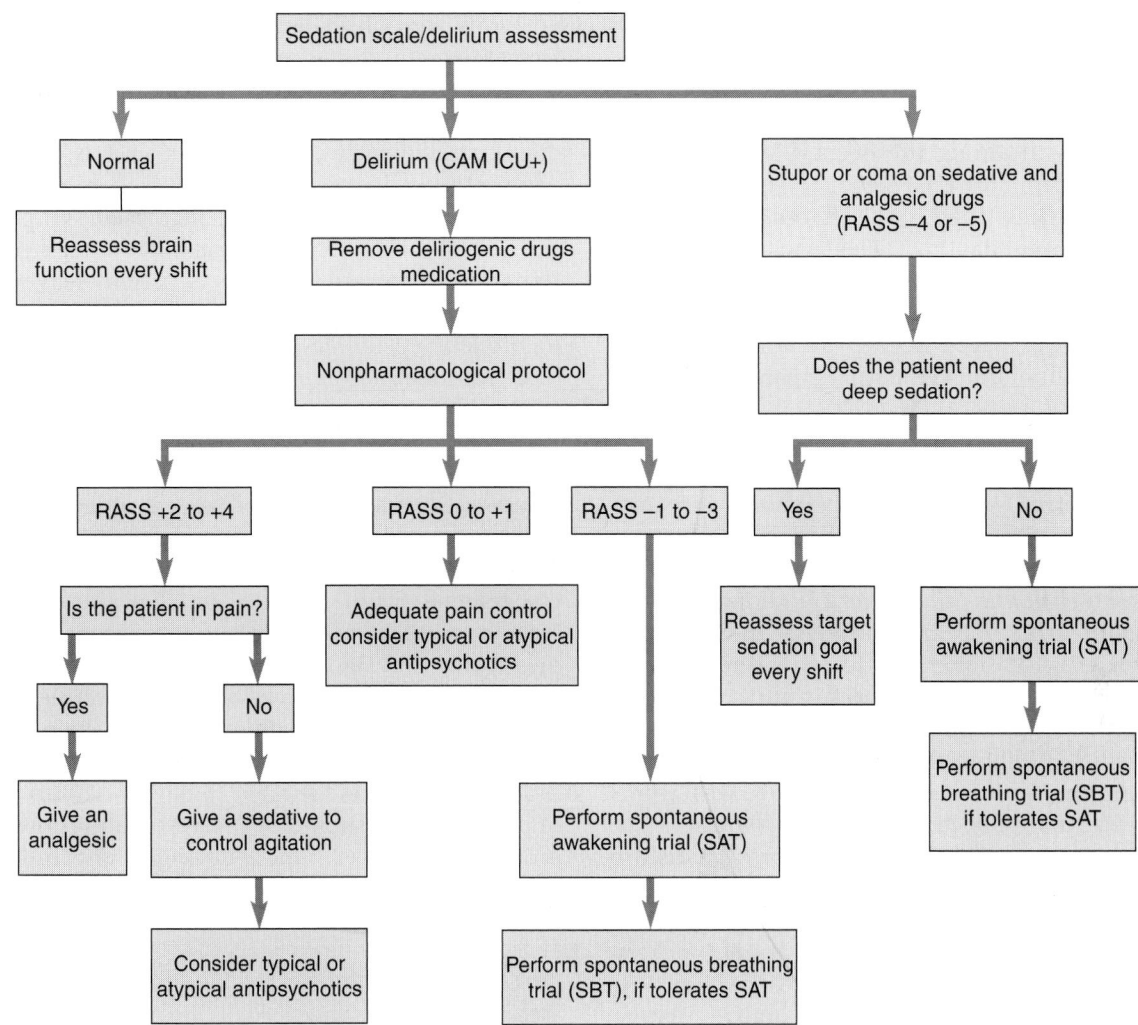

Figure 25-4 *Approach to the sedated or delirious patient.*

of clinical parameters should be implemented. Environmental control entails reestablishing sleep hygiene, through control of excessive noise and staff disturbances at night and ensuring lights are on in the daytime and off at night. Sleep agents may be added to assist with sleep onset, depth, and duration. Increasing daytime communication with family and friends, increasing physical activity, and ensuring replacement of eyeglasses and hearing aids is vital to achieving reorientation of the delirious patient.

Pharmacologic Management of Delirium

Haloperidol: Haloperidol is the agent most often used at our institution as it has few anticholinergic effects, few active metabolites, and mild sedating side effects. It is available in oral and intramuscular forms, but we typically use it intravenously (although not FDA-approved) because of its rapid onset and control of agitation.

Atypical antipsychotics: In patients with enteral access, risperidone, olanzapine, quetiapine, and ziprasidone are available and have been used at our institution. These medications, however, often require titration to higher doses and increased frequency, but are associated (as with haloperidol) with arrhythmias, including QTc prolongation and Torsades de pointes. Use of these medications has, in our experience, been associated with better tolerance of treatment and fairly quick return to the patient's baseline mental status.[37] Improved sensorium and resolution of delirium symptoms appear to coincide with the reestablishment of the sleep-wake cycle. Unless delirium is felt to be the result of sedative or alcohol withdrawal, benzodiazepine monotherapy should be avoided.[36]

SLEEP

Sleep is a basic need for human survival and is essential to healing and recovery from illness and injury. As well, many vital physiological processes are defined in terms of their relationship to a circadian rhythm and are thus intimately involved in the sleep state.

However, sleep disturbances are all too common in hospitalized patients, with repeated arousals and disruptions occurring, on average, every 20 minutes in the ICU setting.[38] As a consequence, these patients have difficulty attaining the deepest stages of sleep (delta wave sleep) and REM sleep. To compensate for these disturbances, these patients often attempt to sleep during the daytime. Daytime sleep, which accounts for over 50% of sleep attained in the critically ill, is unfortunately lacking in REM and delta wave sleep. The deeper stages of sleep are noted for physiological stability and sympathetic-parasympathetic balance.[25]

SOURCES OF SLEEP DISTURBANCES

Although internal factors (pain, discomfort, and anxiety) have been shown to result in sleep deprivation, external factors (lights on at night, staff noise) have been shown to be the primary reason for arousals and sleep fragmentation.[25,38] Evaluations of the ICU have consistently noted staff noise levels in the range of 70-80 decibels or greater. To put this in perspective, a power lawn mower's noise levels are in the range of 65-95 decibels.[39] Nighttime staff communication is the most disruptive noise, as sounds associated with words or meanings are more likely to result in awakenings. Numerous medications have been shown to disturb sleep, mostly through excessive daytime somnolence and disturbances of REM. These include beta-blockers, diuretics, ACE-inhibitors, calcium channel blockers, and benzodiazepines. Additionally, each nighttime diagnostic test, nursing intervention and respiratory evaluation and treatment causes arousal and disturbance of sleep.[25]

CONSEQUENCES OF SLEEP DISTURBANCES

Although the neurocognitive consequences (delirium, anxiety, and irritability) are most obvious, sleep deprivation can lead to increased energy expenditure, lowered seizure threshold, and an inability to regulate body temperature.[25,38,39] Sleep deprivation suppresses antibody responses and cell-mediated immunity. Decreased functional vital capacity, blunted hypercapnic and hypoxic ventilatory responses, and impaired respiratory muscle endurance have been demonstrated with sleep deprivation. Loss of normal day-night cues from sleep deprivation results in disturbed heart rate variability, increased sympathetic activity, and elevated blood pressure. Once sleep patterns return toward normal (as patient leaves ICU), REM rebound occurs with its associated hemodynamic lability, increase in arrhythmias, and myocardial ischemia.[40] This may explain, or contribute to, early postoperative myocardial infarction and death.

PREVENTION OF SLEEP DISTURBANCES

Conversations at night near patient rooms should be minimized. Bedside alarms should not be placed at the head of the bed or in patient room, but rather at central telemetry type stations so that these frequent "false alarms" are not audible to the patient. Routinely measuring vital signs throughout the night and early morning chest radiographs and phlebotomies should be abandoned in the patient who is not unstable or deteriorating. Scheduled baths and linen changes at night should be rescheduled to daytime hours. Lights in patient rooms should be turned off and those in the units should be dimmed during nighttime hours (make day, day and night, night).

PHARMACOLOGICAL MANAGEMENT OF SLEEP

A list of agents used for sleep in hospitalized patients is provided in Table 25-5.

BENZODIAZEPINES

Benzodiazepines, although available in short-acting formulations, have significant effects on the respiratory system and suppress deep stages of sleep. These agents are especially worrisome in patients with chronic

Table 25-5	Agents Used for Sleep in the Hospitalized Patient			
	Initial dosing	Renal dosing	Hepatic dosing	Adverse events/comments
Chloral hydrate	500 mg qhs (may increase to 1000 mg)	Avoid with CrCL < 50	Avoid with severe impairment	Leukopenia, GI distress
Zolpidem	5 mg qhs (may increase to 10 mg)	Not defined	Start at 5 mg with severe impairment	Depression, aggressive behavior, myalgias, amnesia
Mirtazapine	15 mg qhs (may increase to 30 mg)	Not defined	Avoid with severe impairment	Available as dissolvable tablet; avoid with acute depressive disorder; increased appetite, mild anxiolytic effect
Trazodone	50 mg qhs (may increase to 100 mg)	Not defined	Avoid with severe impairment	Avoid with acute depressive disorder; neutropenia, anemia, extrapyramidal symptoms

obstructive pulmonary disease and or hypoventilation syndromes. Benzodiazepines may exacerbate underlying hypercapnia, induce upper airway hypotonia, and increase the number of duration of apneic events.

DIPHENHYDRAMINE

Diphenhydramine is an antihistamine and sedating drug with strong anticholinergic properties and is the agent most likely to be associated with adverse events when utilized for sleep promotion. Paradoxical excitement, visual hallucinations, and delirium are the most common adverse events associated with its use.[25,39-41] As well, the increased daytime somnolence and decreased overall alertness following its nighttime use, should limit the use of this agent to severe pruritus and anaphylaxis.

CHLORAL HYDRATE

Chloral hydrate has been used for years to sedate children for prolonged imaging studies, as well as inducing sleep for polysomnography in both children and adults.[41] This agent induces sleep effectively and without respiratory depression at hypnotic dosing. Given the absence of effect on respiratory rate, $PaCO_2$, PaO_2, it is a preferred sleep agent in our surgical and trauma ICUs.

ZOLPIDEM

Zolpidem, a nonbenzodiazepine hypnotic, has several characteristics that make it useful for the short-term use on an inpatient setting. Zolpidem preserves stages 3 and 4 sleep, as well as REM, and has no significant residual (or "hangover") effects.[41,42] It has also less cognitive impairment and memory loss than the benzodiazepines.

MIRTAZAPINE

Mirtazapine, a noradrenergic, serotonin-2 ($5-HT_2$) antidepressant, has been shown to have excellent sleep promoting effects.[43] Its stimulation of the $5-HT_2$ receptor is thought to mediate its effect on sleep promotion and restoration of sleep architecture. Improved sleep latency, increased time spent in deep stages of sleep, and increased total sleep time has been demonstrated.

TRAZODONE

Trazodone is another antidepressant shown to markedly improve sleep quality (even in nondepressed individuals) by both subjective measures as well as EEG. In addition, it has demonstrated excellent restoration of sleep hygiene in those experiencing posttraumatic stress disorders.[44]

PROCEDURAL SEDATION

Over the last decade, the frequency of "bedside" operative procedures has increased considerably. The factors behind this include the increasing acceptance of staged (or damage control) strategies for managing severe abdominal, soft tissue, and orthopedic pathology, advances in endoscopic and percutaneous techniques, increasing competition for operating room space, and difficulty of transporting severely critically ill patients. As a result, a considerable number of procedures are now being performed at the bedside (specifically in the ICU) that historically had been strictly performed in the operating theater.

PRECAUTIONS

Protocols and safety practices specifically for bedside operative procedures should be in place to ensure the ability to perform these procedures safely. All patients should have blood pressure, electrocardiographic monitoring, and pulse oximetry routinely monitored throughout the procedures. Adequate personnel must be present to allow performance of the procedure, monitoring of sedation/anesthesia, medication administration, manipulation of ventilation if required, and documentation. In addition to the careful development of a bedside procedure protocol, we have implemented the use of a designated "proceduralist" for all bedside surgical procedures. These individuals are senior ICU nurses, trained in the assistance of bedside procedures, airway management, and intravenous anesthetic administration.

PHARMACOLOGICAL MANAGEMENT

FIRST-LINE AGENTS

For procedural sedation, bolus administration of midazolam is preferred, given its rapid onset, depth of sedation, and amnestic effect. For analgesia, fentanyl is utilized at doses dependent on the patient's weight, tolerance, and hemodynamic status. For the deep sedation required for all abdominal bedside surgical procedures, we utilize propofol in larger doses than those employed for continuous sedation.

KETAMINE

Ketamine is also used and is generally well tolerated. We tend to reserve it for complex wound care and dressing changes. Because of its risk of emergence delirium and emesis, it is usually administered with midazolam and metoclopramide. All of the agents mentioned here are titrated to achieve their preset end points as the patient's hemodynamic status allows.

NEUROMUSCULAR BLOCKERS

With regard to neuromuscular agents, we prefer to use vecuronium (Table 25-6) or, in those with renal impairment, cisatracurium. Neuromuscular agents are employed in the majority of bronchoscopies and major bedside operative procedures and in all "open abdomen" procedures.

Table 25-6   Agents Used for Procedural Sedation and "Bedside Anesthesia"

	Initial/ bolus dosing	Maintenance dosing	Renal dosing	Hepatic dosing	Precautions/comments
Fentanyl	50-100 mcg IV	Repeat bolus q 15 min, increase dose as blood pressure allows	Decrease dosing by 25% for CrCL < 50	Not defined	Significant respiratory depression when administered with benzodiazepines
Midazolam	1.0-2.0 mg IV	Repeat doses q 5-15 min as respiratory and hemodynamic status permit.	Decrease dose by 50% with CrCL <10	Use with caution in hepatic failure	Significant respiratory depression when administered with opiates; beware hypotension with boluses
Propofol	10-20 mg IV	0.2 mg/kg/min IV; may repeat bolus of 20 mg as needed	Not defined	Not defined	Reduce dose by 25% and avoid rapid boluses in elderly, debilitated, or head injury patients; beware hypotension
Dexmedetomidine	1 mcg/kg IV bolus	0.2-0.7 mcg/-kg/hr IV	Reduce bolus by 50% or avoid bolus dosing	Reduce bolus by 50% or avoid bolus dosing	Beware hypotension and bradycardia especially with bolus dosing
Ketamine	2 mg/kg IV	0.1-0.5 mg/min IV; may also use repeat boluses of 2-4 mg/kg IV	Not defined	Decrease infusion or repeat boluses by 50%	Low doses benzodiazepineslimit hallucinations, emergence delirium; gastric decompression, metoclopramide, head of bed elevation lowers aspiration risk
Vecuronium	0.1-0.15 mg/kg IV	Repeat dosing q 30-45 min with 0.15 mg/kg	Consider cisatracurium at same dosing	Not defined	Established airway presumed; remember to change to assist mode of ventilation

Cardiac and respiratory monitoring are mandatory with all of these agents and an established airway is presumed.

REFERENCES

1. Jacobi J, Gilles LF, Coursin DB, et al. Clinical guidelines for the sustained use of sedatives and analgesics in the critically ill adult. *Crit Care Med* 2002;30:119-141.
2. Saunders KD, Mc Ardle P, and Lang JD. Pain in the intensive care unit: recognition, measurement, management. *Seminars in Respiratory and Critical Care Medicine* 2001;22:127-135.
3. Sessler CN, Grap MJ, Brophy GM. Multidisciplinary management of sedation and analgesia in critical care. *Seminars in Respiratory and Critical Care Medicine* 2001;22:211-225.
4. Desbiens N, Wu A, Broste, et al. Pain and satisfaction with pain control in seriously ill hospitalized adults: findings from the SUPPORT research investigations. *Crit Care Med* 1996;24:1953-1961.
5. Marco CA, Plewa MC, Buderer N, et al. Self-reported pain scores in the emergency department: lack of association with vital signs. *Acad Emerg Med* 2006;13: 974-978.
6. Logan HL, Sheffield D, Lutgendorf S, et al. Predictors of pain during invasive medical procedures. *J Pain* 2002;3:211-217.
7. Aw T, Haas SJ, Liew D, et al. Meta-analysis of cyclooxygenase-2 inhibitors and their effects on blood pressure. *Arch Intern Med* 2005;165:1-7.
8. Peduta VA, Ballabio M, Stefanini S. Efficacy of propacetamol in the treatment of postoperative pain. *Acta Anaesthesiol Scand* 1998;42:293-298.
9. Khan ZP, Ferguson N, Jones RM. Alpha-2 and imidazoline receptor agonists: their pharmacology and therapeutic role. *Anaesthesia* 1999;54:146-165.
10. Visser E, Schug SA. The role of ketamine in pain management. *Biomed & Pharmacother* 2006;60:341-348.
11. Karmakar MK, Ho AM. Acute pain management of patients with multiple fractured ribs. *J Trauma* 2003;54:615-625.
12. Cotton BA. Achieving adequate pain control in patient's with rib fractures. In: Marcucci L et al (eds.)

Avoiding Common ICU Errors. Philadelphia, PA: Lippincott Williams & Wilkins; 2006.

13. McCaig LF, Burt CW. National Hospital Ambulatory Medical Care Survey: 2002 *Emergency Department Summary: Advance Data from Vital and Health Statistics; No. 340*. Hyattsville, MD: National Center for Health Statistics; 2004.

14. Gallagher EJ, Esses D, Lee C, et al. Randomized clinical trial of morphine in acute abdominal pain. *Ann Emerg Med* 2006;48:150-160.

15. Thomas SH, Silen W, Cheema F, et al. Effects of morphine analgesia on diagnostic accuracy in emergency department patients with abdominal pain: a prospective randomized trial. *J Am Coll Surg* 2003;196:18-31.

16. Mitra S, Sinatra RS. Peri-operative management of acute pain in the opioid-dependent patient. *Anesthesiol* 2004;101:212-27.

17. Mehta V, Langford RM. Acute pain management for opioid dependent patients. *Anaesthesia* 2006;61: 269-276.

18. Olorunto WA, Galandiuk S. Managing the spectrum of surgical pain: Acute pain management of the chronic pain patient. *J Am Coll Surg* 2006;202:169-175.

19. Ely EW, Truman B, Shintani A, et al. Monitoring sedation status over time in ICU patients: Reliability and validity of the Richmond Agitation-Sedation Scale (RASS). *JAMA* 2003;289:2983-2991.

20. Sessler CN, Gosnell M, Grap MJ, et al. The Richmond Agitation-Sedation Scale: validity and reliability in adult intensive care unit patients. *Am J Resp Crit Care Med* 2002;166:1338-1344.

21. Kress JP, Pohlman AS, O'Connor MF, et al. Daily interruption of sedative infusions in critically ill patients undergoing mechanical ventilation. *N Engl J Med* 2000;342:1471-1477.

22. Kress JP, Gehlbach B, Lacy M, et al. The long term psychological effects of daily sedative interruption on critically ill patients. *Am J Resp Crit Care Med* 2003;168:1457-1461.

23. Hall RI, Sandham D, Cardinal P, et al. Propofol versus midazolam for ICU sedation : a Canadian multi-center randomized trial. *Chest* 2001;119:1151-1159.

24. Siobal MS, Kallet RH, Kivett VA, et al. Use of dexmedetomidine to facilitate extubation in surgical intensive-care-unit patients who failed previous weaning attempts following prolonged mechanical ventilation: a pilot study. *Respiratory Care* 2006;51:492-496.

25. Cotton BA. *Sedation, Pain, Sleep, and Delirium in the Trauma Patient*, 2005. VUMC, Department of Surgery, Division of Trauma-Surgical Critical Care. http://www.mc.vanderbilt.edu/surgery/trauma/mdprotocolstyle.htm (accessed 10/01/2006).

26. Mantel M, Sterzinger A, Miner J, et al. Management of the acute undifferentiated agitation in the emergency department: a randomized double-blind trial of droperidol, ziprasidone, and midazolam. *Acad Emerg Med* 2005;12:1167-1172.

27. Yildiz A, Sachs GS, Turgay A. Pharmacological management of agitation in emergency settings. *Emerg Med J* 2003;20:339-346.

28. Kemp CD, Johnson JC, Cotton BA. How we die: the impact of non-neurological organ dysfunction following traumatic brain injury. *J Am Coll Surg* 2006;203:S36.

29. Cotton BA, Snodgrass KB, Fleming SB, et al. Beta-blocker exposure is associated with improved survival following severe traumatic brain injury. *J Trauma* 2007.

30. Dissanaike S, Halldorsson A, Frezza EE, et al. An ethanol protocol to prevent alcohol withdrawal syndrome. *J Am Coll Surg* 2006;203:186-191.

31. Dobrydnjov I, Axelsson K, Berggren L, et al. Intrathecal and oral clonidine as prophylaxis for postoperative alcohol withdrawal syndrome: a randomized double-blinded study. *Anesth Analg* 2004;98:738-744.

32. Ely EW, Inouye SK, Bernard GR, et al. Delirium in mechanically ventilated patients: validity and reliability of the confusion assessment method for the intensive care unit (CAM-ICU). *JAMA* 2001; 286:2703-2710.

33. Ely EW, Shintani A, Truman B, et al. Delirium as a predictor of mortality in mechanically ventilated patients in the intensive care unit. *JAMA* 2004;291:1753-1762.

34. http://www.icudelirium.org/delirium/ (accessed 10/01/2006).

35. Pandharipande P, Cotton BA, Shintani A, et al. Prevalence and Risk Factors for Development of Delirium in Surgical and Trauma Intensive Care Unit Patients. *J Trauma* 2008;65: pp 28-35.

36. Kress JP, Pohlman AS, O'Connor MF, et al. Daily interruption of sedative infusions in critically ill patients undergoing mechanical ventilation. *N Engl J Med* 2000;342:471-477.

37. Schwartz TL, Masand PS. The role of atypical antipsychotics in the treatment of delirium. *Psychosomatics* 2002;43:171-174.

38. Freedman NS, Gazendam J, Levan L, et al. Abnormal sleep/wake cycles and the effect of environmental noise on sleep disruption in the intensive care unit. *Am J Respir Crit Care Med* 2001;163:451-457.

39. http://www.epa.gov/topics/noise (accessed 10/01/2006).

40. Peruzzi WT. Sleep in the intensive care unit. *Pharmacotherapy* 2005;25:34-39.

41. Cotton BA. Sleep disturbances in the ICU. In: Marcucci L. et al (eds.) *Avoiding Common ICU Errors*. Philadelphia, PA: Lippincott Williams & Wilkins; 2006.

42. Steens RD, Pouliot Z, Millar TW, et al. Effects of zolpidem and triazolam on sleep and respiration in mild to moderate chronic obstructive pulmonary disease. *Sleep* 1993;16:318-326.

43. Aslan S, Isik E, Cosar B. The effects of mirtazapine on sleep: a placebo controlled, double-blind study in young healthy volunteers. *Sleep* 2002;25:677-679.

44. Maher MJ, Rego SA, Asnis GM. Sleep disturbances in patients with post-traumatic stress disorder: epidemiology, impact and approaches to management. *CNS Drugs* 2006;20:567-590.

Chapter 26

VENTILATOR MANAGEMENT

Nabil Issa, MD, and Lena M. Napolitano, MD

MECHANICAL VENTILATION AND ACUTE RESPIRATORY FAILURE

Mechanical ventilation is the mainstay of therapy for the treatment of acute respiratory failure and airway protection. Acute respiratory failure is severe respiratory dysfunction resulting in abnormalities of oxygenation or CO_2 elimination with the potential risk of impairing the function of other vital organs. Acute respiratory failure is an end result of different diseases, each with its own pathophysiologic processes. Common etiologies of respiratory failure in the emergency surgery patient include abdominal sepsis, atelectasis, pneumonia (aspiration and bacterial), pulmonary edema, traumatic pulmonary contusions and pulmonary embolus (Table 26-1).

Patients with acute respiratory failure usually present with increased work of breathing manifested by tachypnea, use of accessory muscles, paradoxical breathing, hypoxemia, or cyanosis. Effective strategies in mechanical ventilation must ensure alveolar ventilation and reduce the patient's work of breathing without further damaging the lungs by the treatment itself. In patients who require short-term mechanical ventilation for acute respiratory failure due to etiologies with rapid resolution, such as pulmonary edema, many ventilatory strategies are effective.

ALI AND ARDS

Acute lung injury (ALI) and acute respiratory distress syndrome (ARDS) constitute the main reasons for prolonged mechanical ventilation requirements in surgical patients. The American-European Consensus Committee on ARDS in 1994 defined ALI as "a syndrome of inflammation and increased permeability that is associated with a constellation of clinical, radiologic, and physiologic abnormalities that cannot be explained by, but may coexist with, left atrial or pulmonary capillary hypertension."[1]

The clinical criteria for ALI include the following: acute onset of pulmonary failure, hypoxia with a PaO_2/FiO_2 ratio < 300 mm Hg, bilateral chest infiltrates visible on a chest radiograph and a pulmonary artery occlusion pressure of 18 mm Hg and no clinical evidence of increased left atrial pressure. ARDS is defined as a more severe form of ALI with the same criteria, except the ratio of PaO_2/FiO_2 is defined as < 200 mm Hg, regardless of the positive end-expiratory pressure (PEEP) level used on the ventilator.

A recent prospective population-based study documented a crude incidence of acute lung injury of 78.9 per 100,000 person-years with an in-hospital mortality rate of 38.5%. Most importantly, the mortality rate increased with increasing age. These data suggest an estimated 190,600 cases of ALI annually in the United States, which is associated with 74,500 deaths and 3.6 million hospital days.[2] A recent single-center 5-year observational study reported that the rate of ARDS in trauma has decreased significantly, with a > 50% reduction in the incidence of ARDS after injury, despite similar patient demographics and injury severities.[3]

ARDS and ALI are associated with pathologically complex changes in the lung with diffuse alveolar damage. This state includes alveolar flooding and creation of the characteristic hyaline membranes, as a result of injury to the endothelial and epithelial layers of the alveolar-capillary membrane, with resultant loss of the gas exchange and barrier functions of the lung. (Fig. 26-1).

The syndrome is manifested by an early acute *exudative* phase followed by *proliferative* and *fibrotic* phases.[4] The acute inflammatory/exudative state leads to an increased capillary permeability and the accumulation of proteinaceous pulmonary edema, interfering with oxygen diffusion through the alveolar membrane, and leading to hypoxemia. Hypoxia may further aggravate parenchymal lung injury as well the potential of multiorgan dysfunction. Some patients quickly recover from this first phase; many others progress after about a week into the *proliferative* phase, in which the structural elements in the lungs proliferate in response to the initial injury, including development of fibroblasts and the lung tissue appears densely cellular. Some patients will progress to the *fibrotic*

Table 26-1 Common Indications for Mechanical Ventilation

- Apnea or respiratory arrest
- Tachypnea (respiratory rate > 30 breaths per minute) or bradypnea
- Vital capacity < 15 mL/kg, < 1.0 L or < 30% predicted
- Minute ventilation > 10 L/min
- Hypoxemia
- Hypercarbia
- Exacerbation chronic obstructive pulmonary disease
- Respiratory muscle fatigue
- Neuromuscular diseases
- Obtundation or coma
- Acute lung injury (ALI)
- Acute respiratory distress syndrome (ARDS)

phase, which can occur early or late in the course of ARDS. This fibrosing alveolitis is thought to be a maladaptive fibroproliferative repair response to injury to the alveolar components and seems to result from interactions among myofibroblasts, fibroblasts, acute inflammatory cells, and epithelial cells along with cytokines, growth factors, colony stimulating factors and fibrin. The finding of fibrosing alveolitis on lung biopsy correlates with increased mortality from ALI and ARDS.

It is important to remember that these seemingly "diffuse" parenchymal injuries actually have marked regional differences in the degree of inflammation present and thus the degree of mechanical abnormalities that exist.[5] This heterogeneity can have a significant impact on the effects of a particular mechanical ventilation strategy. It is well recognized that delivered gases preferentially go to the pulmonary regions with the highest compliance and the lowest resistance (ie, the more normal regions) rather than to more diseased areas and can produce regional overdistention.[6]

The treatment of ALI and ARDS is supportive care, including optimized mechanical ventilation, nutritional support, maintenance of optimal fluid balance, source control and treatment of sepsis, and prevention of intervening medical complications. Paramount in the support of the patient with severe respiratory failure and ALI/ARDS is the use of mechanical ventilatory support.

Mechanical ventilatory support can also be injurious and lead to additional lung injury, ie, ventilator-induced lung injury, when used at the extremes of pulmonary physiology.[7] There are a number of mechanisms that can lead to the development of ventilator induced lung injury, including barotrauma, diffuse alveolar injury resulting from overdistention (volutrauma), injury caused by repeated cycles of recruitment/derecruitment (atelectrauma), and the most subtle form of injury related to the release of local mediators in the lung (biotrauma).[8]

Clinical studies in which a single variable is manipulated and tested for its effect on outcome in severe respiratory failure have had disappointing results, with a few rare exceptions. It has become apparent that

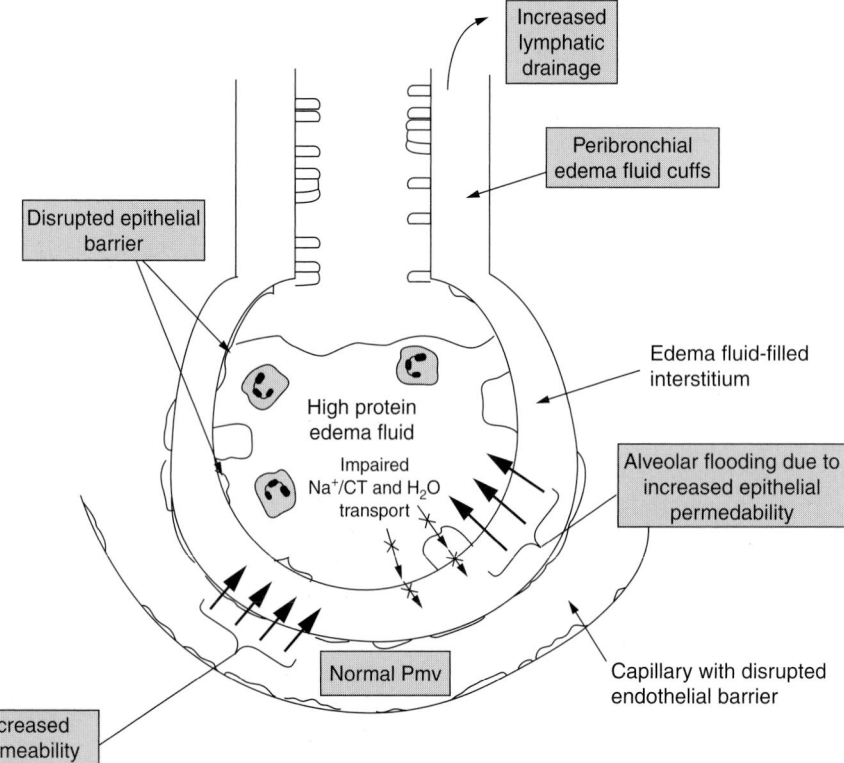

Figure 26-1 *Pathophysiology of acute lung injury and the acute respiratory distress syndrome. From Ware LB. Pathophysiology of acute lung injury and the acute respiratory distress syndrome. Semin Respir Crit Care Med 2006; 27(4): 337-349.*

successful advances in the treatment of severe respiratory failure will involve the implementation of algorithms or strategies that take advantage of multiple techniques to provide effective mechanical ventilatory support, while minimizing ventilator-induced lung injury and improving oxygenation/ventilation.

TRADITIONAL MECHANICAL VENTILATION STRATEGIES

In patients with acute respiratory failure, controlled mechanical ventilation is generally used in the initial phase to ensure adequate alveolar ventilation, arterial oxygenation and to reduce work of breathing without causing further damage to the lung, but more recent studies suggest that early conversion to spontaneous breathing during mechanical ventilation, and partial ventilator support modes, may be beneficial and may promote alveolar recruitment.

Many different strategies of positive-pressure ventilation are available; these are based on various permutations of triggered volume-cycled and pressure-cycled ventilations. Ventilatory strategies have been devised for different disease processes to protect pulmonary parenchyma while maintaining adequate gas exchange. Pressure and volume control refer to the type of breath delivered, not the mode of ventilation. The pressure- or volume-cycled breaths can be delivered via three traditional modes of mechanical ventilation, which include controlled (CMV), assist-controlled (AC) or synchronized intermittent mandatory ventilation (SIMV).

VOLUME-CYCLED (VOLUME CONTROL, VC)

Inhalation proceeds until a set tidal volume (TV) is delivered and is followed by passive exhalation. A feature is that gas is delivered with a constant inspiratory flow pattern, resulting in peak pressures applied to the airways higher than that required for lung distension (plateau pressure). Because the volume delivered is constant, applied airway pressures vary with changing pulmonary compliance (plateau pressure) and airway resistance (peak pressure). A major disadvantage is that high airway pressures may be generated, potentially resulting in barotrauma.

PRESSURE-CYCLED (PRESSURE CONTROL, PC)

A set peak inspiratory pressure (PIP) is applied and the pressure difference between the ventilator and the lungs results in inflation until the peak pressure is attained, and passive exhalation follows. The delivered volume with each respiration is dependent on the pulmonary and thoracic compliance. A theoretical advantage of pressure-cycled breaths is a decelerating inspiratory flow pattern, in which inspiratory flow tapers off as the lung inflates. This usually results in a more homogeneous gas distribution throughout the lungs. A major disadvantage is that dynamic changes in

pulmonary mechanics may result in varying tidal volumes, and with decreased pulmonary compliance rapid reduction in tidal volume and minute ventilation may precipitate acute respiratory acidosis. This necessitates close monitoring of minute ventilation, careful setting of appropriate alarms, and limits the usefulness of this mode in many emergency department patients. Monitoring for intrinsic- or auto-PEEP is also necessary (Fig. 26-2).

PRESSURE-CYCLED (PRESSURE REGULATED VOLUME CONTROL, PRVC)

The ventilator guarantees that the patient will receive the set tidal volume in a pressure-control breath. Constant pressure is applied throughout inspiration (like pressure control), but the ventilator adjusts pressure from breath to breath, as the patient's airway resistance and respiratory system compliance changes, in order to deliver the set tidal volume.

Traditional modes of mechanical ventilation include the following.

Controlled Mechanical Ventilation Mode (CMV)

The ventilator guarantees that the patient will receive the set minimum number of breaths and can be used to achieve normocapnic ventilation. Prolonged CMV results in diaphragmatic inactivity and promotes

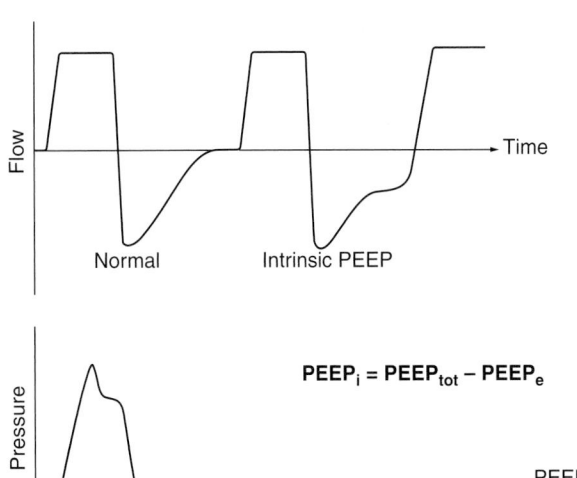

Figure 26-2 *Intrinsic- or Auto-PEEP. Examination of the flow-time curve from the ventilator gives an indication that there is intrinsic PEEP but does not give an indication of the magnitude. The patient does not need to be apneic. A quantitative measurement of intrinsic PEEP can be obtained in an apneic patient by using the expiratory pause hold control on the ventilator. This allows equilibration of pressures between the alveoli and the ventilator allowing the total PEEP to be measured. The value for total PEEP can be read from the PEEP display. Intrinsic PEEP = Total PEEP − Set PEEP.*

atrophy and contractile dysfunction in this important inspiratory muscle.

Assist-Control Ventilation Mode (A/C)

The ventilator guarantees that the patient will receive the set minimum number of breaths, although the patient is able to demand (trigger) more. The ventilator delivers preset breaths in coordination with the respiratory effort of the patient. With each inspiratory effort, the ventilator delivers a full assisted tidal volume. Spontaneous breathing independent of the ventilator between A/C breaths is allowed. A/C ventilation, is a full support mode in that the ventilator performs most, if not all, of the work of breathing. These modes are beneficial for patients who require high minute ventilation. Full ventilatory support reduces oxygen consumption and CO_2 production of the respiratory muscles. A potential drawback of A/C ventilation in the patient with obstructive airway disease is worsening of air trapping and breath stacking.

Synchronous Intermittent Mandatory Ventilation Mode (SIMV)

The ventilator delivers preset breaths in coordination with the respiratory effort of the patient. Spontaneous breathing is allowed between breaths, and is usually assisted with pressure support. Synchronization attempts to limit barotrauma that may occur with IMV when a preset breath is delivered to a patient who is already maximally inhaled (breath stacking) or is forcefully exhaling.

Pressure Support Ventilation (PSV)

For the spontaneously breathing patient, pressure support ventilation (PSV) has been advocated to limit barotrauma and to decrease the work of breathing. Pressure support differs from A/C and IMV in that a level of support pressure is set (not TV) to assist every spontaneous effort. Airway pressure support is maintained until the patient's inspiratory flow falls below a certain cutoff (eg, 25% of peak flow). With some ventilators, there is the ability to set a backup IMV rate should spontaneous respirations cease.

The variables that can be adjusted for mechanical ventilation beside the chosen mode of ventilation are the tidal volume (Vt), respiratory rate (RR), supplemental oxygen (FiO_2), inspiration/expiration ratio (I:E), inspiratory flow rate, pressure support (PS), positive end-expiratory pressure (PEEP), trigger sensitivity (how easy it is for the patient to trigger the ventilator to deliver a breath), rise time (determines speed of rise of flow or pressure in each breath), and, finally, the temperature and humidity of inspired air.

Oxygen uptake via the lungs is dependent on both PaO_2 (which can be manipulated by alterations in inspired oxygen concentration and alveolar pressure) and ventilation-perfusion matching (which can be optimized by reopening collapsed alveoli, thereby reducing intrapulmonary shunting). To improve oxygenation, three main strategies are utilized: (1) increase FiO_2; (2) increase mean alveolar pressure by increasing mean airway pressure (increase PEEP or increase I:E ration, increase inspiratory time); and (3) alveolar recruitment with PEEP. Carbon dioxide elimination via the lungs is largely dependent on alveolar ventilation [alveolar ventilation = respiratory rate x (tidal volume – dead space)]. Methods to improve CO_2 elimination include increasing minute ventilation by increased in tidal volume or respiratory rate.

SYSTEMIC EFFECTS OF MECHANICAL VENTILATION

PULMONARY EFFECTS

Barotrauma may result in pulmonary interstitial emphysema, pneumomediastinum, pneumoperitoneum, pneumothorax, and/or tension pneumothorax. Alveolar cellular dysfunction occurs with high airway pressures. The resultant surfactant depletion leads to atelectasis, which requires further increases in airway pressure to maintain lung volumes. High-inspired concentrations of oxygen (fraction of inspired oxygen, $FiO_2 > 0.5$) result in free-radical formation and secondary cellular damage. These same high concentrations of oxygen can lead to alveolar nitrogen washout and secondary absorption atelectasis.

CARDIOVASCULAR EFFECTS

The heart, great vessels, and pulmonary vasculature reside within the thoracic cavity and are subject to the increased intrathoracic pressures associated with mechanical ventilation. The result is a decrease in cardiac output due to decreased venous return to the right heart, right ventricular dysfunction, and altered left ventricular distensibility. The decreased cardiac output from reduction in right ventricular preload is more pronounced in the hypovolemic patient and those with a low ejection fraction.

RENAL, HEPATIC, AND GASTROINTESTINAL EFFECTS

Positive-pressure ventilation is responsible for an overall decline in renal function with decreased urine volume and sodium excretion. Hepatic function is adversely affected by decreased cardiac output, increased hepatic vascular resistance, and elevated bile duct pressure. The gastric mucosa does not have autoregulatory capability. Thus, mucosal ischemia and secondary bleeding may result from decreased cardiac output and increased gastric venous pressure.

MECHANICAL VENTILATION STRATEGIES FOR ALI AND ARDS

A number of recent advances have been made in development of protective mechanical ventilation strategies for patients with severe respiratory failure, including ALI and ARDS.[9]

LOW TIDAL VOLUME VENTILATION

The use of high tidal volumes or high ventilator pressures in an attempt to ventilate the patient with worsening respiratory failure can result in compromise of cardiopulmonary function and the development of ventilator induced lung injury. There is increasing evidence that alveolar stretch induced by large inspired tidal volumes plays a significant role in the development of ventilator induced lung injury through the incitement of an exaggerated alveolar inflammatory response, which is associated with systemic inflammation as well.[10]

In ARDS, large proportions of the lung alveoli become consolidated and are not available for gas exchange. The resulting available lung units are small in number and give the patient a functional lung that is analogous to a "baby lung" in size. Attempting to force adult magnitude tidal volume breaths into this "baby lung" can result in overdistention of the remaining open alveoli with high distending pressures and significant lung injury may happen due to this alveolar over distention. This can result in the clinical presentation of pneumothorax, pneumomediastinum, pneumoperitoneum, subcutaneous emphysema, and air embolism. It is estimated that barotraumas happens in 13% of ARDS patients and results in a mortality of < 2% of the patients.[11,12] High plateau and peak pressures have been proven to be detrimental to lung function in animal models.[13,14] Only high levels of PEEP have been associated with an increased risk of barotraumas, whereas peak, mean, and plateau pressure have not.[15]

Human and animal studies, have demonstrated a significant association of multiple cytokines and chemokines during ventilator induced or ventilator associated lung injury. Furthermore, proof of concept studies with animal models have demonstrated specific cytokines and chemokines mediating the leukocyte activation and recruitment during ventilator associated lung injury and these cytokines/chemokines may perpetuate ALI/ARDS and MODS (Fig. 26-3).[16] This was further illustrated during the ARDS-Network study. Plasma levels of two pro-inflammatory cytokines, interleukin (IL)-8 and IL-6, and one regulatory cytokine, IL-10, were measured at baseline and 3 days. These markers were chosen because they were known to be increased in ALI, in previous smaller clinical trials they were variably associated with mortality, and increasing evidence suggested they were likely to be affected by mechanical ventilation. In a large, well-characterized population randomized to a ventilation strategy using tidal volumes of 6 or 12 mL/kg of predicted body weight. By day 3, the 6 mL/kg strategy was associated with a greater decrease in interleukin-6 and interleukin-8 levels. There was a 26% reduction in interleukin-6 (95% confidence interval, 12%-37%) and a 12% reduction in interleukin-8 (95% confidence interval, 1%-23%) in the 6 mL/kg group compared with the 12 mL/kg group (Table 26-2.).

The ARDS-Network trial conclusively demonstrated the clinical value of a low tidal volume versus high tidal volume approach in the mechanical ventilatory support of patients with sever respiratory failure secondary to ARDS.[17] This landmark trial was a multicenter,

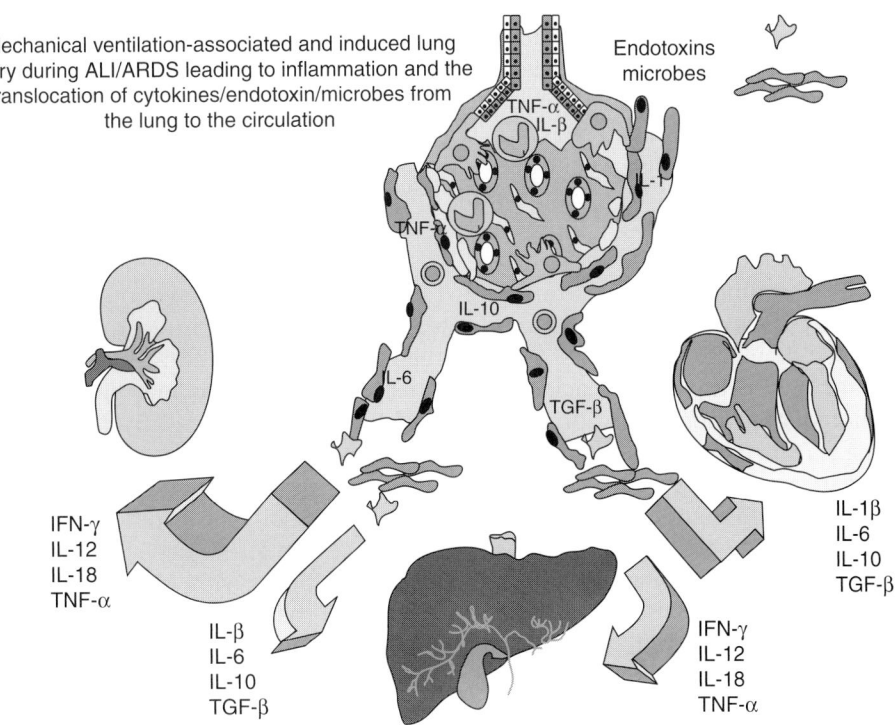

Figure 26-3 *Pathogenesis of ventilator-associated and ventilator-induced lung injury. From Belperio JA, Keane MP, Lynch JP III, Strieter RM. The role of cytokines during the pathogenesis of ventilator-associated and ventilator-induced lung injury. Semin Respir Crit Care Med 2006;27(4):350-364.*

Table 26-2   Low vs High Tidal Volume Strategy and Cytokine Levels

Measurement	6 mL/kg		12 mL/kg		Total	
	n	Median (IQR)	n	Median (IQR)	n	Median (IQR)
IL-6, pg/mL						
Day 0	393	264 (109-766)	388	284 (109-1069)	781	273 (109-899)
Day 3	364	96 (46-213)	354	126 (49-388)	718	104 (47-291)
IL-8, pg/mL						
Day 0	393	43 (0-93)	387	41 (0-114)	780	42 (0-101)
Day 3	364	32 (0-73)	354	35 (0-83)	718	34 (0-77)
IL-10, pg/mL						
Day 0	302	18 (0-57)	291	24 (0-71)	593	19 (0-63)
Day 3	278	1 (0-30)	266	1 (0-36)	544	1 (0-32)

From: Parsons PE, Eisner MD, Thompson BT, et al. AP. NHLBI Acute Respiratory Distress Syndrome Clinical Trials Network. Lower tidal volume ventilation and plasma cytokine markers of inflammation in patients with acute lung injury. *Crit Care Med* 2005;33(1):1-6; discussion 230-232.

randomized, controlled study that compared a tidal volume of 6 mL/kg ideal body weight (and a plateau pressure < 30 cm H_2O) with a tidal volume of 12 mL/kg ideal body weight (and a plateau pressure < 50 cm H_2O). The trial was stopped after the fourth interim analysis when a total of 861 patients were enrolled and the data analysis showed a significantly lower mortality, 31% versus 40%; $p = .007$, in the low tidal volume group. The number of ventilator-free days in the first 28 days was significantly higher in the group treated with low tidal volumes (12+/−11 versus 10+/−11; $p = .007$) as was the number of days without failure of non-pulmonary organs or systems (15+/−11 vs 12+/−11; $p = .006$). The incidence of barotraumas was similar in the two groups, at 10% to 11%. A secondary analysis of a subgroup from this randomized trial confirmed that intrinsic PEEP was significantly higher in patients randomized to the 6 mL/kg protocol group, but the difference of median intrinsic PEEP between the groups was < 1 cm H_2O, and it is unlikely that this was clinically important.[18]

There continues to be some barriers to wider implementation of the low tidal volume ventilation strategy, particularly with regard to patient discomfort and tachypnea as well as concerns about hypercapnia, acidosis, and hypoxemia. In a recent study low tidal volume ventilation strategy was found not to increase sedation use.[19] The recent publication of the *Guidelines for Mechanical Ventilation of the Trauma Patient* from the participants of the "Inflammation and host Response to Injury Large Scale Collaborative Research Program" is an important step forward in standardizing clinical management in trauma patients to ensure that a low tidal volume, lung-protective strategy is used for the ventilation of patients who meet the criteria for ALI and ARDS. This statement also provides guidelines for the use of PEEP in patients with ALI and guidelines to ensure that discontinuation of mechanical ventilation and that extubation occurs at the earliest possible time[20] (Fig. 26-4).

PERMISSIVE HYPERCAPNIA

Mechanical ventilatory strategies to reduce tidal volumes and, thereby, reduce volutrauma can result in an inadequate lung ventilation. Permissive hypercapnia is a consequence of a ventilator strategy that accepts deliberate hypoventilation in an effort to reduce pulmonary over distention and high transalveolar pressures within the compliant noncollapsed lung in patients with ARDS. This technique induces the side effect of hypercarbia and respiratory acidosis, which are managed medically. The tidal volume is gradually reduced to allow a progressive rise in the $PaCO_2$, not to exceed 10 mm Hg/h, to a maximum of 80-100 mm Hg. This is done to keep the static peak airway pressure < 40 cm H_2O and maintain the arterial oxygenation saturation (SaO_2) > 90%, while tolerating a pH as low as 7.15 before initiating administration of intravenous buffering agents.[21] Buffering agents such as $NaHCO_3$ (50 mEq/L) or THAM (36 g/L, tromethamine) can be administered as a continuous intravenous infusion if the arterial pH falls less than 7.15 in asthma patients or 7.28 in patients at risk for simultaneous metabolic acidosis.[22] Higher levels of sedation may be required to offset the respiratory drive induced by hypercapnia and to avoid patient discomfort. The effects of hypercapnia may worsen intracranial pressure, and this technique should potentially be avoided in trauma patients with evidence of brain injury.

Mortality in adult patients with ARDS was reduced to 26%, compared with the expected mortality of 53% based on Acute Physiology and Chronic Health Evaluation II scores, when low tidal volume, pressure-limited ventilation with permissive hypercapnia was

[i] **Mechanical Ventilation Protocol-Inflammation and the Host Response to Injury**
In patients with ALI or established ARDS (PaO_2/FiO_2 300 or PaO_2/FiO_2 200, respectively, with bilateral pulmonary infiltrates) aim for the following within 24 hours of meeting criteria:
(1) Initial tidal volumes may be set at 8 mL/kg predicted body weight (PBW); tidal volumes should be reduced by 1 mL/kg at intervals of < 2 hours until the tidal volume = 6 mL/kg. Tidal volume calculations are based on predicted body weight as follows:
For Males: PBW (kg) = 50 + 2.3 {height (inches) − 60}
For Females: PBW (kg) = 45.5 + 2.3 {height (inches) − 60}
(2) PaO_2 55–80 mm Hg or SpO_2 88%–95% FiO_2/PEEP ratio should be 5 and PEEP must be 35 cm H_2O
(3) Arterial pH 7.25–7.45 with RR < 35 and $PaCO_2$ 25. HCO_3 infusion may be given if necessary. If pH < 7.15 then Vt may be increased by 1 mL/kg to pH 7.15 and target plateau pressures (see below) may be exceeded.
(4) Plateau pressures (PP) 30 cm H_2O reduce Vt to no less than 4 mL/kg.
If Vt < 6 mL/kg and PP < 25 then increase Vt until PP = 25–30 or Vt = 6 mL/kg.
Patients not meeting ALI/ARDS criteria can be ventilated using the mode, rate, and tidal volume chosen at the treating physician's discretion.
[ii] **Patients should undergo a daily assessment of their readiness for a spontaneous breathing trial (SBT):**
(a) Resolution or stabilization of the underlying disease process
(b) No residual effects of neuromuscular blockade
(c) Exhibiting respiratory efforts
(d) Hemodynamically stable
(e) FiO_2 0.5 and PEEP 8 cm H_2O
(f) $PaO2$ > 70 mm Hg
(g) Ve < 15 L/min
(h) Arterial pH between 7.30–7.50
(i) ICP < 20 cm H_2O. If not ready for an SBT, then return to a comfortable, nonfatiguing mode of ventilator support and reassess daily.
If ready, then the patient should receive **a trial of spontaneous breathing (SBT) on CPAP for 30–90 minutes.**
Criteria for failure of a SBT:
(a) RR > 35 for 5 min
(b) SpO_2 < 90% for 30 seconds
(c) HR > 140 or increase or decrease of 20% from baseline
(d) SBP > 180 mm Hg or < 90 mm Hg
(e) Sustained evidence of respiratory distress
(f) Cardiac instability or dysrhythmias;
(g) Arterial pH 7.32
(h) ICP 20 cm H_2O.
If any criteria are met, the CPAP trial is terminated and patient returned to a nonfatiguing mode of support and rested overnight. Repeat CPAP in the morning.
If patient completes CPAP trial, the following criteria should be assessed to determine readiness for extubation and patient extubated if possible:
(a) Does not require suctioning more than Q 4 hours
(b) Good spontaneous cough
(c) Endotracheal tube cuff leak
(d) No recent upper airway obstruction or stridor
(e) No recent reintubation for bronchial hygiene

Figure 26-4 *Pocket card summary of mechanical ventilation of the trauma patient. ALI, acute lung injury, ARDS, acute respiratory distress syndrome; PEEP, positive end-expiratory pressure; RR, relative risk; Vt, tidal volume; Ve, minute volume or expired volume per min; ICP, intracranial pressure; CPAP, continuous positive airway pressure; Q, every. Adapted from Nathens AB, Johnson JL, Minei JP, et al. Inflammation and the Host Response to Injury Investigators. Inflammation and the Host Response to Injury, a large-scale collaborative project: Patient-Oriented Research Core—standard operating procedures for clinical care. I. Guidelines for mechanical ventilation of the trauma patient. J Trauma 2005;59(3):764-769.*

prospectively applied to 64 patients with ARDS.[23] Most recently, a secondary analysis of the ARDS Network low tidal volume multicenter trial (n = 861) documented that hypercapneic acidosis was associated with a reduced 28-day mortality (adjusted odds ratio, 0.14; 95% CI, 0.03– 0.70; *p*= .016) in the 12 mL/kg predicted body weight tidal volume group after controlling for comorbidities and severity of lung injury, but no difference was identified in the 6 mL/kg tidal volume group.[24] These results are consistent with a protective effect of hypercapneic acidosis against ventilator-induced lung injury that was not found when the further ongoing injury was reduced by 6 mL/kg predicted body weight tidal volumes.

OPEN LUNG STRATEGY

Depletion of surfactant and low levels of PEEP can lead to cyclic atelectasis with repeated collapse and opening of those few functional alveoli that remain in severe ARDS. This cycling of alveoli opening and closing can lead to activation of neutrophils, promote additional lung injury, and lead to loss of functional residual lung capacity (FRC). One of the more common means of recruiting collapsed alveoli and increasing FRC is to use increased levels of PEEP. By not allowing all the pressure in the lung to escape during exhalation, alveoli that are unstable and prone to collapse cannot do so. This technique can be thought of as holding the lung partially open so that the next breath is not starting from total collapse in a noncompliant lung.

The optimal level of PEEP to use is difficult to determine, but emerging evidence suggests that maximum recruitment and maintenance of lung volume occurs when the PEEP is set at a level just above the lower inflection point (P_{flex}) on the pressure-volume curve in a patient with ARDS.[25,26] A single breath compliance curve with tidal volume plotted against static airway pressure will demonstrate two inflection points (Fig. 26-5). The lower one represents the theoretical critical opening pressure of most alveoli available for recruitment, and the upper point represents the loss of elastic properties on the lung secondary to over distention. Setting the PEEP slightly higher than the Pflex, will result in maintenance of alveolar distention throughout the ventilatory cycle.

The anticipated end result is an increase in the recruitment of functional residual capacity, decreased intrapulmonary shunting, and improved arterial blood oxygenation. Combining the use of low-volume tidal volume strategies, with the application of PEEP at levels above the lower inflection point, and permissive hypercapnia has been termed the "open-lung approach." Amato et al describe a technique in which PEEP is maintained above the lower inflection point of the pressure-volume curve, tidal volume is kept at < 6 mL/kg, static peak pressure is < 40 cm H_2O, permissive hypercapnia is allowed, and the stepwise use of pressure limited modes of ventilation are used. Using this technique in a prospective study vs conventional mechanical ventilation in ARDS yielded improved survival at 28 days (62% vs 29%; p = .001), a higher rate of weaning from mechanical ventilation, and a lower rate of barotraumas in the open-lung or protective strategy group. There was no difference in the overall hospital mortality between groups, and the high 28-day mortality in the conventional mechanical ventilatory group raises concern about the overall impact of this strategy.[27]

The extent to which tidal volumes and inspiratory airway pressures should be reduced to optimize clinical outcomes is a controversial topic. A recent study examined all patients with plateau pressures (P_{plat}) in the ARDS network lower tidal volume trial (Fig. 26-6)[28] demonstrates the relationship of mortality versus plateau pressure for all patients and shows decreasing mortality as day 1 P_{plat} declines from high to low levels. It does not reveal a safe P_{plat} threshold within the range of day 1 P_{plat} levels measured in patients with ALI/ARDS. Bivariate analysis also demonstrated that lower P_{plat} quartiles were associated with reduced mortality when compared with higher P_{plat} quartiles (p = .039) (Fig. 26-7). The ARDS Network volume and pressure limited strategy used a tidal volume goal of

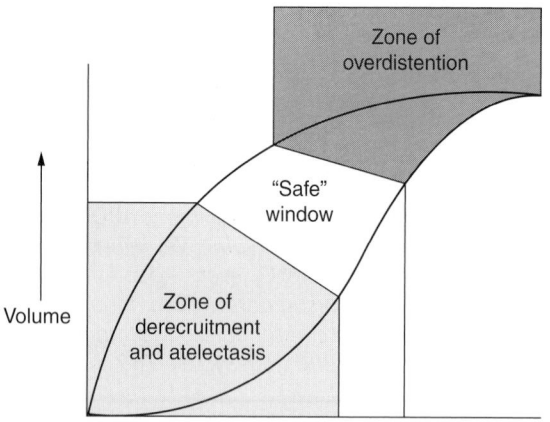

Figure 26-5 *Pressure-volume curve of a moderately diseased lung, such as one with adult acute respiratory distress syndrome. Two hazard zones exist: overdistention and derecruitment and atelectasis. High end-expiratory pressures and small tidal volumes are needed to stay in the "Safe" window. High-frequency oscillatory ventilation may have a larger margin of safety in keeping the lung open within the desired target range of alveolar overdistention. Reprinted with permission from Imai Y, Slutsky AS. High-frequency oscillatory ventilation and ventilator-induced lung injury. Crit Care Med 2005;33(3 Suppl):S129-S134.*

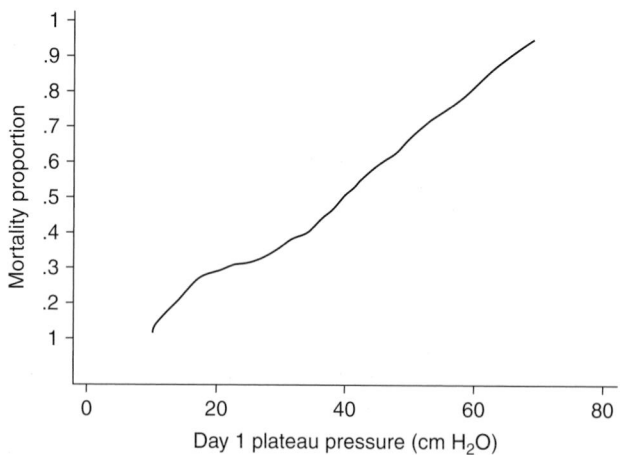

Figure 26-6 *Relationship between mortality and day 1 plateau pressures. Reprinted with permission from Hager et al. Tidal volume reduction in patients with acute lung injury when plateau pressures are not high. Am J Respir Crit Care Med 2005;172(10):1241-1245.*

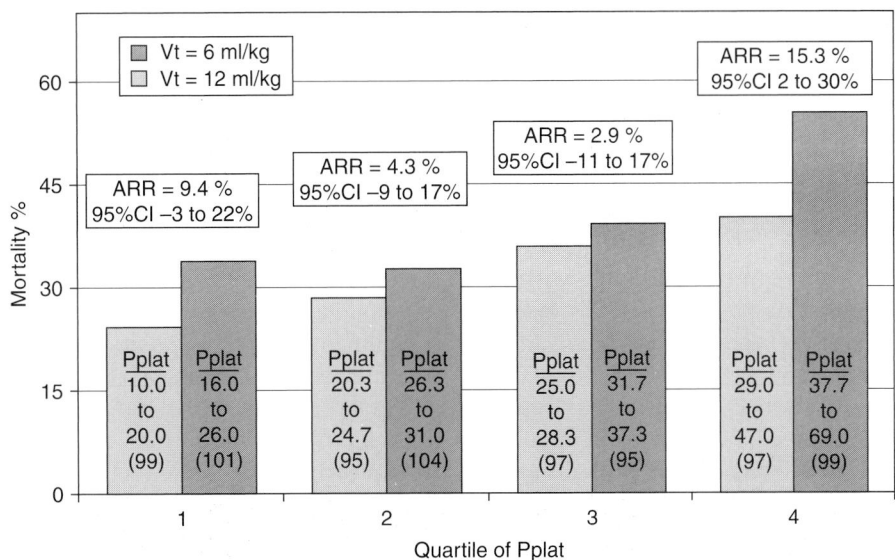

Figure 26-7 *Mortality differences based on day 1 plateau airway pressures. Vt, tidal volume; ARR, absolute risk reduction; CI, confidence interval; Pplat, plateau pressure. Reprinted with permission from Hager et al [27]* [1]*Amato MB, Barbas CS, Mederios DM, et al: Effect of a protective-ventilation strategy on mortality in the acute respiratory distress syndrome.* N Engl J Med *1998; 338:347-354.*

6 mL/kg per predicted body weight, and with this approach, mean P_{plat} was approximately 25 cm H_2O. This additional analysis does not substantiate the widespread belief that tidal volume reduction is without benefit when P_{plat} is already < 30-35 cm H_2O.

AIRWAY PRESSURE RELEASE VENTILATION

Airway pressure release ventilation (APRV) is a pressure-limited, time-cycled mode of mechanical ventilation that allows a patient unrestricted spontaneous breathing during the application of continuous positive airway pressure. It is an alternative approach to open-lung ventilation. Although recruitment maneuvers may be effective in improving gas exchange and compliance, these effects may not be sustained and may require repeated maneuvers. APRV may be viewed as a nearly continuous recruitment maneuver, with high-pressure providing 80% to 95% of the cycle time, creating a stabilized open lung while facilitating spontaneous breathing. The ventilator maintains a high-pressure setting for the bulk of the respiratory cycle, which is followed by a periodic release to a low pressure setting analogous to PEEP.[29]

Patients who are not receiving neuromuscular blockade can spontaneously breathe on top of this form of continuous positive airway pressure, which is periodically lowered to allow ventilation and CO_2 clearance. The spontaneous breathing allowed during APRV can decrease intrathoracic pressure, as inspiration by the patient results in periodic cycles of negative pressure from the diaphragm and chest wall excursion. APRV is no different from pressure-controlled inverse ratio mechanical ventilation in patients receiving neuromuscular blockade.

HIGH-FREQUENCY OSCILLATORY VENTILATION

High-frequency oscillatory ventilation (HFOV) involves the use of a piston pump-driven diaphragm to deliver small tidal volumes at frequencies between 3 and 15 Hz. HFOV is unique in that expiration is active in addition to inspiration, with this component created by the backward movement of the diaphragm, which generates negative pressure. Oxygenation is manipulated by adjusting mean airway pressure, which controls lung inflation in a manner similar to the use of PEEP in conventional mechanical ventilation (CMV). Changing the tidal volume also known as the amplitude or power controls ventilation and carbon dioxide elimination.

In addition to the FIO2, there are only a total of four variables to manipulate when using HFOV:

1. Mean airway pressure is initiated at 1-2 cm H_2O higher than for CMV in premature newborns, 2-4 cm H_2O higher than CMV in full-term newborns and children, and 5 cm H_2O higher than CMV in adults.
2. Frequency (Hz) is set at 12 Hz in premature infants and 5-10 Hz in all others. Lowering the frequency will result in an increase in the tidal volume and a decrease in the $PaCO_2$.
3. Inspiratory time is usually set at 33%, but it may be lengthened to increase the tidal volume.
4. Amplitude or power is set to achieve appropriate chest wall movement and adequate CO_2 elimination. HFOV was initially used as a rescue strategy when other modes of mechanical ventilation had failed.[30,31]

The MOAT (Multicenter Oscillatory Ventilation for Acute Respiratory Distress Syndrome Trial) compared HFOV with a pressure-controlled ventilation strategy (n = 148). HFOV was associated with early (< 16 hrs) improvement in PaO_2/FiO_2 compared with the conventional ventilation group ($p = .008$); however, this difference did not persist beyond 24 hours. The oxygenation index decreased similarly during the first 72 hours in both groups. Thirty-day mortality was 37% in the HFOV group and was 52% in the conventional ventilation group ($p = .1$). No differences were identified in the percentage of patients alive without mechanical ventilation at day 30 (36% HFOV vs 31% conventional; $p = .7$). There were no significant differences in hemodynamic variables, oxygenation or ventilation failure, barotrauma, or mucus plugging between treatment groups. The authors concluded that HFOV is a safe and effective mode of ventilation for the treatment of ARDS in adults.[32]

A similar multicenter randomized trial (n = 61) comparing HFOV with conventional ventilation in adult ARDS was conducted in Europe but was stopped prematurely because of a low inclusion. A review of the clinical experience with HFOV in Toronto (n = 156) in severe ARDS patients (mean PaO_2/FiO_2 ratio, 91+/−48 mm Hg) concluded that HFOV had beneficial effects on oxygenation and may be an effective rescue therapy for adults with severe hypoxemia and that the early institution of HFOV may be advantageous.[33]

HFOV is, in theory, the ideal "lung protective" method, and may have a larger margin of safety in keeping the lung open within the desired target range of alveolar over distention in heterogeneously injured ARDS lungs, but outcome benefits have not yet been proven in a large prospective, randomized trial.[34] Because it has been suggested that the early initiation of HFOV in patients with severe ARDS may be important to successful outcomes, the active identification of patients with ARDS who may be potential candidates for HFOV is important. Although the exact severity threshold at which to initiate a trial of HFOV remains unclear, an emerging approach includes the following severity criteria:[35]

■ $FiO_2 > 0.60$ and $SpO_2 < 88\%$ on CMV with PEEP > 15 cm H_2O, or
■ Plateau pressures > 30 cm H_2O, or
■ Mean airway pressure 24 cm H_2O, or
■ Airway pressure release ventilation with high pressure 35 cm H_2O.

RECRUITMENT STRATEGIES

Alveolar recruitment is one of the primary goals of respiratory therapy for ALI and ARDS. It is aimed at improving pulmonary gas exchange, preventing ventilator-induced lung injury, atelectasis, and "atelectrauma."[36] PEEP may decrease ventilator-induced lung injury by keeping lung regions open that otherwise would be collapsed. Recruitment maneuvers can be used to increase alveolar functional residual capacity.[37] A recent study documented that the percentage of

potentially recruitable lung (mean +/−, SD 13 +/−11) varied widely in patients with ALI or ARDS and that, on average, 24% of the lung could not be recruited. Furthermore, patients with a higher percentage of potentially recruitable lung (which was strongly associated with a favorable response to PEEP) had poorer oxygenation and higher rates of death than patients with a lower percentage of potentially recruitable lung.[38]

Effective recruitment maneuvers and sustained levels of PEEP to avoid derecruitment may obviate the need for the prone position in ARDS for alveolar recruitment.[39] A large amount of experimental data suggests that alveolar recruitment is beneficial in ALI and ARDS. However, there is no single clinical study that clearly proves the effectiveness of alveolar recruitment for lung protection and survival. The combination of recruitment maneuvers (initial cycle of up to three sustained inflation recruitment maneuvers of 40 cm H_2O for 40 seconds) and HFOV in a prospective, multicenter clinical trial "Treatment with Oscillation and an Open Lung Strategy"-TOOLS Trial resulted in a rapid and durable improvement in oxygenation and was well-tolerated, feasible, and physiologically sound.[40]

PRONE POSITIONING

Changes in patient positioning can have a dramatic effect on oxygenation and ventilation in severe ARDS. Changing the patient position to prone or a steep lateral decubitus position can improve the distribution of perfusion to ventilated lung regions, decreasing intrapulmonary shunt and improving oxygenation.[41] The use of intermittent prone positioning can significantly improve oxygenation in 60% to 70% of patients.[42,43]

A multicenter randomized trial of conventional treatment vs placing patients in a prone position for 6 or more hours daily for 10 days was conducted on patients 16 years of age or more with ALI or ARDS.[44] No differences in mortality or complications were identified for the prone versus conventional positioning group at any time point during the study, with up to 6 months follow-up. The mean increase in the PaO_2/FIO_2 ratio was greater in the prone than supine group (63 +/− 67 vs 45 +/− 68; $p = .02$). Of note is that the mean PaO_2 of 85-88 mm Hg and mean PaO_2/FiO_2 ratio of 125:129 are still high for patients with severe ARDS, and, therefore, these patients may not have been likely to benefit considerably by the prone intervention with regard to mortality. A retrospective analysis of patients in the pronation arm of this study revealed that ALI/ARDS patients who responded to prone positioning with a reduction in their $PaCO_2$ 1 mm Hg showed an increase in survival at 28 days with a decrease in the mortality rate from 52% to 35%.[45]

A recent multicenter, randomized, controlled clinical trial of supine vs. prone positioning in 102 pediatric patients failed to demonstrate a significant difference in the main outcome measure, which was ventilator-free days to day 28. There were also no differences in the secondary endpoints study conducted including proportion alive and ventilator free on day 28, mortality, the time to recovery from lung injury, organ failure free days, and functional health.[46]

A prospective, randomized study (n = 136), with guidelines established for ventilator settings and weaning, examined the efficacy of the prolonged prone position (continuous prone position for 20 hours daily) in severe ARDS patients with 48 hours of tracheal intubation. Multivariate analysis documented that randomization to the supine position was an independent risk factor for mortality (odds ratio, 2.53; p = .03). These authors concluded that prone ventilation is feasible and safe and may reduce mortality in patients with severe ARDS when it is initiated early and applied for most of the day.[47]

Prone positioning is labor-intensive with associated risks, including inadvertent extubation. It also requires the use of appropriate cushioning of the dependent portions of the body to avoid pressure ulcerations. However, the technique can be performed safely by a trained and dedicated nursing staff, who are aware of its potential benefits in critically ill patients with severe pulmonary failure in conjunction with judicious use by ICU physicians. In our experience, prone positioning is a useful tool for treatment of hypoxemia, can prevent the need for extracorporeal life support (ECLS), and is used for lung recruitment in patients undergoing ECLS. We do not, however, use prone positioning until the PaO_2/FiO_2 ratio is significantly < 100. One technique involves alternating prone with supine positioning every 6 hours. Patients will often experience an initial worsening in their respiratory status with each change in position, but this passes quickly in the first 15-30 minutes to eventual improvement in oxygenation and ventilation, with 70% of the overall improvement occurring in the first hour of pronation. Prone positioning, although not associated with a significant survival advantage, may serve a role as rescue therapy for patients with ARDS and refractory life-threatening hypoxemia.

EXTRACORPOREAL LIFE SUPPORT (ECLS)

In patients who have acute and severe respiratory failure who are failing all advanced modes of mechanical ventilation, the use of extracorporeal life support (ECLS) is an option. ECLS is a proven modality for the treatment of severe respiratory failure in the neonate.[48,49] Its use in adults remains controversial, but ongoing clinical trials and research have indicated a possible benefit for its use to salvage those patients failing aggressive conventional therapy. For infant, pediatric, and adult patients with severe ARDS, ECLS therapy has produced respective survival rates of 85%, 74%, and 52% in these patients.[50]

Referral to an ECLS center should occur early if there is a suspected need for this technology. This will allow safe transport of the patient and avoidance of the "crash on" with all of its inherent complications. The technique of ECLS for patients with severe respiratory failure involves a venovenous or venoarterial life support circuit with a membrane oxygenator to temporarily take over the function of the lung. While on ECLS, mechanical ventilator settings are adjusted to minimize ventilator-induced lung injury and to maximize the recruitment of FRC. The treatment program for adults involves an algorithm that aims to normalize body physiology, aggressively recruit FRC, and minimize barotrauma. This algorithm used in 141 patients with respiratory failure referred for consideration of ECLS yielded a survival rate of 62% in patients with severe ARDS (median initial PaO_2/FiO_2 ratio of 66).[51]

The primary indication for the use of ECLS in patients with severe respiratory failure is when the risk of dying from ARDS is considered > 80% after optimal ventilator and medical management. This translates to an alveoli-arterial oxygen gradient > 600 mm Hg or a PaO_2/FiO_2 ratio of < 70 on 100% oxygen. Patients should also have a transpulmonary shunt fraction > 30%, despite maximal conventional therapy. Adult patients are typically cannulated percutaneously with large 21- to 23-Fr catheters for drainage and infusion of blood. Anticoagulation is necessary and is titrated by measurement of whole blood-activated clotting time. ECLS allows for a decreasing of mechanical ventilator settings to nondamaging "rest" levels while maintaining FRC recruitment measures. Once the patient's native lung function has improved, the patient is weaned off of ECLS at moderate ventilator settings that allow for potential increases in therapy (eg, FiO₂ 0.5– 0.6). If the weaning of ECLS is successful, the cannulas are removed and recovery continues.

In a series of 255 adult patients who were placed on ECLS for severe ARDS refractory to all other treatment, 67% were weaned off ECLS and 52% survived to hospital discharge.[52] Multivariate analysis identified age, gender, pre-ECLS pH < 7.10, pre-ELCS PaO_2/FiO_2 ratio, and pre-ECLS ventilator days, to all be significant independent variables influencing outcome. None of the patients who survived required permanent mechanical ventilation or supplemental oxygen therapy. Patients who can be successfully decannulated from ECLS have a 77% chance of being discharged from the hospital alive and a complete recovery.

The CESAR (Conventional Ventilation or ECMO for Severe Adult Respiratory Failure) trial is a prospective, randomized trial underway in the United Kingdom in adults with severe acute respiratory failure. The primary hypothesis for this trial is that "for patients with severe, but potentially reversible, respiratory failure, ECMO will increase the rate of survival without severe disability by 6 months post-randomization." The findings from this important pivotal trial will provide critical information regarding the efficacy of ECLS in adult patients with ARDS but will need to be interpreted carefully, because all patients allocated to the ECLS arm of the trial will be transported by an experienced ECMO transport team) to a single center (Glenfield Hospital in Leicester), which is one of the most experienced ECMO centers in the world. The conventional mechanical ventilation arm of the trial can include any treatment modality thought appropriate by the patient's intensivist (excluding ECMO). Intensivists will have full discretion to treat patients as they think appropriate. It will be recommended that intensivists adopt the low-volume ventilation strategy. Adherence to this strategy is defined for the purposes of CESAR as a plateau pressure < 30 cm H_2O (or if plateau pressure is not measured the peak inspiratory pressure). This will usually mean a tidal volume of 4-8 mL/kg body weight as defined in the low tidal volume ventilation strategy according to the ARDS Network group.

Most recently, case reports of the use of a pumpless extracorporeal lung assist device (arterial cannula inserted into the femoral artery, membrane oxygenator with venous cannula return to the femoral vein, driving the force is the patient's blood pressure) have been published in the treatment of severe ARDS to review its efficacy, limitations, and associated adverse events.[53-55]

PHARMACOLOGIC STRATEGIES

Multiple pharmacologic interventions including prostaglandins, prostacyclin, lisofylline, ketoconazole, N-acetylcysteine, corticosteroids, and nitric oxide have been investigated in the treatment of ALI and ARDS, but none as yet has demonstrated improved survival.[56] Two pharmacologic strategies (ketoconazole and lisofylline) were investigated by the ARDS Clinical Trials Network, and both studies were stopped by the Data Safety and Monitoring Boards for futility at interim analyses.[57,58]

A Cochrane Database Systematic Review of pharmacologic therapy for adults with ALI and ARDS reviewed 33 trials that randomized 3272 patients and concluded that two interventions were beneficial in single small trials: corticosteroids given for late-phase ARDS reduced hospital mortality (n = 24) and pentoxifylline reduced 1-month mortality (n = 30). Individual trials of nine additional pharmacologic interventions failed to show a beneficial effect, concluding that effective pharmacotherapy for ALI and ARDS is extremely limited.[59]

Pulmonary coagulopathy may be a prominent feature of ARDS and ventilator-induced lung injury, just as microvascular thrombosis is a common feature of sepsis. Most recently, alterations in coagulation and fibrinolysis in the pathogenesis of ALI and ARDS have been examined, particularly related to alveolar fibrin deposition. Increased local tissue factor mediated thrombin generation and depression of local fibrinolysis related to increased plasminogen activator inhibitors have been reported.[60]

CORTICOSTEROIDS

Because ARDS is pathologically associated with persistent inflammation and excessive fibroproliferation,

previous studies investigated the use of corticosteroids. Four trials of high-dose, short-course corticosteroids for early ARDS failed to show improvements in survival.[61-64] In contrast, several small case series reported improved lung function and survival with moderate-dose corticosteroids, for 7 days, in patients with persistent ARDS.

The multicenter trial (n = 180) from the National Heart, Lung and Blood Institute ARDS Clinical Trials Network randomized patients with ARDS of at least 7 days duration to receive either methylprednisolone or placebo in a double-blind manner.[65] Methylprednisolone therapy was associated with increased ventilator-free and shock-free days, improved oxygenation, and improved pulmonary compliance during the first 28 days. There was no significant difference in 60-day (28.6% vs 29.2%) and 180-day mortality (31.9% vs 31.5%) rates in the entire study cohort. As compared with placebo, methylprednisolone was associated with significantly increased 60 and 180 day mortality rates in patients enrolled at least 14 days after the onset of ARDS and with a higher rate of neuromuscular weakness and increased blood glucose concentrations; however, no increase in infectious complications was identified. These results do not support the routine use of methylprednisolone for persistent ARDS.

SURFACTANT THERAPY

Regardless of the cause, a common pathophysiologic feature of patients with ARDS is a dysfunction of the endogenous surfactant system. Exogenous surfactant therapy is an effective standard of care in neonates with ARDS.[66,67] No similar current effective surfactant therapy exists for adult patients with ARDS; however, ongoing and future research efforts suggest that this may eventually be feasible.[68,69]

A multicenter, randomized, blinded trial of calfactant (a natural lung surfactant containing high levels of surfactant specific protein B compared with placebo in 153 infants, children, and adolescents with respiratory failure from ALI documented that calfactant acutely improved oxygenation and significantly decreased mortality, although no significant decrease in the course of respiratory failure (duration of ventilation, ICU, or hospital stay) was observed.[70] Exogenous surfactant may improve oxygenation, but all clinical studies to date have demonstrated no significant effect on the death rate or length of use of mechanical ventilation in adults.

NITRIC OXIDE

Inhaled nitric oxide is a selective pulmonary vasodilator, resulting in decreased pulmonary vascular resistance, pulmonary arterial pressure, and right ventricular afterload. The selectivity of nitric oxide for the pulmonary circulation is the result of rapid hemoglobin-mediated inactivation of nitric oxide. Two small single-center studies and four multicenter, randomized, placebo-controlled trials have failed to determine the therapeutic role of inhaled nitric oxide in patients with acute respiratory failure. Low-dose inhaled nitric oxide in ALI and ARDS has been associated with improved short-term oxygenation but has had no substantial impact on the duration of mechanical ventilatory support or on mortality.[71,72,73,74]

The improvement in oxygenation associated with inhaled nitric oxide has not been able to be translated into improved clinical outcome. This may be related to the fact that ARDS is a heterogeneous condition with multiple causes, pulmonary and extrapulmonary and that only a small minority of patients with ARDS die of respiratory failure—the majority die of multiple organ dysfunction and failure. These data do not support the routine use of inhaled nitric oxide in the treatment of ALI or ARDS, but it may be considered as a salvage therapy in patients who continue to have life-threatening hypoxemia, despite optimization of all other treatment strategies.

INCREMENTAL APPROACH TO THE MANAGEMENT OF SEVERE ARDS

Development of protocols in the ICU setting is important for the management of complex patients. Protocols reduce undesirable variability, mandate the use of best evidence, impose timeliness, facilitate communication and improve education of health care staff.

In patients with severe refractory hypoxemia, there is potential utility in the incremental approach to ARDS management. Implementation of the specific strategies we have discussed above may result in improved oxygenation, improved pulmonary compliance, and ultimately, survival in individual patients. There is also the possibility that some of these interventional strategies may have additive effects.

It is important to have full knowledge of the results of prospective, randomized trials that have carefully assessed the impact of these treatment strategies on patient outcome in ALI and ARDS. However, faced with an individual patient with refractory hypoxemia resulting from severe ARDS, it is also important to be comfortable with appropriate bedside implementation of these potential treatment strategies for ALI and ARDS.

VENTILATOR STRATEGY ALGORITHM

The initial choice for ventilator setting should bear in mind the primary pathology for which the patient was admitted for. Patients with respiratory failure secondary to acute exacerbations of chronic obstructive airway disease,[75-77] cardiogenic pulmonary edema,[78,79] immunocompromised patients with acute respiratory failure[80,81] and selected patients with difficulty weaning from the ventilator, will benefit from noninvasive positive pressure ventilation (NIV). By contrast, current evidence suggests that patients with ARDS patients are unlikely to have any significant benefits on outcome when noninvasive positive pressure

ventilation is added to standard therapy of low tidal volume, low plateau pressure ventilation.[82-84]

In ARDS patients, after initiation of mechanical ventilation, initial tidal volumes should be set at 8 mL/kg of predicted body weight (PBW); tidal volumes should be reduced by 1 mL/kg at intervals of 2 hours until the

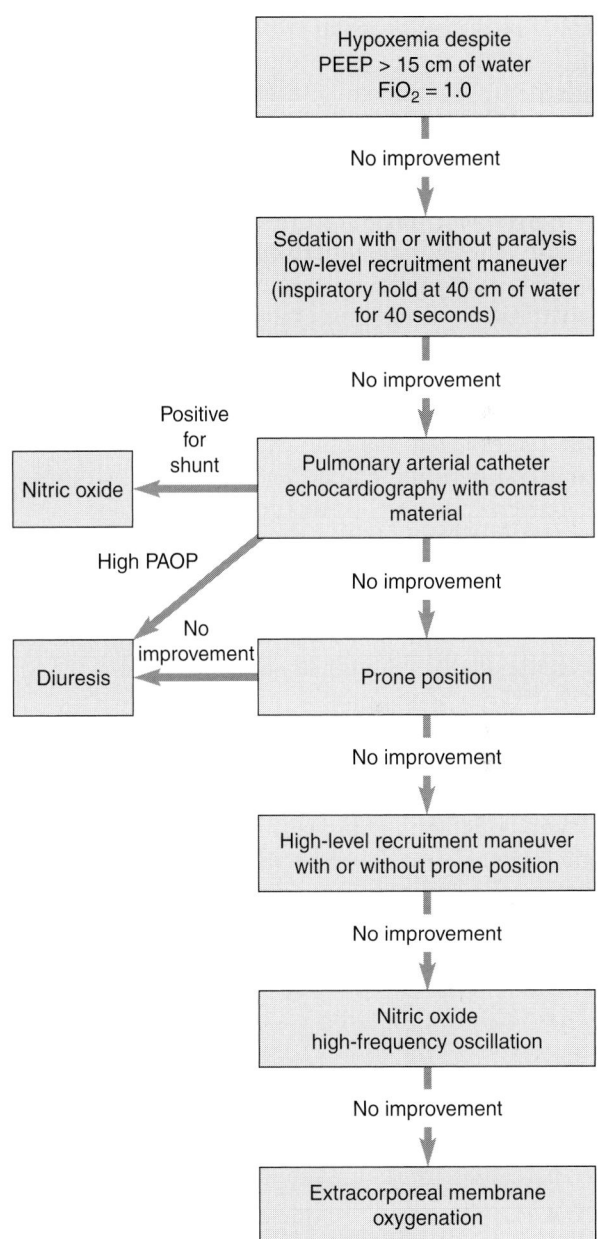

Figure 26-8 *An incremental approach to the management of catastrophic acute respiratory distress syndrome. A high-level recruitment maneuver is used only in patients that are without neurologic disease and bacterial pneumonia and that have adequate blood pressure, filling pressures, and cardiac output. PEEP, positive end-expiratory pressure; PAOP, pulmonary artery occlusion pressure. Reprinted with permission from Case records of the Massachusetts General Hospital. Case 17-2005. A 22-year-old woman with back and leg pain and respiratory failure. N Engl J Med 2005;352(23):2425-2434.*

tidal volume is set at 6 mL/kg. Appropriate sedation to overcome patient anxiety is given and adequate pain control is confirmed. The goal is to achieve appropriate oxygenation with SpO_2 88%-95% and PO_2 55-80 mm Hg while maintaining plateau pressures less than 30 cm H_2O while using FiO_2 of < 0.5%.

If the patient continues to show no improvement, FiO_2 should be increase to 100% and recruitment maneuvers with PEEP of 40 cm H_2O for 40 seconds should be done. If the patient demonstrates improved oxygenation during recruitment maneuvers, the PEEP should be increased until the optimal PEEP is achieved. Diuretics should be used if the patient has objective evidence of pulmonary edema.

If the patient shows no improvement, evaluation for a possible intracardiac shunt or pulmonary hypertension should be initiated. Diagnostic strategies include pulmonary artery catheter placement or transthoracic or transesophageal echocardiogram. If the pulmonary hypertension is confirmed, inhaled nitric oxide should be considered as a therapeutic strategy to improve arterial oxygenation.

If there is still no improvement in oxygenation, prone positioning could be tried and recruitment maneuvers continued. At this point, potential transfer of the patient to a tertiary care center with experience in other ARDS treatment modalities, including airway pressure release ventilation (APRV), high frequency oscillation (HFOV) and possibly extracorporeal membrane oxygenation (ECMO) should be considered (Fig. 26-8).[85]

WEANING STRATEGIES

Invasive mechanical ventilation is lifesaving for patients with acute respiratory failure, but it is also associated with potential for substantial risks. Therefore, once adequate recovery occurs, efforts should focus on liberation from mechanical ventilation as expeditiously as possible. It is estimated that more than 40% of the time that a patient receives mechanical ventilation is spent trying to wean the patient.[86]

Controversy still exists over how to proceed during spontaneous breathing trial (SBT), and which criteria should be fulfilled to start it. Single weaning parameters used to predict extubation success seem to have a rather low accuracy, and some may even have a low negative predictive value. Moreover, authors still disagree about the validity of standard respiratory functional variables determined prior to weaning and supposed to represent prediction criteria for a successful extubation. Therefore, multiple prospective and randomized protocol-directed weaning studies have assessed weaning readiness by means of a structured evaluation.[87-92] Prior to the weaning trial, the patients had to pass a collection of standardized readiness criteria that focused on: (a) reversal of the causative process for ventilatory support, (b) respiratory and ventilatory patterns, (c) ability to protect the airway, and (d) stability of hemodynamic and metabolic parameters. Although these criteria may be helpful in predicting successful extubation, they are not perfect, and the patient's tolerance of an SBT remains the most reliable criterion.

The use of a nursing-directed or respiratory therapist-directed protocol in intensive care units for weaning from mechanical ventilation is associated with a shorter duration of ventilation and length of stay in the ICU.[93-95] Most protocols share two formal components: daily screening of a set of simple observations or interventions to identify readiness to proceed, followed by a spontaneous breathing trial that tests the patient's ability to breathe independently. Daily screening is designed to identify potential barriers regarding medical stability, level of consciousness, oxygenation, ventilation, and airway patency and protection. However, one must avoid selecting criteria that are too restrictive, potentially delaying the discontinuation of ventilation. Patients should undergo daily assessment of their readiness for a spontaneous breathing trial (SBT) once the previously discussed criteria have been assessed and confirmed (Fig. 26-4).

REFERENCES

1. Bernard GR, Artigas A, Brigham KL, Carlet J, Falke K, Hudson L, et al. Report of the American-European consensus conference on ARDS: definitions, mechanisms, relevant outcomes and clinical trial coordination. *Intensive Care Med* 1994;20:225-232.
2. Rubenfeld GD, Caldwell E, Peabody E, et al. Incidence and outcomes of acute lung injury. *N Engl J Med* 2005;353(16):1685-1693.
3. Martin M, Salim A, Murray J, Demetriades D, Belzberg H, Rhee P. The decreasing incidence and mortality of acute respiratory distress syndrome after injury: a 5-year observational study. *J Trauma* 2005;59(5): 1107-1113.
4. Ware LB, Matthay MA. The acute respiratory distress syndrome. *N Engl J Med* 2000;342(18): 1334-1349.
5. Gattinoni L, Pesenti A, Torresin A, et al. Adult respiratory distress syndrome profiles by computed tomography. *J Thorac Imaging* 1988;3:59-64.
6. Gattinoni L, Pesenti A, Baglioni S, et al. Inflammatory pulmonary edema and PEEP: correlation between imaging and physiologic studies. *J Thorac Imaging* 1988;3:59-64.
7. Tremblay LN, Slutsky AS. Ventilator-induced lung injury: from the bench to the bedside. *Intensive Care Med* 2006;32(1):24-33.
8. dos Santos CC, Slutsky AS. The contribution of biophysical lung injury to the development of biotrauma. *Annu Rev Physiol* 2006;68:585-618.
9. Hemmila MR, Napolitano LM. Severe respiratory failure: Advanced treatment options. *Crit Care Med* 2006;34 Suppl(9):S278-S290.

10. Ranieri VM, Suter PM, Tortorella C, et al. Effect of mechanical ventilation on inflammatory mediators in patients with acute respiratory distress syndrome: a randomized controlled trial. *JAMA* 1999;282(1): 54-61.

11. Schnapp LM, Chin DP, Szaflarski N, Matthay MA. Frequency and importance of barotrauma in 100 patients with acute lung injury. *Crit Care Med* 1995;23(2):272-278.

12. Eisner MD, Thompson BT, Schoenfeld D, Anzueto A, Matthay MA. Acute Respiratory Distress Syndrome Network. Airway pressures and early barotrauma in patients with acute lung injury and acute respiratory distress syndrome. *Am J Respir Crit Care Med* 2002;165(7):978-982.

13. Webb HH, Tierney DF. Experimental pulmonary edema due to intermittent positive pressure ventilation with high inflation pressures. Protection by positive end-expiratory pressure. *Am Rev Respir Dis* 1974;110(5): 556-565.

14. Dreyfuss D, Basset G, Soler P, Saumon G. Intermittent positive-pressure hyperventilation with high inflation pressures produces pulmonary microvascular injury in rats. *Am Rev Respir Dis* 1985;132(4): 880-884.

15. Weg JG, Anzueto A, Balk RA. The relation of pneumothorax and other air leaks to mortality in the acute respiratory distress syndrome. *N Engl J Med* 1998;338(6): 341-346.

16. Belperio JA, Keane MP, Lynch JP 3rd, Strieter RM. The role of cytokines during the pathogenesis of ventilator-associated and ventilator-induced lung injury. *Semin Respir Crit Care Med* 2006;27(4):350-364.

17. Ventilation with lower tidal volumes as compared with traditional tidal volumes for acute lung injury and the acute respiratory distress syndrome. The Acute Respiratory Distress Syndrome Network. *N Engl J Med* 2000;342(18):1301-1308.

18. Hough CL, Kallet RH, Ranieri VM, Rubenfeld GD, Luce JM, Hudson LD. Intrinsic positive end-expiratory pressure in Acute Respiratory Distress Syndrome (ARDS) Network subjects. *Crit Care Med* 2005;33(3):527-532.

19. Kahn JM, Andersson L, Karir V, Polissar NL, Neff MJ, Rubenfeld GD. Low tidal volume ventilation does not increase sedation use in patients with acute lung injury. *Crit Care Med* 2005;33(4):766-771.

20. Nathens AB, Johnson JL, Minei JP, et al. Inflammation and the host response to injury investigators. Inflammation and the host response to injury, a large-scale collaborative project: Patient-Oriented Research Core-standard operating procedures for clinical care. I. Guidelines for mechanical ventilation of the trauma patient. *J Trauma* 2005;59(3):764-769.

21. Hickling KG, Henderson SJ, Jackson R. Low mortality associated with low volume pressure limited ventilation with permissive hypercapnia in severe adult respiratory distress syndrome. *Intensive Care Med* 1990;16(6):372-377.

22. Bulger EM, Jurkovich GJ, Gentilello LM, et al. Current clinical options for the treatment and management of acute respiratory distress syndrome. *J Trauma* 2000;48:562-572.

23. Hickling KG, Walsh J, Henderson S, et al. Low mortality rate in adult respiratory distress syndrome using low-volume, pressure-limited ventilation with permissive hypercapnia: A prospective study. *Crit Care Med* 1994;22:1568-1578.

24. Kregenow DA, Rubenfeld GD, Hudson LD, et al. Hypercapnic acidosis and mortality in acute lung injury. *Crit Care Med* 2006;34:229-231.

25. Roupie E, Dambrosio M, Servillo G, et al. Titration of tidal volume and induced hypercapnia in acute respiratory distress syndrome. *Am J Respir Crit Care Med* 1995;152:121-128.

26. Artigas A, Bernard GR, Carlet J, et al. The American-European consensus conference on ARDS, part 2: Ventilatory, pharmacologic, supportive therapy, study design strategies and issues related to recovery and remodeling. *Intensive Care Med* 1998;24:378-398.

27. Amato MB, Barbas CS, Mederios DM, et al. Effect of a protective-ventilation strategy on mortality in the acute respiratory distress syndrome. *N Engl J Med* 1998;338:347-354.

28. Hager DN, Krishnan JA, Hayden DL, et al. Tidal volume reduction in patients with acute lung injury when plateau pressures are not high. *Am J Respir Crit Care Med* 2005;172:1241-1245.

29. Habashi NM. Other approaches to openlung ventilation: Airway pressure release ventilation. *Crit Care Med* 2005;33(Suppl): S228-S240.

30. Fort P, Farmer C, Westerman J, et al. high frequency oscillatory ventilation for adult respiratory distress syndrome: A pilot study. *Crit Care Med* 1997;25:937-947.

31. Mehta S, Lapinsky SE, Hallett DC, et al. Prospective trial of high-frequency oscillation in adults with acute respiratory distress syndrome. *Crit Care Med* 2001;29:1360-1369.

32. Derdak S, Mehta S, Stewart TE, et al. High frequency oscillatory ventilation for acute respiratory distress syndrome in adults: a randomized controlled trial. *Am J Resp Crit Care Med* 2002;166:801-808.

33. Mehta S, Granton J, MacDonald RJ, et al. High-frequency oscillatory ventilation in adults: the Toronto experience. *Chest* 2004;126:518-527.

34. Imai Y, Slutsky AS. High-frequency oscillatory ventilation and ventilator-induced lung injury. *Crit Care Med* 2005;33(3 Suppl):S129-S134.

35. Higgins J, Estetter B, Holland D, et al. High-frequency oscillatory ventilation in adults: Respiratory therapy issues. *Crit Care Med* 2005;33(Suppl):S196-S203.

36. Mols G, Priebe HJ, Guttmann J. Alveolar recruitment in acute lung injury. *Br J Anaesth* 2006;96:156-166.

37. Slutsky AS, Hudson LD. PEEP or No PEEP—lung recruitment may be the solution. *N Engl J Med* 2006;354:1839-1841.

38. Gattinoni L, Caironi P, Cressoni M, et al. Lung recruitment in patients with the acute respiratory distress syndrome. *N Engl J Med* 2006;354:1775-1786.

39. Lim CM, Jung H, Koh Y, et al. Effect of alveolar recruitment maneuver in early acute respiratory distress syndrome according to antiderecruitment strategy, etiological category of diffuse lung injury, and body position of the patient. *Crit Care Med* 2003;31:411-418.

40. Ferguson ND, Chiche JD, Kacmarek RM, et al. Combining high-frequency oscillatory ventilation and

recruitment maneuvers in adults with early acute respiratory distress syndrome. *Crit Care Med* 2005;33: 479-486.

41. Richter T, Bellani G, Scott Harris R, et al. Effect of prone position on regional shunt, aeration, and perfusion in experimental acute lung injury. *Am J Respir Crit Care Med* 2005;172:480-487.

42. Piehl MA, Brown RS. Use of extreme position changes in acute respiratory failure. *Crit Care Med* 1976;4:13-14.

43. Douglas WW, Rehder K, Beynen FM, et al. Improved oxygenation in patients with acute respiratory failure: The prone position. *Am Rev Respir Dis* 1977;115: 559-566.

44. Gattinoni L, Tognoni G, Pesenti A, et al. Effect of prone positioning on the survival of patients with acute respiratory failure. *N Engl J Med* 2001;345: 568-573.

45. Gattinoni L, Vagginelli F, Carlesso E, et al. Decrease in PaCO2 with prone position is predictive of improved outcome in acute respiratory distress syndrome. *Crit Care Med* 2003;31:2727-2733.

46. Curley MA, Hibberd PL, Fineman LD, et al. Effect of prone positioning on clinical outcomes in children with acute lung injury: A randomized controlled trial. *JAMA* 2005;294: 229-237.

47. Mancebo J, Fernandez R, Blanch L, et al. A multicenter trial of prolonged pron ventilation in severe acute respiratory distress syndrome. *Am J Respir Crit Care Med* 2006 Jun 1;17(11):1233-9.

48. Bartlett RH, Roloff DW, Cornell RG, et al. Extracorporeal circulation in neonatal respiratory failure: A prospective randomized study. *Pediatrics* 1985;76:479-487.

49. UK Collaborative ECMO Trial Group. UK collaborative randomized trial of neonatal extracorporeal membrane oxygenation. *Lancet* 1996;348:75-82.

50. *Extracorporeal Life Support Organization: Annual ECMO Registry Report.* July 2003; http://www.elso.med.umich.edu.

51. Rich PB, Awad SS, Kolla S, et al. An approach to the treatment of severe adult respiratory failure. *J Crit Care* 1998;13:26-36.

52. Hemmila MR, Rowe SA, Boules TN, et al. Extracorporeal life support for severe acute respiratory distress syndrome in adults. *Ann Surg* 2004;240: 595-607.

53. Reng M, Philipp A, Kaiser M, et al. Pumpless extracorporeal lung assist and adult respiratory distress syndrome. *Lancet* 2000;356(9225):219-220.

54. Ruettimann U, Ummenhofer W, Rueter F, et al. Management of acute respiratory distress syndrome using pumpless extracorporeal lung assist. *Can J Anaesth* 2006;53:101-105.

55. Zimmerman M, Bein T, Philipp A, et al. Interhospital transportation of patients with severe lung failure on pumpless extracorporeal lung assist. *Br J Anaesth* 2006;96:63-66.

56. Adhikari N, Burns KE, Meade MO. Pharmacologic treatments for acute respiratory distress syndrome and acute lung injury: Systematic review and meta-analysis. *Treat Respir Med* 2004;3:307-328.

57. ARDS Network. Ketoconazole for the early treatment of acute lung injury and acute respiratory distress syndrome: A randomized controlled trial. *JAMA* 2000;283:1995-2002.

58. ARDS Network. Randomized, placebocontrolled trial of lisofylline for the early treatment of acute lung injury and acute respiratory distress syndrome. *Crit Care Med* 2002;30:1-6.

59. Adhikari N, Burns KE, Meade MO. Phmarcologic therapies for adults with acute lung injury and acute respiratory distress syndrome. *Cochrane Database Syst Rev* 2004;18:CD004477.

60. Schultz MJ, Haitsma JJ, Zhang H, et al. Pulmonary coagulopathy as a new target in therapeutic studies of acute lung injury or pneumonia-a review. *Crit Care Med* 2006;34:871-877.

61. Bone RC, Fisher CJ Jr, Clemmer TP, et al. Early methylprednisolone treatment for septic syndrome and the adult respiratory distress syndrome. *Chest* 1987;92:1032-1036; erratum: *Chest* 1988;94:448.

62. Luce JM, Montgomery AB, Marks JD, et al. Ineffectiveness of high-dose methylprednisolone in preventing parenchymal lung injury and improving mortality in patients with septic shock. *Am Rev Respir Dis* 1988;138:62-68.

63. Bernard GR, Luce JM, Sprung CL, et al. High-dose corticosteroids in patients with the adult respiratory distress syndrome. *N Engl J Med* 1987;317: 1565-1570.

64. Weigelt JA, Norcross JF, Borman KR, et al. Early steroid therapy for respiratory failure. *Arch Surg* 1985;120: 536-540.

65. Steinberg KP, Hudson LD, Goodman RB, et al. Efficacy and safety of corticosteroids for persistent acute respiratory distress syndrome. *N Engl J Med* 2006;354: 1671-1684.

66. Stevens TP, Blennow M, Soll RF. Early surfactant administration with brief ventilation vs selective surfactant and continued mechanical ventilation for preterm infants with or at risk for RDS. *Cochrane Database Syst Rev* 2002;(2):CD003063.

67. Sinha SK, Lacaze-Masmonteil T, Valls I, et al. A multicenter, randomized, controlled trial of lucinanctant versus poractant alfa among very premature infants at high risk for respiratory distress syndrome. *Pediatrics* 2005;115:1030-1038.

68. Spragg RG, Lewis JF, Walmrath HD, et al. Effect of recombinant surfactant protein C-based surfactant on the acute respiratory distress syndrome. *N Engl J Med* 2004;31:884-892.

69. Baudouin SV. Exogenous surfactant replacement in ARDS—one day, someday, or never *N Engl J Med* 2004;351:853-855.

70. Wilson DF, Thomas NJ, Markovitz BP, et al. Effect of exogenous surfactant (calfactant) in pediatric acute lung injury: A randomized controlled trial. *JAMA* 2005;293:470-476.

71. Taylor RW, Zimmerman JL, Dellinger RP, et al. Low-dose inhaled nitric oxide in patients with acute lung injury: A randomized controlled trial. *JAMA* 2004;291:1603-1609.

72. Payen D, Vallet B. l'ARDS GdEdNd. Results of the French prospective multicentric randomized double-blind placebocontrolled trial on inhaled nitric oxide (NO) in ARDS. *Abstr. Intensive Care Med* 1999;25:S166.

73. Sokol J, Jacobs SE, Bohn D. Inhaled nitric oxide for acute hypoxic respiratory failure in children and adults: A metaanalysis. *Anesth Analg* 2003;97:989-998.

74. Griffiths MJ, Evans TW. Inhaled nitric oxide therapy in adults. *N Engl J Med* 2005;353:2683-2695.

75. Schettino G, Altobelli N, Kacmarek RM. Noninvasive positive pressure ventilation reverses acute respiratory failure in select "do-not-intubate" patients. *Crit Care Med* 2005;33(9):1976-1982.

76. Carratu P, Bonfitto P, Dragonieri S, et al. Early and late failure of noninvasive ventilation in chronic obstructive pulmonary disease with acute exacerbation. *Eur J Clin Invest* 2005;35(6):404-409.

77. Confalonieri M, Garuti G, Cattaruzza MS, et al. Italian noninvasive positive pressure ventilation (NPPV) study group. A chart of failure risk for noninvasive ventilation in patients with COPD exacerbation. *Eur Respir J* 2005;25(2):348-355.

78. Park M, Lorenzi-Filho G. Noninvasive mechanical ventilation in the treatment of acute cardiogenic pulmonary edema. *Clinics* 2006;61(3):247-252.

79. Park M, Sangean MC, Volpe Mde S, et al. Randomized, prospective trial of oxygen, continuous positive airway pressure, and bilevel positive airway pressure by face mask in acute cardiogenic pulmonary edema. *Crit Care Med* 2004;32(12):2407-2415.

80. Karzai W, Huttemann E. Noninvasive ventilation in immunosuppressed patients. *N Engl J Med* 2001;344(26):2027; author reply 2028.

81. Hilbert G, Gruson D, Vargas F, et al. Noninvasive ventilation in immunosuppressed patients with pulmonary infiltrates, fever, and acute respiratory failure. *N Engl J Med* 2001;344(7):481-487.

82. Garpestad E, Hill NS. Noninvasive ventilation for acute lung injury: How often should we try, how often should we fail *Crit Care* 2006;10(4):147.

83. Caples SM, Gay PC. Noninvasive positive pressure ventilation in the intensive care unit: A concise review. *Crit Care Med* 2005;33(11):2651-2658.

84. Agarwal R, Reddy C, Aggarwal AN, Gupta D. Is there a role for noninvasive ventilation in acute respiratory distress syndrome? A meta-analysis. *Respir Med* 2006;Dec;100(12):2235-8

85. Medoff BD, Shepard JO, Smith RN, et al: Case 17-2005: A 22-year-old woman with back and leg pain and respiratory failure. *N Engl J Med* 2005;352:2425-2434.

86. Esteban A, Alía I, Ibañez J, Benito S, Tobin MJ, Spanish Lung Failure Collaborative Group. Modes of mechanical ventilation and weaning: A national survey of Spanish hospitals. *Chest* 1994;106:1188-1193.

87. Esteban A, Alia I, Gordo F, et al. Extubation outcome after spontaneous breathing trials with T-tube or pressure support ventilation. *Am J Respir Crit Care Med* 1997;156:459-465.

88. Brochard L, Rauss A, Benito S, et al. Comparison of three methods of gradual withdrawal from ventilatory support during weaning from mechanical ventilation. *Am J Respir Crit Care Med* 1994;150:89.

89. Esteban A, Frutos F, Tobin MJ, Alia I, Solsona JF, Vallverdù I, Fernandez R, De la Cal MA, Benito S, Tomas R, Cariedo D, Macias S, Blanco J. A comparison of four methods of weaning patients from mechanical ventilation. *N Engl J Med* 1995;332:345-350

90. Ely EW, Baker AM, Dunagan DP, et al. Effect of the duration of mechanical ventilation of identifying patients capable of breathing spontaneously. *N Engl J Med* 1996;335:1864-1869.

91. Kollef MH, Shapiro SD, Silver P, et al. A randomized, controlled trial of protocol-directed versus physician-directed weaning from mechanical ventilation. *Crit Care Med* 1997;25:567-574.

92. Esteban A, Alia I, Tobin MJ, et al. Effect of spontaneous breathing trial duration on outcome of attempts to discontinue mechanical ventilation. *Am J Respir Crit Care Med* 1999;159:512-518.

93. Tonnelier JM, Prat G, Le Gal G, et al. Impact of a nurses' protocol-directed weaning procedure on outcomes in patients undergoing mechanical ventilation for longer than 48 hours: a prospective cohort study with a matched historical control group. *Crit Care* 2005;9(2): R83-R89.

94. Ramachandran V, Grap MJ, Sessler CN. Protocol-directed weaning: a process of continuous performance improvement. *Crit Care* 2005;9(2):138-140.

95. McLean SE, Jensen LA, Schroeder DG, Gibney NR, Skjodt NM. Improving adherence to a mechanical ventilation weaning protocol for critically ill adults: outcomes after an implementation program. *Am J Crit Care* 2006;15(3):299-309.

Part III
TRAUMA

Chapter 27

TRAUMA TO THE HEAD, FACE, AND NECK

Stephen C. Gale, MD, and Kenneth L. Mattox, MD

INTRODUCTION

Many different disciplines and specialties are involved in the evaluation and treatment of patients with head, face, and neck injuries. The acute care surgeon, however, is often charged with the initial evaluation, stabilization, and treatment of emergent conditions of these areas. Because of the critical nature of this anatomic region, the acute care surgeon must be able to quickly assess and treat many of these conditions. Unlike urgent conditions sustained in other areas of the body, emergent conditions of the head and neck often do not allow the surgeon the luxury of waiting for other specialists to arrive, or even a moment to consult reference materials, before decisions must be made. Therefore, the acute care surgeon must understand the anatomy, physiology, and basic evaluation and treatment algorithms of these conditions and be facile with stabilization techniques before the patient ever arrives to his or her care.

This chapter discusses each of several specific anatomic areas and injuries individually. Many evaluation and treatment schemas overlay these injuries. Numerous acceptable algorithms exist, and often local custom will have unique acceptable approaches to these injuries based on the experiences and training of the component members of the multidisciplinary trauma team.

TRAUMATIC BRAIN INJURY

EPIDEMIOLOGY

Traumatic brain injury (TBI) is very common in patients sustaining blunt trauma and is a leading cause of death from injury. Furthermore, the societal burden of head injury is enormous—not only due to acute care expenses but also from the loss of productivity and the cost of rehabilitation and long-term care. The estimated financial cost to the United States alone is $100 billion annually.[1]

TBI is classified both by the specific anatomic lesion and the patient's clinical neurologic function. While effective treatment is based on both components, the latter is more predictive of neurologic outcome. While abnormal neurological findings are helpful in predicting the need for head computed tomography (CT), a completely normal physical examination does not exclude intracranial pathology.[2] Therefore, all patients who have constitutional signs and/or symptoms suspicious of TBI (headache, somnolence, mental status changes, confusion, nausea/emesis, seizures, perseveration, neurologic deficit, double vision, vertigo, or hemotympanum) require both a complete neurological examination and a noncontrast head CT as soon as possible after arrival to the trauma center.[3,4]

The neurological examination includes a pupillary and cranial nerve evaluation, a search for focal neurological deficits, and an assessment of the patient's level of consciousness. The Glasgow Coma Scale (GCS) (Table 27-1) is used to assess consciousness and forms the basis for the clinical classification of TBI: mild (13-15), moderate (9-12), and severe (≤8).[5,6] The motor component of the GCS is the most important predictor of neurologic recovery.[7,8] Patients with mild TBI generally have had a brief loss of consciousness but no focal neurologic deficit; prognosis is excellent and mortality is rare. Moderate TBI patients often have confusion and occasionally focal neurologic findings. However, they are usually able to follow simple commands and have an overall good prognosis with <10% mortality.[9] Patients with coma (GCS ≤8) have suffered severe TBI. Mortality approaches 40%, and most survivors have a significant persistent neurologic deficit. Intracranial pressure monitoring is often required in these patients because the clinical exam cannot be followed.[1,10,11]

Parenchymal lesions are diagnosed anatomically based on CT scan findings. Concussion is the *absence* of parenchymal damage in a patient with a documented loss of consciousness. This is a clinical diagnosis with variable neurologic symptoms. Postconcussive symptoms are common and include headaches, inattention,

Table 27-1   The Glasgow Coma Scale

Eye opening		Verbal response		Motor response	
Spontaneous	4	Oriented	5	Follows simple commands	6
To voice	3	Confused	4	Localizes (purposeful)	5
To pain	2	Inappropriate words	3	Withdraws (pain)	4
None	1	Incomprehensible	2	Decorticate (flexion to pain)	3
		None	1	Decerebrate (extension to pain)	2
				None	1

short-term memory loss, and mood swings.[6,12] Although the symptoms rarely persist for more than a few months, patients and their families must be warned of these potential sequelae before discharge.

A cerebral contusion is essentially a "bruise" with localized intracerebral hemorrhage and edema adjacent to an area of impact. Depending on the trauma sustained, these lesions can enlarge with time and may coalesce into an intracerebral hematoma with resulting mass effect. Similarly, subarachnoid hemorrhage is often localized anatomically but more often represents a shearing mechanism with local vascular disruption. These lesions typically do not cause mass effect.[13]

Space-occupying hematomas are usually characterized by their relation to the dura as epidural (above the dura) or subdural (below the dura). Epidural hematomas are often seen after a direct lateral impact to the temporal region with skull fracture and laceration to the middle meningeal artery. Blood accumulates between the skull and the dura. There is often little direct trauma to the brain parenchyma, and parenchymal injury is typically secondary to elevated intracranial pressure. Classically, patients experience a brief loss of consciousness with a subsequent lucid interval, before again losing consciousness as the lesion expands and eventual intracranial hypertension develops. In practice, however, this presentation is rare. Clinically, ipsilateral pupillary dilation indicates impending uncal herniation secondary to elevated intracranial pressure and occurs due to direct compression of cranial nerve III. Immediate evacuation is indicated in any patient with altered mental status, a lesion > 1 cm in size, or with evidence of a midline shift on CT scan. With early evacuation, prognosis can be excellent and depends mostly on the degree of underlying cerebral trauma and the time delay to hematoma evacuation.[1,13]

Subdural hematomas accumulate between the dura and the brain itself. The shearing or tearing of dural bridging veins is the most common underlying cause and generally implies a significant force of impact. In addition to the parenchymal compression of the hematoma, significant direct brain injury and axonal shearing are also usually present.[1] Therefore, patients with subdural hematomas have a comparatively worse prognosis and greater residual functional deficits even with small accumulations or early evacuation.

Occasionally, patients will present in coma (GCS ≤ 8) but have minimal findings on initial CT scan. These patients may have suffered a diffuse axonal injury (DAI): an axonal shearing due to rapid deceleration.[14] There may be little or no evidence of injury on CT scan. Some patients with DAI will have scattered punctate hemorrhages, loss of gray–white matter differentiation, diffuse edema with brainstem compression and loss of basolateral cisterns, or compression of the cerebral gyri/sulci. The prognosis for DAI is extremely poor with a high incidence of residual neurologic deficit and a high mortality.[1]

These various lesions describe the primary brain injury sustained by the patient during the traumatic event. That event cannot be altered. The basic management of TBI strives to prevent *secondary* injury that might further compromise neural tissue and further limit neurologic recovery. Independent of its precipitating cause, secondary injury is the result of ischemia at the tissue level either from hypoxia or impaired perfusion due to pressure.[15] Treatment strategies emphasize prevention of hypoxia at the cellular level and center on the concept that the cranium is a closed space with a fixed volume.[1,10,16] Typically intravascular blood, brain tissue, and cerebrospinal fluid (CSF) are the only intracranial contents. Swelling or mass lesions, such as hematomas, occupy space and volume. Once a critical volume has been reached, autoregulation mechanisms fail and intracranial pressure (ICP) increases markedly.[16] An ICP > 20 mm Hg is typically an indication for treatment.[1,10]

Cerebral perfusion pressure (CPP) is the differential between mean arterial pressure (MAP) and ICP (CPP = MAP – ICP). As ICP increases for a given MAP, CPP falls.[1,10,17] Below a CPP of 60 mm Hg, tissue hypoxia appears to occur and can cause secondary brain injury.[17] Furthermore, conditions that lead to increased cellular metabolism may lead to a relative hypoxia as demand surpasses supply. These metabolic alterations must be controlled. Table 27-2 summarizes the various causes of primary and secondary brain injury after trauma.

Table 27-2 Primary and Secondary Causes of Traumatic Brain Injury

Primary Brain Injury

- Diffuse
  - Diffuse axonal injury (DAI)
- Focal
  - Vascular injury
    - Intracerebral hemorrhage
    - Subdural hemorrhage
    - Epidural hemorrhage
    - Subarachnoid hemorrhage
  - Parenchymal
    - Contusion
    - Laceration

Secondary Brain Injury

- Intracranial causes (compression)
  - Hemorrhage (mass effect)
  - Swelling
    - Venous congestion
    - Edema
  - Infection
- Extracranial causes
  - Hypoxia
  - Hypotension
  - Hyponatremia
  - Hyperthermia
  - Hypoglycemia

After the initial resuscitation, management of elevated ICP involves evacuating clinically significant hematomas, preventing hematoma expansion, reducing intracranial swelling, and optimizing cerebral perfusion. Euvolemia is an important goal, and normal saline has been the maintenance fluid of choice; hypotonic solutions are contraindicated in TBI resuscitation because they increase cerebral edema.[1] Low-volume hypertonic saline solutions are increasingly being used for resuscitation and treatment in patients with TBI to limit volume loading and to improve cerebral perfusion by recruiting interstitial and intracellular fluid from the intracranial tissues.

In addition, the head of the patient's bed should be elevated to 30° to augment venous drainage. Constrictive or circumferential neck dressings must be avoided, as should overly compressive cervical collars. Because pain and anxiety increase ICP, adequate analgesia and sedation must be given. Hypothermia must be corrected, and coagulopathy from factor consumption, preinjury medications, or chronic disease must be rapidly and aggressively reversed.

Chronic prolonged hyperventilation should not be used to control ICP; a $PaCO_2$ of 35-40 mm Hg should be a maintained.[1,16] While hyperventilation does decrease ICP, it does so through vasoconstriction at the expense of cerebral blood Flow.[10] Of note, hyperventilation does have a role in the *acute* setting of an elevated ICP with clinical deterioration and can be used as a bridge to operative decompression.[1,16]

If the clinical exam cannot be followed due to coma or anesthesia in a patient with intracranial pathology, then ICP must be monitored and is accomplished with either an intraventricular (ventriculostomy) or extradural (bolt) monitor either in the ICU or in the operating room.[11] Ventriculostomy has the advantage of allowing not only ICP monitoring but also ICP treatment by CSF drainage.

Pharmacologic reduction of intracranial swelling is achieved with hyperosmolar agents—either mannitol or hypertonic saline.[18] Mannitol is administered as a large bolus (1-2 g/kg) in the acute setting and is supplemented with smaller boluses (0.25 g/kg) every few hours as needed.[10] Serum osmolarity must be closely monitored and maintained below 320 mOsm. Hypertonic saline is administered either as 30 cc boluses of 7.5% solution or a continuous infusion of 3% solution with a goal of maintaining serum sodium around 155-160 mEq/L.[19] Hypertonic saline has the advantage of maintaining intravascular volume, whereas mannitol can lead to hypovolemia due to osmotic diuresis thereby compromising cerebral perfusion.[18]

In the most severe cases of intractably elevated ICP, adjunctive measures such as vasopressor agents (dopamine or norepinephrine) to increase MAP, as well as neuromuscular blockade and barbiturate coma to reduce cerebral metabolism, are also used. Decompressive craniectomy may have a role in the treatment of selected patients with severe intracranial hypertension[20,21] but has not yet been rigorously studied. Figure 27-1 summarizes the basic management of traumatic brain injury; Figure 27-2 outlines a common approach to managing elevated intracranial pressure.

While anticonvulsants such as phenytoin are often administered during the first week of TBI treatment, this therapy should not exceed seven days.[22,23] Corticosteroids have no role in TBI management.[1,10,24]

PENETRATING TBI

Due to the variability in injury patterns, the optimal management of penetrating injuries to the brain is less well established. Shockwaves created by the passing missile cause significant cavitation and severe parenchyma disruption away from the missile tract. Subsequent edema is often the cause of fatal elevated intracranial hypertension with herniation. Transcranial tracts that damage both hemispheres cause devastating injury with early herniation and carry an extremely high mortality rate.

Early CT is indicated to assess trajectory and to gauge prognosis. Plain films are not indicated if CT is available. Other modalities, such as MRI and ultrasound, are rarely used. Trajectories nearing vascular structures at the base of the skull may be an indication for angiography to assess vascular integrity.[25]

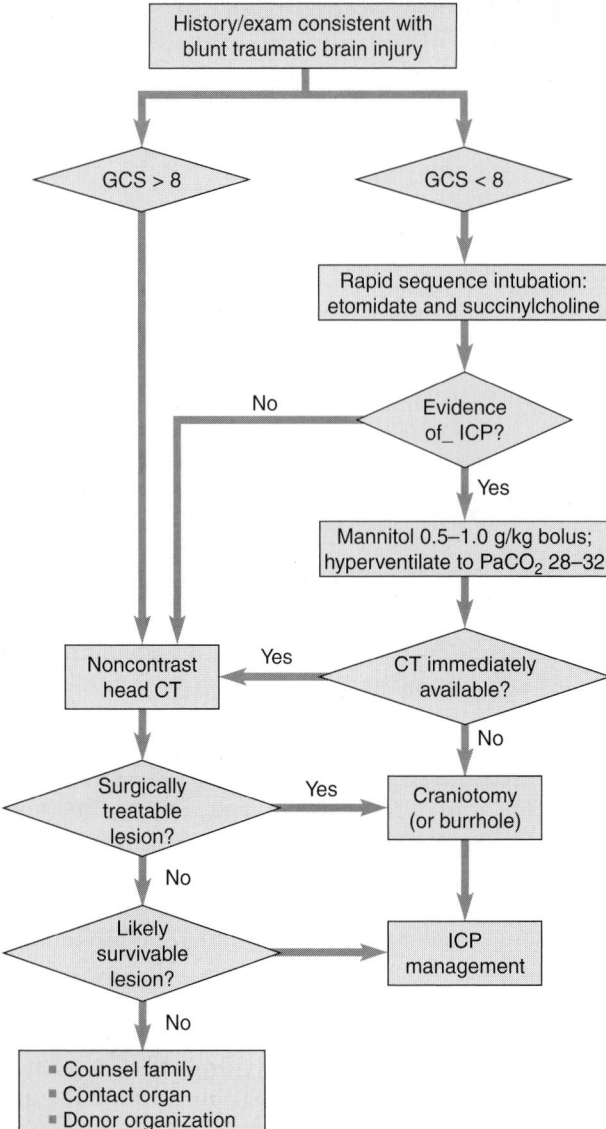

Figure 27-1 *Initial management of blunt traumatic brain injury.*

In penetrating brain injury, surgical intervention is indicated to evacuate hematomas caused by the laceration of cerebral vessels, to debride devitalized tissues, and to remove bone fragments from the wound. Extensive debridement or tract exploration, however, is discouraged because it may cause further neurologic damage. In general, bullets are not retrieved unless they are infected or are very easily accessible.

CRANIOFACIAL TRAUMA

SCALP LACERATIONS
Preoperative Valuation
Although lacerations to the scalp are very common after blunt injury and are often overlooked, their importance should not be underestimated. Injuries to this highly vascular area can result in rapid and

large-volume blood loss; in children they can lead to exsanguination.

Scalp lacerations are best evaluated only after quickly shaving the hair from the involved and surrounding areas. This maneuver not only provides exposure but also aids in cleaning the wound and avoiding subsequent wound infection. Failure to shave scalp lacerations often leads to inadequate hemostasis and poor wound approximation.

Operative Management
With hemorrhage possible in the setting of multiple injuries, rapid control of bleeding must often be achieved before a formal or "cosmetic" closure. Hemostasis can be achieved by a continuous interlocking closure, by suturing individual bleeding vessels, or by applying a Raney clip to the wound edges. The interlocking closure is the most widely used with removal and revision of the closure after the patient is stabilized.

Closure techniques vary depending on the depth and complexity of the wound. Linear, superficial lacerations that do *not* involve the galea aponeurotica can be simply approximated with skin staples. However, if the galea is lacerated, it must be repaired with absorbable suture followed by either stapled or sutured skin closure. Staples or sutures may be removed in 10-14 days. Wound infections are rare but do occur in heavily contaminated wounds or after poor surgical technique.

FACIAL LACERATIONS
Preoperative Valuation
Facial lacerations are common after blunt trauma and can usually be repaired in the emergency department without difficulty. However, it is not uncommon for these wounds to be associated with an underlying bony injury. Therefore, before proceeding with repair, fractures should be excluded either by thorough physical examination, radiography, or both.[26] If fractures are present, soft tissue repair is usually delayed until bony fixation is complete.

Similarly, lacerations close to vital structures, such as the salivary glands, the parotid duct, and the facial nerve and its branches require a proper assessment prior to closure. Injuries to the parotid duct require repair to prevent fistula formation.[27] Because this duct runs parallel to the buccal branch of the facial nerve, paralysis in its distribution suggests likely parotid duct injury and should prompt a thorough evaluation. Inserting a small silastic tube or blunt metallic probe into the oral opening adjacent to the second molar will assist in identifying the transected distal lumen. The proximal lumen will be seen to have saliva emanating from it. The duct can be repaired over the silastic tube using a fine monofilament suture (8-0 nylon) using magnification.[27] Injuries to the facial nerve and its named branches posterior to the line of the lateral

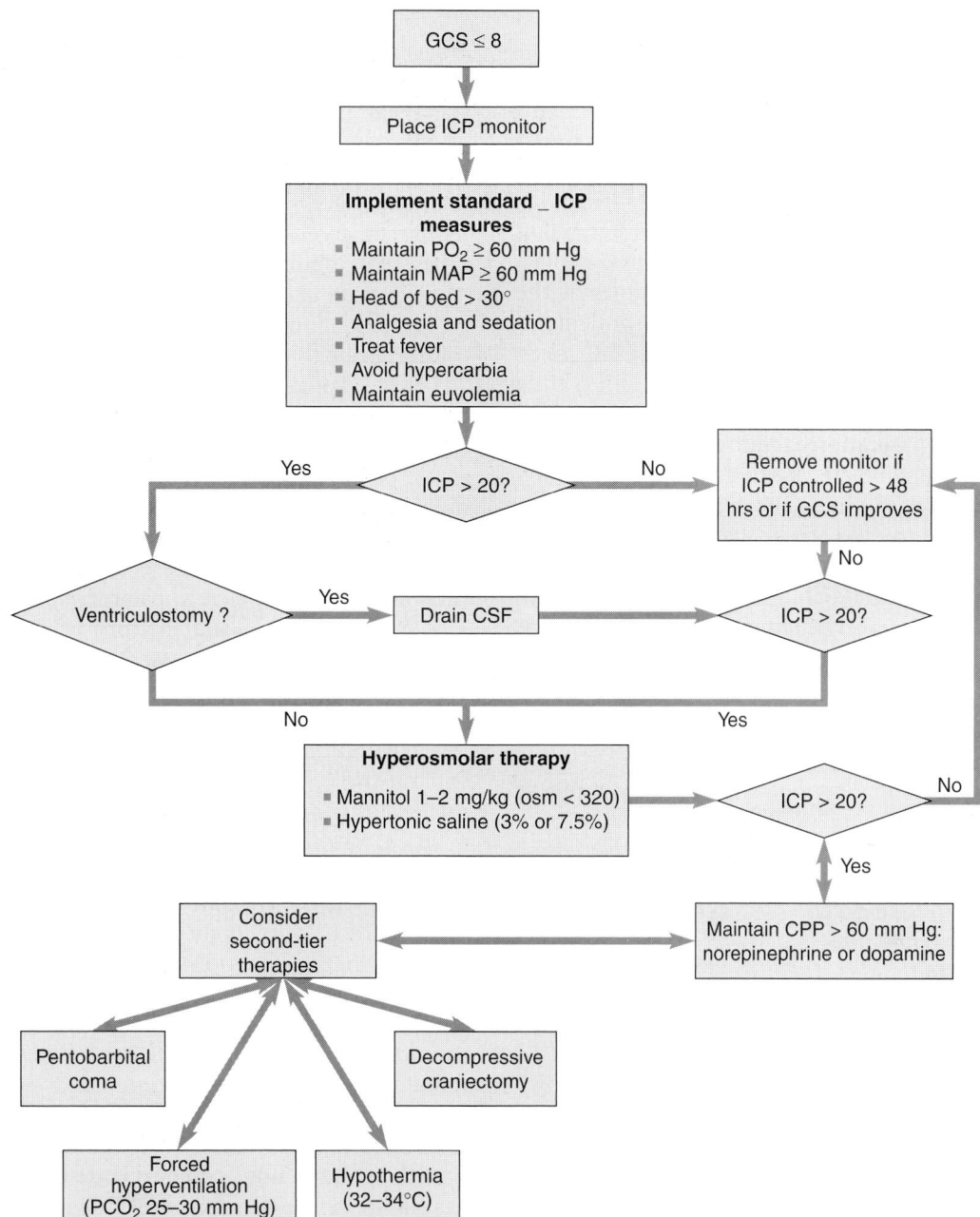

Figure 27-2 *Management of elevated intracranial injury.*

canthus of the eye should also be repaired. Consultation with a plastic surgeon or otolaryngologist may be indicated to achieve proper approximation of these injuries and for effective follow-up.

Operative Management

In the absence of underlying injury, repair of simple lacerations may proceed. The region must be properly anesthetized with a local or regional block (lidocaine or benzocaine). Thorough irrigation with saline, cleansing with an antibacterial soap (ie, Hibiclens), removing foreign bodies, and debriding devitalized tissue are all required to decrease the risk of wound infection. At times, highly contaminated wounds may be best treated by delayed primary closure after

a few days of attentive wound care and systemic antibiotics. Layered closures are indicated with muscle, fascia, and subcutaneous tissues being sequentially approximated as necessary with absorbable suture. This technique reduces tension on the skin closure and prevents the skin from adhering to deeper layers leading to poor cosmesis. Skin approximation can be accomplished with either interrupted or continuous 6-0 monofilament nonabsorbable suture (nylon or Prolene). Facial sutures should be removed in 3-5 days to avoid excessive scarring. Antibiotic ointment should be applied liberally at the time of repair and for the following 14 days with gentle massaging to prevent desiccation and to reduce scarring.

Lacerations to the lip, ear, and nose require special consideration. For lip lacerations, the vermillion-cutaneous border is approximated first with a single nonabsorbable suture in the skin at their junction. This technique provides proper alignment for subsequent muscle approximation with a 3-0 or 4-0 absorbable suture. Intraoral skin/mucosa is then repaired with interrupted absorbable suture, and the facial skin repair is completed with a 6-0 nonabsorbable suture. Ear lacerations are often associated with lacerations of the underlying cartilage. After cleansing and debridement, the cartilage is reapproximated with a 5-0 *clear*, monofilament nonabsorbable suture. The skin is then repaired over it with a 6-0 nonabsorable suture. Full thickness nasal lacerations require precise anatomic realignment. These repairs are performed in three layers. The mucosa is closed with a 4-0 absorbable suture, the cartilage is repaired with a 6-0 clear monofilament nonabsorbable suture, and the skin is closed with a 6-0 monofilament nonabsorbable suture. Table 27-3 summarizes the suture repair of lacerations to various areas of the head and face.

Table 27-3   Principles of Laceration Repairs

● **Scalp**
- ■ Liberally shave surrounding area
- ■ Control bleeding temporarily with Raney clips, interlocking sutures or direct vascular ligation
- ■ Always repair the Galea (absorbable suture)
- ■ Close the skin with nonabsorbable suture or staples

● **Face**
- ■ Exclude underlying fractures or injuries to vital structures
- ■ Debride thoroughly but conservatively
- ■ Close muscle and fascia (absorbable suture) separate from skin
- ■ Use 6-0 monofilament nonabsorbable (nylon or Prolene) for facial skin
- ■ Remove sutures in 3-5 days to avoid scarring

● **Lip**
- ■ First align vermillion–cutaneous border with a "key suture"
- ■ Then close labial muscle with absorbable suture
- ■ Repair mucosa with absorbable suture
- ■ Repair facial skin last with 6-0 nonabsorbable suture

● **Ear**
- ■ Re-approximate cartilage with 5-0 clear monofilament nonabsorbable suture
- ■ Close skin with 6-0 nonabsorbable suture

● **Nose**
- ■ Realign precisely and close in 3 layers
- ■ Repair nasal mucosa with 4-0 absorbable suture
- ■ Repair cartilage with 6-0 clear monofilament nonabsorbable suture
- ■ Repair nasal skin with 6-0 monofilament nonabsorbable suture

---

OCULAR TRAUMA

Preoperative Evaluation

Ocular trauma is very common and is a major cause of visual loss in the United States.[28] While nearly all ocular injuries will require evaluation by an ophthalmologist, the acute care surgeon is often the first team member to evaluate them.[29] Although few eye injuries require emergent intervention, recognizing those that do is the responsibility of the acute care specialist. Also, outside of major academic centers, general surgeons may be required to evaluate and stabilize these injuries prior to transfer to a higher level of care.

In evaluating ocular trauma, the goal for the acute care surgeon is to recognize sight-threatening injuries and to prevent secondary injury.[29] The most important aspect of ocular evaluation is the history. What was the mechanism? Blunt mechanisms such as motor vehicle crashes, assaults, and sports injuries typically cause very different injuries than penetrating mechanisms such as explosions, tool impalements, and shotguns. The patient's own ocular history is also important. Does the patient wear glasses or contacts? Has the patient had previous laser corrective *surgery* or cataract removal? Finally, what was the patient's visual quality immediately after the injury? These elements will help explain the findings on physical exam and will guide further testing and therapy.

In examining the eye after trauma, the single most important question that must be answered is, "Is this an open globe?" Penetrating injuries are, by definition, open globe injuries. If the globe is definitely or likely violated, the examination should stop. The eye should be covered with a metal or other hard patch for protection and immediate ophthalmologic consultation should be obtained. The patient should be given systemic antibiotics (ceftriaxone and vancomycin), tetanus prophylaxis, and analgesics and the patient's head should be elevated 30°.[30]

If the globe is not open or if the status is unknown, examination should proceed. While pain and swelling may limit the extent of examination, topical anesthetics and systemic analgesics can help significantly. After inspecting the eye and excluding a grossly open globe, the patient's visual acuity should be tested. This "vital sign of the eye" should be tested for each eye individually, must be accurately documented, and may require repeated evaluation. Acuity is often tested by using written materials. If the patient has visual loss and cannot see print, judge their ability to see larger objects by counting fingers. In more severe cases, assess more grossly such as testing the patient's ability to discriminate movement or whether or not the patient can detect light. The ocular examination continues by testing the pupils for reactivity to light. An appropriate bilateral response to a unilateral stimulus indicates an intact optic nerve in the setting of severe visual loss.

External assessment will identify lacerations to the eyelids and the periorbital tissues as well as corneal abrasions, subconjunctival hemorrhages, and hyphemas. While each of these conditions is relatively benign, they may indicate underlying bony injury or suggest more severe trauma to the eye itself. Intraocular foreign bodies should be noted and superficial ones removed. Extraocular movements must be tested in each direction to exclude entrapment of the extraocular muscles. The presence of enophthalmos or exophthalmos may also suggest more serious injury such as orbital blowout fracture or retrobulbar hemorrhage, respectively. Finally, if available, slit-lamp examination with fluorescein dye will identify corneal abrasions or small punctuate globe penetrations. [30]

The initial secondary examination of choice for all ocular and orbital injuries is thin-cut computed tomography. With 1-mm cuts and multiplanar reconstruction, the optic nerve, globe, orbit, and periorbital soft tissues can be assessed accurately. Plain films have little or no role in the modern evaluation of ocular trauma.

Operative Management

After excluding severe ocular trauma requiring ophthalmologist consultation, minor injuries can be managed by the evaluating acute care surgeon. Superficial corneal foreign bodies should be removed by gentle irrigation and/or with a soft cotton swab. Minor corneal abrasions are self-limited and require only topical antibiotic ointment for comfort. A patch is typically not required and follow-up with an ophthalmologist is only needed if symptoms last > 48 hours. Isolated subconjunctival hemorrhage also requires no specific treatment.[30]

While periorbital lacerations can be repaired similar to other facial lacerations, those full thickness injuries involving the upper eyelid, the cartilaginous tarsal plate, or the medial canthus (due to possible lacrimal duct injury) should be evaluated and repaired by an ophthalmologist. Similarly, imbedded foreign bodies, even in the absence of full thickness globe violation, will be best evaluated and treated by an experienced ophthalmologist.

Postoperative Care

There are a number of considerations in preparing to transport a patient with an ocular injury to a higher level of care. First, be sure to fully document the history, your physical examination, and the patient's visual acuity at the time of transfer. Carefully cover the eye with a metal patch. If a patch is not available, the bottom of a Styrofoam cup can be taped to the face to cover the eye. Pressure dressings should never be used. Supplemental oxygen should be supplied, especially if the patient is being transported by air. Systemic antibiotics and tetanus should be administered before transport if there is suspicion of an open globe. Antiemetics

and analgesics may be required. The patient's head should be elevated 30° (or reverse Trendelenberg if the spine is immobilized) to decrease swelling. Large, impaled foreign bodies such as knives or ice picks should not be removed prior to transport but rather carefully secured and stabilized for removal at the accepting facility.

MAXILLOFACIAL FRACTURES
Preoperative Evaluation

Facial fractures are common after blunt trauma. While dramatic in appearance and in presentation, they are not usually life threatening. More importantly, the acute care surgeon must recognize that facial fractures serve as a marker for a significant craniofacial impact and suggest the possibility of injury to adjacent neurologic, ocular, or cervical structures. On occasion, however, these injuries may lead to airway compromise or to life-threatening hemorrhage. The acute care surgeon must be able to accurately assess these injuries, recognize the implications to surrounding vital structures, and stabilize emergent conditions.

Operative Management

Airway compromise from facial injuries is most often due to fractures of the mandible. The muscular attachments to the mandible suspend the tongue anteriorly; loss of this support can result in airway obstruction by the tongue. Combined fractures of the nasal bones, maxilla, and mandible can also obstruct the airway due to a combination of pooling blood and mucous and from soft tissue edema.[31] In the comatose patient, these injuries can rapidly lead to airway loss with catastrophic consequences including anoxic brain injury and severe aspiration. Although rapid orotracheal intubation is the ideal method of securing the airway, the edema and bleeding may make vocal cord visualization more difficult or even impossible. In this setting, the surgeon must not hesitate to create a surgical airway to save the patient's life. A rapid cricothyroidotomy is the procedure of choice (see **Cricothyroidotomy**). Formal or percutaneous tracheostomy are too time consuming and cannot be efficiently performed in the emergency setting.

Severe bleeding from facial fractures is rare but can occur with basilar skull fractures or nasal or maxillary fractures. Nasal bleeding after trauma may require packing for tamponade. Nasal packs can be inserted anteriorly into the nares with forceps to achieve hemostasis. However, if this technique fails, posterior packing is indicated.[32,33] This is accomplished by inserting the end of a rubber catheter into the nares and retrieving it from the pharynx with a forceps or clamp. The string from the nasal pack is then secured to the tip of the catheter, and the catheter is withdrawn firmly from the nares. The string is pulled tight and is secured. Bilateral posterior packing usually controls most nasomaxillary bleeding. When nasal packing is unavailable, urinary balloon catheters (Foley) can be used in a similar fashion by inserting the catheter into the nasopharynx through the nares, inflating the balloon, and withdrawing firmly to tamponade bleeders with the inflated balloon.[32,33] A hemostat may be used to secure the clamp and maintain tension. Recently, commercially produced devices and balloons have become available for anterior and posterior nasal packing.

Postoperative Care

After excluding life-threatening conditions, the secondary survey continues with a comprehensive examination of the facial structures. Initially, inspect for hematomas, asymmetry, and lacerations. Ask the patient to bite down to assess for malocclusion, indicting a likely mandibular fracture. Next gently palpate the orbital ridge circumferentially as well as the maxilla, zygoma, and mandible. Apply bilateral pressure to the maxillae and gently pull on the upper jaw to assess for facial instability.

A complete cranial nerve (CN) examination must be accomplished in all patients with facial fractures or severe facial lacerations. This can even be performed in the comatose patient. CN II and III are evaluated by testing the pupillary response to light. Symmetric constriction indicates intact nerves. CN III, IV, and VI provide extraocular movement and are tested by asking the patient to look in the six cardinal directions. In the comatose patient, the oculocephalic (doll's eyes) and oculovestibular (cold caloric) reflexes also evaluate these nerves in addition to CN VIII. CN V provides facial sensation and innervates the muscles of mastication. CN VII innervates the muscles of facial expression. The corneal reflex tests both CN V and VII in the comatose patient. CN VIII provides hearing as well as the reflexes noted above. CN IX and X elevate the palate when the patient says "Ahh..." and also provide the gag reflex in the comatose patient. CN XI innervates the trapesius and CN XII innervates the muscles of the tongue.[34]

Fine-cut CT is usually the only radiographic study needed to evaluate facial fractures. Three-dimensional images are easily obtained with current multidetector scanners. Neither plain films of the face nor Panorex films provide additional data to the consulting plastic surgeon or otolaryngologist.[31]

Of note, orbital blowout fractures are relatively common after blunt trauma. These fractures occur after a large compressive force is applied to the globe causing increased intraorbital pressure and resulting in a fracture (or "blowout") of either the floor or medial wall of the orbit. The acute care surgeon must recognize that, with these fractures, the eye itself has usually sustained a significant force. Further periorbital tissues such as extraocular muscle and orbital fat often herniate into the adjacent sinuses. The result can be a ruptured or damaged globe, extraocular muscle entrapment, and/or enophthalmos. Because of these potentially devastation sequelae, orbital blowout fractures require ophthalmologic evaluation in addition to an otolaryngologist or plastic surgeon.

GUNSHOT WOUNDS OF THE FACE

Preoperative Evaluation

Gunshot injuries to the face deserve special mention. While often dramatic in appearance, such as with close range shotgun injuries or submandibular suicide attempts, the management of these injuries follows the same basic algorithm as other conditions of the head and neck. Airway control is a priority in this setting. Initially with many injuries there may be little swelling; however, the clinician should consider that with time, the airway may become compromised by edema and bleeding. Here, early orotracheal intubation and sedation is indicated to complete the rest of the workup. In more extensive facial injuries where normal anatomic landmarks are severely distorted or are missing, immediate cricothyroidotomy is the safest and most expeditious method to control the airway. When the face has been "blown away," attempts at orotracheal intubation through the injury should not be attempted and only increase the duration of hypoxia/anoxia.

Operative Management

Once the airway is secure, hemorrhage control follows through a combination of surgical ligation and radiographic embolization. Little debridement should occur during the initial evaluation because reconstructive efforts may be extensive. After hemostasis, the evaluation can continue with a CT of the region (both head and neck) to determine trajectory and to assess the need for further imaging studies such as a four-vessel angiogram. Plain films are superfluous and should not be obtained.

Postoperative Care

Once the initial evaluation is complete, otolaryngologists, oromaxillofacial surgeons, plastic surgeons, and/or ophthalmologists should be consulted as indicated by the extent of injury. This multidisciplinary approach to the facial reconstruction typically lead to the best possible functional and cosmetic outcome in these often-devastating and disfiguring injuries.[35]

BLUNT NECK TRAUMA

LARYNGOTRACHEAL TRAUMA

Preoperative Evaluation

Blunt injuries to the larynx are rare but can occur with a direct impact to the anterior neck; they also occur with attempted hangings. These crushing mechanisms typically result in thyroid cartilage fractures. Tracheal injuries due to blunt mechanisms include cricotracheal separation, tracheal lacerations, and avulsion of a mainstem bronchus.

On presentation, awake patients with laryngotracheal injuries will often position themselves upright and forward in the ambulance and in the emergency center to maintain their airway. In this setting, the patient has discovered on his/her own the position of greatest airway comfort and function. Despite concerns about cervical spine injury and immobilization, the patient must NOT be forced to lay down supine. The airway is the priority. Direct transport to the operating room for intubation or tracheostomy in the upright position may be necessary prior to any further evaluation.

On physical exam there will typically be subcutaneous emphysema with most laryngotracheal injuries. With laryngeal injuries, the thyroid cartilage will have an abnormal contour on palpation. The patient may have dysphonia and hemoptysis may be present. After tracheal injury, pneumothorax is common and tension physiology may develop.[36]

Operative Management

The single most important priority in these patients, once the injury is recognized, is to secure the airway. As the surrounding tissues swell, and as hematoma accumulates, the situation will become more tenuous. Orotracheal intubation can be hazardous in blunt laryngotracheal injuries and may further traumatize the area.[18] If possible, performing an awake tracheostomy in the operating room under local anesthesia is the best option. However, in the emergent situation, cricothyroidotomy is indicated by realizing that the tracheostomy may also worsen the injury. Because the tissue will be distorted, this relatively straightforward procedure will be much more difficult.

The airway is more difficult to secure in distal tracheal injuries. In this setting, careful intubation over a bronchoscope (past the injury) may be the only way to achieve airway control. This technique also allows for selective mainstem intubation opposite to a distal tracheobronchial injury.

After the airway is secure, further management is determined by the extent of the injury. Certain minor laryngeal fractures can be treated nonoperatively after tracheostomy. More complex fractures and certain tracheal injuries require operative repair. Laryngeal and proximal tracheal injuries are typically approached through a collar incision 2 cm above the sternal notch. If needed, the upper sternum can be divided through the collar incision to reach more distant tracheal injuries. For injuries to the distal third of the trachea or to either mainstem, a right posterolateral thoracotomy is used.

Laryngotracheal injuries in the neck should be approached anteriorly by splitting the thyroid gland longitudinally.[36,37] Avoid lateral or circumferential dissection; the recurrent laryngeal nerves should *not* be sought out nor identified because this has been shown to increase the incidence of nerve injury.[18,38] Fractures to the larynx are repaired using a perichondral nonabsorbable suture (ie, Prolene) or small metal plates.[36] Tracheal lacerations and laryngeal mucosal tears are repaired with interrupted absorbable sutures (ie, Maxon or polydioxanone, PDS), ensuring that knots are on the outside. Avoid performing a tracheostomy in the injured area.

BLUNT CEREBROVASCULAR INJURY

Since their recognition more than 30 years ago, blunt cerebrovascular injuries (BCVI) had long been considered rare and enigmatic clinical entities. Due a generally low index of suspicion and a lack of efficient screening exams, these injuries typically presented only after the development of neurological symptoms and irreversible damage.[39-43] Given this approach, devastating neurological outcomes were essentially unavoidable. More recently, studies have provided evidence that early screening and treatment of BCVI is justified and can improve neurologic outcomes.[28,42,44-47]

Epidemiology

Classically, three fundamental mechanisms of injury lead to BCVI: direct force to the neck, laceration by bony fragments from adjacent fractures, and hyperextension during contralateral head rotation.[39,41] The latter is the most common cause of carotid artery injury due to stretching of the vessel over the C1-C3 articular processes. Carotid artery injuries after blunt trauma have stroke rates as high as 50%. Clinically these ischemic events typically cause contralateral sensorimotor deficits. Vertebral artery injuries are most often due to associated fractures of the transverse processes of the cervical vertebrae where a combination of direct injury and stretching is to blame. These injuries result in stroke in 25% of cases and manifest mainly as vestibular symptoms such as ataxia, nausea/vomiting, and dizziness, as well as visual field defects.[41] Independent of the mechanism, in BCVI intimal disruption occurs, which leads to platelet aggregation potentially leading to emboli or to complete vascular thrombosis.

Preoperative Evaluation

While some patients develop symptoms from BCVI early in their presentation, most arrive asymptomatic and exhibit a "silent period." This phase is variable in duration but typically lasts from 10 to 72 hours before the onset of neurological symptoms. It is this asymptomatic period that forms the justification for modern screening protocols.[42,48] Criteria for screening have

Table 27-4   Indications for screening for Blunt Cerebrovascular Injury (BCVI)

Injury-Based Risk Factors for BCVI
- LeForte II or III facial fracture
- Cervical spine fractures: C1-C3
- Cervical spine fractures extending into transverse foramina.
- Cervical spine subluxation
- Basilar skull fracture involving the carotid canal
- Near hanging
- Diffuse axonal injury with coma
- Seatbelt sign across neck

Signs or Symptoms of BCVI
- Bleeding or expanding cervical hematoma
- Carotid bruit
- Neurological exam inconsistent with CT findings
- Stroke on delayed head CT

Table 27-5   Denver Grading Scale for BCVI

Grade I	Irregularity of the vessel wall or a dissection/intramural hematoma with less than 25% luminal stenosis
Grade II	Intraluminal thrombus or raised intimal fLap; dissection/intra-mural hematoma with 25% or more luminal narrowing
Grade III	Pseudoaneurysm
Grade IV	Vessel occlusion
Grade V	Vessel transaction

been established (Table 27-4), including signs or symptoms of BCVI or risk factors for BCVI based on injury patterns.[41,45,46,48] While four-vessel cerebral angiography remains the gold standard for diagnosis in most institutions, increasingly computed tomographic angiography (CTA) is being used as a screening tool.[41,49-52] However, the accuracy of CTA is yet to be correlated to the gold-standard arteriogram. While initial reports of CTA were disappointing, with sensitivities < 70%,[50] improved multislice detector technology and increasing experience with this modality has greatly enhanced its usefulness. Using four- and eight-slice detector CT scanners, Bub and colleagues[50] reported sensitivities of 83%-92% for carotid artery injuries in a retrospective comparison of CTA versus four-vessel angiography; sensitivity for vertebral artery injuries was 80%. Interestingly, using 4- and 16-slice detector CT scanners, Berne et al[51] demonstrated 100% sensitivity for BCVI using CTA. The decision to utilize 4-vessel angiogram versus CTA in screening for BCVI is based on the equipment available and experience of the neuroradiologists and surgeons at an individual institution. Magnetic resonance angiography (MRA) may also be an emerging screening tool; however, the prolonged examination time and incompatibility of some equipment with the magnetic field limits its use.[53] Duplex ultrasound is not a sensitive-enough imaging modality to screen for BCVI.[54]

Management

Once the diagnosis is made, management is based on the grade of the injury and the patient's overall medical condition. Table 27-5 shows the Denver Grading Scale for BCVI.[41,55] In the absence of complete occlusion, anatomically accessible lesions of the carotid may be treated surgically with resection and interposition graft. If there are no contraindications to anticoagulation, the remaining patients are treated with an antithrombotic regimen.[47] Both systemic heparinization with transition to warfarin and antiplatelet therapy with aspirin and clopidogrel have been successfully used to treat patients with BCVI; either regimen appears efficacious, significantly reducing stroke rates and improving neurologic outcomes in some series.[41,47] While endovascular stents have been used in BCVI, complication rates due to stroke and vascular occlusion appear prohibitive at this time.[41,56] A useful algorithm for diagnosis and treatment of BCVI is given in Fig. 27-3. Because standardized meanings have not been established between surgeons and their neuroradiology colleagues, for some acute care surgeons, even these recommendations require further study and specific delineation as to efficacy among multiple centers.

PENETRATING NECK TRAUMA

The neck is a highly complex anatomic region with critical aerodigestive, vascular, and neurologic structures concentrated in a very small area and volume. The evaluation and management of penetrating injury to this region is challenging to trauma surgeons and continues to evolve. The key to evaluating any gunshot or stab victim is reliably tracking the tissues penetrated by the missile or blade. The inability to determine "trajectory" by examination alone leads to clinical uncertainty and is the crux of controversies surrounding the evaluation and treatment of patients with these complex wounds. Because missed injuries or delays in diagnosis lead to increased morbidity and mortality with penetrating neck trauma, surgeons do agree on the importance of rapid and confident injury identification and exclusion of life-threatening cervical injuries.[57]

PREOPERATIVE EVALUATION

The initial evaluation of patients with penetrating neck trauma is largely dependent on the physical

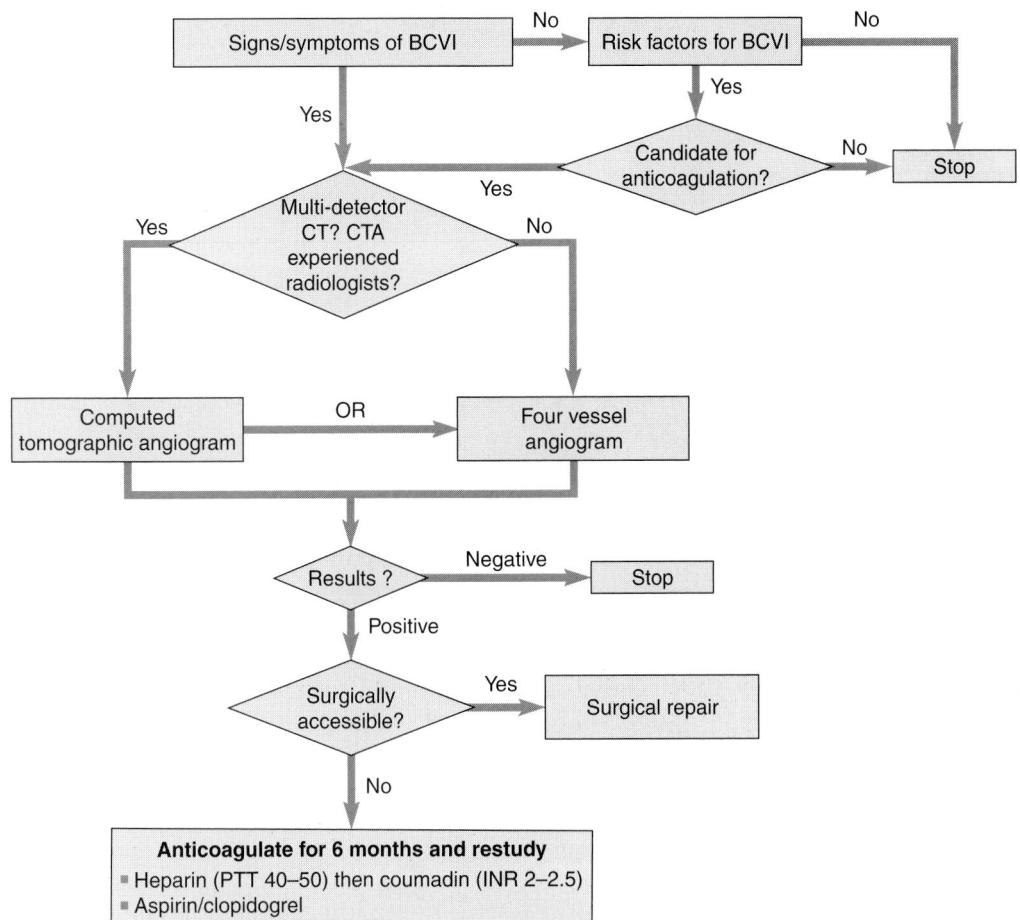

Figure 27-3 *Screening and management of BCVI.*

examination and physiologic status of the patient. Hemodynamic instability or hard signs of injury (Table 27-6) to vital structures mandate immediate operative exploration and repair. So-called "hard signs" of vascular injury include pulsatile bleeding, expanding hematoma, bruit, or unilateral upper extremity pulse deficit. Hard signs of aerodigestive injury are subcutaneous emphysema, wound bubbling,

hoarseness, stridor, or airway compromise. There is no place for secondary testing early in the evaluation of these patients. Thorough operative exploration is indicated with repair or control of all injured structures.

HEMODYNAMICALLY NORMAL PATIENTS

Traditional Approach

The traditional approach to managing hemodynamically normal patients with penetrating anterior neck trauma utilizes the classical neck "zones" as described by Roon and Christensen in 1979.[58] Based largely on the experience of Fogelman and Stewart in 1956,[59] subplatysmal penetrations to Zone II (between the cricoid and the angle of the mandible) have classically mandated complete operative exploration to evaluate the vasculature, trachea, and esophagus in all patients. With Zone I injuries (below the cricoid) and Zone III injuries (above the angle of the mandible), due to the complexity of operative exposure, traditional evaluation relies upon angiography to interrogate the vasculature as well as endoscopy and contrast radiography to evaluate the aerodigestive tract.

Table 27-6	Indications for Immediate Surgery after Penetrating Neck Trauma

- Shock
- Pulsatile bleeding
- Expanding hematoma
- Unilateral extremity pulse deficit
- Audible bruit or palpable thrill
- Airway compromise
- Wound bubbling
- Extensive subcutaneous emphysema
- Stridor
- Hoarseness

Selective Approach

While there has been little controversy surrounding the management of Zone I or Zone III injuries, which are not amenable to accurate physical examination, the management of Zone II penetrations has continued to evolve. In 1994, Atteberry[60] and others described 53 patients with penetrating injury to Zone II. Of these patients, 19 underwent immediate operation based on physical signs. The remaining 34 were managed selectively based on physical exam: 6 patients had angiograms, 18 had carotid duplex, and the others were observed. There were no missed vascular injuries. This report was followed in 1997 by Demetriades[61] and others who prospectively evaluated 223 patients with penetrating neck trauma and included injury to any zone. They compared physical examination findings with the results of angiography, duplex exam, and esophagram and concluded that physical examination could be used to triage patients for further vascular or esophageal studies. They also noted that duplex was a reliable alternative to angiography. In 2003, Azuaje[62] and others reinforced the sensitivity of physical exam to identify vascular injuries requiring repair. They retrospectively reviewed 152 stable patients who underwent four-vessel angiogram after penetrating neck injury. Of the 89 patients who had no physical examination findings suggesting vascular injury, only 3 had positive angiograms, none of whom required operative intervention. They reported a sensitivity of 93% and negative predictive value of 97% for physical exam to identify and exclude vascular injury after penetrating neck trauma and recommended a selective approach based on physical examination findings.

While certainly well described and apparently supported by the literature, few modern trauma surgeons would rely entirely on physical examination to exclude an injury in patients with penetrating neck injuries, regardless of the zone involved. The more commonly accepted application of a "selective management" strategy, and the one most commonly taught to surgeons-in-training, applies the same diagnostic approach to all three cervical zones based on penetration of the platysma, normal hemodynamics, and the absence of "hard" signs of injury. In this scheme, all patients who do not require immediate operation undergo vascular and aerodigestive interrogation with angiography, bronchoscopy, and esophagoscopy and/or esophagography to exclude injury.[63-68] Operative strategies are then directed at specific identified injuries.

This nonspecific algorithm is certainly accurate and reliable to identify and exclude injury. However, this approach does have very real disadvantages. First, this strategy is labor and resource intensive, often requiring input from multiple specialties. Also, as many authors have indicated, the overall diagnostic yield is low with only 10% of patients who undergo selective management having findings on angiography or endoscopy that requires operative intervention.[61] Next, this approach is expensive with costs in excess of $2000 per patient.[61] Finally, these diagnostic procedures are invasive and carry a small but real risk of complications.[69] Interestingly, Meyer[69] and others prospectively evaluated the "selective approach" versus mandatory exploration. Arteriography, panendoscopy, and esophagography were performed in 113 patients with Zone II penetrations, followed by mandatory exploration. Meyer[69] and others identified six major vascular or visceral injuries that were missed using the selective approach.

In the search for less invasive diagnostic techniques, Montalvo et al[70] and Demetriades et al[61] found color duplex ultrasonography to be an accurate alternative to angiogram for arterial evaluation in Zone II or Zone III penetrations. However, this modality is of limited availability, is operator dependent, and requires specialist expertise for interpretation. Ultrasound is further inhibited by patient body habitus, its inability to image the skull base, and its lack of impact on the need for aerodigestive tract evaluation.

Modern Approach

With these different issues in mind, surgeons continue to question whether rigid algorithmic protocols involving multiple invasive studies should apply to the evaluation of all stable patients who sustain penetrating neck injuries. Coupled with the increasing incidence of multizone penetrations, the profession-wide trend toward less invasive diagnostic (and therapeutic) approaches, and the ever-increasing speed and improving resolution of multidetector computed tomography (CT) scanners, newer algorithms are beginning to include helical CT in their diagnostic approach.

In addition to being entirely noninvasive, helical CT with timed contrast injection has the advantage of providing information on all vital neck structures. Not only are the arterial[71] and aerodigestive structures imaged, but major venous, nervous, and bony injuries can also be assessed as well. Trajectory is often clearly demonstrated by this modality: most clearly show ballistic trauma but often with stab wounds as well. When helical CT clearly visualizes trajectory and excludes important structures from the path of injury, no further imaging is needed. In patients where the wounding trajectory is in proximity to a vital structure or where trajectory is unclear, helical CT serves as a triage tool to select those structures that require further individualized invasive diagnostic evaluation.

There is a growing body of literature to support the use helical CT angiography to evaluate patients after penetrating neck trauma. Ofer[72] studied 16 patients with potential carotid artery injuries and determined that CT angiography is highly accurate in diagnosing vascular injury and allowing successful nonoperative management in patients with negative CT scans. In 2001, Mazolewski[73] prospectively compared trauma surgeon–evaluated neck CT with mandatory operative exploration after Zone II penetration and found a sensitivity of 100% for identifying injuries that would require operative intervention. That same year Gracias[75] reported a retrospective series of 23 patients and found that CT was a safe and effective modality "to direct or eliminate further invasive studies in selected stable patients with penetrating neck injury."

In 2002, a prospective study by Munera[76] evaluated 175 patients with penetrating neck injury by CT angiography. The authors were able to characterize vascular injuries accurately in 27 (15.6%) patients and direct them to appropriate therapy. The other 146 patients were successfully observed without further intervention and without missed injury. In 2003, Gonzalez[77] prospectively evaluated a helical CT scan with oral but no IV contrast versus oral contrast esophagography to detect esophageal injuries in stable patients who sustained penetrating neck trauma. The study reported equivalent accuracy of these modalities in the evaluation of penetrating injury to the cervical esophagus and noted that the sensitivity of helical CT was similar to physical examination. Of note, 86% of the patients were stab victims. Certainly one of the recognized limitations of the use of CT in penetrating neck trauma is its difficulty in detecting the trajectory of knife penetrations. In particular, small pharyngoesophageal knife injuries are difficult to detect with CT scan. The conclusions of this study and the limitations it identifies do not apply to patients with ballistic trauma.

Based on the current evidence, there is an increasingly defined role for the use of helical CT in evaluating stable patients with penetrating trauma to the neck who do not have hard signs of vascular or aerodigestive injury. Regardless of the zone of penetration, using this technology is an acceptable method to determine trajectory and thereby triage patients to the operating room, to further specific invasive studies, or to observation and serial examination.[72,75,76,78] If helical CT is not immediately available, if the findings on helical CT are inconclusive, or if the findings do not match the clinical picture, traditional methods of evaluating penetrating neck trauma with angiography, panendoscopy, esophagography, or operative exploration should be pursued. As helical CT technology continues to improve and as surgeons become more comfortable with its use, the role of CT in evaluating stable patients with penetrating injuries will continue to expand.[72,79] Figure 27-4 summarizes the early evaluation and management of penetrating neck injuries.

NECK EXPLORATION FOR PENETRATING TRAUMA

While a specific case can be made for the extensive and complex diagnostic workup for penetrating neck injury, many surgeons make a strong case that the quickest and most expeditious approach to penetrating neck trauma is an immediate neck exploration. The operative management of penetrating injuries of the neck is daunting in that many delicate structures are packed together in a very small space. Furthermore, unlike elective Surgery, hematoma typically distorts the tissue planes and makes an elegant dissection impossible. In operating on the neck, knowledge of its anatomy and its exposure is key. Consider that proximal or distal control may require access to the skull base or chest; therefore, prep and drape accordingly. Also, consider placing a roll under the shoulders to extend the neck, thus improving exposure.

A longitudinal incision on the anterior border of the sternocleidomastoid provides the best exposure for the potential vascular or aerodigestive injuries that may be encountered. Hirschberg and Mattox[80] recommended following the "Trail of Safety," discussed in their recent book *Top Knife*. After entering the platysma, find and stay anterior to the anterior border of the sternocleidomastoid. Failure to do so will result in significant muscle bleeding. Retracting the sternocleidomastoid posteriorly while dissecting its anterior border will lead directly to the internal jugular (IJ) vein. Bleeding is easily stopped with direct pressure. Injuries can be controlled with side-biting vascular clamps and repaired with 5-0 polypropylene. Alternatively, in the extreme situation, the IJ can be ligated with impunity.

Once the IJ is identified, the facial vein will be noted superiorly on its anterior aspect. This is "gatekeeper of the neck" and usually lies directly over the carotid bifurcation.[80] Dividing the facial vein(s) will allow the IJ to be retracted from the underlying carotid artery. The periadventitial plane is the safest area for vascular dissection; gain this plane on the artery's anterior surface where there are no branches. As in elective *Surgery*, gaining proximal and distal control in an uninjured area is the ideal in approaching any vascular injury. This may require extending the incision or even a sternotomy. In some cases, however, such control may not be possible. In this setting, attack the injury straight on and use a finger to gain temporary control while an assistant dissects the rest of the vessel.

Once the vessel is isolated, control can be gained with atraumatic clamps, Rummel tourniquets, or intraluminal balloon catheters. Repair is usually accomplished by resecting the injured segment and placing a synthetic graft. Remember to thrombectomize the vessel before repair. Local or systemic heparinization

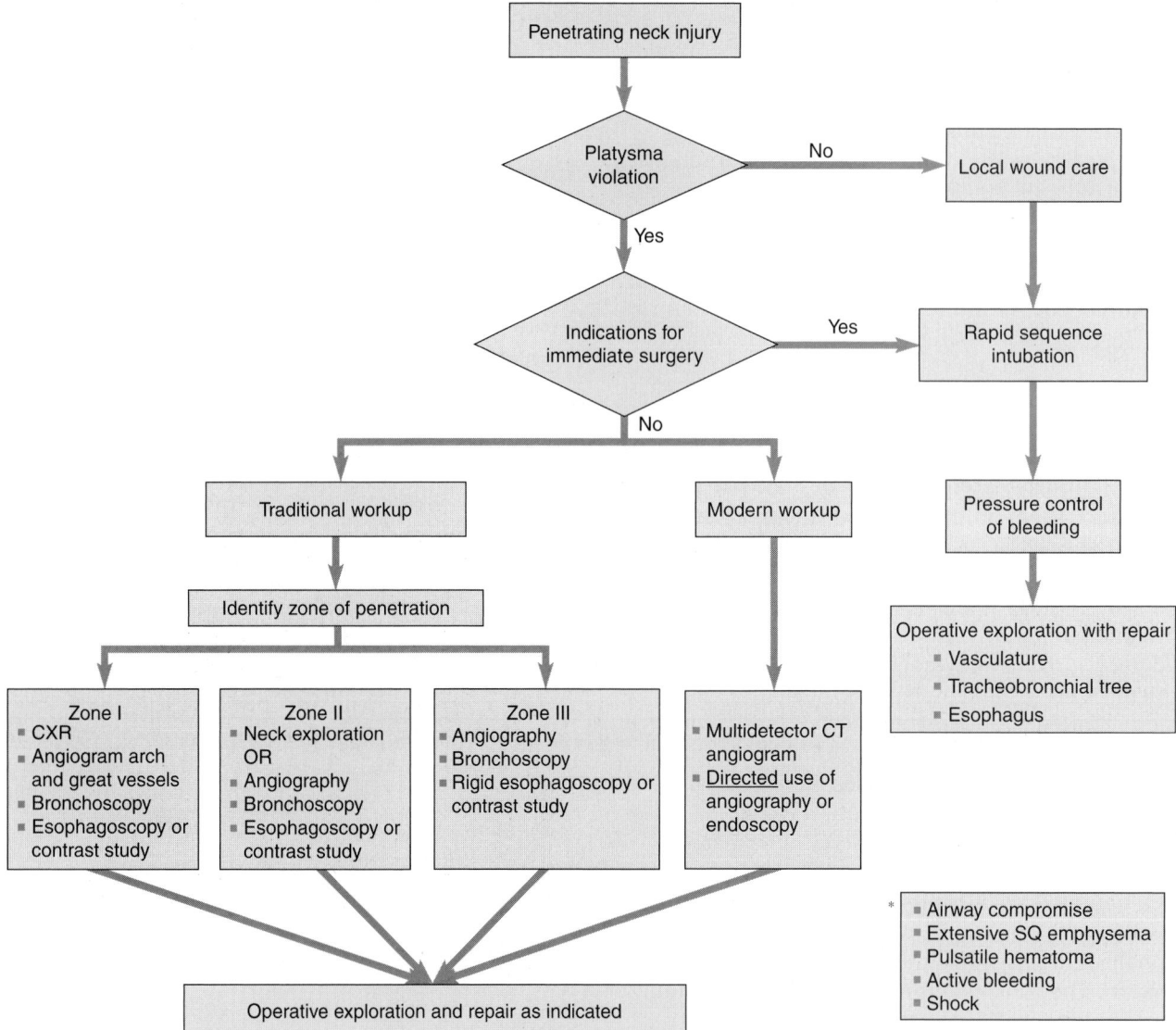

Figure 27-4 *Evaluation and management of penetrating neck injury.*

should be used during occlusion if the patient's condition allows. Damage control options (in extreme settings) for carotid injuries include temporary shunts and ligation.

The esophagus lies medial to the carotid just behind the trachea. A nasogastric tube placed by the anesthesiologist can help identify this structure. To get complete exposure of the cervical esophagus, one must retract the thyroid gland medially. Dividing the omohyoid muscle, the middle thyroid vein, and the inferior thyroid artery will give complete access to the entire cervical esophagus.[80] After debridement, a single layer of full-thickness monofilament absorbable sutures is typically adequate for the repair of most injuries. A closed suction drain is recommended and is typically left in place until after a barium esophagram at 1 week confirms the absence of a leak.[81] Tracheal injuries are typically repaired with 3-0 monofilament absorbable sutures.

In any combined injury to the vessels, esophagus, and/or trachea interpose well-vascularized tissue such as strap muscles, omohyoid, or sternocleidomastoid in between the structures to prevent fistula formation. For transcervical injuries, create a trap door–type incision by connecting bilateral sternocleidomastoid incisions with a horizontal incision below the thyroid cartilage. This U-shaped incision will give great exposure to the entire anterior neck. Finally, an unanticipated injury to the vertebral artery should prompt an effort to temporize the injury while waiting for definitive *angiographic* control. A large balloon catheter (Foley) or bone wax is often effective measures. Attempts to gain direct operative control of vertebral artery injuries are fraught with disaster.

CRICOTHYROIDOTOMY

Although it has often been described in complex terms using various instruments and devices, in reality, the cricothyroidotomy requires only a No. 11 scalpel and a 6 Fr endotracheal tube (ETT). The surgeon should avoid using retractors, hemostats, tracheostomy hooks, or any other instrument. In most patients the cricothyroid membrane is less than 1 cm below the skin. Even in an obese patient, a knowledgeable finger is better than any other instrument.

The procedure is usually emergent, and sterility is not a factor, as the airway itself is not sterile. The landmarks are palpated with the cricothyroid membrane being the *second* depression caudal to the mandible. We mention this because a common mistake made by novices is to confuse the thyrohyoid membrane for the cricothyroid membrane. Once the cricothyroid membrane is palpated, a small (1 cm) transverse incision is made directly over the cricothyroid membrane. The small size of this incision is the key. It only needs to be large enough for an index finger. Larger incisions lead to bleeding from anterior jugular veins laterally.

After incising the skin, insert an index finger both to confirm the position of the cricothyroid membrane and to bluntly dissect the soft tissues from on top of it. Spreading with hemostats or other devices is not necessary and leads to bleeding by damaging adjacent veins. Once the soft tissues have been bluntly swept from on top of the membrane, the No. 11 blade is inserted vertically directly into the membrane. It is removed and inverted so that the handle of the scalpel can be inserted next and rotated 180°—again to bluntly spread open the cricothyroid membrane. No other instrument should be used. The scalpel handle is removed and is simultaneously exchanged for the index finger of the nondominant hand. This move allows one to absolutely confirm that the proper structure is entered. Finally, the index finger is exchanged for the 6 Fr ETT. Alternatively, a 6 Fr tracheostomy tube can be used, but it is much harder to manipulate in the emergent setting. The airway is then secured to the skin on both sides with 2-0 nylon or polypropylene.

NONTRAUMATIC HEAD/NECK EMERGENCIES

EPISTAXIS

Preoperative Evaluation

Occasionally, the acute care surgeon will be asked to evaluate a patient with nontraumatic epistaxis. While rarely life threatening, this common clinical problem does, on occasion, present with airway compromise or hemodynamic instability. Such severe uncontrolled epistaxis is typically present in the setting of a significant concomitant systemic illness (eg, cirrhosis, hemophilia, or leukemia) or with the use of systemic anticoagulants (eg, antiplatelet drugs or warfarin).

Operative Management

Most commonly, epistaxis occurs in the anterior nares from Kiesselbach plexus along the nasal septum. Its presentation is usually clinically obvious with blood dripping from the affected nares. The bleeding site can usually be visualized with a nasal speculum and a penlight. In contrast, posterior epistaxis arises from the sphenopalatine arteries located in the superior aspect of the posterior nasal cavity. Its presentation is varied, ranging from nausea and anemia to hematemesis, hemoptysis, or melena. It may be impossible to discern which side is bleeding with posterior epistaxis.

As with any emergency medical condition, a stable airway must be secured. With airway compromise, brisk nasopharyngeal bleeding may make orotracheal intubation challenging; however, with proper suctioning and good technique, a surgical airway is usually avoided. Anterior bleeding is usually controlled by simple compression of the nares. If bleeding continues after 5 minutes of compression, it should be followed by tamponade with nasal packing consisting of decongestant-soaked (phenylephrine or oxymetolazone) gauze. If these generalized measures fail, an attempt should be made to identify the source of bleeding by direct visualization using a nasal speculum. Once identified, the area can be cauterized with either a silver nitrate stick (applied for 30 seconds) or electrocautery.[33]

Posterior bleeding is more difficult to control, and early consultation from an otolaryngologist is recommended. If temporizing measures are necessary, posterior nasal packing is accomplished by inserting a rubber catheter into the nares and retrieving the tip from the oral cavity with a forceps or clamp. Commercially available or improvised gauze packs are then secured by a string or umbilical tape to the catheter and pulled into the mouth and drawn tight against the posterior nasal cavity with firm, persistent tension. Balloon tamponade with a 10-14 French Foley catheter is also effective and is accomplished similarly by inserting the catheter into the bleeding nares and visualizing the tip in the oropharynx, filling the balloon with 10 cc of saline, and withdrawing the catheter firmly. Tension is maintained on either the gauze packing or the balloon catheter by applying a padded clamp at the level of the nares or by tying another gauze pack to the external portion of the string or catheter with a 0 silk suture. Bilateral packing may be necessary if the exact bleeding site is unknown.[33]

Postoperative Management

Persistent bleeding despite these techniques requires a search for other correctable factors such as coagulopathy from illness or medications, uncontrolled hypertension, or improper packing techniques. In extreme cases, bleeding vessels may require angiographic embolization by an interventional radiologist or operative ligation by an otolaryngologist.

AIRWAY OBSTRUCTION

Preoperative Management

Aside from traumatic causes of airway compromise, the acute care surgeon may become emergently involved in the care of patients with airway obstruction from other causes. These etiologies are most commonly aspiration of foreign bodies (including vomitus), oropharyngeal or cervical soft tissue infections, and anaphylaxis. Other causes include tumors of the head and neck and postsurgical bleeding with external compression.

The findings on physical exam will differ depending on the level and extent of obstruction. With total obstruction, regardless of level, there will be no air movement and no coughing. Inspiratory stridor indicates a glottic or supraglottic obstruction, while expiratory stridor typically indicates a subglottic or intrathoracic lesion. Patients nearing complete obstruction will have suprasternal or intercostal retractions, indicating a very high work of breathing; fatigue is inevitable with eventual decompensation. Cyanosis is a late sign indicating severe respiratory distress and impending loss of airway.

Operative Management

In the emergent situation, there is usually little time for ancillary studies. If the clinical situation permits and the cause of airway compromise in unknown, however, a chest radiograph and CT from the nasopharynx to the lower chest can help identify correctable lesions such a foreign body aspiration or deep neck abscess. Patients should be accompanied to the radiology suite by a physician who has the equipment and skill needed in the setting of acute airway decompensation.

In the more emergent setting, proceeding directly to endoscopy can be both diagnostic and therapeutic. Direct laryngoscopy and/or rigid bronchoscopy can be used to simultaneously establish an airway, identify the underlying cause of obstruction, and, in cases of a foreign body, provide definitive treatment. Rapid sequence intubation is usually accomplished by preoxygenating and then administering etomidate (20 mg) and succinylcholine (1.5 mg/kg). Laryngeal mask airway and Combitubes are alternatives that can be effective temporary measures until further expertise arrives. Of note, however, these devices are less effective protection from aspiration.

If airway control cannot be achieved, a surgical airway is indicated. Cricothyroidotomy can be quickly accomplished by an experienced surgeon; in this setting, however, this tissue may be distorted by the underlying process (eg, abscess or tumor). Awake tracheostomy is another option if the airway can be temporized and if the patient's pain and anxiety can be controlled safely.

Postoperative Care

Adjunctive measures in specific airway obstructive disorders include inhaled racemic epinephrine for airway edema due to infectious processes such as croup or epiglottitis. Systemic corticosteroids are occasionally needed. The need for airway control is rare but should be recognized early to avoid unnecessary morbidity and mortality. For anaphylaxis, intravenous epinephrine, inhaled beta agonists, systemic corticosteroids (intravenous methylprednisolone), and histamine blocking agents (both H1 and H2) should be given rapidly. Also, the causative agent (medications, blood products, etc) should be immediately withdrawn. Airway control should be considered early because orotracheal intubation may become impossible as swelling progresses.

REFERENCES

1. Marik PE, Varon J, Trask T. Management of head trauma. *Chest* 2002;122(2):699-711.
2. Stein SC, Spettell C, Young G, Ross SE. Limitations of neurological assessment in mild head injury. *Brain Inj* 1993;7(5):425-430.
3. Falimirski ME, Gonzalez R, Rodriguez A, Wilberger J. The need for head computed tomography in patients sustaining loss of consciousness after mild head injury. *J Trauma* 2003;55(1):1-6.
4. Cushman JG, Agarwal N, Fabian TC, et al. Practice management guidelines for the management of mild traumatic brain injury: the EAST practice management guidelines work group. *J Trauma* 2001;51(5):1016-1026.
5. Teasdale G, Jennett B. Assessment of coma and impaired consciousness. A practical scale. *Lancet* 1974; 2(7872):81-84.
6. Kelly D, Doberstein C, Becker DP. General principles of head injury management. In: Narayan R, Wilberger J, Povlishock J, eds. *Neurotrauma*. New York: McGraw-Hill, 1996; pp. 71-101.
7. Meredith W, Rutledge R, Hansen AR, et al. Field triage of trauma patients based upon the ability to follow commands: a study in 29,573 injured patients. *J Trauma* 1995;38(1):129-135.
8. Ross SE, Leipold C, Terregino C, O'Malley KF. Efficacy of the motor component of the Glasgow Coma Scale in trauma triage. *J Trauma* 1998;45(1): 42-44.
9. Udekwu P, Kromhout-Schiro S, Vaslef S, et al. Glasgow Coma Scale score, mortality, and functional outcome in head-injured patients. *J Trauma* 2004;56(5): 1084-1089.
10. Vincent JL, Berre J. Primer on medical management of severe brain injury. *Crit Care Med* 2005;33(6): 1392-1399.
11. The Brain Trauma Foundation. The American Association of Neurological Surgeons. The Joint Section on Neurotrauma and Critical Care. Indications for intracranial pressure monitoring. *J Neurotrauma* 2000;17(6-7):479-491.

12. Mittenberg W, Strauman S. Diagnosis of mild head injury and the postconcussion syndrome. *J Head Trauma Rehabil* 2000;15(2):783-791.

13. Valadka A. Injury to the Cranium. In: Moore E, Feliciano D, Mattox K, eds. *Trauma.* New York: McGraw-Hill, 2004.

14. Smith DH, Meaney DF, Shull WH. Diffuse axonal injury in head trauma. *J Head Trauma Rehabil* 2003;18(4):307-316.

15. Miller JD, Becker DP. Secondary insults to the injured brain. *J R Coll Surg Edinb* 1982;27(5):292-298.

16. Stocchetti N, Maas AI, Chieregato A, van der Plas AA. Hyperventilation in head injury: a review. *Chest* 2005; 127(5):1812-1827.

17. The Brain Trauma Foundation. The American Association of Neurological Surgeons. The Joint Section on Neurotrauma and Critical Care. Guidelines for cerebral perfusion pressure. *J Neurotrauma* 2000;17(6-7):507-511.

18. Ogden AT, Mayer SA, Connolly ES, Jr. Hyperosmolar agents in neurosurgical practice: the evolving role of hypertonic saline. *Neurosurgery* 2005;57(2):207-215; discussion 207-215.

19. Hartl R, Ghajar J, Hochleuthner H, Mauritz W. Hypertonic/hyperoncotic saline reliably reduces ICP in severely head-injured patients with intracranial hypertension. *Acta Neurochir Suppl* 1997;70:126-9.

20. De Luca GP, Volpin L, Fornezza U, et al. The role of decompressive craniectomy in the treatment of uncontrollable post–traumatic intracranial hypertension. *Acta Neurochir Suppl* 2000;76:401-404.

21. Albanese J, Leone M, Alliez JR, et al. Decompressive craniectomy for severe traumatic brain injury: Evaluation of the effects at one year. *Crit Care Med* 2003;31(10):2535-2538.

22. Temkin NR, Dikmen SS, Wilensky AJ, et al. A randomized, double–blind study of phenytoin for the prevention of post-traumatic seizures. *N Engl J Med* 1990; 323(8):497-502.

23. The Brain Trauma Foundation. The American Association of Neurological Surgeons. The Joint Section on Neurotrauma and Critical Care. Role of antiseizure prophylaxis following head injury. *J Neurotrauma* 2000;17(6-7):549-553.

24. Gomes JA, Stevens RD, Lewin JJ, 3rd, et al. Glucocorticoid therapy in neurologic critical care. *Crit Care Med* 2005;33(6):1214-1224.

25. Neuroimaging in the management of penetrating brain injury. *J Trauma* 2001;51(2 Suppl):S7- S11.

26. Holmgren EP, Dierks EJ, Assael LA, et al. Facial soft tissue injuries as an aid to ordering a combination head and facial computed tomography in trauma patients. *J Oral Maxillofac Surg* 2005;63(5):651-654.

27. Steinberg MJ, Herrera AF. Management of parotid duct injuries. Oral Surg Oral *Med Oral Pathol Oral Radiol Endod* 2005;99(2):136-141.

28. Miller PR, Fabian TC, Bee TK, et al. Blunt cerebrovascular injuries: diagnosis and treatment. *J Trauma* 2001; 51(2):279-85; discussion 285-286.

29. Pelletier CR, Jordan DR, Braga R, McDonald H. Assessment of ocular trauma associated with head and neck injuries. *J Trauma* 1998;44(2):350-354.

30. Kleinman D. Injury to the Eye. In: Moore E, Feliciano D, Mattox K, eds. *Trauma.* New York: McGraw-Hill, 2004.

31. Seyfer A, Hansen J. Facial trauma. In: Moore E, Feliciano D, Mattox K, eds. *Trauma.* New York: McGraw-Hill, 2004.

32. Tan L, Calhoun K. Epistaxis. *Med Clin North Am* 1999; 83:43-56.

33. Kucik CJ, Clenney T. Management of epistaxis. *Am Fam Physician* 2005;71(2):305-311.

34. Katzen JT, Jarrahy R, Eby JB, et al. Craniofacial and skull base trauma. *J Trauma* 2003;54(5):1026-1034.

35. Dolin J, Scalea T, Mannor L, et al. The management of gunshot wounds to the face. *J Trauma* 1992;4:508-514.

36. Atkins BZ, Abbate S, Fisher SR, Vaslef SN. Current management of laryngotracheal trauma: case report and literature review. *J Trauma* 2004;56(1):185-190.

37. Schaefer S. Laryngeal and esophageal trauma. In: Cummings C, Fredericks J, Harker L, et al., eds. *Otolaryngology Head and Neck Surgery.* St. Louis, MO: Mosby, 1998; pp. 2001-2012.

38. Mathisen DJ, Grillo H. Laryngotracheal trauma. *Ann Thorac Surg* 1987;43(3):254-262.

39. Crissey MM, Bernstein EF. Delayed presentation of carotid intimal tear following blunt craniocervical trauma. *Surgery* 1974;75(4):543-549.

40. Perry MO, Snyder WH, Thal ER. Carotid artery injuries caused by blunt trauma. *Ann Surg* 1980;192(1):74-77.

41. Cothren CC, Moore EE. Blunt cerebrovascular injuries. *Clinics* 2005;60(6):489-496.

42. Biffl WL, Moore EE, Elliott JP, et al. The devastating potential of blunt vertebral arterial injuries. *Ann Surg* 2000;231(5):672-681.

43. Berne JD, Norwood SH, McAuley CE, et al. The high morbidity of blunt cerebrovascular injury in an unscreened population: more evidence of the need for mandatory screening protocols. *J Am Coll Surg* 2001;192(3):314-321.

44. Cothren C, Moore E, Ray C, Jr. Carotid artery stents for blunt cerebrovascular injury. *Perspect Vasc Surg Endovasc Ther* 2006;18(1):73.

45. Cothren CC, Moore EE, Ray CE, Jr., et al. Screening for blunt cerebrovascular injuries is cost-effective. *Am J Surg* 2005;190(6):845-849.

46. Miller PR, Fabian TC, Croce MA, et al. Prospective screening for blunt cerebrovascular injuries: analysis of diagnostic modalities and outcomes. *Ann Surg* 2002; 236(3):386-93; discussion 393-395.

47. Cothren CC, Moore EE, Biffl WL, et al. Anticoagulation is the gold standard therapy for blunt carotid injuries to reduce stroke rate. *Arch Surg* 2004;139(5):540-5; discussion 545-546.

48. Biffl WL, Moore EE, Offner PJ, et al. Optimizing screening for blunt cerebrovascular injuries. *Am J Surg* 1999; 178(6):517-522.

49. Rogers FB, Baker EF, Osler TM, et al. Computed tomographic angiography as a screening modality for blunt cervical arterial injuries: preliminary results. *J Trauma* 1999;46(3):380-385.

50. Bub LD, Hollingworth W, Jarvik JG, Hallam DK. Screening for blunt cerebrovascular injury: evaluating the accuracy of multidetector computed tomographic angiography. *J Trauma* 2005;59(3):691-697.

51. Berne JD, Norwood SH, McAuley CE, Villareal DH. Helical computed tomographic angiography: an excellent screening test for blunt cerebrovascular injury. *J Trauma* 2004;57(1):11-17; discussion 17-19.

52. Biffl WL, Egglin T, Benedetto B, et al. Sixteen-slice computed tomographic angiography is a reliable noninvasive screening test for clinically significant blunt cerebrovascular injuries. *J Trauma* 2006;60(4):745-751; discussion 751-72.

53. Bok AP, Peter JC. Carotid and vertebral artery occlusion after blunt cervical injury: the role of MR angiography in early diagnosis. *J Trauma* 1996;40(6):968-972.

54. Mutze S, Rademacher G, Matthes G, et al. Blunt cerebrovascular injury in patients with blunt multiple trauma: diagnostic accuracy of duplex Doppler US and early CT angiography. *Radiology* 2005;237(3):884-892.

55. Biffl WL, Moore EE, Offner PJ, et al. Blunt carotid arterial injuries: implications of a new grading scale. *J Trauma* 1999;47(5):845-853.

56. Cothren CC, Moore EE, Ray CE, Jr., et al. Carotid artery stents for blunt cerebrovascular injury: risks exceed benefits. *Arch Surg* 2005;140(5):480-485; discussion 485-486.

57. Shama DM, Odell J. Penetrating neck trauma with tracheal and oesophageal injuries. *Br J Surg* 1984;71(7): 534-536.

58. Roon AJ, Christensen N. Evaluation and treatment of penetrating cervical injuries. *J Trauma* 1979;19(6): 391-397.

59. Fogelman MJ, Stewart RD. Penetrating wounds of the neck. *Am J Surg* 1956;91(4):581-593; discussion, 593-596.

60. Atteberry LR, Dennis JW, Menawat SS, Frykberg ER. Physical examination alone is safe and accurate for evaluation of vascular injuries in penetrating Zone II neck trauma. *J Am Coll Surg* 1994;179(6):657-662.

61. Demetriades D, Theodorou D, Cornwell E, et al. Evaluation of penetrating injuries of the neck: prospective study of 223 patients. *World J Surg* 1997;21(1):41-7; discussion 47-48.

62. Azuaje RE, Jacobson LE, Glover J, et al. Reliability of physical examination as a predictor of vascular injury after penetrating neck trauma. *Am Surg* 2003;69(9): 804-807.

63. Back MR, BaumgarTNer FJ, Klein SR. Detection and evaluation of aerodigestive tract injuries caused by cervical and transmediastinal gunshot wounds. *J Trauma* 1997;42(4):680-686.

64. BifFL WL, Moore EE, Rehse DH, et al. Selective management of penetrating neck trauma based on cervical level of injury. *Am J Surg* 1997;174(6):678-682.

65. Klyachkin ML, Rohmiller M, Charash WE, et al. Penetrating injuries of the neck: selective management evolving. *Am Surg* 1997;63(2):189-194.

66. van As AB, van Deurzen DF, Verleisdonk EJ. Gunshots to the neck: selective angiography as part of conservative management. *Injury* 2002;33(5):453-456.

67. Asensio JA, Valenziano CP, Falcone RE, Grosh JD. Management of penetrating neck injuries. The controversy surrounding zone II injuries. *Surg Clin North Am* 1991;71(2):267-296.

68. Eddy VA. Is routine arteriography mandatory for penetrating injury to zone 1 of the neck? Zone 1 Penetrating Neck Injury Study Group. *J Trauma* 2000;48(2):208-213; discussion 213-214.

69. Meyer JP, Barrett JA, Schuler JJ, FLanigan DP. Mandatory vs selective exploration for penetrating neck trauma. A prospective assessment. *Arch Surg* 1987;122(5):592-597.

70. Montalvo BM, LeBlang SD, Nunez DB, Jr., et al. Color Doppler sonography in penetrating injuries of the neck. *AJNR Am J Neuroradiol* 1996;17(5):943-951.

71. Ofer A, Nitecki SS, Braun J, et al. CT angiography of the carotid arteries in trauma to the neck. *Eur J Vasc Endovasc Surg* 2001;21(5):401-407.

72. Nunez DB. Jr., Torres–Leon M, Munera F. Vascular injuries of the neck and thoracic inlet: helical CT–angiographic correlation. *Radiographics* 2004: 24(4):1087-1098; discussion 1099-1100.

73. Mazolewski PJ, Curry JD, Browder T, Fildes J. Computed tomographic scan can be used for surgical decision making in zone II penetrating neck injuries. *J Trauma* 2001;51(2):315-319.

74. Noyes LD, McSwain NE, Jr., Markowitz IP. Panendoscopy with arteriography versus mandatory exploration of penetrating wounds of the neck. *Ann Surg* 1986;204(1):21-31.

75. Gracias VH, Reilly PM, Philpott J, et al. Computed tomography in the evaluation of penetrating neck trauma: a preliminary study. *Arch Surg* 2001;136(11):1231-1235.

76. Munera F, Soto JA, Palacio DM, et al. Penetrating neck injuries: helical CT angiography for initial evaluation. *Radiology* 2002;224(2):366-372.

77. Gonzalez RP, Falimirski M, Holevar MR, Turk B. Penetrating zone II neck injury: does dynamic computed tomographic scan contribute to the diagnostic sensitivity of physical examination for surgically significant injury? A prospective blinded study. *J Trauma* 2003;54(1):61-64; discussion 64-65.

78. Woo K, Magner DP, Wilson MT, Margulies DR. CT angiography in penetrating neck trauma reduces the need for operative neck exploration. *Am Surg* 2005;71(9):754-758.

79. Munera F, Soto JA, Nunez D. Penetrating injuries of the neck and the increasing role of CTA. *Emerg Radiol* 2004;10(6):303-309.

80. Hirschberg A, Mattox K. *The Neck: Safari in Tiger Country.* Top Knife: The Art & Craft of Trauma Surgery. Shrewsbury, UK: tfm Publishing, Ltd., 2005.

81. Britt L. Neck Injuries: Evaluation and management. In: Moore E, Feliciano D, Mattox K, eds. *Trauma.* New York: McGraw-Hill, 2004.

Chapter 28

THORACIC TRAUMA

George D. Garcia, MD, and Juan A. Asensio, MD

INTRODUCTION

Thoracic injury accounts for approximately 25% of all trauma in the United States.[1,2,3] Thoracic injuries are estimated to occur with a frequency of 12 patients per million population. It is estimated that approximately 16,000 deaths occur from thoracic injury every year in the United States.[2] Most patients sustaining severe injury succumb at the scene of the traumatic incident. In a study of 2895 trauma deaths in the county of Los Angeles, 1929 (67%) were pronounced dead at the scene or at the nearest nontrauma hospital.[4] In a review of mortality from San Francisco trauma system, Baker[1] reported that 53% of all deaths from thoracic trauma occurred at the scene. In a comparison between an urban and rural trauma system, mortality figures reported were 40.5% in San Diego and 72% in Vermont.[5] Needless to say, the cost to society in health care dollars is staggering.

The vast majority of blunt and penetrating thoracic injuries do not require thoracotomy for definitive treatment. In fact, most thoracic injuries can be managed by tube thoracostomy alone.[6] The prognosis for patients sustaining severe thoracic injury, however, is grim. In a recent review of 2648 trauma deaths,[7] the thorax was the site of critical injury in 28%. Thoracic injuries, along with penetrating trauma and age greater than 60, were found to be significant risk factors for arriving without vital signs at trauma centers. Thoracic trauma is a contributing factor in 50% of all civilian trauma deaths.[8] Furthermore, patients with significant thoracic trauma were more likely to succumb within the first 60 minutes than patients with severe abdominal or head injury (17% vs 11% vs 7%, respectively). The mortality of patients sustaining thoracic injuries rises significantly if the patient arrives at a trauma center with either respiratory distress or shock. Freedland[9] reported that 11% of all thoracic trauma patients arriving at the trauma center required endotracheal intubation at arrival, and of these, 58% died. In addition if shock was present, mortality rose to 73%.

PREOPERATIVE MANAGEMENT

INITIAL ASSESSMENT AND MANAGEMENT

All patients admitted to a trauma center should be evaluated and resuscitated in accordance with Advanced Trauma Life Support (ATLS) protocols.[10] Patients sustaining penetrating thoracic injuries arriving in cardiopulmonary arrest with short transport times will require Emergency Department resuscitative thoracotomy (EDT). In all others, a rapid and thorough initial physical exam should focus on identifying and treating life-threatening injuries.[11] Assessment of the airway assumes priority with the establishment of a definitive airway as needed. Orotracheal intubation with in-line cervical stabilization is the preferred route. If the patient cannot be intubated, a surgical airway via cricothyroidotomy should be rapidly performed. Primary assessment continues with evaluation of breath sounds. Absent or diminished breath sounds mandate tube thoracostomy for decompression of a pneumo or hemothorax. For hemothoraces, the quantity of blood evacuated from the hemithoracic cavity, as well as the rate of evacuation will signal the need for an emergency thoracotomy.

Rapid restoration of intravascular volume is the next priority. Large bore peripheral intravenous lines are started. If needed, an 8.5 French introducing catheter placed in the femoral vein provides an additional route for the rapid volume infusion. Rapid infusers should be used as they can rapidly deliver large volumes of warm intravenous fluids and blood to prevent hypothermia.

Immediately after life-threatening injuries have been identified and addressed during the primary survey, the secondary survey is begun, this includes a thorough "head-to-toe" physical exam followed by appropriate imaging studies in the hemodynamically stable patient. The thoracic cage is examined for tenderness, crepitus, and presence of flail segments. Palpation of all pulses comparing one side to the other and upper extremity to lower extremity can alert the examiner to the presence of thoracic vascular injury.

The chest is again carefully auscultated to assess breath sounds and to evaluate heart sounds. The goal of the secondary survey is to identify all injuries, especially those that are potentially life-threatening if missed.[11]

DIAGNOSTIC INTERVENTIONS

The chest is the easiest of body cavities to initially assess. A plain anteroposterior (AP) radiograph can provide evidence of many injuries as well as alert the trauma surgeon the presence of hemorrhage into either hemithorax. A simple pneumothorax is often not detected on physical exam but may be identified on plain radiography. The radiograph allows evaluation to detect fracture of the clavicles, ribs and occasionally, the sternum, scapula, and thoracic vertebrae.

A chest roentgenogram may also occasionally detect diaphragmatic injuries. For instance, the presence of hollow viscera or coiled nasogastric tube in the left hemithorax is pathognomonic for the presence ruptured diaphragm.[10] In the absence of this finding, the diagnosis of diaphragmatic rupture can be difficult to make. Computed tomography (CT) does not reliably demonstrate the injury. Murray[12] has reported a 42% incidence of diaphragmatic injuries after penetrating left thoracoabdominal injury. Diagnostic laparoscopy is the diagnostic method of choice in stable patients to diagnose penetrating diaphragmatic injuries.

If a widened mediastinum is visualized, further investigations are warranted to exclude significant thoracic vascular injury. Arteriographic evaluation of the aorta remains the "gold standard" to detect thoracic aortic injury; however, use of spiral or helical computed tomography has largely replaced this invasive procedure. Aortography is most often used when helical CT is equivocal. A ruptured thoracic aorta may be present despite a normal chest radiograph in a small minority of patients. Helical computed tomography is frequently ordered based on mechanism of injury alone.

For patients that have sustained significant anterior impacts to the thorax and present with abnormal electrocardiograms on admission, the presence of blunt cardiac injury/myocardial contusion (BCI) must be entertained. The subcostal window of the Focused Assessment with Sonography for Trauma (FAST) exam allows evaluation of the pericardium to exclude pericardial tamponade. A formal two-dimensional echocardiogram is the test of choice for the structural assessment of the heart if there is evidence or strong clinical suspicion for the presence of, blunt cardiac injury.

OPERATIVE MANAGEMENT

EMERGENCY DEPARTMENT THORACOTOMY (EDT)

The left anterolateral thoracotomy, was first described by Spangaro[13] in 1906. Approximately 50 years later, Beall[14] proposed that patients experiencing cessation of cardiac function should undergo immediate resuscitative thoracotomy and open cardiac massage whether in the emergency department (ED), operating room (OR) or recovery room and was the first to perform this procedure. In 1966 Beall[15] advocated for the use of immediate cardiorrhaphy in the Emergency Department (ED) and was the first to perform this procedure successfully.

Emergency Department (ED) thoracotomy is a surgical procedure of great value if undertaken following strict indications for its performance. This procedure is routinely performed in urban trauma centers that receive patients "in extremis." This technically complex and challenging procedure should be performed by trauma surgeons who are familiar with the management of penetrating cardiothoracic injuries. As emergency medical services (EMS) of many large cities continue to apply the principles of "load and go"; many of these patients reach urban trauma centers in need of immediate control of exsanguinating hemorrhage secondary to penetrating injuries to the heart and major thoracic blood vessels.

When performed in an expedient fashion, Emergency Department thoracotomy (EDT), aortic cross-clamping and cardiography is successful in salvaging approximately 10% of all penetrating cardiac injuries. Open cardiopulmonary massage after definitive repair of penetrating cardiac injuries is more effective in producing a greater ejection fraction. Similarly, lacerations of major thoracic blood vessels can also be controlled by means of vascular clamps.

Prehospital factors predictive of poor outcome include absence of vital signs, fixed and dilated pupils, absence of cardiac rhythm, and absence of motion in the extremities. Similarly, the absence of a palpable pulse and the presence of cardiopulmonary arrest are predictors of poor outcome.

Generally accepted indications for this procedure include cardiopulmonary arrest secondary to penetrating thoracic injuries and profound shock with systolic blood pressures of less than 60 mm Hg due to either exsanguinating hemorrhage or pericardial tamponade. Cardiopulmonary arrest secondary to blunt injury is generally a contraindication to the performance of this procedure.

The objectives to be achieved with this procedure include resuscitation of agonal patients arriving with penetrating cardiothoracic injuries, evacuation of pericardial tamponade, control of massive intrathoracic hemorrhage secondary to cardiovascular injuries, prevention of air emboli, and restoration of cardiac function using open cardiopulmonary massage. Other objectives accomplished include definitive repairs of penetrating cardiac injuries and control of exsanguinating thoracic vascular injuries. Similarly, cross-clamping of the descending thoracic aorta, redistributing the remaining blood volume to perfuse the carotid and coronary arteries, is achieved with this technique.

Emergency Department thoracotomy (EDT) should be performed simultaneously with the initial assessment evaluation and resuscitation, using the Advanced Trauma Life Support (ATLS) protocols of the American College of Surgeons (ACS). Similarly, immediate venous access with simultaneous use of rapid infusion techniques complements the resuscitative process. Simultaneous placement of a chest tube in the right hemithoracic cavity is also recommended, as the output, if significant, may indicate extension into a right anterolateral thoracotomy.

Patients are generally transferred to the Emergency Department (ED) gurney on arrival. The left arm is elevated and the entire thorax is prepped rapidly with an antiseptic solution. A left anterolateral thoracotomy commencing at the lateral border of the left sternocostal junction and inferior to the nipple at the fifth intercostals space is carried out and extended laterally to the latissimus dorsi. In females, the breast is retracted cephalad. This incision is rapidly carried through skin and subcutaneous tissue and the serratus anterior until the intercostal muscles have been reached. The three layers of these interdigitated muscles are sharply transected with Brown or Metzenbaum scissors. Occasionally, the left fourth and fifth costochondral cartilages may be transected to provide greater exposure. A Finochietto retractor is then placed to separate the ribs. At that time, the trauma surgeon should evaluate the extent of hemorrhage present within the left hemithoracic cavity. Exsanguinating hemorrhage with almost complete loss of the patient's intravascular volume is a reliable indicator of poor outcome.

The left lung is then elevated medially and the thoracic aorta is located immediately as it enters the abdomen via the aortic hiatus. The aorta should then be palpated to assess the status of the remaining blood volume. It can also be temporarily occluded digitally against the bodies of the lower thoracic vertebrae. To fully cross-clamp the aorta, a combination of sharp and blunt dissection commencing at both the superior and inferior borders of the aorta is performed, so that the aorta may be encircled between the thumb and index fingers, this facilitates the aortic cross-clamp to be placed safely. Inexperienced surgeons often mistakenly clamp the esophagus, which is located superior to the aorta. A nasogastric tube previously placed can serve as a guide in differentiating the esophagus from an often empty and nonpulsating thoracic aorta. The aorta should not be cross-clamped until after the cardiac injury is repaired.

Trauma surgeons should then observe the pericardium and search for the presence of a pericardial injury. The pericardium, is usually tense and discolored in the presence of tamponade. The phrenic nerve must be identified and preserved. A longitudinal opening in the pericardial sac is then made anterior to the phrenic nerve and extended both inferiorly and superiorly. Opening the pericardium can be challenging.

Often the sac is quite tense. Injudicious opening with a scalpel may iatrogenically lacerate the underlying myocardium. Usually it is necessary to grasp the pericardium with two Allis clamps to steady it and then make a small, one- or two-centimeter incision sharply, followed by opening the pericardium with Metzenbaum scissors, first cephalad and then caudad.

After opening the pericardium, clotted blood is evacuated. The trauma surgeon should immediately note the presence or absence, and type of underlying cardiac rhythm as well as location of the penetrating injury or injuries. Immediate digital control is necessary to prevent ongoing hemorrhage. An attempt must be made to elucidate the trajectory of the wounding agent, as missiles often enter in one area and migrate to adjacent areas such as the contralateral hemithoracic cavity. Similarly, the trauma surgeon should also estimate the blood volume remaining within the cardiac chambers. The finding of a flaccid heart, devoid of any effective forward pumping motion is a strong predictor of poor outcome. Other predictors of poor outcome are empty coronary arteries and presence of air, indicating air emboli which at times may be seen in the coronary veins, but not the coronary arteries given their thick walls.

Digital control of penetrating ventricular injuries as they are simultaneously sutured prevents further hemorrhage. We generally recommend the use of monofilament suture, such as 2-0 polypropylene, we use the MH needle. Lacerations of the atria can be controlled with a partial occlusion vascular clamp such as a Satisnky clamp prior to definitive cardiorrhaphy. If the injury or injuries are quite large, balloon tamponade using a Foley catheter can temporarily arrest the hemorrhage either to allow the performance of cardiorrhaphy or to gain time so that the patient may be transferred expediently to an operating room for a more definitive surgical procedure; although we do not recommend this technique except for unusually large myocardial lacerations. We do not recommend the use of bioprosthetic materials such as Teflon patches in the Emergency Department (ED). This is a time-consuming technique that, if needed, should be performed in the operating room.

The use of a skin stapler to temporarily occlude lacerations in the myocardium has been used, so as to allow expedient transfer to the operating room for definitive cardiorrhaphy; however, it is recommended that these staples be removed and replaced with sutures. In some cases, they have been left in place with no untoward effects. In our experience, staples do not effectively control hemorrhage, tend to enlarge the cardiac injury, and prove to be rather difficult to remove, and, therefore, we do not recommend their routine use.

Although successful repairs are denoted by cessation of bleeding and progressive filling of the cardiac chambers, they may be effectively accomplished without the heart being able to recover its rhythm. Strict pharmacologic manipulation coupled with directly delivered countershocks of 20 to 50 joules is frequently needed to restore a normal sinus rhythm. If a sinus rhythm cannot be quickly restored despite multiple attempts, the prognosis is grave and the outcome is poor. At times a rhythm can be restored, but no effective pumping mechanism is observed. In these situations, no pulsations are detected in the descending thoracic aorta. Progressive myocardial death can be witnessed, first by dilatation of the right ventricle with accompanying cessation of contractility and motion, followed by the same process in the left ventricle. Restoration of a synchronized rhythm with either a ventricular and in some cases an atrioventricular (A-V) pacemaker has been attempted by the authors with very poor results.

There is certainly no shortage of literature regarding the use of emergency department thoracotomy. Despite this extensive body of literature, most series are retrospective and many are from institutions that use the technique infrequently, leaving many questions regarding the use of this technically demanding procedure unresolved. This led Asensio, Wall, and others[16] working with ad hoc subcommittee on outcomes of American College of Surgeons Committee on Trauma (ACS-COT) to review the available literature and to determine outcomes and develop practice management guidelines for the use of this procedure.

In their analysis Asensio, Wall, and others[16] analyzed 42 selected series dealing with emergency department thoracotomy (EDT). A total of 7035 emergency department thoracotomies were performed with 551 survivors. This results in an overall survival rate of 7.83%. When stratified by mechanism of injury, there were 4482 thoracotomies for penetrating injury with 500 survivors for a survival rate of 11.16%. For blunt injury, 2193 thoracotomies were performed, and 35 patients survived for a survival rate of 1.6%. In a sublet analysis of series specifically addressing penetrating cardiac injury, 363 patients survived 1,165 emergency department thoracotomies, yielding a survival rate of 31.1%. This figure must be viewed with caution as all but one of the series were retrospective.

These figures led Asensio, Wall et al[16] to formulate the following recommendations as the ACS practice management guidelines.

1. Emergency department thoracotomy should be performed rarely in patients sustaining cardiopulmonary arrest secondary to blunt injury. It should be limited to those arriving with vital signs and experiencing a witnessed arrest.
2. Emergency department thoracotomy is best applied to patients sustaining penetrating cardiac injury who arrive after a short transport time with witnessed signs of life: pupillary response, spontaneous ventilation, presence of carotid pulse, measurable or palpable blood pressure, extremity movement, and cardiac electrical activity.
3. Emergency department thoracotomy should be performed in patients sustaining penetrating noncardiac thoracic injuries, but these patients generally experience a low survival rate.
4. Emergency department thoracotomy should be performed in patients sustaining exsanguinating abdominal vascular injury, but these patients generally experience a low survival rate. The procedure should be used as an adjunct to definitive repair of their abdominal vascular injury.

Emergency Department thoracotomy remains a powerful tool in the trauma surgeon's armamentarium. It should be employed wisely and with appropriate indications. Finally, it should be performed only by trauma surgeons and surgeons properly trained and able to address any potential injury that may be found.

MANAGEMENT OF SPECIFIC INJURIES

Sternal Fractures

Fracture of the sternum accounts for approximately 5% to 10% of all thoracic injuries. Direct impacts between the sternum and the steering wheel of an automobile involved in a deceleration crash remain the classic mechanism causing this injury. Most sternal fractures involve the midbody followed by the manubrium. Comminuted fractures account for less than 10%. Individuals particularly prone to sternal fracture include patients over the age of 50, those using shoulder harness restraints, and women.

The diagnosis of sternal fracture should be suspected in patients that complain of anterior chest pain and manifest tenderness over the sternum. Associated physical finding may include ecchymosis, erythema, swelling, and palpable deformities. A freely mobile sternum confirms the diagnosis of central flail chest. Diagnosis can be confirmed with a chest radiograph. A cross lateral film may be obtained to detect posterior displacement of the sternum. CT scans provide greater detail.

Given the magnitude of force required to fracture the sternum, associated injuries are common. These injuries include rib fractures in approximately 40% or patients along with long bone fractures in 25% and closed head injuries in nearly 20% of patients. The association between sternal fractures and myocardial contusion has been variably reported. The incidence ranges from as low as 4%[17] when determined by electrocardiogram and cardiac enzyme levels to as high as 91%[18] when defined as abnormalities on radionucleotide angiography (RNA) used in the past. The incidence of cardiac abnormalities requiring treatment is very low. Fracture of the sternum should alert the clinician to search for associated injuries. However, if a sternal fracture occurs as an isolated injury, the clinical course is benign. Brookes and coworkers,[19] in a series of 272 patients with sternal fractures, reported an overall mortality rate of 0.74%. Among 124 patients with isolated fractures of the sternum, mortality was zero.

Initially, the treatment of patients with fractures of the sternum centers on identification and stabilization of associated injuries. Treatment of sternal fractures consists primarily of pain relief. In rare instances, such as severe pain or displacement of the sternum with impingement of the right ventricle, operative repair may be required to elevate the sternum. Operative reduction and internal fixation can be accomplished with either plates or wires.

Rib Fractures and Flail Chest

The ribs are the commonly injured component of the thoracic cage, especially in patients that sustain blunt trauma. The most common cause of rib fractures are motor vehicle accidents (MVAs). Significant pain is associated with these fractures leading to inability or unwillingness to produce a deep inspiratory effort. Pain, combined with an underlying pulmonary contusion, leads to alterations in both dynamic and static compliances. The underlying contusion renders a portion of the lung edematous with variable degrees of hemorrhage and necrosis. The injured lung is thus unavailable for effective gas exchange resulting in significant decreases in alveolar ventilation along with ventilatory perfusion mismatch and shunts. In the multiply injured patient and in the elderly, this often results in significant morbidity. It has been recommended that patients with three or more rib fractures be hospitalized, whereas elderly patients with six or more rib fractures should be admitted to a Surgical Intensive Care Unit (SICU). Overall trauma-related mortality is considerably higher in elderly patients with rib fractures; while mortality increases linearly with an increasing number of fractured ribs.[20,21]

The initial diagnostic test of choice is the chest radiograph. However, it is estimated that up to 60% of the time, rib fractures will not be visualized on plain films. Fractures of the upper four ribs are particularly hard to detect initially and may not be seen until callous develops in 1 to 2 weeks. A history of significant trauma to the thoracic cage coupled with clinical finding of tenderness to palpation of the thoracic cage supports the diagnosis.

Because of the heavy musculature overlying the first three ribs, it requires a force of significant magnitude to fracture them. Given the severity of trauma required to fracture the first ribs, associated injuries to other ribs and organ systems are not uncommon. Pulmonary injury to some extent is almost universal. The most significant injuries associated with upper rib fractures are injuries to the thoracic vasculature. First rib fracture, regardless of mechanism is associated with a relatively low incidence of vascular injury, although, with displacement, the incidence appears to be slightly higher. However, when due to a traumatic cause, the incidence is much higher. In a review of 730 patients with thoracic traumas, first rib fracture with concomitant head, thoracic, abdominal, or long bone fractures was associated with vascular injury in 24% of cases.[22] Indications for arteriogram or helical computed tomography include widened mediastinum on chest radiography, upper extremity pulse deficit, and posteriorly displaced first rib fracture.

Fractures of the fourth through ninth ribs are most common. Direct force applied to these ribs can cause inward protrusion of the fractured segment lacerating both the visceral and parietal, the pleuras and lung. This results in a pneumothorax or hemothorax. The application of force in the anteroposterior direction causes an outward bowing of the ribs with resultant fractures, making laceration of the lung less likely.

The 10th through 12th ribs protect the solid abdominal organs. Fractures of these ribs are associated with injury to the liver and spleen. Associated injury of the liver can be seen up to 10% of the time with fractures of the right lower rib cage.[23] In a recent prospective observational study of patients presenting to a Level I trauma center,[24] 7.2% of patients with left lower rib pain or tenderness had associated splenic injuries. An additional 2.3% were found to have left renal injuries.

Flail chest is a very severe form of chest wall injury. The incidence of flail chest amongst patients with chest wall injury ranges between 5 and 13%[2]. By definition, a flail chest occurs when a patient sustains at least three consecutive rib fractures, each in two places. The result is a discontinuity of a segment of the thoracic wall, leading to paradoxical movement of the affected section of the thoracic cage during both the inspiratory and expiratory phases. The generation of negative pleural pressure during inspiration results in inward movement of the flail segment while the rest of the chest wall moves outward. In the past, it was this paradoxical movement described as "Pendelluft: that was thought to be the primary cause of the hypoxemia that accompanies flail chest." In fact, it is the underlying pulmonary contusion that is predominantly responsible due to impaired gas exchange as described earlier.

The cornerstone of treatment for all rib fractures is pain control. Pain secondary to rib fractures adversely affects pulmonary function. Pain can be managed with intravenous analgesia, either nonsteroidal anti-inflammatories or narcotics, intercostals nerve blocks with local anesthetic, or intrapleural or epidural catheters. Intercostal nerve blocks, while offering excellent analgesia, require reinjection every 4 to 6 hours and may cause iatrogenic pneumothorax. Epidural analgesia for rib fractures has been shown to be superior to intravenous analgesia and has been shown to be an independent predictor of decreased mortality and pulmonary complications.[25] Regardless of the route chosen, analgesia must be adequate to allow adequate ventilation and preservation of a cough mechanism adequate to clear pulmonary secretions.

Given the magnitude of injury resulting in a flail chest, a significant number of patients will require intubation, mechanical ventilation, and positive pressure for reasons other than the flail chest, predominantly for their severe underlying pulmonary contusion. Positive pressure results in internal stabilization of the flail segment. Controversy still exists regarding the use of surgical stabilization versus conservative management in the presence of a flail segment. Sixty-eight percent of patients requiring intubation for flail chest are extubated by the third day.[26] However, selected patients may be considered for operative stabilization of the flail segment for pain control and failure to wean from mechanical ventilation amongst the most common causes sited. A nonrandomized comparison of patients with flail segments undergoing operative fixation versus those treated conservatively found a significant reduction in the mean length of mechanical ventilation required.[27] The same study, however, found that patients with an accompanying pulmonary contusion probably do not benefit from operative stabilization.

Scapular and Clavicular Fractures

The scapula is well protected by a large overlying muscle mass and is relatively mobile around the postero-lateral chest wall. As a result, fractures of the scapula are relatively uncommon. Most fractures of the scapula involve the body and neck. Fractures of the glenoid fossa, coracoid process, and the acromion occur with lesser frequency. If the diagnosis of scapular fracture is established, the trauma surgeon must assume the thoracic wall has absorbed a tremendous amount of energy. When a scapular fracture is present, associated injuries are the rule; these associated injuries occur with an incidence of 80% to 98%.[28,29] There is a 54% incidence of associated pulmonary contusions. Rib fractures are equally frequent. The clavicle is fractured along with the scapula 27% of the time. Brachial plexus injury is found in 13% of patients and associated vascular injury is estimated to be present in 11% of patients. A significant number of associated craniocerebral injuries and abdominal injuries may also be associated with scapular fractures.[28]

Because of the frequency and severity of associated injuries, scapular fractures are often overlooked in the initial management of the multiply injured patient. Clinical findings that suggest the presence of a scapular fracture include tenderness, edema, and crepitus. Scapular fractures are visible on initial plain radiographic studies in 88% of patients but may be overlooked in up to 35% of patients.[30] Treatment consists of simple immobilization with a sling and adequate pain control. Open reduction and internal fixation is uncommonly required.

Scapulothoracic dissociation is a rare injury caused by lateral or rotational displacement of the shoulder resulting in severe soft tissue injury. It is characterized by a complete disruption of the scapulothoracic articulation with lateral scapular displacement and intact skin. It is associated with massive musculoskeletal injury and often includes injury to the subclavian or axillary vessels and partial or complete avulsion of the brachial plexus. If the neurovascular injury is severe, for all practical purposes, it is essentially a closed forequarter amputation. Lateral displacement of the scapula on a chest radiograph is pathognomonic. Diagnosis or suspicion of this injury mandates selective arteriography, as associated vascular injuries are present in up to 88% of patients.[31] If vascular injury is identified and neurologic compromise is incomplete or unclear, the extremity should be revascularized in a period of 4 to 6 hours. In patients with complete avulsion of the brachial plexus, early above-elbow amputation is most appropriate.

In contrast to fractures of the scapula, clavicular fractures commonly occur as an isolated injury. The middle third of the clavicle is the site of fracture in 75% to 80% of patients, following a fall or blow with lateral force applied to the shoulder. Fractures of the proximal and distal third of the clavicle are unusual and occur after application of a direct downward force to the top of the shoulder. Associated injuries can include rib fractures, upper extremity injuries, and pneumothorax. Injury to the subclavian and axillary vessels has also been reported.[32,33] Clinical findings include pain, tenderness over the clavicle, and deformity. A plain radiograph of the chest confirms the diagnosis. Open fixation is rarely indicated. Treatment consists of immobilization in a sling and pain control.

The sternoclavicular joint is anchored by substantial ligamentous support. Disruption is uncommon; however, traumatic dislocation occurs after a substantial force has been directed to this area. Anterior dislocation occurs more frequently than posterior dislocation. The diagnosis is based on physical exam. Generally, the patient complains of pain with arm motion or lateral compression of the shoulder. In anterior dislocations, the medial end of the clavicle appears prominent. In cases of posterior dislocations, a hollow may be palpated at the lateral edge of the sternum. Posterior dislocations can be associated with compression of the trachea, injury to the brachial plexus and injury to the subclavian artery or vein.[34] The presence of a palpable pulse after a posterior dislocation does not exclude an intimal tear of the subclavian artery. In these cases, arteriography should be considered. Treatment of both anterior and posterior dislocation is closed reduction. Operative reduction is reserved for those that fail closed reduction.

Pneumothorax and Hemothorax

A pneumothorax occurs when air from lacerated or injured pulmonary parenchyma escapes into and is trapped within the pleural space. A pneumothorax may be caused by both blunt and penetrating trauma.

Mechanisms include fractured ribs piercing the pulmonary parenchyma, deceleration injury resulting in tearing, direct injury to the pulmonary parenchyma by missiles or stab wounds and alveolar rupture secondary to acute increases in intrathoracic pressure. Gray and coworkers[35] reported, an 8% incidence of pneumothorax and a 42% incidence of hemopneumothorax in a series of 2917 patients sustaining penetrating trauma; while Harrison and coworkers[36] reported a 24% incidence of pneumothorax and 55% incidence of hemopneumothorax in a series of 203 patients sustaining blunt thoracic trauma. Pneumothoraces are classified in three types: simple, tension, and open.

The pathophysiology of a simple pneumothorax is based on compression by the air trapped in the pleural space on the ipsilateral lung. Tidal and total lung volumes are decreased and the patient's ability to oxygenate and ventilate is impaired. Clinical findings of simple pneumothorax include shortness of breath, chest pain, decreased breath sounds, and hyperresonance to percussion on the affected side. Treatment consists of evacuating the trapped air via closed tube thoracostomy.

Tension pneumothorax occurs when a pulmonary injury allows air to continue to escape into the pleural space but not exit the thoracic cavity. The continuing accumulation of air into the pleural space eventually leads to total collapse of the affected lung. As air continues to escape, the mediastinal structures are displaced to the contralateral side. This result is compression of the unaffected lung leading to progressively deteriorating ventilatory function. In addition, the vena cava is displaced and twisted in its axis thus causing a decrease in venous return to the heart resulting in hypotension. Tension pneumothorax is a rapidly fatal condition that requires urgent decompression with needle thoracostomy followed immediately by tube thoracostomy or immediate chest tube insertion. Because clinical signs may not be readily evident in the often chaotic setting of the resuscitation area of a trauma center, any suspicion of tension pneumothorax mandates immediate decompression. Decompression should never be delayed for confirmatory diagnostic tests.

Injuries that result in an open defect in the chest wall are defined as an open pneumothorax, or "sucking chest wound." The opening in the chest wall allows for equilibration between the positive atmospheric and negative intrathoracic pressures. The result is immediate collapse of the ipsilateral lung. If the chest wall defect is large enough, air will flow preferentially from the trachea through the defect. This obviously leads to elimination of the ability to oxygenate or ventilate with resultant profound hypoxia leading to cardiopulmonary arrest. Management of an open pneumothorax consists of covering the defect with a dressing and securing it on three sides. This allows air to flow freely from the unsecured side during exhalation but prevents the inflow of air during inspiration. Tube thoracostomy should then be performed at a site remote from the defect. Surgical reconstruction of the chest wall defect is required.

A hemothorax is defined as an accumulation of blood within the pleural cavity. Penetrating trauma is the most common cause. The pathophysiology of hemothorax mirrors that of pneumothorax, except that compression of the lung occurs by the accumulated blood rather than air. Physical findings are the same with the exception that dullness to percussion will be noted on the affected side, rather than the hyperresonance seen with pneumothorax. A volume of 200 to 300 ml of blood must be present in the pleural space for a hemothorax to be visible on chest radiograph. Treatment consists of draining the blood from the pleural space with closed tube thoracostomy. Most patients can be managed with closed tube thoracostomy alone and will not require operative intervention. However, if the initial chest tube output exceeds 1000 to 1500 ml or bleeding continues at a rate of 200 ml per hour for a period of 4 hours, immediate thoracotomy is required. Mortality has been shown to increase linearly with volume of hemorrhage after thoracic injury[37] with the risk of death at 1500 ml or blood loss three times greater that at 500 ml. Bleeding of this volume generally indicates significant damage to the pulmonary parenchyma, hilar pulmonary vessels, or other thoracic vascular structures that are unlikely to spontaneously stop bleeding. In the rare situation in which a large quantity of blood is evacuated and its flow is continuous, the chest tube should be clamped and the patient transferred immediately to the operating room for an emergency thoracotomy.

Traumatic Asphyxia

A syndrome originally described *masque ecchymotique* and comprised of craniocervical and thoracic cyanosis, facial edema, petechiae, and subconjunctival hemorrhage was first reported in 1837 noted on autopsy studies of people trampled by crowds in Paris.[38] This syndrome occurs when the thoracic cage or upper abdomen is subjected to a direct pressure transmitted by a large weight load, resulting in a large amount of positive pressure being transmitted to the mediastinum. Blood is then forced out of the right atrium into the valveless innominate vein, jugulars, and other veins of the head and neck; pressure is then also transmitted to the capillaries of the head and neck, which become engorged and rupture leading to the classical physical findings described earlier. Treatment is largely supportive and directed at ensuring adequate oxygenation and attending to any associated injuries. Elevation of the head of the bed is recommended. The outcome is generally good and is related to the length and extent of asphyxia and to associated injuries.

Pulmonary Injury
Pulmonary Contusion

Pulmonary contusion should be suspected in any patient that sustains a direct, high-energy blunt impact to the chest. Pulmonary contusion consists of a direct bruise of the lung followed by alveolar hemorrhage surrounded by a zone of peripheral edema rendering the affected area of the lung ineffective for gas exchange. The clinical presentation of patients with pulmonary contusion ranges from benign to severe hypoxia due to respiratory failure. Focal or diffuse areas of opacification on chest radiography are the mainstay of diagnosis; however, the radiographic findings are not always immediately. The mean time to opacification is 6 hours, although it may take up to 48 hours for the contusion to be visible on chest radiograph.[39]

The treatment of pulmonary contusion is largely supportive. Associated injuries should be identified and treated with tube thoracostomy to evacuate an associated hemopneumothorax and pain control for chest wall injury. Supplemental oxygen is given as required to the hypoxic patient. Prophylactic intubation in the absence of respiratory failure is not indicated. The injured lung is well known to be highly susceptible to both over- and underperfusion. The effect of fluid administration on an experimental model of pulmonary contusion was shown to worsen hypoxia due to an increase in the zone of edema,[40] suggesting that the contused lung is at risk during aggressive fluid resuscitation. Prospective studies have failed to substantiate this risk.[41,42] Patients with pulmonary contusions should receive necessary fluid resuscitation to obtain euvolemia by judicious intravenous fluid replacement. There is no role for the use of steroids in the treatment of pulmonary contusion.[43] Antibiotics should be used only in the case of confirmed superimposed pneumonia. The use of empiric antibiotics is not indicated and only contributes to the selection of resistant organisms.

Penetrating Pulmonary Injury

The majority of injuries to the lung can be managed by tube thoracostomy alone. Low pulmonary arterial pressures, lung expansion, and high concentrations of tissue thromboplastin combine to limit blood loss in most cases. Of all penetrating pulmonary injuries, approximately 10% to 15% will require thoracotomy.[6] Penetrating injury to the lung may be divided into high and low velocity wounds. Stab wounds and most civilian gunshot wounds are considered to be low velocity wounds. In these cases, there is no associated blast injury and damage is limited to the dissipated energy in the missile tract. High-velocity gunshot wounds, generally defined as missiles traveling at a velocity that exceeds 1500 to 2500 feet per second, cause far more extensive damage. The damage is compounded by blast injury, the effect of the projectile tumbling, and secondary projectiles generated by injured bone fragments. Although the majority of high velocity injuries are still managed with tube thoracostomy alone, these injuries are much more likely to require operative intervention.

Although 10%-15% of patients will require thoracotomy, it is estimated that 20% of these will require some form of pulmonary resection.[44,45] Historically, anatomic lobectomies or pneumonectomies were the resective procedures performed. High mortality rates, up to 55% for anatomic lobectomy and up to 100% for pneumonectomy[46,47] prompted the development of simpler techniques. Pulmonary tractotomy, opening of the pulmonary injury tract over vascular clamps and selective ligation of bleeding vessels, was described by Wall[48] as a safe and straightforward procedure. Asensio[49] described the technique of using a linear stapler to open the missile tract to perform selective deep vascular ligation, bronchial repairs, or ligation as a tissue-sparing procedure. Other techniques including partial lobectomy and pneumonorrhaphy have been described to allow rapid and minimal resections.[50] A recent 4-year, multicenter review[46] of patients that underwent pulmonary resection following trauma revealed that 75% of patients requiring resection were treated with "minor" resection, defined as pneumonorrhaphy, tractotomy, and wedge resection. Major resection was defined as anatomic lobectomy and pneumonectomy. Regression analysis found that increasing amount of lung resection was an independent predictor of mortality, along with blunt mechanism and low blood pressure at the time of thoracotomy. Pneumonorrhaphy was associated with 9% mortality, tractotomy with 13% mortality, wedge resection with 30% mortality, lobectomy with 43% mortality, and pneumonectomy with 50% mortality.

AIRWAY OBSTRUCTION AND INJURY TO THE TRACHEA AND TRACHEOBRONCHIAL TREE

In the unconscious trauma patient, the airway may become obstructed as the tongue falls backward, occluding the airway. Airway obstruction may also result from foreign objects or direct trauma to the larynx or trachea from either penetrating or blunt injury. The simplest way to relieve airway obstruction is to perform the chin lift or jaw thrust maneuver as described in the Advance Trauma Life Support manual,[10] maneuvers that all trauma surgeons should be able to perform. If obstruction is due to foreign bodies, the obstructing body is removed during direct laryngoscopy and the airway secured via endotracheal intubation.

If the airway is obstructed secondary to direct injury to the larynx or trachea, orotracheal intubation is the preferred method of airway control. If the injury is severe enough to prevent adequate visualization of the vocal cords, intubation may be performed with the aid of fiberoptic bronchoscopy. If damage to the airway is extensive enough to prevent orotracheal intubation, lifesaving cricothyroidotomy must be performed. Tracheostomy should not be used for this purpose.

Complete transection of the cervical trachea or cricotracheal separation is a rare injury that usually results in death or negative sequelae including cerebral anoxia if diagnosis or treatment is delayed. The cricotracheal junction is a relative weak point and shear forces created by sudden deceleration injures may tear the junction completely. The usual causative mechanism is a clothesline injury sustained while riding a motorcycle or a direct impact of the neck against the steering wheel or dashboard.[51,52] Other mechanisms include direct impact from contact sports such as martial arts or strangulation.[53,54] In the rare case of cricotracheal separation, securing the airway requires the performance of an immediate, lifesaving tracheostomy, one of the rare occasions in which this procedure is needed. Orotracheal intubation is possible if the ends of the airway are in close approximation; however, the creation of a false passage is possible with resultant worsening of respiratory distress.

Tracheal and tracheobronchial tree ruptures are uncommon. Injuries to the trachea and tracheobronchial tree may occur from blunt or penetrating trauma. Bertelsen and Howitz[55] found in a review of 1178 patients dying of traumatic injuries, that only 33 (2.8%) patients had tracheobronchial injury. Of these 33 patients, however, 27 (82%) died almost instantaneously. Asensio[56] confirmed the low incidence of this injury in a review of 4193 patients presenting with penetrating injury to the neck. Only 331 patients (8%) demonstrated tracheobronchial injury. The diagnosis of tracheobronchial injury requires prompt diagnosis, skillful airway management, and prompt surgical repair. The diagnosis of tracheobronchial injury in blunt trauma is not always straightforward and can easily be missed in the patient with multiple injuries. Associated injuries have been reported in 69% of patients with blunt tracheobronchial injury and 58% of those with penetrating injuries.[57]

In a review of 32 patients with tracheobronchial injury over 28 years,[57] the most common physical findings were air escaping from the wound in the case of cervical injury and massive air leaks and mobility to expand the lung after placement of a chest tube in patients with mediastinal or main bronchus injury. Of 15 patients with a distal bronchial injury, 2 had a minimal air leaks and only 1 (7%) failed to demonstrate an air leak after placement of a chest tube. Twenty-eight (88%) of 32 patients in this series had an abnormal chest radiograph. The most common findings were pneumothorax and pneumomediastinum. In an earlier series,[58] the most common findings on chest radiograph were subcutaneous emphysema, pneumothorax, pneumomediastinum, and air surrounding the main-stem bronchi.

Treatment priority in these patients includes securing an airway. This is no small task in patients sustaining significant airway injury. If the diagnosis of airway injury is known or suspected, orotracheal intubation must be attempted with great caution. The use of sedatives or paralytics on an awake patient may cause the loss of an airway that was being spontaneously protected. Passage of the endotracheal tube may create a false passage. The use of fiberoptic bronchoscopy requires equipment and experience that may not always be available in the trauma resuscitation area. Urgent tracheostomy or cricothyroidotomy in the operating room is advocated by many as the safest option for airway control. Once the airway is secured, associated injuries can be evaluated and treated.

Nonoperative management of tracheobronchial injuries is reserved for a select few patients with small defined as less than one-third circumference injuries. In addition, the lung must fully expand and any air leak present must stop shortly after tube thoracostomy. In general, patients requiring positive pressure ventilation are not candidates for nonoperative management. With the exception of these few patients, treatment of injuries to the tracheobronchial tree consists of thoracotomy and primary repair.

CARDIAC AND THORACIC VASCULAR INJURIES
Penetrating Cardiac Injury

With the description of the death of Sarpedon in the *Iliad*,[59] Homer provides the earliest description of death from an exsanguinating cardiac injury. Beck[60] classifies the history of wounds of the heart into three historical periods. The first is the period of mysticism in which cardiac wounds were described, but were considered uniformly fatal. This belief continued into the 17th century and was followed by the period of observation and experimentation. The period of suture began with Block[60] in 1882. He successfully repaired cardiac injuries created in a rabbit model. The animals survived and, for the first time the possibility that a human could survive this injury was considered. Cappelen[60] in 1895 was the first surgeon to repair a right ventricular injury and ligate the distal third of the left anterior descending coronary artery. The patient survived but died in sepsis 3 days later. Rehn[60] successfully repaired an injury to the right ventricle resulting in the patient's survival. Hill was the first to successfully repair left ventricular injury. Cardiac surgery was born.

The clinical presentation of patients sustaining penetrating injury to the heart can vary from hemodynamically stability to cardiopulmonary arrest. Their clinical presentation depends on multiple factors including mechanism, extent of injury and transport time to the trauma center. Patients sustaining high-velocity gunshot wounds, patients who arrive late to a trauma center having experienced cardiopulmonary arrest for prolonged periods, and those with massive and exsanguinating blood loss into the left hemithoracic cavity invariably have little chance of survival. It is well known, however, that the muscular left ventricular wall and, to a lesser extent, the right ventricular wall can seal small wounds and prevent exsanguination, allowing patients to arrive at the trauma center alive.

The most helpful diagnostic findings of penetrating cardiac injury are hemodynamic instability and a penetrating wound to the precordium, epigastrium, or superior mediastinum. Cardiac injury may be present in the absence of Beck triad: hypotension muffled heart sounds and distended neck veins. Those are the classic signs of pericardial tamponade. It should be remembered, however, that pericardial tamponade is a unique manifestation of cardiac injury. The fibrous pericardium is relatively inelastic. Rapid accumulations of even a small volume of blood results in increased intrapericardial pressures. This increase in pressure results in compression of the thin-walled right ventricle leading to decreased left ventricular end diastolic volume, thus lowering the cardiac output.

It has been suggested, however, that the effects of pericardial tamponade after cardiac injury are not uniformly negative. Moreno et al,[61] in a retrospective study, demonstrated that cardiac tamponade after penetrating cardiac injury may have a protective effect. One hundred consecutive patients presenting with acute cardiac injuries were reviewed, of which 77 presented with pericardial tamponade. Patients were stratified according to injury mechanism, wound site, vital signs on presentation, and the presence or absence of cardiac tamponade. The presence of cardiac tamponade significantly improved survival following stab wounds, gunshot wounds, right and left chamber wounds, and overall in patients arriving with vital signs. These findings led the authors to conclude that pericardial tamponade is protective after penetrating cardiac injury.

Conversely, Buckman and Asensio,[62] in a prospective study of 66 penetrating wounds of the heart, did not find pericardial tamponade to be an independent factor for survival. Similarly, Asensio[63] in a 1-year prospective pilot study of 60 penetrating injuries of the heart, failed to identify pericardial tamponade as a predictor of survival. And again, in a 2-year prospective study of 105 patients presenting after penetrating injury to the heart, Asensio[64] did not find pericardial tamponade associated with improved survival. It is not necessarily clear, then, if pericardial tamponade is protective or not. Most likely, there is a transient protective effect that may allow the patient to survive long enough to reach the trauma center. How long the potentially protective effect of pericardial tamponade lasts, however, is not well defined.

Cardiac injuries must always be considered in patients sustaining penetrating precordial wounds presenting with hemodynamic instability, although a fraction of patients, present awake, alert, hemodynamically stable, and with penetrating precordial injury. As previously stated, signs of pericardial tamponade may not be evident. If an injury exists, continued bleeding may lead to tamponade. The delayed presentation of pericardial tamponade is potentially disastrous. The options available for the diagnosis of these occult cardiac injuries are the subxiphoid pericardial window and echocardiography. It should be noted that pericardiocentesis has no role in the evaluation of cardiac trauma caused by an unacceptably high incidence of both false positives and false negatives.

The original technique of pericardial window was described by Larrey in the 1800s. It is remarkable, that only small variations in the original technique have been added to this procedure. This technique, although routinely employed in patients with penetrating precordial injury, has seen a marked diminution in its role during recent times due to the advent of 2-dimensional echocardiography as part of the FAST exam. Nevertheless, it is a technique that is still widely employed in many countries that do not have access to ultrasound equipment. Its use still remains valid in a very selected subset of patients. In the past, it was used liberally to evaluate patients sustaining penetrating injury in the area defined as inferior to the clavicles, superior to the costal margins, and medial to the midclavicular lines. This technique evaluates for the presence of blood in the pericardium. It is indicated for penetrating trauma in proximity to the heart and is considered simple to perform, safe, and accurate.

All trauma surgeons should be familiar with this technique, albeit will employ it uncommonly. Pericardial window must be performed in an operating room under general anesthesia. As it is routine with all trauma patients, the patient's entire torso must be prepped from neck to midthighs. A 10-centimeter incision is made in the midline over the xiphoid process. This incision is then carried through skin and subcutaneous tissue and hemostasis controlled with electrocautery. Electrocautery can also be used to directly dissect around the xiphoid process. Utilizing a combination of blunt and sharp dissection, the xiphoid process is isolated, dissected, grasped by Allis clamps and displaced cephalad; blunt dissection with a Kittner dissector will separate the adipose tissue often adherent beneath the xiphoid. Furthermore, blunt and sharp dissection after digitally palpating the transmitted cardiac impulses is used to locate the pericardium, which is then isolated by the utilization of Kittner dissectors separating the pericardial fat until the fibrous sac of the pericardium is visualized. The pericardium is then grasped between two Allis clamps and placed under gentle downward traction. If the patient's hemodynamic state allows it, the patient may be placed in the reverse Trendelenburg position to allow for the pericardium to descend and thus become more accessible.

A better grasp is usually obtained by replacing the Allis clamps and regrasping the pericardium. After this has been done, the area is gently lavaged with saline to remove any blood or clots that have resulted from dissection that may bias the results of the window. Hemostasis is once again checked. A longitudinal incision measuring approximately 1 to 2 centimeters is made in the pericardium sharply, with meticulous care taken to avoid creating an iatrogenic injury to the underlying myocardium. After this longitudinal aperture is made, fluid in the pericardium will escape, the field is either flooded with clear straw-colored pericardial fluid, which signifies a negative window or with blood, indicative of a positive window, and, thus, an underlying cardiac injury. A positive pericardial window mandates proceeding with median sternotomy. Finally, the field may remain dry, if blood has clotted within the pericardium. This is a common pitfall that often vexes inexperienced surgeons which are misled into thinking that there's no underlying cardiac injury. For these uncommon situations, we recommend passing a suction catheter through the previously made incision which will, after application of suction, liberate pericardial clots, thus allowing blood to escape rendering the window positive. Frequent pitfalls faced by inexperienced surgeons are mistaking the central tendon of the diaphragm for the pericardium and repeatedly incising it, causing bleeding and requiring further dissection. Although the subxiphoid window is accurate, it is an invasive procedure. The emergence of ultrasonography in the evaluation of trauma patients has diminished its use; however, subxiphoid window remains an important technique and should be at the disposal of all trauma surgeons and surgeons receiving for trauma patients.

The use of echocardiography in the evaluation of cardiac trauma was evaluated by Meyer et al[65] in a prospective study of 105 hemodynamically stable patients with thoracic injury. The patients each underwent two-dimensional echocardiography followed by subxiphoid pericardial window. For the entire group, subxiphoid window had a sensitivity of 100%, specificity of 92%, and accuracy of 92%. In the presence of hemothorax, echocardiography had a reported sensitivity of 56%, specificity of 93%, and accuracy of 90%. However, sensitivity, specificity, and accuracy of echocardiography improved to 100%, 89%, and 91% in patients without hemothorax. In patients without hemothorax, echocardiography missed no significant injury and proved to be an acceptable diagnostic option for patients with penetrating injury in proximity to the heart.

Since its description by McKenney,[66] the bedside Focused Assessment with Sonography for Trauma (FAST) exam has become increasingly standard in U.S. trauma centers.[67] Four sonographic windows are obtained in the exam—the subcostal window, the right upper quadrant window, the left upper quadrant window, and the suprapubic window—allowing the detection of significant amounts of free fluid. The subcostal window provides a view of the heart and pericardium allowing for the evaluation of pericardial effusion and tamponade. In a prospective study of 247 patients with penetrating chest injury, Rozycki[68] was able to demonstrate a 100% sensitivity and specificity for hemopericardium with the use of the FAST exam. In a later multi-institutional study involving five Level I trauma centers with 209 patients, Rozycki and colleagues[69] demonstrated a sensitivity of 100%, specificity of 96.9%, and an accuracy of 97.3% with sonography for pericardial fluid in patients with precordial or transthoracic wounds.

The five most common incisions used in the management of penetrating thoracic wounds are (1) the median sternotomy, (2) the "book" thoracotomy, (3) the left anterolateral thoracotomy, (4) the bilateral anterolateral thoracotomy, and (5) the posterolateral thoracotomy. Unlike abdominal trauma in which all injuries can be accessed via laparotomy, thoracic injuries require sound judgment in choosing the approach. Given the gravity of the potential wounds, a second choice is not always available.

The median sternotomy is the incision of choice for penetrating precordial injuries. The "book" thoracotomy was described by Steenburg and Ravitch for the management of injuries to the thoracic inlet particularly for left subclavian vessel injuries. This incision has largely been abandoned. The left anterolateral thoracotomy is the incision of choice for those patients that arrive in extremis after cardiac injury. It is most often used in the Emergency Department (ED) for resuscitative purposes. It is also the incision of choice in patients undergoing celiotomy that deteriorate secondary to an occult cardiac injury. The left anterolateral thoracotomy can be extended across the midline in the event that injuries traverse the midline into the right hemithoracic cavity. The classic posterolateral thoracotomy is not employed in the management of cardiac injuries. It is better suited to the management of noncardiac thoracic injuries such as pulmonary, esophageal, or aortic.

Atrial injuries can be controlled with the use of a Satinsky clamp, allowing the trauma surgeon to repair the atrial wound. The repair is executed with a 2-0 polypropylene monofilament suture in an interrupted or running fashion without the use of Teflon pledgets.[70] We prefer to use the MH needle. The walls of the atria are very thin, demanding precise technique. Ventricular wounds require digital occlusion of the defect. Repair of the wound is, again, carried out with 2-0 polypropylene monofilament suture in a simple interrupted, horizontal mattress, or running pattern.[70] Gunshot wounds tend to produce some degree of blast effect that can lead to the breakdown of a repair as the myocardium becomes increasingly friable. When this occurs, prosthetic Teflon pledgets are used to buttress the suture line. The repair of ventricular wounds in proximity to coronary arteries deserves special mention. Misplacing a suture may lead to myocardial infarction by occluding the artery. It is recommended that sutures be placed underneath the bed of the coronary artery.[70]

The use of autogenous material to buttress suture lines is well known. A small flap of pericardium can be elevated and used in the same manner as Teflon pledgets. Although many trauma surgeons have been trained to use Teflon pledgets to strengthen myocardial suture lines, as first described by Mattox,[71] there is no evidence in the literature to suggest that this technique increases tensile strength of repaired myocardium. The routine use of Teflon pledgets cannot be recommended based on available evidence and is left to the discretion of the operating surgeon.

Blunt Cardiac Injury

Historically, the term "myocardial contusion" was used to describe the entire spectrum of myocardial injury that can occur with nonpenetrating trauma to the chest. Because there is no agreed-on definition of the term, the true incidence of myocardial injury after blunt chest trauma is difficult to discern. The reported incidence of myocardial contusion ranges from 17% to 70% in different study populations despite similar mechanisms of injury.[72,73] Mattox,[72] in a consensus statement, recommended the replacement of the term "myocardial contusion" with "blunt cardiac injury" with a specific descriptor (ie, blunt cardiac injury with septal rupture) to allow less ambiguity when dealing with these injuries and their sequelae.

The majority of blunt cardiac injuries are the result of motor vehicle collisions. However, falls, blast injuries, and other blunt mechanisms have also been described.[74] The injured myocardium is characterized by muscle necrosis, edema, and hemorrhagic infiltrates. The outcomes of these injuries range from electrocardiographic changes that are asymptomatic to cardiogenic shock and death. Despite this, there are few reliable signs or symptoms that are specific for blunt cardiac injury and well-defined, universally accepted diagnostic criteria do not exist. Many patients have signs of external chest trauma. Chest pain is common in patients subjected to blunt chest trauma and only the occasional patient will describe anginal type pain that is not relieved by nitrates. In patients with an appropriate mechanism of injury or those with an unexpectedly poor cardiovascular response to associated injuries, the index of suspicion must remain high. The frequency with which the diagnosis of blunt cardiac injury is made will be directly proportional to the aggressiveness with which it is sought.

An electrocardiogram should be performed on all patients in whom blunt cardiac injury is suspected. There are, however, no findings on electrocardiogram that are pathognomonic for blunt cardiac injury. When all electrocardiographic changes such as tachycardia and nonspecific changes are included in the workup of blunt cardiac injury, the sensitivity of ECG for diagnosing blunt cardiac injury approaches 96% but with a specificity of only 47%.[75,76] The most common finding is sinus tachycardia, followed by premature atrial or ventricular contractions. Other abnormalities, in order of frequency are T wave changes, atrial fibrillation or flutter, ST elevation or depression, conduction delays, ventricular dysrhythmias, and new Q waves. In a large meta-analysis of blunt cardiac injury, Maenza[77] found that on 2.6% of patients with blunt cardiac injury developed complex tachycardias requiring intervention. Several studies[78-80] have concluded that hemodynamically stable patients with normal ECGs require no additional studies to evaluate for blunt cardiac injury.

Although there are studies to suggest that CPK isoenzyme levels may be useful in determining which patients would benefit from imaging studies to evaluate for blunt cardiac injury, the overwhelming majority of available studies conclude that CPK isoenzyme analysis is not warranted.[81] CK-MB has been isolated in skeletal muscle, lung, stomach, pancreas, liver, small bowel, and colon. The release of CK-MB from other organs and tissues during trauma will confound the interpretation of the values. Likewise, circulating cardiac troponin-T has no important clinical value in the diagnosis of blunt cardiac injury.[82] Troponin-I, in contrast to CK-MB, is found only in the cardiac myocyte and offers the opportunity to selectively screen patients with blunt cardiac injury. Even moderated elevations of troponin-I have been shown to correlate with a four-fold increase in mortality in surgical patients.[83] A prospective review of 333 blunt thoracic patients[84] identified 13% with significant blunt cardiac injury, defined as hypotension in the absence of bleeding or neurogenic cause, cardiac arrhythmias, posttraumatic echocardiographic abnormality, or cardiac index less than 2.5 l/min/m². By combining ECG and troponin I at 8 hours, a negative predictive value of 100% was obtained, eliminating patients without significant blunt cardiac injury.

Echocardiography is the primary exam for the structural assessment of the heart. Echocardiographic exam, however, adds little to the evaluation of the hemodynamically stable patient that is suspected of having blunt cardiac injury. In a prospective analysis of 105 patients with severe blunt chest trauma, Karalis[85] found that routine echocardiography was of no value as most patients remained asymptomatic. The authors did state, however, that a transthoracic echocardiogram (TTE) should be performed in any patient who develops symptoms or has a physical exam that suggests underlying cardiac disease. Whereas transthoracic echocardiogram was useful most of the time, in 19% of patients its results are suboptimal secondary to chest wall injury, pleural tubes, mechanical ventilation, or body habitus. Therefore, Karalis[85] recommended that a transesophageal echocardiogram (TEE) be obtained if transthoracic echocardiography is suboptimal. Echocardiography has proven to have diagnostic utility in the unstable or complicated blunt cardiac injury patient. Applications such as M-Mode and Doppler add information not available on the FAST exam. Structural abnormalities such as wall motion defects and valvular incompetence are easily recognized.

The use of the pulmonary artery (PA) catheter has value in the critical patient with blunt cardiac injury. Evidence of hemodynamic instability, age greater than 60, abnormal ECG, and future surgical intervention have been described as indications for its use.[75] The pulmonary artery catheter can provide continuous information regarding preload, afterload, and ventricular function. In the resuscitation of the multiple injured patient with significant blunt cardiac injury, these values may be useful and the use of the PA catheter should be considered in these patients.

In summary, signs and symptoms suspicious for blunt cardiac injury warrant expeditious workup. ECG remains a sensitive test for blunt cardiac injury, but all ECG changes must be considered to avoid missed injuries. The addition of troponin-I may serve to identify those patients at increased risk. Patients with ECG abnormality and troponin-I elevation should be admitted for continuous ECG monitoring for 24 to 48 hours. Conversely, if the admission ECG is normal, the risk of having blunt cardiac injury requiring treatment is insignificant and pursuit of the diagnosis should be halted. Echocardiography should be reserved for those patients with undifferentiated clinical scenarios that warrant investigation and hemodynamic instability to diagnose life-threatening injuries. If optimal transthoracic echocardiography (TTE) cannot be performed, transesophageal echocardiography (TEE) should be obtained. Pulmonary artery catheter placement can be considered in a select subgroup of patients.

Injury of the Great Vessels

Vesalius, in 1557, first reported case of a ruptured thoracic aorta, on a patient being thrown from a horse.[86] Thoracic aortic injuries can occur following both penetrating and blunt trauma. Over 90% of thoracic great vessel injuries are the result of penetrating trauma.[87] Most patients with penetrating injury to the aorta, or other thoracic great vessels, succumb from exsanguination at the scene, or they arrive at the trauma center "in extremis" to undergo resuscitative thoracotomy. The survival rate of these patients is very low. Blunt injury to the aorta is responsible for approximately 8000 deaths each year in the United States.[88] This injury most commonly is the result of motor vehicular collisions but may also result from falls from great height, crushing thoracic injuries, or pedestrians struck by vehicles. Although most of these patients will also die at the scene of the injury, up to 15% will arrive at the trauma center with signs of life.[89] These patients have a reasonably good chance of survival, provided that their injury is diagnosed and treated without delay.

Suspicion for blunt aortic injury should be high with a history of significant deceleration injury. Although most patients with traumatic aortic injury present with multiple associated injuries, up to 30% will show no external signs of chest trauma[90] and may have a completely normal physical exam.[91] Most patients, however, will have clinical findings that suggest injury to the aorta. These include external evidence of chest trauma, sternal fracture, thoracic inlet hematoma, and systolic murmur in the precordial or intrascapular area. The chest radiograph is the first screening exam and should be obtained in all trauma patients. Findings on chest radiography that are considered strongly suggestive of aortic injury are widened mediastinum of greater than 8 cm or mediastinal/chest width ratio of > 0.38,[92] an indistinct or obliterated aortic knob, depression of the left main-stem bronchus, deviation of the nasogastric tube to the right, which is the least frequently seen but most reliable finding,[10] loss of the aortopulmonary window, widened paraspinous or paratracheal stripe, and apical capping.

Patients with any of these radiographic abnormalities should undergo aggressive investigation with either aortography or computed tomography (CT) of the chest. Angiography has long been considered the "gold standard" diagnostic test for traumatic injury of the aorta. However, this test is often not immediately available. The use of CT to a great extent has supplanted the use of aortic angiography in many cases. When conventional scanners are used, aortography is reserved for those with abnormal CT findings. A potential pitfall with this approach is that aortography and, potentially, diagnosis and treatment if further delayed. With the advent of helical or spiral CT scanners, this problem is resolved as they are far more sensitive and appear to have a 100% negative predictive value.[93,94] When helical or spiral CT is used, angiography need only be obtained in those patients with equivocal exams.

Once the diagnosis of aortic injury is made, prompt surgical repair is mandated. Immediate repair, however, may not be possible in all patients such as those that are unstable as a result of associated intra-abdominal injuries requiring immediate laparotomy or those that require emergent craniotomy for severe closed head injury. In these cases, control of blood pressure with beta blockers or nitroprusside is indicated until other injuries are controlled.[94] There have been a number of different surgical techniques reported for the repair of blunt aortic injury. They have included direct suture repair for simple injuries, the use of passive shunt bypass[95] such as the Gott shunt, cardiopulmonary bypass,[96] and the "clamp and sew" technique.[97] Whatever the technique used, the most feared complication is paraplegia. Prolonged ischemic time of the spinal cord must be avoided at all costs. It is well known that if cross-clamp time exceeds thirty minutes the incidence of paraplegia is 5% to 10%.[89]

Injuries to other major thoracic blood vessels require proximal and distal control. Injuries to the innominate artery can be repaired primarily if small or bypassed with a prosthetic graft. Repair of injuries to the common carotid arteries mirrors that of the innominate artery. Because of the difficult approach to the subclavian arteries, injuries to these vessels are particularly challenging. In most instances, repair includes either lateral arteriorrhaphy or interposition graft. Injuries to the internal mammary or verterbral arteries are managed with ligation.

Isolated injury to the suprahepatic inferior vena cava or the superior vena cava is infrequent and requires primary repair. Injury to the pulmonary veins is difficult to manage via an anterior incision. Control may require clamping of the entire pulmonary hilum. If ligation of a pulmonary vein is required, resection of the corresponding lobe is mandatory. Injury of the subclavian vein is managed with lateral venorrhaphy, if possible, or ligation. The azygous vein is not usually considered along with the thoracic great vessels; however, injury can prove fatal.[98] When injured, it is best managed by suture ligation of both proximal and distal ends.

ESOPHAGEAL INJURY

Esophageal injuries are uncommon, most series report fewer than nine patients per year with esophageal injury.[99] Thoracic esophageal injury is rare; the majority occur secondary to penetrating trauma. Blunt injury of the thoracic esophagus is extremely rare. Blunt injuries occur almost exclusively in the neck; however, if the intrathoracic portion is injured, it usually occurs just proximal to the esophagogastric junction on the left side. The signs and symptoms of thoracic esophageal injury are nonspecific, pain and fever most commonly, and take several hours to develop. Associated injury to vital structures is common and addressing these injuries, by necessity, takes precedence. The diagnosis and definitive therapy of thoracic esophageal injuries is, therefore, often delayed. Unfortunately, delay in diagnosis and treatment of these injuries results in a higher incidence of mediastinitis, thoracic sepsis, and death.[99]

The two primary diagnostic tools to evaluate for the presence of esophageal injury are contrast esophagography and esophagoscopy. The combination of contrast esophagography and esophagoscopy reliably identifies injuries with a sensitivity and specificity approaching 100%. Once the diagnosis is made, treatment includes immediate thoracotomy with debridement and primary repair of the injury if the injury has been detected early. Various tissue flaps are used to buttress the repair, including pericardium and pleura,[100] to improve anastomotic outcome. In a review of 43 penetrating esophageal injuries, Asensio[99] found that if primary repair was attempted after sixteen hours the incidence of complications rose sharply. If diagnosis and repair is not completed within this time frame, primary repair is discouraged. In these cases, esophageal diversion and wide drainage of the pleural spaces and mediastinum are required.

DIAPHRAGMATIC INJURY

Diaphragmatic injury is uncommon. In a study[101] spanning 9 years, 60 blunt diaphragmatic injuries were detected among 7500 trauma patients for an incidence of 0.8%. Injury to the diaphragm is most commonly seen on the left and has been reported to have a left to right ratio of up to 25 to 1.[102] Blunt trauma typically produces large diaphragmatic tears, whereas penetrating trauma results in small perforations. The appearance of hollow viscera or nasogastric tube in the left hemithoracic cavity generally establishes the diagnosis. However, the diagnosis may be difficult as initial radiographic findings may be deceiving. In fact, initial chest radiographs may be interpreted as normal in up to 50% of patients.[103] Computed tomography is often not diagnostic. In the hemodynamically stable patient, an upper gastrointestinal study (UGI) generally identifies the stomach displaced into the left chest. In patients without indication for laparotomy, diagnostic laparoscopy has been shown to reliably detect occult diaphragmatic injuries.[12]

All injuries to the diaphragm should be repaired. After displaced abdominal organs are reduced, the edge of the defect is debrided of any devitalized tissue and the defect is repaired primarily. The repair not only restores the normal continuity and motion of the diaphragm; it also prevents later herniation and possible incarceration and strangulation of abdominal organs.

REFERENCES

1. Baker C, Oppenheimer L, Stephens B, et al. Epidemiology of trauma deaths. *Am J Surg* 1980;140: 144-150.
2. LoCicero J, Mattox K. Epidemiology of chest trauma. *Surg Clin North Am* 1989;69:15-19.
3. Shorr R, Crittendan M, Indeck M, et al. Blunt thoracic trauma: analysis of 515 patients. *Ann Surg* 1987;206:200-205.
4. Demetriades D, Murray J, Sinz B, et al. Epidemiology of major trauma deaths in Los Angeles County. *J Am Coll Surg* 1998;187:373-383.
5. Rogers F, Shackford S, Hoyt D, et al. Trauma deaths in a mature urban vs rural trauma system. A comparison. *Arch Surg* 1997;132:376-382.
6. Mattox K. Approaches to trauma involving the major vessels of the thorax. *Surg Clin North Am* 1989;69: 77-91.
7. Demetriades D, Murray J, Charalambides C, et al. Trauma fatalities: timing and location of hospital deaths. *J Am Coll Surg* 2004;198:20-26.
8. Hunt P, Greaves I, Owens W. Emergency thoracotomy in thoracic trauma—a review. *Injury* 2006;37:1-19.

9. Freedland M, Wilson R, Bender J, et al. The management of flail chest injury: factors affecting outcome. *J Trauma* 1990;12:1460-1468.

10. American College of Surgeons Committee on Trauma. *Advanced Trauma Life Support Faculty Manual.* 7th ed. Chicago: ACS; 2004.

11. Yamamoto L, Schroeder C, Morley D, et al. Thoracic trauma: the deadly dozen. *Crit Care Nurs Q* 2005;28: 22-40.

12. Murray J, Demetriades D, Cornwell E, et al. Penetrating left thoracoabdominal trauma: the incidence and clinical presentation of diaphragm injuries. *J Trauma* 1997;43:624-626.

13. Spangaro S. *Sulla tecnica da seguire negli interventi chirurgici per ferrite del cuore e su di un nuovo processo di toracotomia. Clin Chir* 1906;14:227 in Beck C. Wounds of the heart. The technique of suture. *Arch Surg* 1926;13: 205-227.

14. Beall A, Oschner J, Morris G, et al. Penetrating wounds of the heart. *J Trauma* 1961;1:195-207.

15. Beall A, Dietrich E, Crawford H, et al. Surgical management of penetrating cardiac injuries. *Am J Surg* 1966;112:686-691.

16. Working Group, AD Hoc Subcommittee on Outcomes, American College of Surgeons—Committee on Trauma. Practice management guidelines for emergency department thoracotomy. *J Am Coll Surg* 2001;193:303-309.

17. Athanassiadi K, Gerazounis M, Moustardas M, et al. Sternal fractures: retrospective analysis of 100 cases. *World J Surg* 2002;26:1243-1246.

18. Harley D, Mena I. Cardiac and vascular sequelae of sternal fractures. *J Trauma* 1986;26:553-555.

19. Brookes J, Dunn R, Rogers I. Sternal fractures: a retrospective analysis of 272 cases. *J Trauma* 1993;35:46-54.

20. Sirmali M, Turut H, Topcu S, et al. A comprehensive analysis of traumatic rib fractures: morbidity, mortality and management. *Eur J Cardiothorac Surg* 2003;24: 133-138.

21. Stawicki S, Grossman M, Hoey B, et al. Rib fractures in the elderly: a marker of injury severity. *J Am Geriatr Soc* 2004;52:805-808.

22. Gupta A, Jamshidi M, Rubin J. Traumatic first rib fracture: is angiography necessary? A review of 730 cases. *Cardiovasc Surg* 1997;5:48-53.

23. Shweiki E, Klena J, Wood G, et al. Assessing the true risk of abdominal solid organ injury in hospitalized rib fracture patients. *J Trauma* 2001;50:684-688.

24. Holmes J, Ngyuen H, Jacoby R, et al. Do all patients with left costal margin injuries require radiographic evaluation for intraabdominal injury? *Ann Emerg Med* 2005;46:232-236.

25. Wisner DH. A stepwise logistic regression analysis of factors affecting morbidity and mortality after thoracic trauma: effect of epidural analgesia. *J Trauma* 1990;30:799-805.

26. Richardson JD, Adams L, Flint LM. Selective management of flail chest and pulmonary contusion. *Ann Surg* 1982;196:481-487.

27. Voggenreiter G, Neudeck F, Aufmkolk M, Obertacke U, Schmit-Neuerburg KP. Operative chest wall stabilization in flail chest—outcomes of patients with or without pulmonary contusion. *J Am Coll Surg* 1998;187: 130–148.

28. McGahan J, Rab G, Bublin A. Fractures of the scapula. *J Trauma* 1980;20:880-883.

29. Thompson D, Flynn T, Miller P, et al. The significance of scapular fractures. *J Trauma* 1985;25:974-977.

30. Harris R, Harris J. The prevalence and significance of missed scapular fracture in blunt chest trauma. *Am J Roentgenol* 1988;151:747-750.

31. Brucker P, Gruen G, Kaufmann R. Scapulothoracic dissociation: evaluation and management. *Injury* 2005;36(10):1147-1155.

32. Poole G. Fracture of the upper ribs and injury to the great vessels. *Surg Gynecol Obstet* 1989;169:275-282.

33. Costa M, Robbs J. Nonpenetrating subclavian artery trauma. *J Vasc Surg* 1988;8:71-75.

34. Buckerfield C, Castle M. Acute traumatic retrosternal dislocation of the clavicle. *J Bone Joint Surg* 1984;66A:379-385.

35. Harrison W, Gray A, Couves C, et al. Severe nonpenetrating injuries to the chest; clinical results in the management of 216 patients. *Am J Surg* 1960;100: 715-722.

36. Gray A, Harrison W, Couves C, et al. Penetrating injuries to the chest; clinical results in the management of 769 patients. *Am J Surg* 1960;100:709-714.

37. Karmy-Jones R, Jurkovich G, Nathens A, et al. Timing of urgent thoracotomy for hemorrhage after trauma: a multicenter study. *Arch Surg* 2001;136:513-518.

38. Dunne J, Shaked G, Golokovsky M. Traumatic asphyxia: an indicator of potentially severe injury in trauma. *Injury* 1996;27:746-749.

39. Miller P, Croce M, Bee T, et al. ARDS after pulmonary contusion: accurate measurement of contusion volume identifies high risk patients. *J Trauma* 2001;51:223-230.

40. Richardson J, Franz J, Grover F, et al. Pulmonary contusion and hemorrhage—crystalloid vs colloid replacement. *J Surg Res* 1974;16:330-336.

41. Bongard F, Lewis F. Crystalloid resuscitation of patients with pulmonary contusion. *Am J Surg* 1984;148: 145-151.

42. Johnson J, Cogbill T, Winga E. Determinants of outcome after pulmonary contusion. *J Trauma* 1986;26:695-697.

43. Wanek S, Mayberry J. Blunt thoracic trauma: flail chest, pulmonary contusion and blast injury. *Crit Care Clin* 2004;20:71-81.

44. Tominaga G, Waxman K, Scannell G, et al. Emergency thoracotomy with lung resection following trauma. *Am Surg* 1993;59:834-837.

45. Carillo E, Block E, Zeppa R, et al. Urgent lobectomy and pneumonectomy. *Eur J Emerg Med* 1994;1:26-130.

46. Karmy-Jones R, Jurkovich G, Shatz D, et al. Management of traumatic lung injury: a western trauma association multicenter review. *J Trauma* 2001;51:1049-1053.

47. Thompson D, Rowlands B, Walker W, et al. Urgent thoracotomy for pulmonary or tracheobronchial injury. *J Trauma* 1988;28:276-280.

48. Wall M, Hirshberg A, Mattox K. Pulmonary tractotomy with selective vascular ligation for penetrating injuries to the lung. *Am J Surg* 1994;168:665-669.

49. Asensio J, Demetriades D, Berne J. Stapled pulmonary tractotomy: a rapid way to control hemorrhage in penetrating pulmonary injuries. *J Am Coll Surg* 1997;185:486-487.

50. Velmahos G, Baker C, Demetriades D, et al. Lung-sparing surgery after penetrating trauma using tractotomy, partial lobectomy and pneumonorrhaphy. *Arch Surg* 1999;134:186-189.

51. Courard L, Velly J, Martigne C, et al. Post traumatic disruption of the laryngo-tracheal junction. *Euro J Cardiothorac Surg* 1989;3:441-444.

52. Sofferman R. Management of laryngotracheal trauma. *Am J Surg* 1981;141:412-417.

53. Schaefer S, Close L. Acute management of laryngeal trauma update. *Ann Otol Rhinol Laryngol* 1989;98:98-104.

54. O'Connor P, Russell J, Moriarty D. Anesthetic implications of laryngeal trauma. *Anesth Analg* 1998;87:1283-1284.

55. Bertelsen S, Howitz P. Injuries of the trachea and bronchi. *Thorax* 1972;27:188-194.

56. Asensio J, Valenziano C, Falcone R, et al. Management of penetrating neck injuries: the controversy surrounding zone II injuries. *Surg Clin North Am* 1991;71:267-296.

57. Rossbach M, Johnson S, Gomez M, et al. Management of tracheobronchial injuries: a 28 year experience. *Ann Thorac Surg* 1998;65:182-186.

58. Unger J, Schuchmann G, Grossman J, et al. Tears of the trachea and main bronchi caused by trauma. *AJR* 1989;153:1175-1180.

59. Homer. *The Iliad.* Vol. XVI,. London: George Bell & Sons; 1904:299, lines 588-625. Translated by Alexander Pope.

60. Beck C. Wounds of the heart. The technic of surture. *Arch Surg* 1926;13:205-227.

61. Moreno C, Moore E, Majune J, et al. Pericardial tamponade. A critical determinant for survival following penetrating cardiac wounds. *J Trauma* 1986;26:821-825.

62. Buckman R, Badellina M, Mauro L, et al. Penetrating cardiac wounds: prospective factors influencing initial resuscitation. *J Trauma* 1993;34:717-727.

63. Asensio J, Murray J, Demetriades D, et al. Penetrating cardiac injuries: a prospective study of variables predicting outcome. *J Am Coll Surg* 1998;186:24-34.

64. Asensio J, Berne J, Demetriades D, et al. One hundred five penetrating cardiac injuries: a 2-year prospective evaluation. *J Trauma* 1998;44:1073-1082.

65. Meyer D, Jessen M, Grayburn P. Use of echocardiography to detect occult cardiac injury after penetrating thoracic trauma: a prospective study. *J Trauma* 1995;39:902-909.

66. McKenney M, Lentz K, Nunez D, et al. Can ultrasound replace diagnostic peritoneal lavage in the assessment of blunt trauma? *J Trauma* 1994;37:439-441.

67. Patel A, Brenning C, Cotner J, et al. Successful diagnosis of penetrating cardiac injury using surgeon performed sonography. *Ann Thorac Surg* 2003;76:2043-2047.

68. Rozycki G, Feliciano D, Schmidt J, et al. The role of surgeon performed ultrasound in patients with possible cardiac wounds. *Ann Surg* 1996;223:737-744.

69. Meyer D, Jessen M, Grayburn P. Use of echocardiography to detect occult cardiac injury after penetrating thoracic trauma: a prospective study. *J Trauma* 1995;39:902-909.

70. Asensio J, Stewart B, Murray J, et al. Penetrating cardiac injuries. *Surg Clin North Am* 1996;76:685-724.

71. Mattox K, Espada R, Beall A, et al. Performing thoracotomy in the emergency center. *J Am Coll Emerg Phys* 1974;3:13-17.

72. Mattox K, Flint M, Carrico C, et al. Blunt Cardiac Injury. *J Trauma* 1992;33:649-650.

73. Parmley L, Manion W, Mattingly T. Nonpenetrating traumatic injury of the heart. *Circulation* 1958;18:371-396.

74. Tenzer M. The spectrum of myocardial contusion—a review. *J Trauma* 1985;25:620-627.

75. Orliaguet G, Ferjani M, Riou B. The heart in blunt trauma. *Anesthesiology* 2001;95:544-548.

76. Healey M, Brown R, Fleiszer D. Blunt cardiac injury: is this diagnosis necessary? *J Trauma* 1990;30:137-146.

77. Maenza R, Seaberg D, D'Amico F. A meta-analysis of blunt cardiac trauma: ending myocardial confusion. *Am J Emerg Med* 1996;14:237-241.

78. Foil M, Mackersie R, Furst S, et al. The asymptomatic patient with suspected myocardial contusion. *Am J Surg* 1990;160:638-643.

79. Dubrow T, Mihalka J, Eisenhauer D, et al. Myocardial contusion in the stable patient: what level of care is appropriate? *Surgery* 1989;106:267-274.

80. Nagy K, Krosner S, Roberts R, et al. Determining which patients require evaluation for blunt cardiac injury following blunt chest trauma. *World J Surg* 2001;25:108-111.

81. Pasquale M, Nagy K, Clarke J. *Practice Management Guidelines for the Screening of Blunt Cardiac Injury. EAST Practice Parameter Workgroup for Screening of Blunt Cardiac Injury.* 1998. Available at http://www.east.org/tpg/chap2.pdf.

82. Ferjani M, Droc G, Dreux S, et al. Circulating cardiac troponin T in myocardial contusion. *Chest* 1997;111:427-433.

83. Relos R, Hasinoff I, Beilman G. Moderately elevated serum troponin concentrations are associated with increased morbidity and mortality rates in surgical intensive care unit patients. *Crit Care Med* 2003;31:2598-2603.

84. Velmahos G, Karaiskakis M, Salim A, et al. Normal electrocardiography and serum troponin I levels preclude the presence of clinically significant blunt cardiac injury. *J Trauma* 2003;54:45-51.

85. Karalis D, Victor M, Davis G, et al. The role of echocardiography in blunt chest trauma: a transthoracic and transesophageal echocardiographic study. *J Trauma* 1994;36:53-58.

86. Vesalius A. In: Beonetus T (ed). *Sepulchretaum sive Anataomia Practica ex Cad a veribus Morbo.* Geneva; 1700.

87. Mattox K, Feliciano D, Beall A, et al. Five thousand seven hundred sixty cardiovascular injuries in 4459 patients epidemiologic evolution 1958-1988. *Ann Surg* 1989;209:698-705.

88. Nagy K, Fabian T, Rodman G, et al. *Guidelines for the Diagnosis and Management of Blunt Aortic Injury. An EAST Practice Management Guidelines Workgroup.* 2000. Available at http://www.east.org/tpg/chap8.pdf.

89. Fabian T, Richardson J, Croce M, et al. Prospective study of blunt aortic injury: multicenter trial of the

American Association for the Surgery of Trauma. *J Trauma* 1997;42:374-380.

90. Mattox K. Approaches to trauma involving the major vessels of the thorax. *Surg Clin North Am* 1989;69: 77-91.

91. Kram H, Appel P, Wohlmuth D, et al. Diagnosis of traumatic thoracic aortic rupture: a 10-year retrospective analysis. *Ann Thorac Surg* 1989;47:282-286.

92. Avery J, Hall D, Adams J, et al. Traumatic rupture of the thoracic aorta. *South Med J* 1979;72:1238-1240.

93. Mirvis S, Kathirkamuganathas S, Buell J, et al. Use of spiral computed tomography for the assessment of blunt trauma patients with potential aortic injury. *J Trauma* 1998;45:922-930.

94. Fabian T, Davis K, Gavant M, et al. Prospective study of blunt aortic injury: helical CT is diagnostic and antihypertensive therapy reduces rupture. *Ann Surg* 1998;227:666-677.

95. Gott V. Heparinized shunts for thoracic vascular operations. *Ann Thorac Surg* 1972;14:219-220.

96. Pate J, Fabian T, Walker W. Acute traumatic rupture of the aortic isthmus: repair with cardiopulmonary bypass. *Ann Thorac Surg* 1995;59:90-98.

97. Mattox K, Holtzman M, Pickard L, et al. Clamp/repair: a safe technique for treatment of blunt injury to the descending thoracic aorta. *Ann Thorac Surg* 1985;40:456-463.

98. Sydder C, Eyer S. Blunt chest trauma with transaction of the azygous vein: a case report. *J Trauma* 1989;29:889-890.

99. Asensio J, Berne J, Demetriades D, et al. Penetrating esophageal injury: the time interval of safety of preoperative evaluation—how long is safe? *J Trauma* 1997;43:319-324.

100. Grillo H, Wilkins E. Esophageal repair following late diagnosis of intrathoracic perforation. *Ann Thorac Surg* 1975;20:387-399.

101. Rodriquez-Morales G, Rodriquez A, Shatney C. Acute rupture of the diaphragm in blunt trauma: analysis of 60 patients. *J Trauma* 1986;26:438-444.

102. Gravier L, Freeark R. Traumatic diaphragmatic hernia. *Arch Surg* 1963;86:363-373.

103. Miller L, Bennett E, Root H, et al. Management of penetrating and blunt diaphragmatic injury. *J Trauma* 1984;24:403-409.

Chapter 29

THE ABDOMEN

Michael E. Lekawa, MD, and David B. Hoyt, MD

While comprehensive management of the multiple trauma patient is the expertise of the trauma surgeon, many specific injuries are managed by other surgical specialists, particularly orthopedic surgeons and neurosurgeons. Abdominal trauma is unique in that the management of most abdominal trauma is completely within the purview of the trauma surgeon. As such, it is imperative that trauma surgeons remain competent and current in their knowledge of abdominal trauma management.

EPIDEMIOLOGY

In some respects, our approach to abdominal trauma has come full circle since our earliest forays into trauma management. For millennia, nonoperative management of abdominal trauma was the mainstay of therapy. It is likely that many trauma patients with spleen and liver injuries were unwittingly treated well with bed rest and clear liquids. Successful nonoperative management of penetrating abdominal trauma was reported by Ambrose Parè in the 16th century. In the 1885 meeting of the American Surgical Association, 13 of 33 patients sustaining abdominal gunshot wounds (GSW) treated nonoperatively survived. As methods of antisepsis and anesthesia developed, surgeons were no longer satisfied to leave survival from abdominal trauma to chance. Surgical management implementing aggressive operative techniques developed rapidly during the world wars. In the latter part of the 20th century, less debilitating surgical approaches became popularized, including splenorrhaphy and primary colon repair. As our knowledge of the natural course of abdominal trauma has matured, we have become more comfortable with nonoperative management of the majority of blunt abdominal injuries. This concept has spilled over into both knife and even gunshot wounds to the abdomen. The current strategies for nonoperative management are frequently more complex and, in fact, often more labor-intensive for the treating surgeon. The diminished role for operative

intervention has made formal trauma education more important than ever, as the individual surgeon's operative experience in trauma has diminished substantially.

MECHANISM AND ITS RELATIONSHIP TO ABDOMINAL INJURY

The mechanism of injury is often the first clue that leads to the diagnosis of specific abdominal injuries. Although the final diagnosis is normally delineated by other modalities, every experienced trauma surgeon should develop a diagnostic algorithm that begins with the mechanism of injury. Likely abdominal injuries can be predicted based on both the mechanism of injury and the association of specific abdominal injuries with more obvious extra-abdominal injuries. The likelihood of abdominal injuries with many of these mechanisms has led to the liberal use of abdominal computed tomography (CT) scans if the physical examination is impaired, and in many cases even if the exam appears reliable.

It is generally accepted that there are two forces involved in abdominal trauma, compression and shear strain. Direct compression is likely responsible for most solid organ injuries. A liver laceration seen on a driver with same side passenger space intrusion is a good illustration of this. However, shear injuries can also produce significant solid organ injuries. Sudden deceleration will cause tissue near a point of fixation to move at a different rate than free tissue. Front end accidents may produce injuries to the hilum of the spleen or liver lacerations close to the inferior vena cava (IVC) or falciform ligament. Bowel injuries may be caused by either mechanism. Direct compression may cause a sudden increase in intraluminal pressure, which results in an antimesenteric blowout of the bowel. Alternatively, the high incidence of bowel injury near the Ligament of Treitz supports a shear mechanism for blunt bowel injury.

BLUNT TRAUMA MECHANISMS
Motor Vehicle Crash

Patients presenting after a motor vehicle crash (MVC) have somewhat predictable abdominal injuries, depending on details that should be extracted from the paramedics. On-scene mortalities, ejection, depth and location of passenger space intrusion, use of seat belts or airbags, vehicle speed, and site of impact, as well as on-scene vitals are all important details that can influence the diagnostic workup of the injured abdomen. The most common abdominal organs injured in an MVC where the victim is not wearing a seatbelt include the spleen and liver. In patients who are wearing restraints, hollow viscus injury becomes more common, particularly if a shoulder harness is absent. If the physical examination reveals a seatbelt sign, the incidence of abdominal injury has been reported as high as 64% and bowel injury as high as 21%.[1] Patients who sustain side impact crashes will more commonly have solid organ injuries on the same side as the passenger space intrusion. If the MVC involved a rapid deceleration as seen in head on or bridge abutment accidents, mesenteric injuries are common. Patients ejected from a vehicle are at high risk of abdominal injury, though no specific injury is more likely than another.

Falls

Patients who sustain falls greater than 20 feet are more likely to sustain intra-abdominal injuries. It should be noted whether the landing is grass or concrete. In one study, 6% of patients who sustained free falls averaging 29 feet had intra-abdominal injuries, mostly solid organ.[2]

Pedestrian versus Auto

Pedestrians hit by vehicles are more likely to sustain intra-abdominal injuries if the speed is greater than 15 mph. Solid organ injuries will predominate with this mechanism.

Motorcycle Crash

Motorcycle trauma patients have a 4% incidence of severe abdominal injury, most commonly solid organ injury. The presence of significant abdominal abrasions may complicate the accuracy of the physical examination. There is a very high correlation between rib fractures and abdominal injury in motorcycle trauma, with multisystem injury being the rule rather than the exception.[3]

Blast Injury

Blast injuries, although uncommon in civilian trauma, are mostly associated with military and terrorist activities. The recent experience in the Middle East is now illustrating the injuries to be anticipated. Every trauma surgeon should have at least a basic understanding of how blasts can create abdominal injury. The primary blast wave travels through the abdomen and creates shear injuries in solid organs as well as hollow viscus perforations from sudden changes in pressure within the lumen of the bowel. Secondary injuries include penetrating injuries from projectiles moving from the blast source. The tertiary injury is due to the impact of the victim being thrown away from the blast.

Bicycle Accidents

Bicyclists hit by vehicles may suffer the entire spectrum of abdominal injuries, with solid organ injuries being most common. One mechanism worth discussing occurs when the front wheel impacts a curb or a wall and the handlebar is suddenly turned into the upper abdomen. There is a well described relationship with this mechanism causing bowel and pancreatic injury. The point of impact is likely to be a source of focal tenderness, making the physical examination difficult to interpret. Because of the often minor mechanism, these patients may present in a delayed fashion. A thorough search for injuries is important to avoid the significant morbidity of a delayed diagnosis.

PENETRATING TRAUMA MECHANISMS
Stab Wounds

The thoracoabdominal area is defined as that area inferior to the nipples and superior to the costal margin. The major consideration here is the possibility of diaphragmatic injuries with or without intra-abdominal injury.

Patients who present hemodynamically unstable with stab wounds to the back have likely suffered a major vascular injury. In hemodynamically stable patients, retroperitoneal organs are at risk. Due to the thickness of the back musculature, the majority of these patients will nave no intra-abdominal injuries.

Anterior stab wounds have a 33-50% risk of entering the peritoneum. Of those, about half will cause an injury that requires surgical repair. Most of these injuries involve the intestines.

Gunshot Wounds

It has been reported that more than 90% of GSWs that traverse the peritoneum will cause an injury that is amenable to surgical repair.[4] More recent studies have illustrated that close to half of all abdominal gunshot wounds may not involve major hemorrhage or bowel injury and are thus amenable to nonoperative management.

ASSOCIATED INJURIES

RIB FRACTURES

Trauma patients with right rib fractures have triple the risk of liver injuries (10.7%), whereas patients with left rib fractures have a fourfold risk of spleen injuries

(11.3%) as well as an association with diaphragm injuries.[5] Rib fractures are associated with a significant risk of abdominal injury in general. If left rib tenderness is the only finding, there is still a 3% incidence of significant renal or spleen injury.

PELVIC FRACTURES

Blunt trauma patients who sustain pelvic fractures have a 15% incidence of liver injury, a 15% incidence of spleen injury, a 6% incidence of hollow viscus injury, and a 4% risk of renal injury.[6] A CT evaluation of the abdomen and pelvis is essential when a pelvic fracture is identified in order to assist with orthopedic management, identify ongoing pelvic hemorrhage, as well as identify associated abdominal injuries.

SPINE FRACTURES

Lumbar compression fractures (Chance fractures) are more common in MVCs where lap restraints are used and in falls where the victim falls on the feet. They are associated with a 22% risk of bowel or mesenteric injury requiring laparotomy.[7] Transverse process fractures of the lumbar spine are common and are an indicator of significant traumatic force, although the association with abdominal injury is not clear.

DIAGNOSTIC OPTIONS

PHYSICAL EXAMINATION

Although the abdominal examination is a key component of most initial patient evaluations, there are many factors that may compromise its value in trauma. The presence of peritonitis is still considered an absolute indication for laparotomy after trauma. The identification of peritonitis in the examination of the trauma patient should include tenderness to palpation in multiple quadrants apart from any abdominal contusions or open wounds. Rebound tenderness is not a required finding to determine peritonitis and likely represents a more advanced process.

The ability to discern peritonitis is often compromised by other factors in the posttrauma setting. Major closed head injury, spinal cord injury, pharmacologic paralysis, and general anesthesia used to treat other injuries will severely impact the ability to determine the presence of peritonitis. In these settings, the lack of abdominal findings in no way precludes abdominal injury. Other conditions that have traditionally been thought to limit the detection of peritonitis include other extra-abdominal distracting injuries, narcotic administration, or alcohol and drug intoxication. Many investigators have challenged that dogma, and many trauma surgeons feel that the abdominal examination may be followed in many of these settings. Peritonitis may be mimicked by abdominal wall contusions or abrasions (seat belt sign), rectus sheath hematomas, or lower rib fractures. Examiner

experience is an important factor in the accurate identification of mild or moderate peritonitis. The development of peritonitis often occurs in a delayed fashion and may lead to laparotomy hours after the primary injury. The time to develop peritonitis is likely a direct result of the magnitude of peritoneal contamination and can vary widely from patient to patient.

Abrasions and abdominal wall contusions (seatbelt signs) can produce tenderness that may or may not require a laparotomy and can be difficult to discriminate from peritonitis. In this setting, the perceived presence of peritonitis may be one of the more common findings that lead to a nontherapeutic laparotomy. This lack of specificity of the abdominal examination results in most trauma surgeons interpreting the physical examination in the context of other diagnostic approaches, most commonly CT.

PLAIN RADIOGRAPHS

In blunt trauma, plain radiographs of the abdomen have been mostly abandoned. The anterior-posterior AP chest film may have findings indicative of a diaphragmatic injury, particularly if a nasogastric tube is displaced into the left chest. Rarely, free air may be present as well. An AP view of the pelvis has been a mainstay as an adjunct to the primary survey. Its main value was to identify potential sources of hemorrhage as early as possible. In the stable trauma patient, the pelvic film may be safely left out if a pelvic CT scan is planned.[8] Omission of the pelvic x-ray will decrease radiation exposure, cost, and resuscitation time. In penetrating trauma, plain films can be helpful to look for retained opaque foreign bodies. Entry and exit wounds should be marked to improve the yield of these films.

DIAGNOSTIC PERITONEAL LAVAGE

Diagnostic peritoneal lavage (DPL) came into popularity in the 1960s as a useful method to determine the presence of significant abdominal injuries. The concept was that there is a threshold amount of blood that reflects a major solid organ injury in blunt trauma that would require a laparotomy. In penetrating trauma, a smaller amount of blood was evidence of an intraperitoneal injury that was thought to require laparotomy. Over the last few decades, however, nonoperative management of solid organ injury has become a mainstay in blunt trauma. Although a positive DPL may be present, it does not necessarily indicate that a laparotomy will be optimal therapy by today's standards. Similarly, a positive DPL in penetrating trauma is evidence of intraperitoneal penetration, but may not represent an injury that necessitates laparotomy. As a result, the indications for DPL have narrowed considerably. A DPL is still a viable option when the patient is too unstable for CT scanning and an adequate ultrasound evaluation is not possible. More commonly in our institution, DPL is applied after a CT scan to evaluate for bowel injury when the CT scan or abdominal examination findings are suspicious.

Technique of Diagnostic Peritoneal Lavage

There are multiple techniques for performing a DPL, and the approach is usually tailored to the patient's situation and the surgeon's or institution's experience. In patients with evidence of prior abdominal surgery, an open technique is advisable. Otherwise, a semiopen or closed approach is more suitable. Generally, a single lumen catheter with multiple holes is inserted into the peritoneum using a Seldinger technique. In gravid patients, a supraumbilical site is chosen to avoid injury to the uterus. In patients with known pelvic fractures, a supraumbilical site will decrease the risk of releasing an anterior extraperitoneal hematoma freely into the peritoneum. This complication can both increase the hemorrhage as well as give a false-positive study. Otherwise, a site between the umbilicus and the superior pubic rami is chosen. The authors use the immediate infraumbilical site to provide the most reliable entry into the peritoneum. If greater than 10 cc of frank blood are aspirated on entry, the study is considered positive. Otherwise, 1 liter of warm sterile saline is placed into the peritoneum. The speed of this infusion can be improved by using large tubing (not IV tubing) and raising the fluid bag as high as possible with the gurney as low as possible. With care to maintain a fluid column in the tubing, the near empty bag is then lowered to the ground, the gurney is raised as high as possible, and at least 600 cc are removed. This fluid is then evaluated for cell counts, bilirubin, amylase, and Gram stain. Cell count results usually can be expedited by using the urinalysis counter and should be available within 10 minutes.

The cell counts that are considered positive in blunt trauma vary, but 100,000 red blood cells (RBC) or 500 white blood cells (WBC) is the most common standard. RBC counts from 50,000 to 100,000 thousand are relative, and counts less than 50,000 are likely negative. The presence of bilirubin, amylase, or creatinine in values substantially greater than serum values is considered positive. Particulate matter such as food or stool is likewise positive for bowel injury.

The cell count numbers that are considered positive are much lower in penetrating trauma, and in fact really exist to determine if there was substantial peritoneal penetration. RBC counts greater than 10,000 and WBC counts greater than 100 are typically considered positive. Again, elevations in bilirubin, amylase, or creatinine and the presence of particulate matter are all considered positive.

As originally described, a DPL was meant to be performed during the initial trauma resuscitation and the cell count values that determine a positive study were extracted from data using that standard. As the time interval increases between the injury and the DPL, the results and the meaning of those results may change. A DPL done to look for bowel injury may be more effective if it is delayed by 3 hours to allow an inflammatory response to the injury. The results would be interpreted in the context of comparing DPL effluent WBC/RBC to blood WBC/RBC, with ratios > 1 being considered positive.[9]

Focused Abdominal Sonography for Trauma

Over the last 10 years, surgeon-performed abdominal ultrasound has become a mainstay of the trauma resuscitation, though its value varies depending on the experience of the individual examiner. The Focused Abdominal Sonography for Trauma (FAST) exam looks at 4 to 6 compartments and evaluates for the presence or absence of fluid (Fig. 29-1). The pericardial sac, the hepatorenal space (Morison pouch), the splenorenal space, and the pelvis are all evaluated, with some studies including the colic gutters. Volumes as little as 30 cc can be reliably detected by most adequately trained surgeons. The learning curve is relatively short and usually includes 30-100 supervised studies.[10] Pneumothorax or obesity can diminish the quality of the upper abdominal exam and lead to false negative studies.

Ultrasound may be most valuable in the trauma patient who presents in shock with multiple potential sources of hemorrhage. If the ultrasound is negative, the abdomen is unlikely to be a major component of traumatic shock and a search for alternative sources of hemorrhage is indicated. Follow-up ultrasounds performed 5 to 20 minutes after the initial ultrasound may increase the study reliability. A positive ultrasound in an unstable patient would normally indicate the need for laparotomy.

Contrast-enhanced ultrasound is being investigated for use in abdominal trauma. Early investigations have shown a significant increase in the ability to diagnose specific solid organ injuries.[11] How this could be implemented during the initial resuscitation is yet to be seen.

Computed Tomography

CT has evolved to be the primary tool in the evaluation of abdominal trauma. Its role is best established in blunt trauma due to its high specificity and sensitivity for solid organ injury. It has allowed accurate grading of liver and spleen injury and identification of active bleeding. In the past, the reliability of CT for the diagnosis of bowel injury was felt to be poor. Many studies, however, now support the sensitivity of CT for blunt bowel injury, particularly with increasing precision of multidetector scanners.[12]

There are drawbacks to CT as a diagnostic tool; most notable is that the patient must be transported out of the resuscitation room to the radiology department. It can be time consuming, although technical improvements

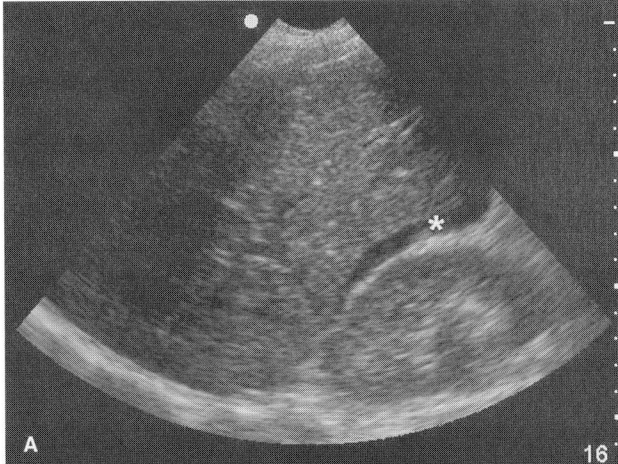

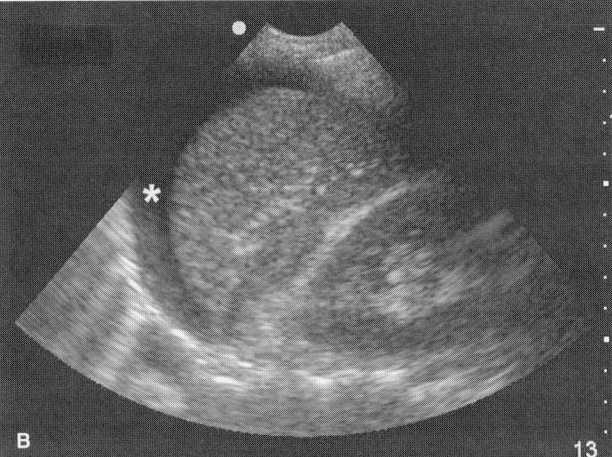

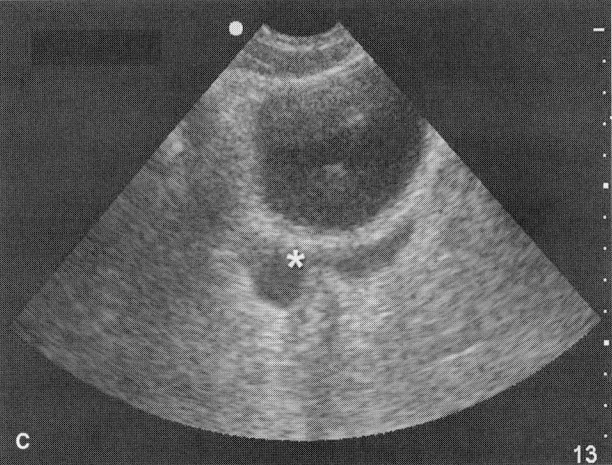

Figure 29-1 *FAST Exam reveals blood in Morrison pouch (A), Splenorenal fossa (B), a pelvis (C).*

have improved the speed dramatically. It is still rather expensive and exposes the patient to some amount of radiation (approximately 2 rads). Intravenous contrast should be given but carries with it the potential for renal insult and allergic reaction.

There is some controversy in the selection process of who should undergo abdominal CT scan. Most surgeons agree that patients subject to significant blunt trauma mechanism who have a compromised examination due to closed head injury, significant intoxication, or spinal cord injury should undergo CT scan of the abdomen. Blunt trauma patients undergoing general anesthesia for urgent extra-abdominal operation should be considered for abdominal CT scan as their examination will be on hold during the perioperative time. The incidence of unexpected injury in this situation is quite low (@1%) but can be serious.[13] Trauma patients with abdominal pain or tenderness, lower rib fractures or tenderness, pelvic fractures, or abdominal seat belt signs should also have CT scans. There is some question as to whether patients should undergo abdominal CT if their physical examination is negative but there is a major mechanism of injury. Several studies supporting the liberal application of chest CT scan have come out over the last decade.[14] These scans are performed primarily for mechanism, not symptoms, including MVC > 35 mph and falls > 15 FT. In these cases, if the IV contrast is already administered for a chest CT scan, there is little downside to obtaining an abdominal CT scan. The additional time, cost, and radiation exposure are rather minimal while the benefits include potential trauma findings as well as nontrauma findings. Perhaps most importantly, a negative study may lead to an earlier discharge with confidence that no abdominal injuries have been missed. This has led some centers to migrate toward applying abdominal CT as part of a "pan scan" based on significant mechanism alone.[15] Although liberal use of CT scan for evaluation of the abdomen is increasingly common, it is still reasonable to evaluate patients with lesser trauma mechanisms with surgeon performed ultrasound and reliable serial abdominal examinations.

There is still some controversy as to the value of oral contrast. Critics have referred to the increased time prior to CT scan as well as an increased risk of aspiration. Centers that use CT to evaluate for blunt bowel injury may rely on the contrast to improve sensitivity. This can be particularly important in identifying duodenal injuries. Proponents point out that aspiration risks are only potential and that rapid protocols are available that add little or no time to the pre-CT scan workup. As the discrimination of multidetector CT scanners increases, the added benefit of contrast may be lost and the question becomes irrelevant. As such, there is a clear trend away from the use of oral contrast, but each institution should review its value with its own radiologists.

Patients should generally undergo CT scan only when hemodynamically stable. However, it is a matter of judgment as to when and for how long a patient should go to the scanner. CT scanners should be located as close as possible to the trauma bay. The trauma resuscitation should continue throughout the CT scan and the trauma service should be in attendance to better monitor the patient's hemodynamic status as well as to immediately review the results. An abdominal injury producing hemodynamic instability does not require a CT scan for diagnosis, as other studies or findings will direct care.

In the 1980s and early 1990s, the use of CT in the evaluation of penetrating trauma was mostly limited to the evaluation of the retroperitoneum after stab wounds to the back. Patients who are hemodynamically stable with injuries limited to between the tip of the scapulas and the pelvic brims, and posterior to the midaxillary lines can be evaluated with triple contrast CT scan. The contrast may improve the ability to discern duodenal and colon injuries. More recently, CT has been used to evaluate intraperitoneal structures. Wounds from trajectories that may be isolated to the liver may be confidently evaluated by CT scan (Fig. 29-2). CT scan may also be useful to evaluate bullet trajectories that are suspected to be subcutaneous (Fig. 29-3). CT evaluation of hollow viscus injuries and diaphragm injuries due to penetrating trauma is a relatively recent development. With increasing precision of multidetector scanners, CT is now being applied to anterior penetrating trauma. CT diagnosis of bowel and diaphragm injuries usually relies on secondary findings such as free fluid and mesenteric stranding. An evaluation of CT in abdominal GSWs has illustrated its utility in determining the bullet trajectory and ruling out hollow viscus injuries.[16] A follow-up trial of 152 patients suffering gunshot and stab wounds to the abdomen who were hemodynamically stable and without peritonitis showed CT to be very accurate in selecting candidates for nonoperative management. Overall, 25%

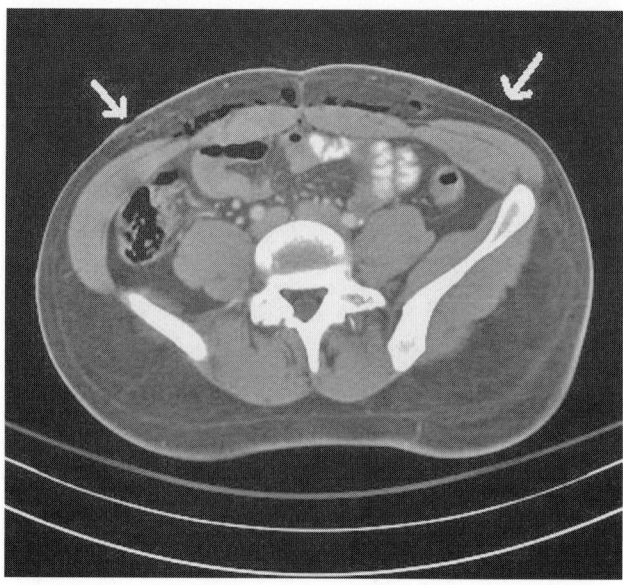

Figure 29-3 *Extraperitoneal trajectory is well illustrated on CT scan. Entry and exit wounds are marked by arrows.*

of these patients were able to avoid nontherapeutic laparotomy.[17] The role of CT in penetrating trauma is clearly expanding and for the time being will rely on institutional expertise and experience.

OPERATIVE MANAGEMENT

LAPAROSCOPY IN TRAUMA
The role of laparoscopy as a diagnostic tool in trauma is mostly limited to stab wounds and tangential gunshot wounds. Although laparoscopy in the emergency department (ED) with local anesthesia has been described, most trauma surgeons will move the patient to the operating room (OR) and proceed under general anesthesia. Peritoneal penetration should be obvious if the injuries are anterior to the posterior axillary lines. Evaluation of the bowel is difficult, and significant miss rates have been reported. Moreover, exposing the entire length of the bowel runs the risk of injury and should be attempted only by a surgeon with appropriate advanced laparoscopic training.

OTHER MODALITIES
The ability of laboratory values to identify abdominal injury in trauma patients is limited. Amylase or lipase is included in many trauma laboratory panels, although its value is questionable. An initially elevated amylase has little correlation to intestinal or pancreatic injury, although an upward trend may be indicative of pancreatic injury. Abnormal values may have a variety of incidental causes and can lead to unnecessary workup. Patients in whom a pancreatic or bowel injury is specifically suspected, it is reasonable to follow amylase or lipase levels.

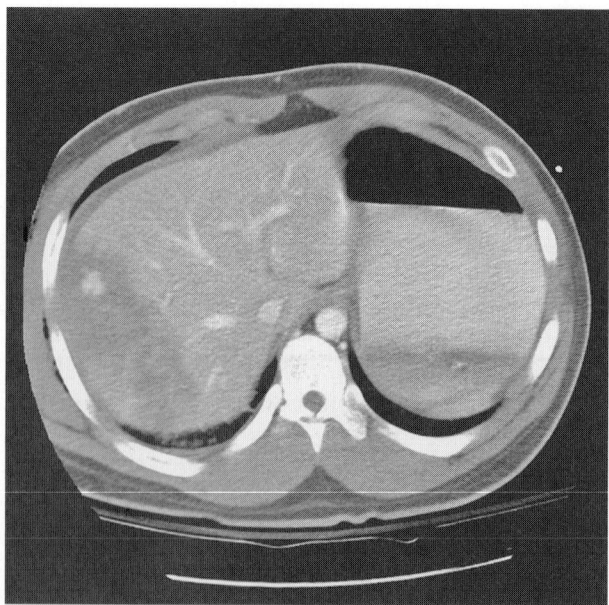

Figure 29-2 *CT scan illustrates wound track of transhepatic GSW. This was successfully managed by transhepatic arterial embolization.*

INITIAL MANAGEMENT OF THE BLUNT ABDOMINAL TRAUMA PATIENT

PREOPERATIVE MANAGEMENT

After the primary survey is completed and the initial resuscitation is underway, specific evaluation of the abdomen takes place as part of the secondary survey. The details of the mechanism of injury are considered along with associated injuries. The physical examination is performed with consideration of any confounding factors. A chest radiograph is completed as well as a pelvic radiograph as indicated. Abdominal ultrasound is routinely performed by the trauma surgeon. In patients identified as seriously injured or at significant risk of abdominal injury, gastric intubation is indicated to decrease the risk of aspiration, to decompress gastric distention that may alter the abdominal examination, and to identify hemorrhage. If the patient has an endotracheal tube placed, an oral route is used for gastric intubation to decrease the risk of epistaxis or delayed sinusitis. Otherwise, a nasogastric tube is indicated. Similarly, if significant injury is suspected or the patient cannot produce a urine sample, the urinary bladder is intubated. This may improve the quality of the abdominal examination, prevent bladder distention, provide a specimen for evaluation of RBC counts, and allow ongoing determination of urine output.

INDICATIONS FOR IMMEDIATE LAPAROTOMY

The two indications for immediate laparotomy after blunt trauma are peritonitis and persistent shock with free abdominal fluid on ultrasound.

As discussed earlier in this chapter, the detection of peritonitis after blunt trauma is often complicated by confounding factors. Nonetheless, if clearly present, peritonitis indicates the need for early laparotomy. If the patient is hemodynamically stable and a CT scan is immediately available, there is likely time to allow for workup of other potentially life-threatening problems (if indicated) while the OR is being prepared, specifically head injury. It is also common that peritonitis after blunt trauma may take hours to develop.

More commonly, immediate laparotomy after blunt trauma is indicated due to hemodynamic instability in concert with some evidence of peritoneal bleeding such as free fluid on ultrasound or a positive DPL. Patients who present with hypotension and evidence of intra-abdominal bleeding usually will undergo some amount of resuscitation. If there is an adequate response to resuscitation, immediate laparotomy is not necessary and alternative evaluation and treatment takes place. There are a variety of standards for how much fluid or blood transfusions should lead to laparotomy; however, each circumstance must be judged on its own merit. For example, if the ultrasound reveals a sliver of fluid in the face of bilateral femur fractures and a hemothorax, giving more blood and fluid may be appropriate prior to the decision to proceed to laparotomy. By contrast, if no other sources of hemorrhage are identified, more concrete standards may be utilized. Patients with no identifiable extra-abdominal source of hemorrhage who require more than 2 units of blood during the initial resuscitation to maintain hemodynamic stability are more likely to fail nonoperative management and should be considered for immediate laparotomy. In the face of multiple injuries, the decision to obtain a CT scan or to proceed directly to the OR is complex and requires the close involvement of an experienced trauma surgeon. Patients with high risk for head injury should obtain a head CT as soon as possible. However, additional hypotension is a major secondary insult that significantly increases the likelihood of poor outcome after head injury. Patients with persistent or recurrent hemodynamic instability should not be taken to the CT scanner. If the patient is hemodynamically unstable, the head CT scan should be delayed until after the operation is completed. This may require intraoperative coordination with a neurosurgeon along with intra-operative intracranial pressure monitoring.

INITIAL MANAGEMENT OF PENETRATING TRAUMA

As our diagnostic and interventional options increase, the decision tree for penetrating abdominal injury has evolved considerably. The history of penetrating trauma management has generally coincided with the history of wartime surgery. The management strategies that developed were based on the injury patterns seen with high-velocity weapons and blasts typical of warfare and were influenced by the limited resources available in the battlefield as well as the goal of returning soldiers to the battlefield. In civilian trauma, lack of resources should not be an issue, the weapons involved produce far less peripheral injury, and returning the victims to the "battlefield" is certainly not a priority. The increase in civilian penetrating injuries over the last several decades has led to the development of alternatives to laparotomy that differ depending on the mechanism of injury.

OPERATIVE MANAGEMENT

INDICATIONS FOR IMMEDIATE LAPAROTOMY

Patients who present with penetrating injuries to the abdomen with hemodynamic instability or peritonitis should undergo immediate laparotomy. A primary and secondary survey should be performed while the operating room is being prepared. Centers with high volumes of penetrating trauma may benefit from a system in which these patients are triaged directly to the operating room for resuscitation. Minimal fluid resuscitation should occur prior to laparotomy to maintain a systolic blood pressure (SBP) above 70 mm Hg. Patients with penetrating abdominal injuries who do not have hemodynamic instability or peritonitis are candidates for further workup and may be able to avoid unnecessary laparotomy

STAB WOUNDS
Back

Stab wounds to the back have a low incidence of producing an intra-abdominal injury requiring operative repair. The frequency of laparotomy is decreasing due to an increased comfort level with nonoperative management of liver and kidneys injuries. Most surgeons, however, will obtain a triple contrast CT scan, as laparoscopy and DPL are both inappropriate for evaluation of retroperitoneal injuries. The organs of specific concern include the diaphragm, the spleen, the liver, the pancreas, the duodenum, the aorta, the kidneys, and ureters.

Thoracoabdominal

Stab wounds below the nipples and above the costal margin, while theoretically thoracic, often penetrate through the diaphragm and create abdominal injury. If the injury is on the right side, the defect in the diaphragm should be protected by the liver and unlikely to allow bowel herniation. If the patient remains hemodynamically stable, the liver injury may be managed nonoperatively just like any stable liver laceration. A CT scan is indicated and the liver will usually illustrate the tract of the wound. If the wound is on the left side, diaphragmatic injury must be ruled out. For wounds anterior to the posterior axillary line, laparoscopy is the study of choice. Although CT scanning is useful to identify some of the associated injuries, it may not be able to discriminate small diaphragm injuries. If the diaphragm is uninjured, intra-abdominal injury is effectively ruled out. If the laparoscopy is positive, the abdomen must be evaluated for associated injuries. Laparoscopic evaluation for penetrating bowel injury may lack sensitivity in most surgeons' hands. Converting to a laparotomy may be most prudent, allowing for an open diaphragm repair and a complete abdominal evaluation. The diaphragm also can be evaluated thoracoscopically (ie, VATS) as well. If an injury is discovered, thorough evaluation of the abdomen would necessitate a laparotomy. An alternative strategy is to delay the laparoscopy by 12-24 hours until a bowel injury is ruled out by physical exam. Then the diaphragm can be approached either laparoscopically or thoracoscopically with the patient in the lateral decubitus position. If an injury is discovered, a minimally invasive repair would be definitive and open laparotomy is avoided.

Anterior

A variety of strategies have been described for the management of anterior abdominal stab wounds.

Admission with serial physical examinations has been shown in many studies to be a safe and effective approach. Although this may lead to a delay in diagnosis, outcomes in patients sustaining bowel injury are comparable. Many surgeons prefer a more definitive management algorithm. Hemodynamically stable patients who sustain anterior stab wounds and have a negative FAST exam can undergo local wound exploration (LWE) in the ED under local anesthesia. In obese patients or patients who sustain multiple stab wounds, LWE may not be viable. If anterior fascial penetration is excluded on LWE, the patient can be discharged home after irrigation and wound repair. If fascial penetration is confirmed or fascia integrity cannot be determined, a DPL can be performed. Thresholds which indicate the need for laparotomy are RBC counts > 100-10,000 and WBC counts > 500. A negative DPL should be followed by 24 hours of observation. Alternatives to DPL include CT scan or serial exams. More recently, anterior stab wounds have been comprehensively evaluated with CT without LWE or DPL.[17] The entrance wounds should be illustrated with radiopaque markers. Only suspected bowel injury or major bleeding would lead to an operation. All other patients are clinically observed for the development of peritonitis or hemorrhage. The results are comparable to observation alone. The advantage is that solid organ injuries can be identified and treated with IR expeditiously.

GUNSHOT WOUNDS

Until recently, patients sustaining gunshot wounds (GSW) with a trajectory that potentially traverses the peritoneal cavity would undergo urgent laparotomy. The rationale for this relates to the thought that 90% of patients who sustain intraperitoneal penetration from a GSW will have injuries amenable to operative repair. However, there is a growing body of evidence that selective nonoperative management may decrease the rate of nontherapeutic laparotomy after abdominal GSW. If peritonitis is absent and the patient is hemodynamically stable, CT scan should be considered. This is particularly true if the trajectory is suspicious for being transhepatic or tangential. Bullet tracts through the liver are illustrated quite well on modern CT scanners. These injuries may be addressed nonoperatively as is done in blunt trauma. GSWs suspicious for being tangential and extraperitoneal may be managed either by diagnostic laparoscopy or by CT scan, which has the significant advantage of being less invasive. The possibility of blast injury must be considered with high velocity weapons. The authors are currently obtaining CT scans for all suspected transhepatic or tangential injuries, though some centers have proposed CT scanning all hemodynamically stable penetrating abdominal injuries (Fig. 29-4). Institutional experiences will determine which approach is optimal. Adequate resources to closely follow the physical

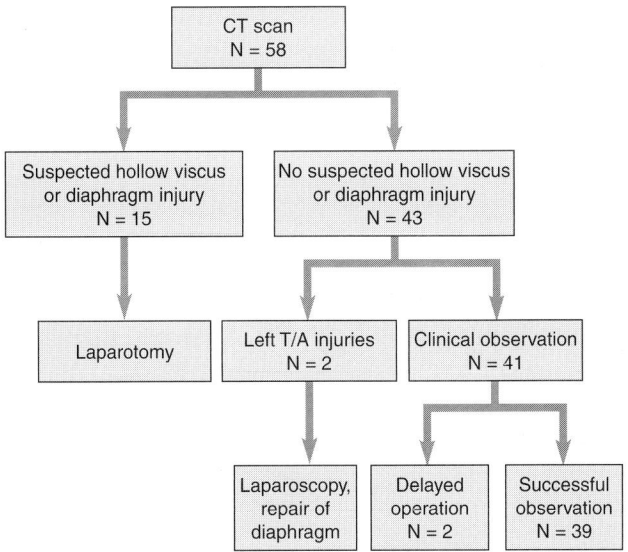

Figure 29-4 *Algorithm for the management of penetrating abdominal trauma (Demetriades).*

examination of patients with abdominal GSWs treated nonoperatively is essential.

Management of shotgun wounds to the abdomen (SGWA) is not well standardized due to their infrequent occurrence. The magnitude of injury is closely related to the distance between the gun and the victim. The greater the distance, the wider the scatter of pellets. In 1963, a scoring system was developed that divides patients into three different management groups depending on distance and penetration. This was revised in 1993 as follows: type 1 has a greater than 25 cm scatter, type 2 has a scatter between 10 and 25 cm, and type 3 has a scatter less than 10 cm indicating a close range injury. In one review, two-thirds of patients with type 1 injuries to the abdomen did not require laparotomy. Those who did had developed peritonitis, distension or increasing tenderness with a known intraperitoneal pellet. Type 2 or 3 patients were all treated with laparotomy. Brackenridge et al reviewed 32 SGWA and found DPL to be an excellent predictor of intra-abdominal injuries requiring operation. More recently, Velhamos et al reviewed 56 SGWA and found the presence of peritonitis to be an excellent predictor of the need for laparotomy.[18] In summary, clinical judgment based on the pellet scatter and, most importantly, the physical examination should be considered in determining whether or not to perform a laparotomy. In borderline cases, DPL may be helpful.

BLAST INJURIES

Recognizing who is at risk of abdominal injuries after a blast is critical. Evaluation of the tympanic membrane may provide a reasonable screen for triaging these patients. The absence of tympanic trauma likely rules out primary injury. Injuries from projectiles should be evaluated the same as any other penetrating trauma, and injury from the resulting fall is managed as in any blunt trauma patient. Those patients who do suffer from tympanic trauma should be evaluated for abdominal trauma by CT scan.

OPERATIVE MANAGEMENT

GASTRIC INJURIES

The vast majority of gastric injuries can be managed with simple closure. The generous and redundant blood supply allows for essentially any technique to be successful. Prevention of gross peritoneal contamination early in the laparotomy is essential. Quick closure with atraumatic clamps will be sufficient initially to allow evaluation of more urgent injuries. Two layered closure of the defect is standard, although a single application of a TIA stapler is more time efficient.

PANCREAS AND DUODENUM

Injury to the duodenum and pancreas is perhaps the most challenging in abdominal trauma. They are well protected in the retroperitoneum, so primary injury is less common. The retroperitoneal location, however, makes diagnosis more complex and surgical access more difficult. The close anatomic relationship with other vital structures makes significant associated injuries very common. Early mortality is usually due to associated injuries, whereas delayed mortality and most morbidity is increased with delayed intervention.

DUODENAL INJURIES

Duodenal hematomas are usually diagnosed by CT scan. They can be subtle or several centimeters in diameter. Symptoms include pain and emesis due to obstruction. If discovered on CT, nasogastric intubation and serial examinations are the best therapy. Resolution occurs in 5 days to 3 weeks and parenteral nutrition may be necessary. Laparotomy is not indicated in the absence of peritonitis from perforation. If a duodenal hematoma is discovered at laparotomy, it is unclear what strategy is best. Opening the hematoma may diminish the obstruction but bears the risk of creating a full-thickness injury. Unless the hematoma is very large (> 4 cm), it is likely most prudent to leave it intact.

Evidence of duodenal perforation on CT scan mandates early laparotomy. Several options have been proposed for managing duodenal injuries. The location of the injury relative to the ampulla of Vater must be considered. In general, clean duodenal injuries involving less than 50% of the circumference may be closed primarily. If more than 50% of the circumference is involved or if the ends cannot be brought together without tension, a roux-en-y duodenojejunostomy may be performed. In cases of primary repair, many options have been suggested to decrease the rate of leakage, although there are few data to support any one as superior. Pyloric exclusion is proposed to decrease the amount of gastric fluid that passes through the injured duodenum. This can be performed with a noncutting TA stapler or by making a proximal gastrotomy and closing the pylorus with running absorbable sutures. Both of these methods will normally open up in one to three weeks. Classically, gastric drainage is provided with a gastrojejunostomy, with a nasogastric tube, and a nasojejunostomy feeding tube. The benefit of pyloric exclusion has been questioned, and a well-placed nasogastric tube without alternative gastric drainage is an acceptable alternative. When this is employed, a retrograde jejunostomy drainage tube with a distal jejunostomy feeding tube should be considered (Fig. 29-5). Regardless of how it is managed, the risk of leakage is significant. Wide drainage should be employed anterior and posterior to the repair to allow for control if a fistula should result. Lateral duodenal fistulas are notorious for their slow closure. Many surgeons will give somatostatin during the first week after injury despite few data to support its use.

Injuries to the duodenum may be combined with pancreatic injury, an association that increases morbidity considerably. Combined injuries usually are a result of penetrating trauma. Whenever possible, primary repair with wide drainage of both the duodenum as well as the pancreas should be performed. Highly destructive injuries, particularly if they involve the distal common bile duct or the ampulla may require a trauma Whipple procedure. This is associated with a significant morbidity and mortality and, as such, should be employed only as a last resort.

PANCREAS

The pancreas acts more like a hollow viscus organ in that outcome after injury is closely related to early diagnosis and intervention. No single diagnostic modality is perfect for the determination of pancreatic injury, and it is often a coalition of findings that lead to the diagnosis. Serum hyperamylasemia has often been used to make the diagnosis, but this is an imprecise method at best. The majority of patients with pancreatic injury will have abnormal initial amylase, and the majority of patients with initially elevated amylase levels do not have pancreatic injuries. Delayed hyperamylasemia is more indicative of a potential pancreatic injury and should be further evaluated by other modalities. In penetrating trauma as well as unstable blunt trauma, the diagnosis or exclusion of pancreatic injury is made at the time of laparotomy. In blunt trauma or in stable stab wounds to the back, the diagnosis of pancreatic injury is most often made by CT. The findings on CT may be vague, and any abnormality should be aggressively pursued by endoscopic retrograde cholangiopancreatography (ERCP) or laparotomy. A negative CT scan does not completely rule out a pancreatic injury, and serial CT scanning may increase the accuracy. Magnetic resonance cholangiopancreatography (MRCP) has been considered, but some have found that it is less accurate in the early setting. In stable patients with positive CT scans or suspicious clinical situations, ERCP is a good option for identifying major duct injuries. Although some pancreatic duct injuries have been managed with stent placement, the results have been disappointing. Significant morbidity, especially major duct strictures,

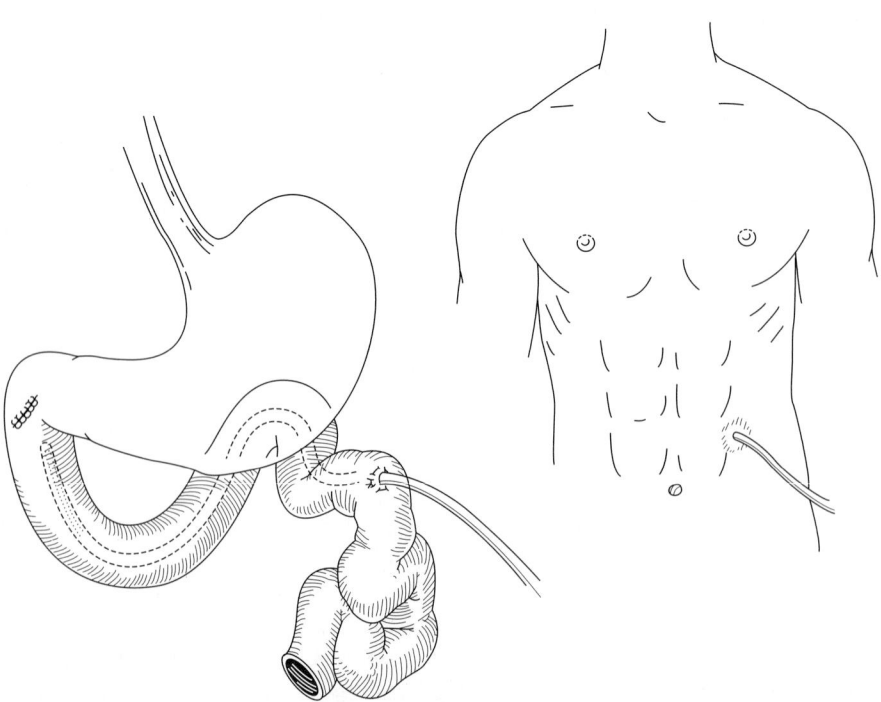

Figure 29-5 *Transjejunal decompression of duodenum injury.*

has been reported. It is likely that this technique will improve, and each institution should cautiously consider its own experience. At this time, the standard of care for pancreatic injury with major duct injury remains laparotomy. If the ERCP does not show a major duct leak, the patient may be managed expectantly, with follow-up CT scans as indicated.

At the time of laparotomy, the pancreas is evaluated anteriorly by opening the gastrocolic ligament and posteriorly with a Kocher maneuver. Lacerations not involving the main duct should be drained. Injuries to the main duct left of the mesenteric vessels are best managed with a distal pancreatectomy, preserving the spleen if possible. Injuries to the main duct to the right of the mesenteric vessels should be repaired if possible and drained widely. A surgical jejunostomy tube should be considered. Whipple procedure should be considered only for destructive injury of the pancreas and duodenum, particularly if it involves the distal common bile duct.[19]

SMALL BOWEL INJURIES

Management of small bowel injuries from penetrating trauma is reasonably straightforward. During the trauma laparotomy, after sites of major hemorrhage are controlled, leakage of intestinal contents should be quickly controlled with the application of atraumatic clamps. Small serosal injuries may be left alone, although significant serosal injuries are best closed in a longitudinal manner with interrupted 3-0 silk sutures. Bowel wall hematomas due to penetrating trauma should be opened to assure mucosal integrity. Very small enterotomies from stab wounds may be closed with a one- or two-layered technique. If the enterotomy is more than minimal or is due to a gunshot wound, simple resection is prudent. One effective way to save time and minimize bowel loss is to use the enterotomy to place a stapler for the anastomosis, and then resect any damaged bowel wall with another stapler. This obviates the need for division and ligation of the mesentery. If multiple enterotomies are encountered in a short segment of bowel, a resection including those enterotomies should be performed. Intestinal injuries with substantial bowel wall or mesenteric injury should be resected en bloc.

The diagnosis of bowel injury after blunt trauma continues to present a difficult challenge to the trauma surgeon. Delays in operative repair can have a profoundly detrimental effect. Although spleen and liver injuries are the most common intra-abdominal organs injured in blunt trauma, patients who are involved in MVCs while wearing seatbelts will often have bowel or mesenteric injuries.

CT Findings of Small Bowel Injury

Historically, CT scan was felt to be insensitive in identifying blunt bowel injury. Many studies now support the efficacy of CT for blunt bowel injury. In a review of our experience, 21 of 22 consecutive blunt bowel injured patients were diagnosed prospectively on CT scan. The one missed injury was identified on review of the preoperative CT after the injury became clinically evident. The CT findings indicating bowel injury included free fluid without solid organ injury, focal bowel wall thickening, contrast extravasation, and free air. Our review of 2800 abdominal CT scans on blunt trauma patients revealed that the occurrence of just one of these findings was associated with a 13% incidence of bowel injury, whereas two or more findings were associated with a 67% incidence of bowel injury. Other investigations have had similar results. If the initial CT scan has only one of the above findings, a follow-up CT scan or DPL in 4 hours is indicated. With two or more findings, it is reasonable to proceed directly to laparotomy. Outcomes for blunt bowel injury do not change if the bowel injury is repaired within 4 to 6 hours of injury. As the interval from presentation to operation increases beyond 8 hours, morbidity may increase substantially.

There is a subset of blunt abdominal trauma patients who have not incurred a bowel perforation at the time of presentation, but perforate later due to necrosis caused by crushing force or from ischemia associated with mesenteric injury. Patients with ongoing symptoms of abdominal pain or emesis should be evaluated by a follow-up CT scan even if the original scan was normal.

COLON INJURIES

The management of colon trauma has evolved greatly over the last few decades. Injuries that in the past were treated with three stage, and later two stage procedures employing colostomy placement are usually managed safely now with single stage procedures. Mortality between single and multiple stage repairs is equal, and the morbidity of patients who have colostomies is higher. When the morbidity from the colostomy takedown is included, the differences are even greater.

As a general rule, almost all civilian injuries to the colon can be managed with resection and primary anastomosis. For patients who have highly destructive injuries, or in whom the laparotomy was delayed and a significant fecal peritonitis is present, resection with end colostomy or resection with primary anastomosis with a proximal protective loop ileostomy may be considered, although there is indeterminate evidence to support this. The advantage to the proximal loop ileostomy is that it can be easily closed with a peristomal incision, avoiding a new midline incision. Shock is no longer an absolute indication for colostomy, as a damage control laparotomy is likely more appropriate. The anastomosis can be fashioned at the time of reoperation.

RECTAL INJURIES

Rectal injuries can be caused by gunshot wounds, transanal foreign bodies, or from major open pelvic fractures with bony penetration into the rectum. Classically, gunshot wounds to the rectum were treated with diversion, presacral drainage and, if possible, primary repair with or without distal washout. There is still debate as to the optimal management, and the optimal approach should be tailored to the specific injury. In general, intraperitoneal rectal injuries should be managed like colon injuries. Extraperitoneal injuries should be repaired transanally if possible. Diversion is not required in this setting. If an injury is identified or highly suspected but not amenable to repair, diversion with presacral drainage is likely the safest approach. Distal washout is not needed in any scenario other than highly destructive injuries.[20,21] Severe perineal injuries or injuries associated with open pelvic fractures should be diverted. Diversion is optimally done as a laparoscopically assisted loop colostomy, avoiding a midline incision. The distal portion of the colostomy can be closed with a noncutting stapler to provide complete diversion. The optimal timing of colostomy takedown varies depending on the injury, but can range from 7 days to 3 months. With the described technique, the takedown can be performed locally through the colostomy site.

LIVER INJURY
Preoperative Management
The liver is the most common organ injured in the abdomen. More than 85% of liver injuries are now managed nonoperatively. Patients with liver injuries who present with hemodynamic instability unresponsive to initial fluid resuscitation and a positive FAST examination will proceed to the operating room for surgical management. The majority of patients, however, will respond to the resuscitation and can thus be evaluated by CT scan. For these patients, nonoperative management is standard treatment, with a failure rate between 2 and 8%. The most important factor in predicting successful nonoperative management (NOM) is hemodynamic status and response to initial fluid resuscitation. Patients with higher grade injuries are more likely to be hemodynamically unstable and therefore have an overall lower rate of being managed nonoperatively. However, high grade injuries in hemodynamically stable patients can still be initially approached nonoperatively. Although the failure rate is still moderately worse in higher than lower grade injuries, the high morbidity and mortality associated with operative intervention make the nonoperative approach more appealing. Another predictor of failure of NOM is active extravasation on CT scan. These patients are best managed by selective arteriography with transcatheter embolization. Continuous monitoring and ongoing resuscitation with a qualified team is critical during these procedures. Patients with injury limited to the liver requiring more than 2-4 units of blood within the first 4 hours or with recurrent hypotension may be considered failures of nonoperative intervention and

an alternative intervention is then indicated. Because of the risk of failure, nonoperative management requires full operative capabilities including an immediately available surgeon, operating room, and scrub team. As such, we recommend that these patients be kept on a surgical service in a verified trauma center.

OPERATIVE MANAGEMENT

The individual surgeon's operative experience with liver injuries has declined substantially due to the expanding indications for nonoperative management. It is thus worthwhile to review the various described techniques for major liver injuries to avoid errors and wasted time when these problems are encountered.

Significant hemorrhage from the liver can come from three sources: hepatic arteries, portal veins, and retrohepatic IVC/hepatic vein injuries. Moderate liver injuries with visible arterial or venous injuries can be directly clamped and ligated, clipped, or suture ligated. If major bleeding is encountered, the liver should be packed, both posterior and anterior as allowed. The falciform ligament is then divided between heavy clamps and ligated with 0 silk ties. The falciform division is then continued superiorly with electrocautery being careful to stop prior to the confluence of the IVC, hepatic, and phrenic veins. The injured lobe should be mobilized by taking down the appropriate triangular and coronary ligaments sharply or with electrocautery. This should allow for better exposure of the injury as well as more effective packing. Again, bleeding vessels may then be directly visualized, clamped, and carefully ligated. Ongoing bleeding may be controlled with digital compression of the porta hepatis (Pringle maneuver). Although other maneuvers such as hepatic bypass are described for hemorrhage that continues during a Pringle maneuver, a retrocaval IVC or hepatic vein injury is likely. At this point it would be appropriate to consider tightly packing the liver and converting to damage control laparotomy, as long as the bleeding is controlled by packing. Better outcomes may be possible with physiological optimization as well as interventional techniques. If this is not effective, control of the suprahepatic and infrahepatic IVC with primary repair of the injury can be attempted.

If there is a significant laceration near the edge of the liver, transhepatic sutures may be placed parallel to the injury with 0 chromic sutures on a blunt liver needle. These sutures may be pledgeted with teflon or omentum and should include the anterior and posterior hepatic capsule. Gunshot wounds that traverse some distance of parenchyma may be managed with a tractotomy. This is particularly useful if the tract runs within 1 or 2 centimeters of the anterior surface. A long clamp is placed into the bullet tract and the liver is divided from the capsule with electrocautery. Significant vessels are ligated or clipped prior to division.

Injuries to bile ducts should be repaired or ligated when identified. Drainage of all significant lacerations is prudent.

Various hemostatic agents (fibrin glue, FloSeal) are available and are helpful to control nonarterial liver bleeding. Instilling these agents just prior to placing packs may diminish hemorrhage and is a reasonable maneuver. Placing a tongue of well-vascularized omentum into a laceration or along a cut liver edge can also reduce hemorrhage and acts well as a physiologic packing. Superficial coagulation of raw liver surfaces can be achieved with an argon beam coagulator. Electrocoagulation of a raw liver surface is most effective by using high energy values and "arcing" the energy to the liver edge without touching the parenchyma.

SPLEEN
Preoperative Management
Patients with any grade spleen injury who are hemodynamically stable may be considered for nonoperative management. As with liver injuries, active extravasation on CT scan should be managed with splenic artery angiography and embolization as needed. Collateral perfusion through the short gastric vessels will normally maintain viability of the spleen.

In the 1980s and 1990s, several novel methods of splenorrhaphy were developed. As nonoperative management of spleen injuries has evolved, the opportunity to apply these has diminished considerably. In laparotomy done for hemodynamic instability, the magnitude of hemorrhage is usually so severe that splenorrhaphy may not be possible. In cases of delayed laparotomy for failed nonoperative management, the integrity of the spleen may be so compromised that splenorrhaphy is often not feasible. Nonetheless, an active trauma surgeon will still be presented with spleen injuries that are amenable to repair.

Operative Management
The first step in operative management is adequate mobilization of the spleen up to the midline to allow better access for splenorrhaphy and more effective packing. In cases where the injury is limited to just one pole, partial splenectomy with horizontal pledgeted mattress sutures can be effective. The addition of hemostatic agents also can be effective. Placing posterior and anterior packs will control most parenchymal bleeding. Care should be taken not to injure the pancreatic tail. If a splenectomy is performed, the splenic bed must be carefully evaluated and all bleeding points ligated. Routine drainage is not indicated and does not lower the incidence of developing a subphrenic abscess; however, closed suction drainage may still be indicated in selected patients to observe for early postoperative bleeding or for suspected distal pancreatic

injury. Historically, prolonged gastric suctioning was used to prevent bleeding from the ligated short gastric vessels, but this is now considered unnecessary. Nonoperative management for penetrating injury to the spleen is applied less frequently due to the risk of associated diaphragm injury.

URINARY TRACT INJURIES
Kidney
Surgical intervention for renal injuries has declined in parallel to liver and spleen injuries. In the stable patient where the renal injury is illustrated by CT scan, there are few indications for operation. Nonenhancement of the kidney on CT scan is indicative of a renovascular injury and is discussed in the vascular trauma section. Major disruption of the renal pelvis and exsanguination are both indications for surgical intervention. Otherwise, most kidney injuries should be initially managed nonoperatively. When surgery is indicated, an attempt to conserve renal tissue is reasonable.

Ureter
The majority of ureteral injuries are due to penetrating trauma. Other than for hematomas, nonoperative management has very limited application and should generally be avoided. Ureteral injuries should be repaired over a ureteral catheter as soon as they are recognized. Proximal and middle ureteral transections are treated by primary repair. When possible, the ends of the ureter are spatulated to avoid stricture. Distal injuries are repaired with reimplantation into the bladder. If there is inadequate length to reach the bladder, the bladder can be brought up toward the ureter using a psoas hitch. This may be augmented by a bladder (Boari) flap. All repairs should be stented with a double J stent. Extensive loss of ureter length may be managed with nephrectomy, though alternative reconstruction options are possible at a later date if a percutaneous drain is placed. In the urgent setting, the uninjured ureter should not be used in the repair to avoid the risk of compromising both kidneys. With proper experience, complex reconstruction with ureteroureterostomy or ileal conduit is possible, and may be performed in a delayed fashion.

Bladder
Bladder injury can result from both blunt and penetrating trauma. Microscopic or gross hematuria is a reasonable screen for this. CT cystogram is the optimal study of choice in the trauma patient. In general, extraperitoneal injuries can be managed with 10 days of catheter drainage without formal repair. Intraperitoneal injury should be repaired with a two-layer absorbable suture repair followed by transurethral drainage for 7 days. Routine cyctography is normally done prior to removal of ureteral catheter. Suprapubic catheters are rarely indicated.[22]

Diaphragm

Diaphragm injury can occur from both blunt and penetrating trauma. The injury tends to be larger with blunt trauma, but the diagnosis can be elusive in both types. All left-sided diaphragm injuries should be repaired to prevent future bowel incarcerations. The true lifetime risk of bowel incarceration for diaphragm injuries is unknown, and a prospective study is unlikely to ever be performed. Diaphragm repair can be done with interrupted or simple prolene suture repair. Pledgets can be used if the suture line integrity is in doubt. If the defect is large and cannot be closed primarily, artificial grafts can be used. Goretex is the most commonly used graft, though biological grafts should be used in cases of abdominal contamination. Right-sided defects that are small can usually be left alone if it is found radiographically; however, they should be repaired if found in the OR. Laparoscopic repair is effective if bowel injury has been excluded.

ABDOMINAL VASCULAR INJURY

Preoperative Management

Injuries to the major vascular structures of the abdomen are usually due to penetrating trauma. These injuries will often cause the patient to present in shock with the specific injury being found at emergent laparotomy. Prolonged preoperative resuscitation is of little value in these patients, and interventions in the resuscitation bay should be as limited as possible. Blood and fresh frozen plasma should be available in the OR and the blood bank should be mobilized to keep up with ongoing needs. A cell saver may be useful, although the high incidence of concomitant enteric injury may diminish its utility. The laparotomy begins with a generous incision, four quadrant packing, and evacuation of the hemoperitoneum. A thorough knowledge of the anatomy and collateral circulation is essential in making the decision to ligate or repair the injury. Limited volume resuscitation should be used until exposure and control of the injury is complete. Patients with abdominal vascular injuries who are hemodynamically stable will likely have some amount of retroperitoneal tamponade. Patients with free intraperitoneal hemorrhage from a vascular injury will present in extremis. In either case, proximal control is indicated with the proximal aorta being the usual site. If a resuscitative thoracotomy is performed in the trauma bay, aortic cross clamping is indicated and may allow transport to the operating room. Prelaparotomy left thoracotomy has been described and is a reasonable maneuver in patients with hypotension and obvious massive hemoperitoneum.

Operative Management

The general approach to hemorrhage or hematoma from abdominal vascular injury corresponds to three anatomic zones. Zone 1 is in the midline, Zone 2 is in the upper lateral retroperitoneum, and Zone 3 is in the pelvis (Fig. 29-6).

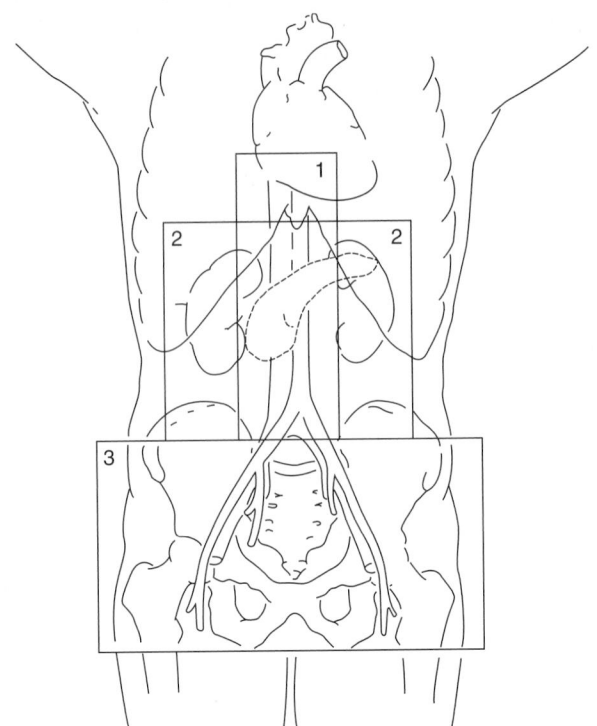

Figure 29-6   *Vascular zones of the abdomen.*

Zone 1

Zone 1 vascular injuries are classically divided between supramesocolic and inframesocolic. All central hematomas should be explored after obtaining proximal and distal (if possible) control. If the patient is stable and the hematoma is contained, the best exposure of the aorta is via a left medial rotation of the spleen, pancreas, colon, and, if needed, kidney. Access to the supraceliac aorta can be improved by incising the aortic crus and placing a vascular clamp on the lower thoracic aorta. If there is active hemorrhage or the patient is unstable, the supraceliac aorta can be accessed quicker by retracting the left lobe of the liver up and to the right, the stomach and esophagus down and to the left, followed by incision of the lesser omentum. The time of aortic clamping and unclamping should be noted by the anesthesiologist.

Injuries to the upper aorta are best treated with lateral aortorrhaphy, with or without a polytetrafluoroethylene (PTFE) patch. More devastating injuries requiring aortic resection are best treated with a synthetic vascular graft (12-16-mm Dacron). The celiac axis may be ligated without reconstruction to allow access to this area. Similarly, injuries to the celiac axis, the splenic artery, the left gastric artery, or the common hepatic artery proximal to the pancreatic-duodenal artery (PDA) may also be ligated without reconstruction. Injury to the proximal superior mesenteric artery (SMA) or vein (SMV) may be above or below the lower margin of the pancreas. If needed for adequate exposure, the pancreas can be divided sharply with meticulous suture homeostasis and closure of the proximal duct. A covered stapler can also be used when appropriate. Ligation of the SMA may or may not cause bowel ischemia depending on the level of distal vasoconstriction, presence of ongoing shock, and the adequacy of collateral circulation through the middle colic and inferior mesenteric arteries. If the patient is stable, repair using a PTFE or reverse saphenous vein is appropriate. Some authors have noted that it may be beneficial to make the anastomosis into the lower aorta to prevent contact with any pancreatic injury. In unstable patients in whom distal bowel viability is in question, an intraluminal shunt may be placed as part of a damage control operation.

Injuries to the SMV should be repaired with lateral venorrhaphy or primary repair when possible. Ligation is tolerated in most patients and should be followed with aggressive postoperative fluid resuscitation.

Injury to the proximal renal arteries may also present with central hematomas. The left renal artery may be accessed via a left medial visceral rotation, whereas the proximal right renal artery is best accessed at the base of the mesocolon between the aorta and the IVC.

Hemorrhage or hematomas in the midline may also present in the inframesocolic area. These are usually due to injuries of the infrarenal aorta or IVC. Exposure in this area is obtained by opening the midline retroperitoneum to identify the left renal vein. The aorta can be clamped at this level, just as is done for controlling the neck of an infrarenal aortic aneurysm. Repairs of lesser injuries can be performed primarily with or without a patch. Larger injuries can be managed with an interposition graft (PTFE or Dacron). Although these injuries often coincide with bowel injury, extra-anatomic bypass is probably not necessary. There is ample evidence that with proper evacuation of enteric contents, and with copious irrigation and control of bowel injury, synthetic grafts are safe. The bowel and vascular repair should be separated by time to prevent cross contamination. The vascular repair should then be protected by closing the retroperitoneum or with an omental pedicle. The IMA may be divided as is needed for repair of the aorta.

The IVC may also be exposed with a right medial visceral rotation. This is the approach more commonly used by most trauma surgeons due to its familiarity and the ability to expose the entire IVC from the liver to the bifurcation. Primary venorrhaphy is preferred; however, the infrarenal IVC may also be ligated with a certain amount of morbidity.

Zone 2

Zone 2 injuries in the upper lateral retroperitoneum may result from renal-vascular injuries. In hemodynamically stable patients, an early CT scan is critical for a timely diagnosis to provide an opportunity for optimal management. In blunt trauma, injury of the renal artery is a rare finding (.05% of blunt traumas) that may be discovered by lack of renal enhancement on CT scan. Although revascularization is possible, it is done in less than 10% of cases with considerable morbidity. Observation with delayed nephrectomy is currently the most common approach. Endovascular interventions including renal artery stents are gaining popularity in some centers with promising results. Blunt renal vein injury is also rare and is best managed by anticoagulation.

Renal vascular injuries are more often seen with penetrating trauma. Other than stab wounds to the back, these will frequently be found without a preoperative CT scan. Renal artery or vein injuries found at laparotomy usually present as a Zone 2 injury but may present as a central hematomas or hemorrhage if the injury is in the proximal vessel. Active extravasation from Zone 2 should be exposed by direct compression with a lateral to medial mobilization of the kidney. Rapidly expanding hematomas can be addressed by first obtaining proximal control of the renal vasculature via an opening of the midline retroperitoneum. Vein injury is best repaired by venorrhaphy. If it is not amenable to repair, the left vein may be ligated proximal to the gonadal and adrenal veins with retention of good renal function. The right renal vein may lack adequate collateral flow and may require nephrectomy. In a damage control procedure, this could be determined at the time of reoperation. Repair of renal artery injuries is difficult due to their small size. Reconstruction with a saphenous vein conduit is optimal. Nephrectomy is also reasonable as long as a normal size contralateral kidney is confirmed.

Zone 3

Zone 3 hematoma or hemorrhage is found in the pelvis. The majority of pelvic hematomas in blunt trauma are due to pelvic fractures and should not be opened as the tamponade will be released and difficult bleeding will ensue from the presacral veins. Hemorrhage from the internal iliac vessels seen on CT scan is best managed by endovascular thrombosis of a branch or the entire vessel. Endovascular techniques are being investigated for injuries to the common or external iliac artery; however, the most common management now is surgical. At laparotomy, iliac artery injury is managed by proximal control just distal to the bifurcation. Distal control is just proximal to the inguinal ligament. Back bleeding from the internal iliac artery is managed by vessel occlusion with a vascular tape or by ligation. The iliac artery must be primarily repaired with or without an intervening graft. Rotation of the internal iliac vessel as a conduit for extensive iliac artery injury has been described. In unstable patients, a temporary shunt can be placed with formal repair within 48 hours. Consideration should be given for a distal ipsilateral four compartment fasciotomy.

Iliac vein injuries can be difficult to manage, particularly on the right side where exposure through the artery may be compromised. Bleeding from these vessels is initially controlled with direct pressure proximally and distally. Lateral venorrhaphy should be attempted if at all possible. Ligation is tolerated with some morbidity, particularly leg swelling. Survival from iliac vessel injury is mostly dependent on the presence of shock due to free hemorrhage into the peritoneum.[23]

SPECIAL CIRCUMSTANCES

PEDIATRICS

Children are more vulnerable to abdominal injury for two major reasons. They tend to have less abdominal fat and lesser developed abdominal musculature, and therefore have less protection. They also have less coverage by the ribs and pelvis, so more of the abdomen is exposed. This makes the liver, pancreas, duodenum and bladder more susceptible to injury.

PREGNANCY

As a general rule, evaluation and management of abdominal trauma in the gravid patient should closely parallel that of any other patient. The increased intravascular volume may affect the appearance of hemodynamic stability, and this must be adjusted for in determining who is a candidate for nonoperative management of solid organ injuries. As the blood supply to the gravid uterus is primarily affected, compensated shock from solid organ injury could put the viability of the fetus at substantial risk. As discussed earlier, DPL catheters and laparoscopes should both be placed in the supraumbilical position. CT scans of the abdomen will generally expose the abdomen to 2 rads of radiation exposure. It is possible that repeated CT scans could have some impact on the fetus, with the greatest risk in the first trimester. CT scans should not be avoided, as a missed abdominal injury will have major implications for the fetus as well as the mother. Nonetheless, abdominal CT scans in pregnant patients should have reasonably clear indications. Uterine rupture from blunt or penetrating trauma is an immediate indication for operation with fetus extraction and uterine repair.

LIVER DISEASE

Patients with significant liver disease are at increased risk of morbidity and death as a result of abdominal injury. This is confounded by the fact that they will also have significantly worse outcomes after a laparotomy. Aggressive medical management of their metabolic derangements with particular attention to correction of their coagulopathy is critical. Appropriate interventional radiology techniques should be aggressively implemented early to avoid laparotomy if possible.

CONDUCT OF TRAUMA LAPAROTOMY
Preoperative Management

The trauma laparotomy has become a less frequent procedure, being practiced regularly by only experienced full-time trauma surgeons. Once a mainstay of surgical training, the increasing role of nonoperative management of abdominal trauma combined with the limitations on resident work hours have significantly decreased the number of trauma laparotomies performed by most chief surgery residents. To accommodate this, it is essential that a clear and standard approach to the trauma laparotomy is utilized by any surgeon who treats trauma patients.

A table-mounted retraction system should be available; however, a Balfour retractor is helpful for an initial evaluation. A large amount of laparotomy pads should be available prior to the incision. Large Richardson retractors and vascular clamps should be included in the setup. An oral-gastric tube and a Foley catheter should be placed prior to incision. The gastric tube can be changed to a nasogastric tube if it is determined to be necessary for prolonged gastric decompression. For as long as the patient is intubated, the oral route is best to decrease the incidence of sinusitis and epistaxis. Patients undergoing laparotomy for trauma are vulnerable to venous thromboembolic complications. Sequential compression devices should be placed prior to induction if possible. Antibiotics should be given intravenously as soon as possible after the decision to go to the OR. A single agent broad spectrum antibiotic is appropriate. If given prior to incision, the wound complication rate will be reduced. The prep and drape for a trauma laparotomy should extend superiorly up to the neck and laterally down to the table to allow for unanticipated tube thoracostomy or sternotomy. One thigh should be included in the prep in case the saphenous vein is needed as a vascular graft. Direct and ongoing communication between the blood bank and the OR team is essential. Blood should be available and in the OR prior to the incision. The patient who undergoes a trauma laparotomy is extremely vulnerable to hypothermia. Hypothermia is a critical factor in the process of coagulation. Coagulopathy can occur at temperatures below 35°C. Coagulation essentially cannot occur at temperatures below 32°C. Every effort should be made to keep the patient warm in the OR, including a fluid warmer, a warm OR, but, most important, limiting blood loss. As the patient's temperature falls, damage control laparotomy should be considered.

Operative Management

The first function of the trauma laparotomy is to control hemorrhage. Laparotomy pads should be packed into all four quadrants to compress the solid organs and to absorb excess blood. Gross contamination from bowel injury should be controlled with bowel clamps followed by careful evaluation of the liver and spleen. The duodenum is evaluated with a Kocher maneuver, and the lesser sac is opened to expose the pancreas and the posterior wall of the stomach. The bowel is run from the ligament of Treitz to the rectum. At this point the packs are removed and a definitive management of solid organ injuries is done (as described earlier). Bowel injuries may be repaired prior to pack removal if hemorrhage is adequately controlled.

DAMAGE CONTROL LAPAROTOMY

The decision to perform a damage control operation may be made at any time when the patient's physiologic status will not support a definitive repair. The one determinate that affects outcome is how long the operation continues prior to the decision to convert to a damage control laparotomy. As a general rule, the earlier the decision, the better the outcome. The decision should be based on the presence of significant hypothermia, acidosis, and coagulopathy that does not respond to initial maneuvers. Perihepatic and perisplenic packs should be placed both posterior and anterior to the affected organ. Compressive packs should be placed anterior to any areas of retroperitoneal and pelvic hemorrhage. All bowel injures should be resected using a stapler. Anastomosis may be fashioned at the time of the initial operation or delayed until the next laparotomy. An oral-gastric tube should be positioned by palpation. Many temporary closures have been described over the last decade, usually made up of drains placed on packs, with a clear sterile cover (eg, Bogata bag) covered again with drains and an adhesive drape. We now employ an abdominal wound vac system, which provides good control of fluids from the abdomen.

Postoperative Management

After the closure, the patient is cared for in the surgical intensive care unit (SICU). During this time, warming measures and blood products are administered. Other diagnostic studies are obtained as indicated, specifically head and spine CT scans as well as extremity films. These are managed as seen fit prior to the second laparotomy. The patient should be returned to the OR about 24 hours after normalization of the coagulopathy, hypothermia, and acidosis. This is most commonly about 72 hours later. Earlier returns may be needed if the wound management system falls apart. The packs are removed and the abdomen is reevaluated. Once the intestinal continuity is restored and ongoing bleeding is controlled, the abdomen is closed as allowed. Repacking may be necessary for persistent bleeding. Multiple return trips to the OR may be needed to close the fascia. Care should be taken to prevent the intestines from having direct contact with the anterior or lateral abdominal wall. After 7-9 days, the formation of granulation tissue may be such that further attempts at primary fascia closure can put the intestines at risk of enterotomy and fistula. In this situation, aggressive attempts to close the abdomen with advancement flaps should be made. If this is not possible, delayed closure techniques can be performed using absorbable mesh or skin grafts directly onto the bowel after an adequate granulation bed is present. More commonly, we now apply acellular skin grafts (Alloderm,® Permocol®) directly over the bowel attached to the native fascia, with skin/subcutaneous advancement flaps. If advancement flaps are not possible, a wound vac® is applied over the grafts.

ABDOMINAL COMPARTMENT SYNDROME

Patients who sustain significant abdominal injuries associated with shock and reperfusion can have significant third spacing into the abdomen. This may be predicted in the operating room during laparotomy. Placement of a temporary abdominal closure can be effective in preventing pathologic elevations of intra-abdominal pressure (IAP). This condition can also result from resuscitated shock states caused by injury remote to the abdomen. In cases where laparotomy has not been performed or if the abdomen has been closed, resuscitation after shock with resulting reperfusion can lead to significant abdominal organ edema with IAP elevation. Bladder pressures can be measured by direct manometry. The classic clinical findings associated with abdominal compartment syndrome include low urine output (UOP). In this clinical setting, when pressures exceed 30 mm Hg, decompressive laparotomy should be considered.[24] The outcome of decompressive laparotomy includes improved UOP and lower IAP. The survival advantage to decompressive laparotomy has yet to be determined.

CONCLUSIONS

The management of abdominal trauma continues to evolve. Diagnostic options have expanded both in the use of ultrasound for rapid evaluation as well as the expanded role of CT for more specific diagnosis. Management options have also blossomed, with a definite trend toward employing operative interventions only when necessary. Endovascular options have revolutionized treatment of vascular and solid organ injuries, whereas damage control surgery has improved survival of major abdominal hemorrhage.

REFERENCES

1. Chandler CF, Lane JS, Waxman KS. Seatbelt sign following blunt trauma is associated with increased incidence of abdominal injury. *Am Surg* 1997; 63(10):885-888.

2. Velmahos GC, Demetriades D, Theodorou D, et al. Patterns of injury in victims of urban free-falls. *World J Surg* 1997; 21(8):816-820; discussion 820-821.

3. Kraus JF, Peek-Asa C, Cryer HG. Incidence, severity, and patterns of intrathoracic and intra-abdominal injuries in motorcycle crashes. *J Trauma* 2002;52(3):548-553.

4. Moore EE, Moore JB, Van Duzer-Moore S, et al. Mandatory laparotomy for gunshot wounds penetrating the abdomen. *Am J Surg* 1980;140(6):847-851.

5. Shweiki E, Klena J, Wood GC, et al. Assessing the true risk of abdominal solid organ injury in hospitalized rib fracture patients. *J Trauma* 2001;50(4):684-688.

6. Killeen KL, DeMeo JH. CT detection of serious internal and skeletal injuries in patients with pelvic fractures. *Acad Radiol* 1999;6(4):224-228.

7. Tyroch AH, McGuire EL, McLean SF, et al. The association between Chance fractures and intra-abdominal injuries revisited: a multicenter review. *Am Surg* 2005;71(5):434-438.

8. Obaid AK, Barleben A, Porral D, et al. Utility of plain film pelvic radiographs in blunt trauma patients in the emergency department. *Am Surg* 2006;72(10):951-954.

9. Fang JF, Chen RJ, Lin BC. Cell count ratio: new criterion of diagnostic peritoneal lavage for detection of hollow organ perforation. *J Trauma* 1998;45(3):540-544.

10. Gracias VH, Frankel HL, Gupta R, et al. Defining the learning curve for the Focused Abdominal Sonogram for Trauma (FAST) examination: implications for credentialing. *Am Surg* 2001;67(4):364-368.

11. McGahan, JP, Horton S, Gerscovich EO, et al. Appearance of solid organ injury with contrast-enhanced sonography in blunt abdominal trauma: preliminary experience. *AJR Am J Roentgenol* 2006; 187(3):658-666.

12. Stuhlfaut JW, Soto JA, Lucey BC, et al. Blunt abdominal trauma: performance of CT without oral contrast material. *Radiology* 2004;233(3):689-694.

13. Schauer BA, Nguyen H, Wisner DH, et al. Is definitive abdominal evaluation required in blunt trauma victims undergoing urgent extra-abdominal surgery? *Acad Emerg Med* 2005;12(8):707-711.

14. Demetriades D, Gomez H, Velmahos GC. Routine helical computed tomographic evaluation of the mediastinum in high-risk blunt trauma patients. *Arch Surg* 1998; 133(10):1084-1088.

15. Salim A, Sangthong B, Martin M, et al. Whole body imaging in blunt multisystem trauma patients without obvious signs of injury: results of a prospective study. *Arch Surg* 2006;141(5):468-473; discussion 473-475.

16. Velmahos GC, Demetriades D, Toutouzas KG, et al. Selective nonoperative management in 1,856 patients with abdominal gunshot wounds: should routine laparotomy still be the standard of care? *Ann Surg* 2001;234(3):395-402; discussion 402-403.

17. Demetriades D, Hadjizacharia P, Constantinou C, et al. Selective nonoperative management of penetrating abdominal solid organ injuries. *Ann Surg* 2006;244(4):620-628.

18. Velmahos GC, Safaoui M, Demetriades D. Management of shotgun wounds: do we need classification systems? *Int Surg* 1999;84(2):99-104.

19. Asensio JA, Petrone P, Roldan G, et al. Pancreaticoduodenectomy: a rare procedure for the management of complex pancreaticoduodenal injuries. *J Am Coll Surg* 2003;197(6):937-942.

20. Gonzalez RP, Phelan H 3rd, Hassan M, et al. Is fecal diversion necessary for nondestructive penetrating extraperitoneal rectal injuries? *J Trauma* 2006;61(4):815-819.

21. Cleary RK, Pomerantz RA, Lampman RM. Colon and rectal injuries. *Dis Colon Rectum* 2006;49(8):1203-1222.

22. Corriere JN Jr, Sandler CM. Diagnosis and management of bladder injuries. *Urol Clin North Am* 2006;33(1):67-71, vi.

23. Haan J, Rodriguez A, Chiu W, et a. Operative management and outcome of iliac vessel injury: a ten-year experience. *Am Surg* 2003;69(7):581-586.

24. De Waele JJ, Hoste EA, Malbrain ML. Decompressive laparotomy for abdominal compartment syndrome—a critical analysis. *Crit Care* 2006;10(2):R51.

Chapter 30

THE PELVIS

*Sharmila Dissanaike, MD, and
Gregory J. Jurkovich, MD*

EPIDEMIOLOGY

Pelvic injury can present both a diagnostic and therapeutic challenge, with injury severity ranging from minor to life-threatening hemorrhage. Falls are the most common cause of pelvic fractures, most notably in the elderly with osteoporosis. However, the majority of severe pelvic trauma results from motor vehicle crashes. Associated closed head injury and long bone fractures are present in 50% of these patients and are obvious contributors to mortality and morbidity.[1,2] Associated injury to the genitourinary or digestive tract occurs in approximately 10% of all pelvic fractures, occasionally difficult to diagnose in the polytrauma patient.[3] Management of combined bony pelvis and anatomically juxtaposed organ injuries presents a particularly serious challenge to prioritizing care and treatment algorithms.

The mortality rate from pelvic fractures is approximately 10%-20%, with death usually due to exsanguinating arterial or venous injury.[1-4] Mortality has decreased substantially over the last half-century, primarily due to improved resuscitation protocols, rapid availability of blood products, and development of techniques to compress the pelvis externally and control exsanguination.

It is important to place the assessment and treatment of pelvic injury within the context of overall resuscitation. Immediate airway control, ensuring adequate ventilation and maintaining effective circulation are the first priorities. Hypovolemia should be initially treated with intravenous crystalloid. Blood should be used early in patients with refractory hypotension after the initial bolus of fluid, or clinical suspicion of hemorrhage. Determining the sources of hemorrhage is crucial in deciding further treatment, especially in the unstable patient with combined torso and pelvic injury. External pelvic stabilization is also important to prevent further injury while the patient is being transported and assessed. These issues will be dealt with in detail throughout the chapter.

Current management of pelvic trauma in North America involves a multidisciplinary team composed of acute care surgeons, emergency physicians, orthopedists, and diagnostic and interventional radiologists. Improved technology has presented the physician with a wide variety of options in controlling hemorrhage associated with pelvic fractures. Developing a systematic approach to the management of pelvic bleeding, fracture stabilization, and associated injuries is crucial in ensuring good outcomes from this potentially fatal injury. This chapter deals with the incidence, mechanisms, and management of pelvic fractures and associated injuries from blunt trauma. Penetrating trauma is discussed in another section of this book.

ANATOMY

The pelvis is a bony ring formed by the sacrum and paired innominate bones. The sacroiliac ligaments anchor the sacrum posteriorly, and the pubic symphysis joins the innominate bones anteriorly. The sacrospinous and sacrotuberous ligaments provide support for the pelvic floor. The pelvic ligaments are important to stability. The sacroiliac, ileolumbar, and sacrospinous ligaments prevent external rotation and "opening" of the pelvis. The sacroiliac, sacrotuberous, and lateral lumbosacral ligaments provide vertical stability.[5] The sacroiliac joint is the strongest in the human body, and provides much of the structural integrity. The pubic symphysis is the weakest link, providing only 15% of inherent pelvic stability.[6]

The pelvis has a rich arterial and venous blood supply. Venous injury is more common than arterial, and it is often self-limiting due to tamponade by the pelvic retroperitoneum.[7] The external and internal iliac veins receive blood from multiple venous plexuses—sacral, pudendal, hemorrhoidal, prostatic, and vesical—in addition to the femoral, gluteal, inferior epigastric, and obturator veins. The pelvic viscera are supplied by multiple branches of the internal iliac (hypogastric) artery, which originates from the common iliac artery opposite the lumbosacral junction, and ends near the sciatic foramen. The dense collateral network on one side ensures that the hypogastric artery or its branches may be ligated if necessary. This also makes unilateral angiographic coil embolization possible with a low risk of pelvic ischemia. The external iliac artery courses obliquely downward and laterally along the medial border of psoas major to emerge below the inguinal ligament as the common femoral artery.

The sacral plexus is formed by the lumbosacral trunk and primarily supplies the pelvic viscera and muscles. It lies posteriorly between the piriformis muscle and the pelvic fascia. The sciatic nerve is the largest nerve in the human body and is formed from the sacral plexus, exiting the pelvis at the greater sciatic foramen. The pudendal plexus is smaller and supplies the genital and anococcygeal region.

CLASSIFICATION

Pelvic fractures are generally classified based on the mechanism of injury and the direction of the applied disruptive forces. Different mechanisms result in distinct fracture patterns that can help predict the likelihood of injury to vessels, nerves, and organs. The primary vectors are (1) anteroposterior compression, (2) lateral compression, and (3) vertical shear forces.[8] The clinician should consider these three major force vector injury patterns when first evaluating a pelvic trauma, bearing in mind that complex fractures involving a combination of these mechanisms are often seen in high-speed motor vehicle collisions.

Anteroposterior injuries commonly occur in head-on motor vehicle collisions, motorcycle crashes, and pedestrians struck by vehicles. These injuries characteristically produce pubic diastasis either at the symphysis or through pubic rami fractures. Widening of the sacroiliac joints may also occur. These changes result in external rotation and opening of the pelvis. This increases pelvic volume and prevents tamponade of bleeding vessels, allowing unabated major hemorrhage. This injury pattern is associated with major torso trauma and a higher incidence of acute respiratory distress (ARDS) syndrome in survivors (Fig. 30-1).[9]

Lateral compression fractures are the most frequently seen pelvic injury (Fig. 30-2). They occur in side-impact ("T-bone") motor vehicle collisions and car–pedestrian accidents. Falls are a common cause of this fracture in the elderly population. Impacted sacral fractures and horizontal pubic rami fractures result in internal rotation of the hemipelvis. This causes a decrease in pelvic volume and is, therefore, less likely to result in exsanguinating hemorrhage. Brain injury is the most common cause of mortality in this group of patients.

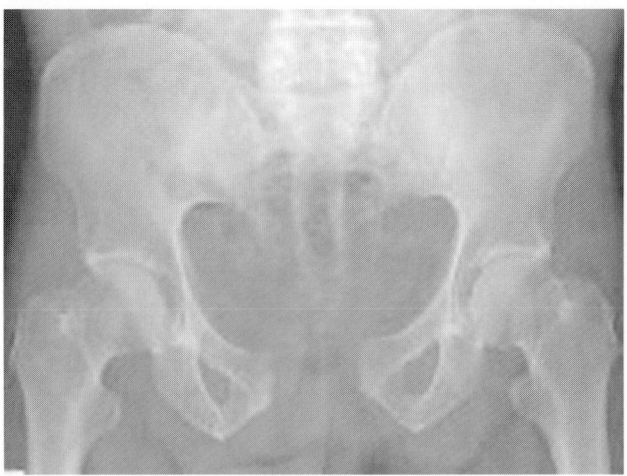

Figure 30-1 *AP fracture with pubic diastasis and "open book" widening.*

Vertical shear injuries usually result from force applied in a craniocaudal direction, such as a fall from a height onto the lower limbs. Pubic rami fractures and disruption of the sacroiliac ligaments may occur. Disruption of the posterior ligaments results in upward displacement of the hemipelvis. These fractures are inherently unstable. The shear mechanism causes disruption of venous plexus as well as tearing of the hypogastric vessels, and is associated with significant bleeding and increased need for transfusion (Fig. 30-3).[10]

The Young–Burgess system is a commonly used classification system for pelvic fractures. It is based on the vector of injury as well as pelvic stability (Table 30-1). The injury severity in each category increases from 1 to 3. The severity of associated injuries also increases with higher grades of injury, reflecting the greater force of impact upon the body. The Tile classification was an earlier attempt at classifying pelvic fractures according to vector of force and is also widely used. This system includes injuries that do not disrupt the pelvic ring,

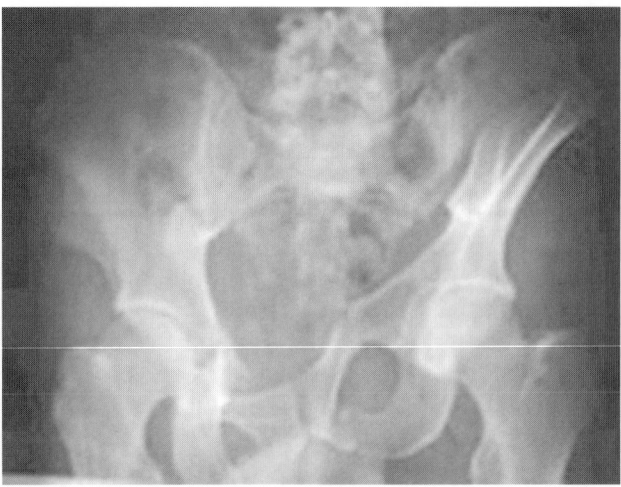

Figure 30-2 *Lateral compression fracture with reduction in pelvic volume.*

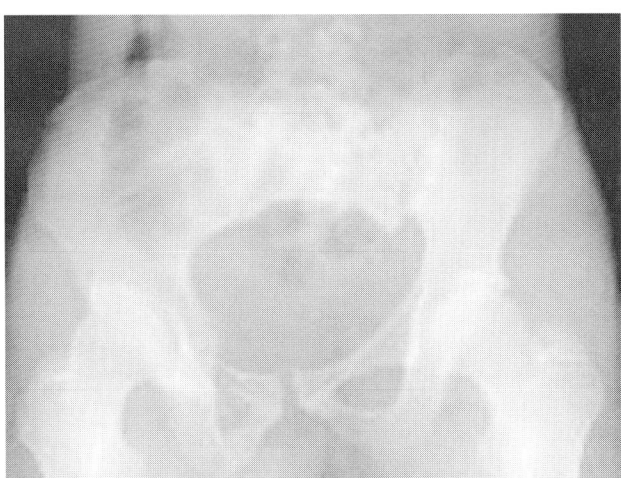

Figure 30-3 *Vertical shear fracture with superior displacement of the hemipelvis.*

such as avulsion fractures of the iliac spines and ischial tuberosities. Pelvic fractures with an intact ring, pure acetabular fractures, "straddle" fractures of the pubic rami, and isolated fractures are classified as stable. Unstable pelvic fractures include all injuries involving the pelvic ring in more than one location, or in which the posterior pelvis, sacrum, and sacroiliac complex are disrupted. Open-book fractures are caused by diastasis of the symphysis pubis and external rotation of the iliac bones, causing widening of the pelvis.[9] These fractures are associated with a higher rate of arterial and visceral pelvic injury.

DIAGNOSIS

Examination of the pelvis is part of the primary survey of the trauma patient. Only one person should perform the clinical exam of the pelvis in order to not continually disrupt pelvic stability and exacerbate bleeding. The pelvis should be compressed to determine stability in both the anteroposterior and mediolateral axis. The examiner should place a hand on each anterior superior iliac spine and gently push medially and then rotate externally. "Springing" the pelvis (rapid compression for a very short time) is painful and should be avoided.

The perineum should be examined for hematoma, active bleeding, or lacerations. Scrotal or labial hematomas are common in anterior compression and straddle injuries. Blood at the urethral meatus is an indicator of potential urethral injury, and a urinary catheter should not be placed blindly in this circumstance. The patient should be log-rolled and a rectal examination performed. Anorectal lacerations or blood on the examining finger should be noted. A high-riding prostate is an indicator of potential urologic injury. In women, vaginal bleeding should prompt a speculum examination to evaluate for lacerations to the vaginal wall or cervix.

Military antishock trousers (MAST), also known as pneumatic antishock garments (PASG), or the currently more popular pelvic stabilizing sheet can be applied by prehospital personnel to help tamponade bleeding and stabilize the pelvis. The MAST garment is largely out of favor in most prehospital systems, but occasionally the acute care surgeon may see one applied prior to a long transfer. The MAST consists of pneumatic compression sleeves that inflate sequentially, to provide support for the lower torso and limbs. Compartments should be decompressed sequentially starting at the abdomen while the patient is receiving adequate resuscitation. There is no reason to remove the sheeted pelvis until adequate imaging studies have been obtained, if MAST has been applied properly.

Application of a folded bed sheet across the greater trochanters is the simplest and most widely available

Table 30-1 Young–Burgess Classification System			
Mechanism and type	Characteristics	Hemipelvis displacement	Stability
AP compression, type I	Pubic diastasis < 2.5 cm	External rotation	Stable
AP compression, type II	Pubic diastasis > 2.5 cm, anterior SI joint disruption	External rotation	Rotationally unstable, vertically stable
AP compression, type III	Type II plus posterior SI joint disruption	External rotation	Rotationally unstable, vertically unstable
Lateral compression, type I	Ipsilateral sacral buckle fracture, ipsilateral horizontal pubic rami fractures (or disruption of symphysis with overlapping pubic bones)	Internal rotation	Stable
Lateral compression, type II	Type I plus ipsilateral iliac wing fracture or posterior SI joint disruption	Internal rotation	Rotationally unstable, vertically unstable
Vertical shear	Vertical pubic rami fractures, SI joint disruption ± adjacent fractures	Vertical (cranial)	Rotationally unstable, vertically unstable

technique to obtain temporary stabilization. The patient should be log rolled while the sheet is positioned underneath the pelvis. When the patient is placed supine, a two-person maneuver is required to adequately tighten the sheet across the pelvis. Traction and countertraction are used to obtain adequate compression across the trochanters. Hemostats or clamps are used to secure the sheet in place (Fig. 30-4). The sheet should be wide enough to distribute force evenly and with a smooth contour to prevent point ischemia. Alternatively, the ends may be knotted and cinched tight with a short rod. This technique decreases pelvic volume and allows for diagnostic peritoneal lavage, angiography, or laparotomy to be performed without the need for sheet removal.[11] There are several commercially available pelvic binders that employ the same principle.[12]

IMAGING

RADIOGRAPHY

The standard trauma series consists of lateral cervical spine, anteroposterior (AP) chest and pelvis radiographs. This is recommended for all trauma patients with multisystem injuries, obvious skeletal injuries, or in whom the physical examination is not completely reliable. Inlet and outlet views of the pelvis often provide further information. These views are taken at 45° angles to the pelvis and enable visualization of injuries that may be missed on the AP film. Inlet views are useful in identifying subtle lateral compression and vertical shear injuries. They also help to better visualize the degree of displacement of anterior pubic fractures. Outlet views better delineate the sacrum and sacroiliac joints. Judet views may also be obtained to visualize the acetabulum.

Computed tomography scan

Computed tomography (CT) scanning has replaced the aforementioned series in many institutions (Figs. 30-5 and 30-6). CT is superior in providing three-dimensional reconstructions of fracture detail, showing precise locations of fracture fragments and better evaluating the degree of displacement and diastases.[13] The ability to detect posterior fractures and determine the stability of pelvic fractures is greatly increased with CT.[14] In several retrospective series, the sensitivity of plain radiographs compared to computed tomography (CT) scanning was between 67 and 75%, respectively. In patients with positive findings on radiography, over 50% were found to have additional fractures or an increase in fracture grade on CT scan.[15] Stable patients with pelvic fractures usually undergo CT scanning to evaluate their abdomens and pelvises for solid or hollow organ injury. Thus, there is often no added time or expenditure in the evaluation of the bony pelvis.

In addition to better definition of bony injury, CT also allows for assessment of vascular injury, in particular arterial injury. Contrast extravasation ("blush") is

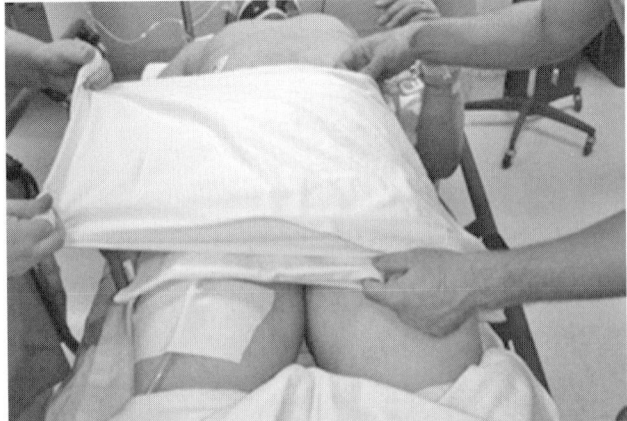
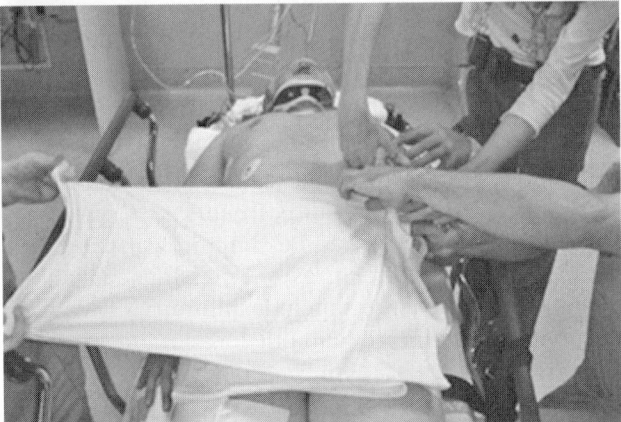
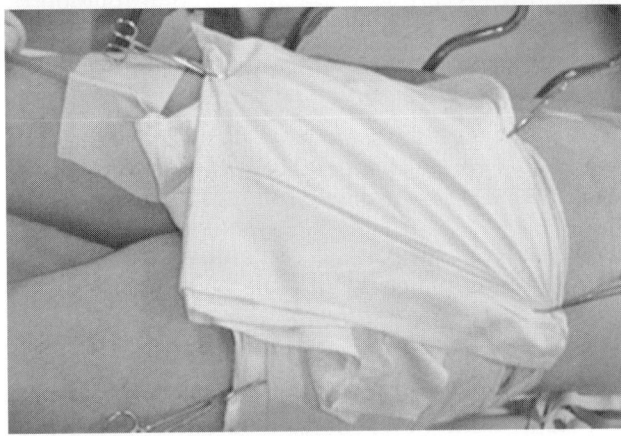

Figure 30-4 *A. Countertraction used to secure sheet across the pelvis. B. Hemostats used to anchor sheet in place. C. Fully sheeted pelvis. (Photographs courtesy of Dave Baker, MD, Harborview Medical Center, Seattle.)*

a strong indicator of active arterial bleeding, and predicts the need for angiography. CT cystogram may also be used as an adjunct to evaluate the lower urinary tract and diagnose bladder rupture, as discussed later in this chapter.

INITIAL ASSESSMENT AND MANAGEMENT

Patients who are determined to have a pelvic fracture either by clinical examination or AP radiograph should continue to be managed according to advanced

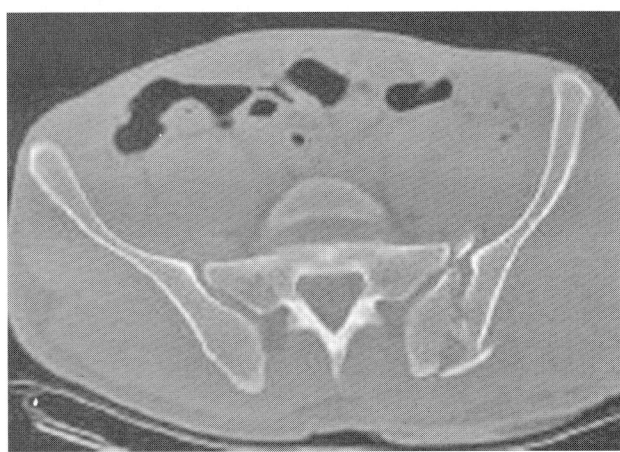

Figure 30-5 *CT scan of vertical shear pelvic fracture.*

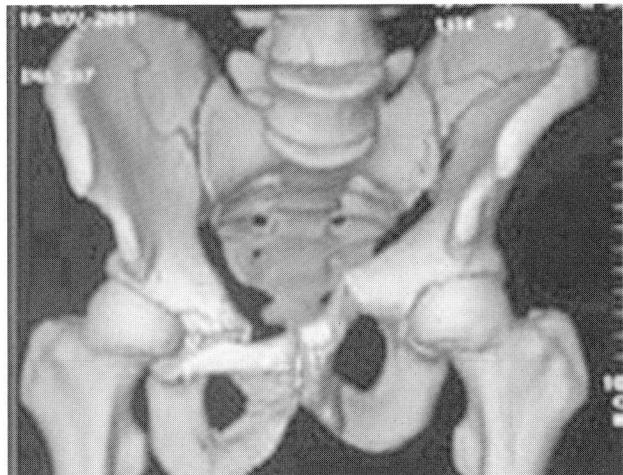

Figure 30-6 *Three-dimensional CT reconstruction of vertical shear fracture.*

trauma life support guidelines. Patients with an unstable pelvic fracture should undergo a temporary stabilization technique as soon as this is recognized while further evaluation or transportation is continued. There are several techniques that may be used for this purpose, as discussed previously.

MANAGEMENT OF MAJOR PELVIC BLEEDING

There is some controversy regarding the best method to control significant pelvic bleeding. An estimated 85% of pelvic vascular injuries are venous in nature. These result from disruption of the venous plexus and oozing from fracture fragments. Due to the low-pressure flow and the propensity for tamponade, these injuries are often self-limiting. Correction of coagulopathy and reduction of pelvic volume by external fixation and alignment of fracture fragments are the mainstays of controlling venous hemorrhage.[16] Orthopedic external fixation is usually applied in the operating room, although some surgeons are able to perform this procedure in the emergency room or intensive care unit.

Proponents of this method cite the greater incidence of venous injuries from pelvic trauma, and reserve angiography for treatment failure.[17-19]

While external stabilization and compression may be effective in reducing bleeding from pelvic venous injuries, patients with recalcitrant bleeding often have arterial injuries best addressed by angiography and embolization.[20,21] In addition, there is little high-level evidence to support that external fixation significantly reduces bleeding and improves survival in hemodynamically unstable patients.

While arterial bleeding is less common, it can be expected in up to 15% of pelvic fractures.[22] Arterial bleeding is certainly the more likely cause of hemodynamic instability. Hemorrhage may result from injury to a major iliac vessel, but more frequently it is due to disruption of a smaller branch of the hypogastric artery, deep in the pelvis and relatively inaccessible by standard surgical techniques. Angiography is commonly accepted as first-line therapy, with selective embolization of bleeding vessels. The results of angiographic embolization for pelvic fractures have steadily improved since the first reports in 1972 where angiography was used as a "last resort" and associated with high mortality.[23]

Since hemodynamically significant bleeding is usually arterial, angiography as first-line treatment prevents delays and potentially reduces blood loss. Noninvasive stabilization techniques (eg, sheeting) can be applied in the emergency room, and venous bleeding may be controlled by this method until arterial injury has been excluded. Additionally, angiography can diagnose and treat hemorrhage from other sources in patients with polytrauma. A large number of reports have demonstrated the safety and efficacy of angiographic embolization.[24] The question facing the surgeon is how to decide which patient would be best served by early angiographic intervention.

Older patients have been shown to require angiography more frequently and for less severe fracture patterns than younger patients.[25] Fracture patterns,[26] hemodynamic profiles, rate and volume of blood transfusions, and CT scan findings have all been studied to determine the likelihood of arterial versus venous injury.[27,28] Hypotension unresponsive to fluid infusion, transfusion requirements greater than four units in 24 hours,[29] and active contrast extravasation[23] on CT scan have been shown to be predictors of arterial bleeding and should warrant strong consideration of angiography. Information about arterial bleeding may also be determined by the volume of hematoma seen on CT scan. A pelvic hematoma larger than 500 ml on CT scan increases the likelihood of arterial injury requiring angiography to almost 50%. This finding also predicts the need for large (greater than six units) blood transfusion. Conversely, patients with less than 200 ml of pelvic blood have only 5% incidence of pelvic arterial bleeding on angiography.[30]

A clinical prediction rule was recently described to help assess which patients would most likely benefit from angiography. Predictors of the need for intervention included pulse greater than 130, emergency department hematocrit less than 30, obturator ring fracture displaced > 1 cm, and pubic symphysis diastasis > 1 cm. The probability of major bleeding ranged from 2% for zero predictors to over 60% for three or more positive predictors.[31]

There are several series documenting success with both angiography and external fixation, and part of the decision should be based on available local resources. While angiography appears to be superior in managing life-threatening hemorrhage, this intervention requires the rapid mobilization of several key resources. Ready availability of a trained interventional radiologist or vascular surgeon, experienced technical support, and an angiography unit equipped with critical care monitoring capability are essential in ensuring successful outcomes.

DEFINITIVE CONTROL OF PELVIC BLEEDING

ANGIOGRAPH

Angiography is usually performed via a femoral approach using a micropuncture (4 or 5 Fr) access system. Abdominal aortography is initially performed, followed by imaging of the bilateral common iliac arteries. The hypogastric arteries are then accessed and explored to identify actively bleeding branches. Embolization is performed to the most distal branches to prevent ischemia to surrounding pelvic structures. With multiple bleeding branches or vasospasm precluding distal catheterization, more proximal branches may need to be coil embolized. The main hypogastric can be embolized unilaterally with low risk of side effects. Completion angiography confirms bleeding cessation (Figs. 30-7 and 30-8). The success rate of angiography in controlling pelvic arterial bleeding is over 90% in most series.[30]

Damage-control angiography

The concept of damage control has become one of the mainstays of initial trauma management. The emphasis on rapid control of hemorrhage, early resuscitation, and delayed definitive treatment has extended to other disciplines including orthopedic surgery. The role of angiography in the unstable patient can also be seen in this light.

Femoral arterial access may be obtained in the emergency room while awaiting mobilization of the angiography team. The interventionalist can obtain rapid control of bleeding through embolization of both internal iliac arteries. This approach avoids the time-consuming selective arterial catheterization and embolization of multiple distal branches. Bilateral embolization should be done with gel foam to allow

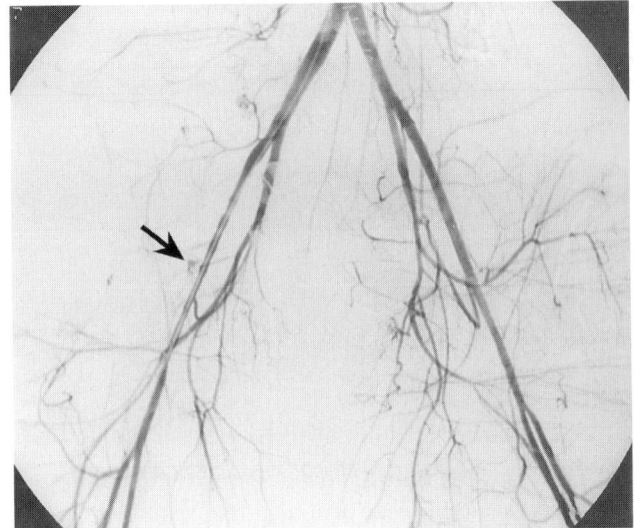
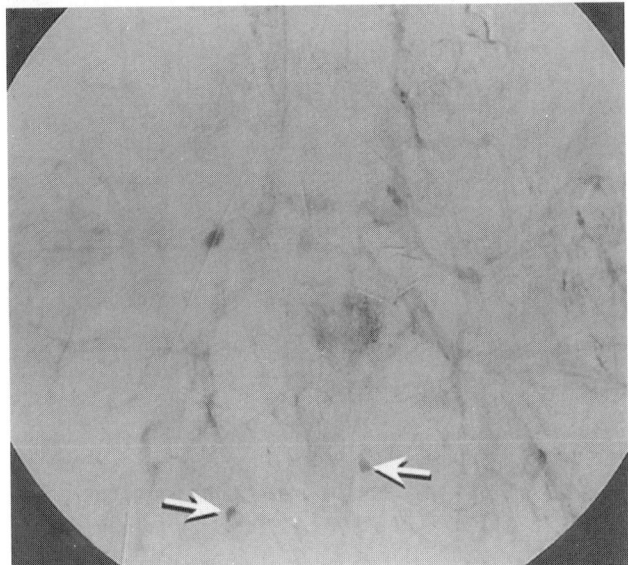

Figure 30-7 *A. Contrast extravasation on angiogram. B. Multiple points of extravasation evident on angiogram.*

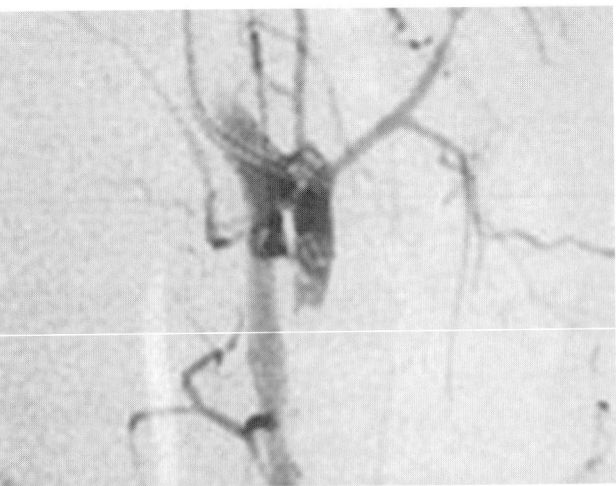

Figure 30-8 *Postembolization angiogram of hypogastric artery.*

for later recanalization and prevent permanent pelvic ischemia. This method rapidly controls life-threatening bleeding, allowing the patient to be immediately mobilized for other interventions.

Finally, the femoral access sheath is left in place when the patient leaves the angiography suite. This allows for quick access while the patient continues to be resuscitated and other injuries treated. Repeat angiography may then be performed should rebleeding occur.[32]

Recurrent bleeding has been reported in approximately 7% of patients. This is often at a new site that was not previously embolized and likely reflects vasospasm of these vessels at the time of initial angiography. Multiple arteries requiring embolization at initial angiography, transfusion rates of greater than two units per hour prior to initial angiogram and pubic symphysis widening have been shown to be associated with recurrent bleeding.[33] Recurrent bleeding may be effectively treated with repeat angiography and embolization.

The complication rate of pelvic angiography is low. In addition to the standard complications of arterial access—pseudoaneurysm, bleeding, and ischemia—several cases of gluteal muscle necrosis have been reported.[34] Gluteal necrosis is more likely to occur with proximal embolization, particularly of the main hypogastric artery. Urologic and sexual dysfunction has not been directly attributed to angiography, although common in patients with pelvic fractures in general.[35]

External fixation

While several authors have shown that external fixation aids hemorrhage control, the mechanism is not completely clear. The rigid framework provides stability and prevents motion of fracture fragments that may cause further bleeding. Closure of pelvic volume resulting in tamponade of venous bleeding is hypothesized as the primary mechanism of reducing blood loss.[36] There are two major types of external fixation: anterior fixation and the posterior pelvic C-clamp.

The anterior external fixator was originally developed for use in open-book pelvic injuries. The device consists of pins inserted into the iliac crest and connected by two anterior horizontal bars. Supraacetabular pin insertion is also used and may provide more biomechanical stability (Fig. 30-9). Anterior fixation may be used to treat rotationally unstable but vertically stable fractures.[37] This method is not effective in treating posterior disruptions of the pelvic ring or vertically unstable shear injuries. It also impairs access to the abdomen should emergent laparotomy become necessary.

The posterior clamp (Ganz or C clamp) was developed to address posterior instability and is effective in preventing motion of fracture fragments and bleeding from the posterior venous plexus.[38] This method has

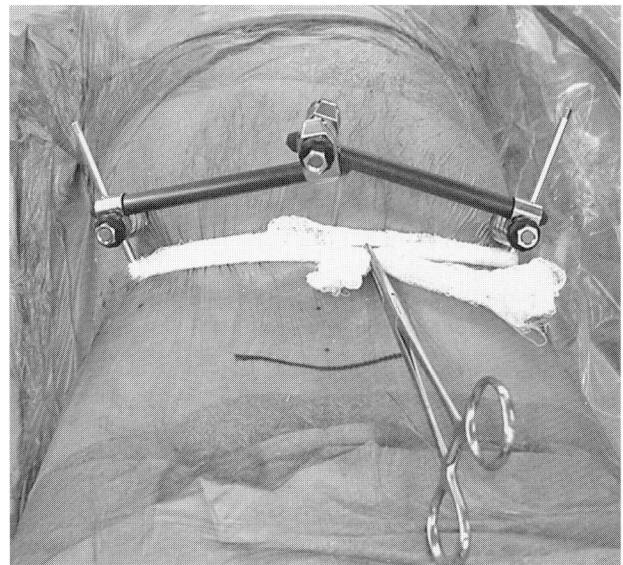

Figure 30-9 *Anterior external fixator.*

been shown to have superior biomechanical stability compared with anterior fixation. It may be applied rapidly in the operating room or in the emergency room. The C-shaped clamp is attached to the pelvis through two anterosuperior iliac pins. The clamp may be rotated cephalad or caudad, allowing unrestricted access to the abdomen.[39]

Several authors have shown that long-term functional results with external fixation are significantly inferior, to open reduction and internal fixation. Therefore, this should be viewed as a temporary means of pelvic stability only.[40,41] Complications of both methods include loosening, displacement, and pin perforation into the pelvis.[42]

Intra-abdominal packing

Direct pelvic packing is not recommended as initial treatment for pelvic bleeding, since there is little data to support the efficacy of this maneuver. However, in patients who require operative intervention for a concurrent intra-abdominal injury, packing may provide temporary stabilization. In the patient undergoing a laparotomy for trauma, the sudden decrease in intra-abdominal pressure may increase pelvic hematoma volume by 15%. The tamponade effect is released, and rebleeding from smaller vessels often occurs.

Packing the pelvis with laparotomy pads can provide direct compression of involved vessels and help restore the tamponade effect.[43] Exploration and direct ligation or repair of bleeding pelvic vessels has also been described. While this method may be effective for injury to the common iliac vessels, the site of bleeding is usually the smaller branches in the distal pelvis, and surgical exposure is extremely difficult. Since prolonged operative times with an open abdomen have been shown to result in hypothermia, acidosis, and coagulopathy, an extensive search for the bleeding artery should be avoided.

In patients with positive laparotomy findings, a damage control approach is a safer alternative. The abdomen and pelvis should be packed, and temporary wound closure performed. If the pelvis is the source of ongoing bleeding, the interventionalist should be alerted, and the patient should be taken to the angiography suite after the operation.

Preperitoneal packing for unstable pelvic fractures has recently been revisited as a surgical technique to control hemorrhage.[44] This approach involves packing the true pelvis with laparotomy pads via an inferior midline incision and extensive preperitoneal dissection. However, in patients undergoing laparotomy, this requires additional dissection and may prolong operative times. The preliminary results are encouraging, and this technique may find a role if angiography is not readily available.

OPEN PELVIC FRACTURES

Open pelvic fractures involve a communication between fracture fragments and the skin, usually through large perineal, groin, or buttock lacerations. These devastating injuries carry a high morbidity and mortality. In historical series, as many as 50% of these patients were nonsurvivors, although more recent literature notes an 18% overall mortality.[45] In one third to one-half of these cases, mortality is directly attributable to the injury itself. The majority of early deaths are due to exsanguination from multiple vessel injuries. Patients with open fractures require approximately four times as many blood transfusions in the first 24 hours than patients with closed pelvic fractures.[46] One-third of later deaths are due to pelvic sepsis, which still carries greater than 50% mortality. The presence of associated intra-abdominal injuries conferred 90% mortality in a recent retrospective series.[47] The principles of treatment illustrated include control of hemorrhage, extensive debridement of devitalized soft tissue, diagnosis, and treatment of associated urogenital and colorectal injuries and fixation of the fracture itself.

Patients should be managed in the emergency room following the same guidelines as for closed pelvic fractures. The perineum should be examined, and a digital rectal examination performed. Speculum examination should also be performed to evaluate for vaginal tears. An initial AP radiograph should be obtained. CT scanning should be utilized in the hemodynamically stable patient, to better delineate the extent of soft-tissue and bony injury. Lacerations and wounds should not be probed or examined extensively in the emergency room, as this is a suboptimal environment to assess the extent of damage and may lead to further bleeding.

The initial step in management is hemorrhage control. The same principles of temporary noninvasive stabilization followed by angiography as needed should be applied. Visible bleeding vessels may be controlled by direct pressure. Large bleeding wounds should be packed and pressure dressings applied. Patients with open fractures should be taken to the operating room as soon as possible for definitive assessment, hemorrhage control, and irrigation and debridement of injuries. The patient should be placed supine in low stirrups to ensure adequate visualization of the entire perineum. Lacerations should be copiously irrigated and examined. Bleeding vessels should be ligated. Laparotomy rarely affords adequate visualization of pelvic injuries and should only be performed for associated intra-abdominal injuries. If control of hemorrhage is unable to be obtained, direct packing and angiography, either on-table or in the angiography suite, may be required.

Following control of bleeding, all lacerated soft tissue should be examined, irrigated, and viability determined. Devitalized tissue and skin should be sharply debrided. Pulsatile lavage technique may help in removing foreign material and ensuring adequate irrigation. Serial debridements are often necessary and have been shown to reduce the incidence of pelvic sepsis.[48] Prophylactic broad-spectrum antibiotic coverage should be initiated early in all patients.[49]

The genitourinary system and colorectal tract must be evaluated for injury in all open pelvic fractures. Depending on patient stability, this can be performed immediately or in a delayed fashion. The diagnosis and management of these injuries will be considered separately.

THE ROLE OF FECAL DIVERSION IN OPEN PELVIC FRACTURES

Due to the high mortality of pelvic sepsis, diversion of the fecal stream has long been considered a mandatory component of the treatment for open pelvic fractures.[50] Recurrent fecal soiling of the perineal wound and fracture fragments was felt to be largely responsible for the infectious mortality and morbidity of these fractures. Several wartime series demonstrated improved survival with routine fecal diversion. However, the efficacy of fecal diversion has never been prospectively evaluated in a randomized controlled fashion, and several recent retrospective reviews have questioned the need for mandatory diversion.[51,52] While the need for diversion in patients with incontinent, full-thickness rectal injuries is uniformly accepted, the benefit in other patients is unclear.

Subsets of patients with buttock and perineal wounds close to the anal sphincter complex have shown a small reduction in infection rates in some series. Patients with anterior and lateral groin wounds have not been shown to benefit from colostomy.[53] In addition, ostomy reversal is associated with a significant complication rate and subjects the patient to an additional procedure with general anesthesia. A recent metanalysis of the English literature revealed no statistically significant benefit in mortality or reduction in infectious complications from the procedure.[54] There is insufficient evidence at this time to recommend routine diversion of the fecal stream in all patients with an open pelvic fracture. However, individual patient assessment is essential to evaluate for full-thickness rectal injury or anal sphincter destruction, both indications for diversion.

RECTAL AND SIGMOID COLON INJURIES

Rectal perforation is an uncommon injury associated with pelvic fractures, occurring in less than 1% of all cases. However, in open pelvic fractures the incidence of anorectal injury approaches 20%.[55] While the mechanism in most cases is direct trauma to the rectum due to displaced fracture fragments, several instances of delayed rectal perforation associated with ischemia have been reported.[56] The rectum has a rich vascular supply with multiple collateral vessels, which likely accounts for the rarity of ischemic injury. Injury to the sigmoid colon usually occurs at the level of the pelvic brim, from a shear injury.

Since unrecognized colorectal injury can be a devastating source of sepsis, all patients with pelvic trauma should undergo a digital rectal examination. Blood in the rectum, lacerations involving the anorectal complex or free air in the peri-rectal tissues on computed tomography mandate further evaluation. Several methods exist for evaluation of the rectum and lower colon. Anoscopy is the first step in evaluation, and can be performed at bedside. CT scan with rectal contrast may be an adjunct in diagnosing full-thickness perforation of the colon and rectum in stable patients with closed fractures.

Direct examination in the operating room should be performed in all open pelvic fractures, and all patients with clinical suspicion for colorectal injury. This is best performed with the patient in lithotomy position. Proctoscopy and sigmoidocopy, using rigid or flexible endoscopes, will enable the surgeon to visualize the mucosa of the colon and rectum. Perforations, tears, or ischemic areas may be identified and require immediate management.

Most of the available data on treating colorectal injuries is derived from penetrating trauma victims. Improvements in mortality in battlefield injuries during World War II and Vietnam led to the widespread use of fecal diversion for these injuries. However, several recent series have demonstrated equivalent or improved outcomes for patients managed with primary repair of colon injuries. Smaller lacerations of the colon may be primarily repaired, while larger lacerations or extensive devitalizations may be better served

with segmental resection. The benefit of primary repair or segmental resection over colostomy has been shown, even in the face of risk factors such as stool contamination, shock, transfusions and location of injury (right versus left colon).[57-59]

The management of rectal injury is controversial, and often depends on location of injury. Intraperitoneal rectal injuries should be primarily repaired, if possible, and successful outcomes with a one-stage repair have been shown. These injuries are treated similar to colonic injuries. The majority of extraperitoneal injuries are not easily accessible for primary repair, and diverting colostomy is indicated in these cases.

The role of presacral drainage is controversial. Patients who have undergone mobilization and exploration of their rectal wound during laparotomy and are able to be primarily repaired are effectively intraperitonealized, and drainage may not add much benefit. Patients who have undergone diversion without exploration of the perirectal tissues may benefit from the drains placed in the closed retrorectal space to prevent closed-space infection. A reduction in pelvic infection with presacral drainage has been shown in several retrospective series. However, the only prospective randomized trial conducted showed no difference in infectious complications.[60]

BLADDER RUPTURE

Bladder rupture occurs in approximately 8-10% of all pelvic fractures. Injury may result from deceleration force on a full bladder, or direct trauma from fracture fragments. The rate of associated injury to other organs is high, approximately 80-90% in some series.[61] Pubic rami and obturator fractures, pubic diastasis greater than 1 cm and widened sacroiliac diastasis are associated with a higher likelihood of bladder rupture.[62]

Patients may complain of symptoms of dysuria, urinary retention, or pain. Gross hematuria is the most common sign of bladder injury, occurring in almost 95% of patients. The combination of pelvic fracture and any degree of hematuria should mandate cystourethrography.[63] While the gold standard for many years has been retrograde cystourethrography with bladder distention and postvoiding views, several authors have shown equivalent or superior results with CT cystography.[64] Characteristic patterns of contrast extravasation can be seen with intraperitoneal and extraperitoneal bladder ruptures in both conventional and CT cystography (Fig. 30-10 through 30-13). Adequate contrast instillation to cause distention of the bladder is important to avoid false-negative results. Most authors recommend 350 ml of contrast, or distention to a bladder pressure of 40 mm Hg.

A comparison of CT cystography findings with intraoperative findings at laparotomy has shown the

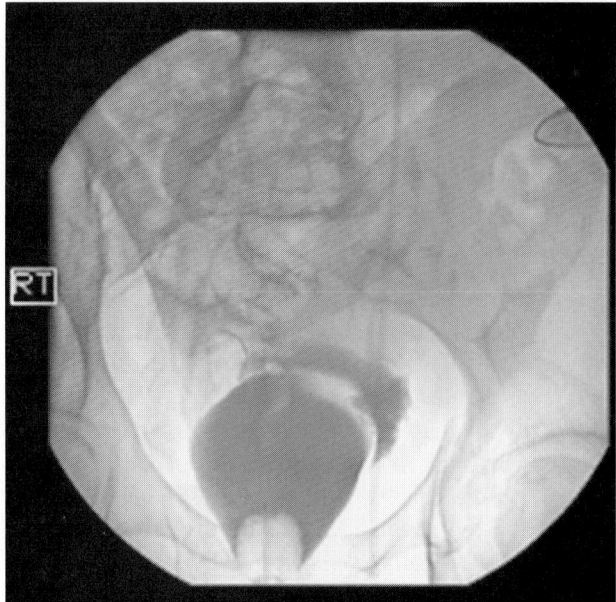

Figure 30-10 *Extraperitoneal bladder rupture on cystogram.*

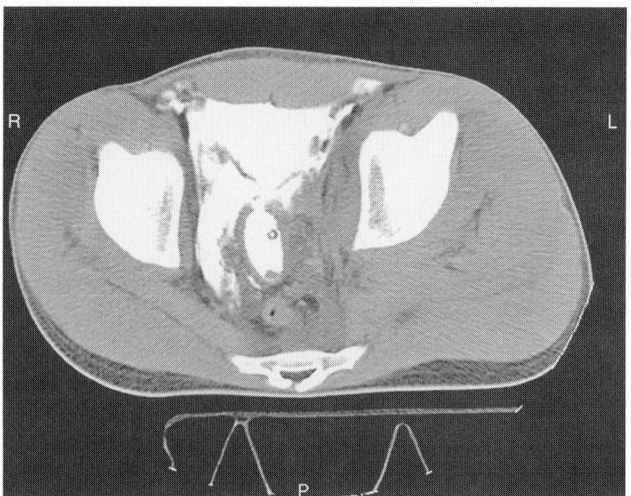

Figure 30-12 *Extraperitoneal bladder rupture on CT.*

sensitivity and specificity for detecting bladder rupture to be 95 and 100%, respectively.[65] CT cystography is more expensive than conventional cystography and delivers a higher radiation dose. However, since the vast majority of trauma patients undergo CT scan of the abdomen and pelvis to evaluate for solid organ and bony injury, CT cystography may be performed at the time of initial evaluation with little additional cost or time expenditure.

Nonoperative treatment of bladder injury was first described in 1975 and became widely accepted in the 1980s.[66,67] Extraperitoneal bladder ruptures are usually managed by catheter drainage alone for approximately 10 days and do not require operative repair. Transurethral catheterization alone is adequate in patients without concomitant urethral injury. A larger diameter catheter (20 Fr) or a three-way irrigation catheter may be used if blood clots are present.

In hemodynamically stable patients undergoing laparotomy for associated injuries, these defects are usually closed via an intraperitoneal approach at the time of surgery. Most extraperitoneal injuries are small in diameter and situated anteriorly. These can be repaired through an extraperitoneal incision in patients undergoing orthopedic fixation of the pelvic fracture. One benefit of primary repair in these patients is the prevention of urine contamination of orthopedic hardware, which can result in infection and the need for hardware removal.

Intraperitoneal bladder rupture is treated surgically, due to the high rate of associated intra-abdominal

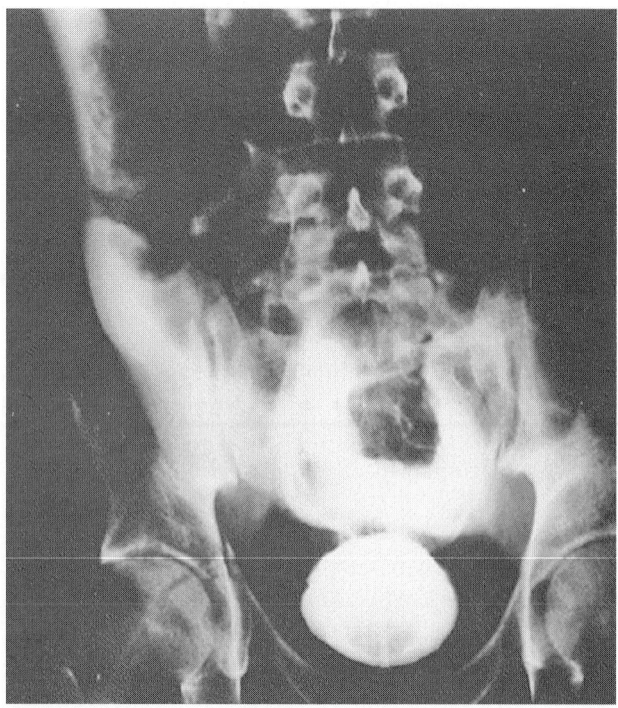

Figure 30-11 *Intraperitoneal bladder rupture on cystogram.*

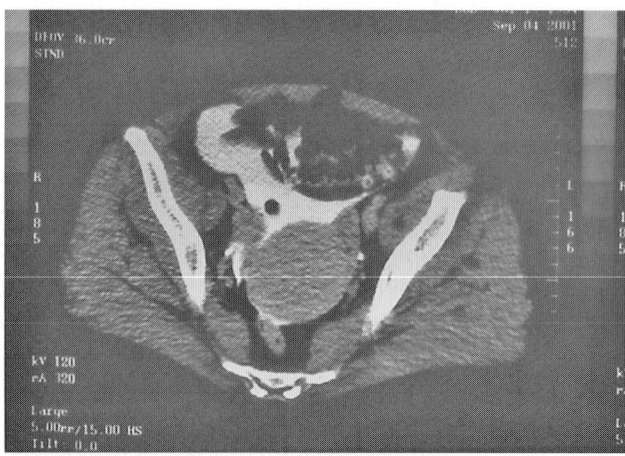

Figure 30-13 *Intraperitoneal bladder rupture on CT.*

sepsis with catheter drainage alone. At laparotomy, these injuries typically present as stellate lacerations of the dome. Since 8% of cases have associated extraperitoneal lacerations, it is recommended that the opening be enlarged to allow thorough inspection of the bladder and avoid missing a concomitant injury.[68] This also facilitates identification of the trigone and inspection of ureteral orifices and the bladder neck. Lacerations are usually closed in two layers with absorbable sutures.

THE ROLE OF SUPRAPUBIC CATHETERIZATION

The principles of bladder repair remain the debridement of devitalized tissue, identification of ureteral orifices, establishment of a watertight closure, and drainage using a catheter. Historically, suprapubic catheter drainage was used extensively in patients undergoing repair of the bladder. This was felt to provide superior drainage and "protect" the bladder repair. However, several recent series have shown that transurethral catheter drainage alone is effective and associated with similar outcomes to suprapubic catheterization alone or combined suprapubic and transurethral catheterization.[69]

Several studies have reported an increase in urinary infection rates with suprapubic catheterization.[70,71] Increased rates of urethral strictures, urinary retention, wound colonization, and difficulty with long-term care patients managed with suprapubic tubes alone have also been reported.[72] Their presence also complicates the management of pubic rami fractures. There does not appear to be a proven benefit for routine suprapubic cystostomy in patients undergoing treatment for bladder rupture.[73]

A recent study found that 23% of urologic injuries at a Level I trauma center had initially missed diagnoses, with a mean delay of 19 hours prior to recognition of intraperitoneal bladder injuries and 7 days for extraperitoneal bladder ruptures. This highlights the need for awareness of urologic injuries in every patient presenting with a pelvic fracture.[74]

URETHRAL INJURY

Urethral injury in blunt trauma occurs in approximately 10% of pelvic fractures in men, while the incidence in women is less than 5%. The longer urethra renders injury more probable in men. Injury usually occurs in the posterior urethra at the prostate–membranous junction. Anterior urethral injuries are less common, and usually the result of a straddle injury.[75] Pubic arch fractures have an increased risk of urethral injury, with likelihood of injury proportional to the number of broken rami. Malgaigne fracture—fracture of both pubic rami with ipsilateral sacral, sacroiliac, or ilium disruption—is associated with a threefold increased risk for urethral injury.[76]

Urinary retention is a common symptom, with inability to void despite the sensation of bladder fullness. Clinical signs include blood at the urethral meatus, which may be present in 55-85% of patients. However, up to 57% of patients do not manifest any clinical evidence of urethral injury.[84] Digital rectal examination should be performed to evaluate prostate position, bulbocavernosus reflex, and anal sphincter function. A retrograde urethrogram is necessary to define the location and extent of the injury (Fig. 30-14).

Historically, the treatment of these injuries has been suprapubic cystostomy followed by delayed urethroplasty 3-6 months after the incident.[77] This approach avoids dissection within acute hematoma and possible damage to pelvic nerves. However, this results in prolonged hospitalization and an almost inevitable urethral stricture formation. The stricture often results in the need for major reconstructive surgery at the time of reoperation.[78] The effect on potency is difficult to assess, since many patients suffer nerve injury at the time of the fracture. Incontinence is reported to be between 5 and 27%, respectively, following reconstruction.[79]

Recent advances in urological surgery have made primary realignment over a catheter the treatment of choice for posterior urethral injuries when feasible. This may be achieved with a magnetic-tipped catheter under fluoroscopic guidance or via transurethral endoscopic catheter stenting, avoiding an open operation and dissection within hematoma. Several studies have shown a significantly reduced stricture rate and improved continence and potency with primary realignment.[80] The patient undergoes fewer procedures and avoids a suprapubic cystostomy.

The urethral stricture rate in one series of early alignment was 40%, all of which responded to internal urethrotomy. Continence is maintained in almost all patients, which compares favorably to the 10% incontinence rate after delayed open reconstruction.[81] While more research is needed on the long-term

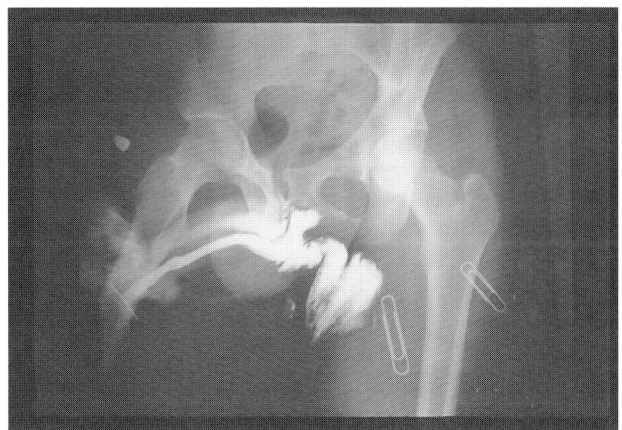

Figure 30-14 *Anterior rupture on retrograde urethrogram.*

effects on sexual function and continence with each approach, early realignment appears to be an effective strategy in stable patients. In cases of orthopedic instrumentation of the pelvis, this approach is preferred because of the lower risk of hardware contamination with a transurethral catheter than a suprapubic cystostomy.[82]

NEUROLOGIC INJURY

While early resuscitation and stabilization have improved outcomes for high-grade pelvic fractures, neurologic injury remains a source of long-term pain and disability. Neurologic injuries are seen in 10-15% of all pelvic fractures. However, this rises to almost 50% in unstable vertical shear injuries.[83] Posterior ring disruption is responsible for the majority of deficits.[84] Electromyographic studies identify a higher prevalence of deficits, although most of these are not clinically significant. Most patients have mixed sensory and motor deficits, and one third have an isolated sensory neuropathy. Although the vast majority of injuries are present on initial arrival to the emergency room, many patients do not receive a thoroughly documented neurological examination until some time after admission.

Injury patterns vary according to the mechanism of injury. Lateral compression fractures often results in entrapment of sacral nerves. Vertical shear injuries are likely to cause stretch and avulsion of nerve roots.[85] Sacral ala and foramina fractures usually cause injury to L5, S1, and S2 nerve roots. Comminuted fractures of the sacroiliac joint commonly result in superior gluteal nerve injury. Fractures medial to the sacral foramina and transverse sacral fractures cause the highest incidence of autonomic dysfunction, increasing the risk of bladder and bowel incontinence and sexual impotency.[86]

Early identification of nerve injury involves a thorough physical examination. Perineal sensation, voiding ability, and anal sphincter tone must be evaluated. Systematic evaluation of lower extremity dermatomes, and myotomes should be performed as soon as the patients' clinical condition permits. Nerve injury is a recognized complication of orthopedic manipulation and fixation of unstable pelvic fractures. Early and accurate documentation of patient's preoperative neurological function is important in avoiding potential medicolegal pitfalls and expediting physical rehabilitation.

The natural history of nerve deficits is continued improvement up to 2 years from the time of injury. Most of the improvement is seen by 1 year, and partial recovery of function is the norm in 60-70% of patients. Early stabilization and reduction of fractures may improve recovery by decompressing entrapped nerve roots and preventing further stretch injury.

SEXUAL DYSFUNCTION

Sexual dysfunction, especially erectile dysfunction, is a well-known consequence of pelvic fractures, especially those associated with posterior urethral injury. The wide range in reported incidence is due to the variability of criteria used to define dysfunction. As many as 70-80% of men with associated urethral injury have some degree of dysfunction 6 months after injury, with 20-40% suffering from impotence.[87] The incidence of symptomatic dysfunction in patients without urethral injury is estimated between 10 and 30%, respectively. Erectile dysfunction after pelvic fracture is due to a combination of neurogenic, vascular, corporal, and psychogenic injury.[88] Investigations in these patients may include nocturnal tumescence testing, pharmacological testing using an agent such as prostaglandin E, and duplex vascular ultrasound. Magnetic resonance imaging may be useful in assessing soft-tissue damage and fibrosis of the corpora cavernosa.

There is no specific treatment of erectile dysfunction postpelvic fracture. Standard treatments include drugs such as phosphodiesterase inhibitors, intracorporal injection, mechanical devices, and prostheses, as used in patients with dysfunction from other causes. In the rare patient who has impotence due to an arterial injury, microsurgical revascularisation has been used with some success.

Sexual dysfunction in women is reported less frequently. A multicenter trauma outcomes study found that symphyseal diastasis was associated with sexual and excretory dysfunction in women, while sacroiliac fractures were associated with a higher risk of dysfunction in men. This led to a significant decrease in health-related quality of life in both groups.[89]

SPECIAL POPULATIONS

PELVIC FRACTURES IN CHILDREN

Children are significantly less likely than adults to suffer pelvic fractures. The incidence of pelvic fractures in pediatric trauma is estimated at between 2 and 5%, respectively, primarily due to motor vehicle–pedestrian crashes. Although uncommon, the morbidity and mortality of these injuries remain high. The high impact required to produce a pediatric pelvic fracture is reflected in the large number of associated injuries, between 70 and 80%, respectively, in most series. The shallow pelvis and relatively large trunk area predisposes these patients to associated solid organ and visceral injuries, which are slightly more common than in adult pelvic fracture patients. Unlike in adults, exsanguination from pelvic fractures is very rare in children.[90,91] The increased elasticity of immature bones and contractility of young vessels may contribute to this protective effect. Lower genitourinary injury is less common (0.9%) in pediatric patients and is not found in patients with a normal clinical examination and no gross hematuria.[92]

Historically, most pediatric pelvic fractures have been treated nonoperatively, with spica cast placement and gradual mobilization. However, in patients with unstable pelvic fractures, open anterior and posterior fixation may be preferred. The principles of treatment are obtaining good fracture reduction and restoring pelvic symmetry. Inadequate reduction may result in long-term complications such as leg length discrepancy, scoliosis, back pain, and limp. While most patients have impaired mobility and self-care at discharge from hospital, a recent study showed a return to near-maximal functional outcome at 6 months regardless of degree of initial injury.[93] A multidisciplinary approach is crucial in providing early rehabilitation, restoring mobility, and minimizing the disruption in school and other activities in these children.

PELVIC FRACTURES IN THE ELDERLY

The elderly population is the fastest-growing demographic in the United States. Trauma is the fifth leading cause of death in patients over 65 years. Pelvic fractures in older patients are often the result of relatively minor trauma, such as standing falls and low-speed motor vehicle accidents. Lateral compression fractures are the most common type, related to the different injury mechanisms compared to younger patients. Although pelvic fracture patterns tend to be less severe, the incidence of blood transfusion and angiography is disproportionately high in elderly patients.[94] In patients undergoing a liberal angiographic strategy, it was found that age over 60 years was associated with a 94% likelihood of positive findings requiring embolization.[95]

Despite these interventions, mortality is four times as high in elderly patients, even after adjusting for overall injury severity.[96] There are several explanations of this effect. The ubiquity of osteoporosis and brittle bones in this population may lead to fractures from minor impacts. The lack of elasticity within soft tissue and poor skin turgor create a greater potential space and minimize the tamponade effect on small venous bleeding. Atherosclerotic vessels are also less likely to contract and spontaneously stop arterial bleeding. The elderly are therefore more likely to bleed copiously from a low-grade pelvic fracture, and thus care providers must have a very low threshold for aggressive intervention aimed at stopping the bleeding early. Comorbidities often confound the treatment and resuscitation and invasive monitoring with careful attention to hemodynamic stability, cardiac stress, temperature, and endocrine function is essential.

The one-year mortality rate for pelvic fractures in elderly patients is approximately 12%, and one-third of patients have reduced ambulatory status after injury.[97] Acute care surgeons should recognize the high risk of death and disability in elderly patients after relatively minor pelvic fractures.

PELVIC FRACTURES IN PREGNANCY

The overall incidence of trauma in pregnancy is approximately 7%. The maternal mortality rate for pelvic fractures is 9%, similar to age and injury severity score–matched nonpregnant controls. The fetal mortality rate is significantly higher at 35-70%. Fetal mortality is higher in pelvic fractures than in other forms of blunt trauma. This is due to maternal instability and hypotension as well as direct uterine and placental trauma. Mortality does not appear to be related to fracture type or trimester of the pregnancy.[98] Treatment of pregnant patients follows the same principles as other adults, and hemodynamic stability of the mother should be the main priority. The fetus should be shielded from radiation using an appropriate device (lead apron) where possible. Angiography and CT scanning should be avoided when possible, especially early in pregnancy. Ultrasonography is the preferred method of immediate abdominal evaluation. Nonoperative management of pelvic fractures with closed stabilization and bed rest has been described in the majority of cases. Continuous external fetal heart rate monitoring is recommended for at least 24 hours.[99]

Since fractures heal in 8-12 weeks, most patients injured early in pregnancy are able to undergo vaginal delivery. Displaced fractures, pubic rami, and lateral compression fractures make vaginal delivery more hazardous and are relative indications for cesarean section. In patients requiring emergency section for maternal or fetal distress, a maternal survival rate of 75% and fetal survival of 45% have been reported.[100]

LONG-TERM OUTCOMES

Improvements in early resuscitation, hemorrhage control, and skeletal fixation have resulted in a marked decrease in the mortality of pelvic fractures. However, many patients suffer significant morbidity in the short and long term. While injuries to the thorax and abdomen increase in-hospital morbidity and mortality, they are less important factors in long-term disability. Inadequate reduction and stabilization of pelvic fractures can lead to pelvic tilt, pain, and scoliosis. This in turn may lead to difficulty with ambulation, causing permanent disability and possible loss of livelihood. Patients with unstable posterior fractures, open fractures, and associated lower extremity injuries tend to have worse outcomes and more residual disability.

Many pelvic trauma patients suffer from chronic or recurrent pain. Pain associated with routine daily activity, standing, or sitting is seen in approximately 25% of patients with treated unstable pelvic fractures.[101] Sacroiliac joint disruptions particularly have a strong propensity toward causing long-term pain and disability. Local injections of analgesic agents into the joint may provide relief in patients with recalcitrant pain. Sacral fractures can be associated with pain that extends to the leg. These patients often have absent ankle reflexes due to radiculopathy.[102] Presence of pain correlates with inability to return to work in many studies.

Approximately half of all male patients suffer from sexual dysfunction one year after injury. Painful erections, complete or partial impotence, and premature ejaculation are common findings. Treatment is most effective in patients with partial deficits, and full return of function is unusual in patients presenting with impotence. Female patients are affected much less frequently and usually complain of dyspareunia.[103] Most patients suffer from moderate depression and anxiety during the first year postinjury. Patients who have chronic pain or sexual dysfunction are more likely to report high levels of anxiety and depression. The ability to return to work inversely correlates with psychosocial dysfunction scores.

Prolonged urinary dysfunction in patients with genitourinary injuries has already been discussed. However, patients without direct injury may also present with increased urinary frequency, multiple episodes of retention, and urinary tract infections within the first year after injury. Patients with open pelvic fractures are more likely to have long-term disability related to voiding and bowel incontinence.[46]

Most pelvic fractures occur in young healthy patients who were previously employed. In one series, 75% of patients were able to return to work within one year, with approximately one quarter requiring job modifications. Perception of secondary gain and pending litigation has been shown to correlate with delayed recovery of function and failure to return to work.[104] Pediatric patients have a higher rate of successful rehabilitation. Injured children without a concomitant head injury have a nearly 100% school return rate.

ALGORITHM FOR MANAGEMENT OF PATIENTS WITH A BLEEDING PELVIC FRACTURE

We have developed an algorithm at our institution to guide management of these complicated patients (Fig. 30-15). Patients undergo chest, lateral cervical spine and pelvis radiographs upon admission to the emergency room. Clinical or radiological suspicion of a hemothorax mandates placement of a tube thoracostomy on that side. Patients who are hemodynamically unstable undergo an immediate diagnostic peritoneal

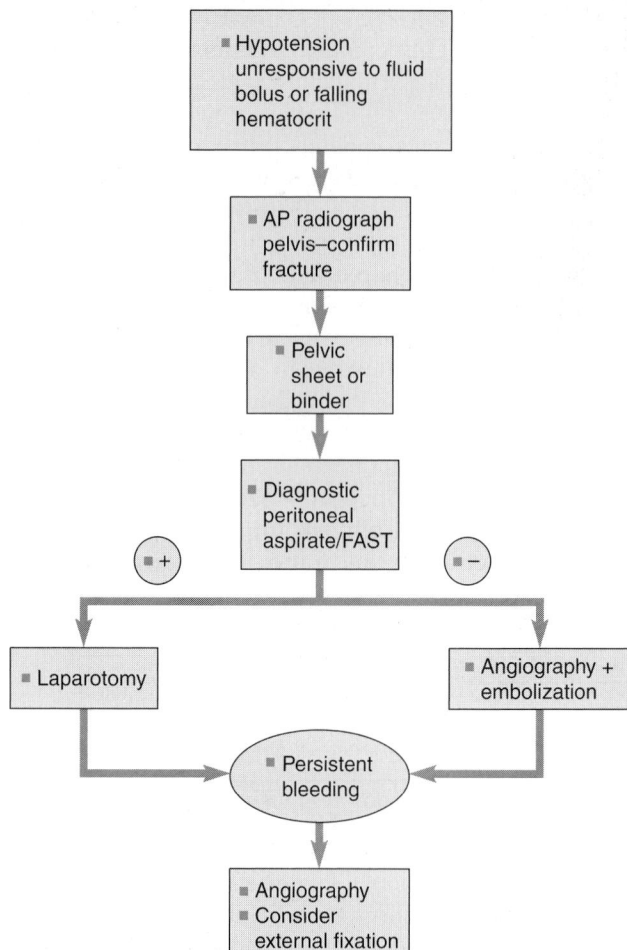

Figure 30-15 *Algorithm for unstable pelvic bleeding.*

aspirate (DPA) in the suprapubic location if a pelvic fracture is evident. A grossly positive DPA, or a hemothorax greater than 1.5 L, results in the patient being taken immediately to the operating room for a thoracotomy or laparotomy. If the chest or abdomen is not the major source of bleeding, yet the patient has clinical evidence of ongoing hemorrhage, the patient taken to the radiology suite for pelvic angiography. Patients with positive findings at laparotomy or thoracotomy continue to be monitored postoperatively. The new or continued onset of hemodynamic instability or a declining hematocrit in these patients prompts angiographic evaluation.

Patients with a negative DPA and documented pelvic fracture undergo angiography as first-line treatment. The patient remains in a sheet or binder during assessment and transport.

REFERENCES

1. Poole GV, Ward EF, Muakkassa FF, et al. Pelvic fracture from major blunt trauma: outcome is determined by associated injuries. *Ann Surg* 1991;213:532-538.

2. Gilliland MD, Ward RE, Barton RM, et al. Factors affecting mortality in pelvic fractures. *J Trauma* 1982;22:691-693.

3. Aihara R, Blansfield JS, Millham FH, et al. Fracture locations influence the likelihood of rectal and lower urinary tract injuries in patients sustaining pelvic fractures. *J Trauma* 2002;52(2):20-208.

4. Parreira J, Coimbra R, Rasslan S, et al. The role of associated injuries on outcome of blunt trauma patients sustaining pelvic fractures. *Injury* 2000;31:677-682.

5. Cryer HM, Miller FB, Evers BM, et al. Pelvic fracture classification: correlation with hemorrhage. *J Trauma* 1988;28:973-980.

6. Durkin AD, Sagi CH, Durham R, et al. Contemporary management of pelvic fractures. *Am J Surg* 2006;192:211-223.

7. Evers BM, Cryer HM, Miller FB. Pelvic fracture hemorrhage. *Arch Surg* 1989;124:422-424.

8. Young JWR, Resnick CS. Fractures of the pelvis: current concepts of classification. *AJR* 1990;155:1169-1175.

9. Burgess AR, Eastridge BJ, Young JW. Pelvic ring disruptions: effective classification system and treatment protocols. *J Trauma* 1990;30(7):848-856.

10. Ben-Menachem Y, Coldwell DM, Young JW, et al. Hemorrhage associated with pelvic fractures: causes, diagnosis and emergent management. *Am J Roentgenol* 1991;157:1005-1014.

11. Heetveld MJ, Harris I, Schlaphoff G, et al. Hemodynamically unstable pelvic fractures: Recent care and new guidelines. *World J Surg* 2004;28:904-909.

12. Krieg JC, Mohr M, Ellis TJ, et al. Emergent stabilization of pelvic ring injuries by controlled circumferential compression: a clinical trial. *J Trauma* 2005;59:659-664.

13. Stewart BG, Rhea JT, Sheridan RL, Novilline RA (2002) Is the screening portable pelvis film clinically useful in multiple trauma patients who will be examined by abdominopelvic CT? Experience with 397 patients. *Emerg Radiol* 2002;9:266-271.

14. Their ME, Bensch FV, Koskinen SK. Diagnostic value of pelvic radiography in the initial trauma series in blunt trauma. *Eur Radiol* 2005;15(8):1533-1537.

15. Guillamondegui OD, Pryor JP, Gracias VH et al. Pelvic radiography in blunt trauma resuscitation: A diminishing role. *J Trauma* 2002;53(6):1043-1047.

16. Gylling SF, Ward RE, Holcroft JE, et al. Immediate external fixation of unstable pelvic fractures. *Am J surg* 1985;150:721-724.

17. Bassam D, Cephas GA, Ferguson KA, et al. A protocol for the immediate management of unstable pelvic fractures. *Am Surg* 1998;64(9):862-867.

18. Goldstein A, Phillips T, Sclafani SJ, et al. Early open reduction and internal fixation of the disrupted pelvic ring. *J Trauma* 1986;26:325-333.

19. Gruen GS, Leit ME, Gruen RJ, et al. The acute management of hemodynamically unstable multiple trauma patients with pelvic ring fractures. *J Trauma* 1994;36:706-713.

20. Panetta T, Sclafani SJA, Goldstein AS, et al. Percutaneous transcatheter embolization for massive bleeding pelvic fractures. *J Trauma* 1985;25:1021-1029.

21. Miller PR, Moore PS, Mansell E, et al. External fixation or arteriogram in bleeding pelvic fracture: initial therapy guided by markers of arterial hemorrhage. *J Trauma* 2003;54:437-443.

22. Huittinen VM, Slatis P. Postmortem angiography and dissection of the hypogastric artery in pelvic fractures. *Surgery* 1973;73:454-462.

23. Margolies MN, Ring EJ, Waltman AC et al. Arteriography in the management of hemorrhage from pelvic fractures. *N Engl J Med* 1972;287:317-321.

24. Agolini SF, Shah K, Jaffe J et al. Arterial embolization is a rapid and effective technique for controlling pelvic fracture hemorrhage. *J Trauma* 1997;43:395-399.

25. Velmahos GC, Toutouzas KG, Vassiliu P et al. A prospective study on the safety and efficacy of angiographic embolization for pelvic and visceral injuries. *J Trauma* 2002;53(2):303-308.

26. Eastridge BJ, Starr AJ, Minei JP, et al. The importance of fracture pattern in guiding therapeutic decision making in patients with hemorrhagic shock and pelvic ring disruptions. *J Trauma* 2002;53:446-451.

27. Blackmore CC, Jurkovich GJ, Linnau KF, et al. Assessment of volume of hemorrhage and outcome from pelvic fracture. *Arch Surg* 2003;138:504-509.

28. Sarin EL, Moore JB, Moore EE et al. Pelvic fracture pattern does not always predict the need for urgent embolization. *J Trauma* 2005;58(5):973-977.

29. Wong YC, Wang LJ, Ng CJ, et al. Mortality after successful transcatheter arterial embolization in patients with unstable pelvic fractures: rate of blood transfusion as a predictive factor. *J Trauma* 2000;49:71-75.

30. Sheridan MK, Blackmore CC, Linnau KF et al. Can CT predict the source of arterial hemorrhage in patients with pelvic fractures? *Emerg Radiol* 2002;9(4):188-194.

31. Blackmore CC, Cummings P, Jurkovich GJ, et al. Predicting major hemorrhage in patients with pelvic fracture. *J Trauma* 2006;61:346-352.

32. Velmahos GC, Chawan S, Vassiliu P et al. Angiographic embolization of bilateral internal iliac arteries to control life-threatening hemorrhage following blunt trauma to the pelvis. *Am Surg* 2000;66:858-862.

33. Gourlay D, Hoffer E, Routt M et al. Pelvic angiography for recurrent traumatic pelvic arterial hemorrhage. *J Trauma* 2005;59:1168-1174.

34. Yasamura K, Ikegami K, Kamohara T et al. High incidence of ischemic necrosis of the gluteal muscle after transcatheter angiographic embolization for severe pelvic fracture. *J Trauma* 2005;58(5):985-990.

35. Ramirez JI, Velmahos GC, Best CR et al. Male sexual function after bilateral internal iliac artery embolization for pelvic fracture. *J Trauma* 2004;56:734-741.

36. Latenser BA, Gentilello LM, Tarver AA, et al. Improved outcome with early fixation of skeletally unstable pelvic fractures. *J Trauma* 1991;31:28-31.

37. Ghanayem AJ, Stover MD, Goldstein JA, et al. Emergent treatment of pelvic fractures: comparison of methods for stabilization. *Clin Orthop* 1995;318:75-80.

38. Heini PF, Witt J, Ganz R. The pelvic C clamp for the emergency treatment of unstable pelvic injuries. A report on clinical experience of 30 cases. *Injury* 1996; 27 Supp 1:S A38-45.

39. Sadri H, Nguyen-Tang T, Stern R et al. Control of severe hemorrhage using C clamp and arterial embolization in hemodynamically unstable patients with pelvic disruption. *Arch Orthop Trauma Surg* 2005;125(7): 443-447.

40. Pennal GF, Massiah KA. Non-union and delayed union of fractures of the pelvis. *Clin Orthop Relat Res* 1980;151:124-129.

41. Wild JJ Jr, Hanson GW, Tullos HS. Unstable fractures of the pelvis treated by external fixation. *J Bone Joint Surg Am* 1982;64(7):110-120.

42. Pohlemann T, Braune C, Gansslen A et al. Pelvic emergency clamps: Anatomic landmarks for a safe primary application. *J Orthop Trauma* 2004;18(2):102-105.

43. Ertel W, Keel M, Eid K, et al. Control of severe hemorrhage using C-clamp and pelvic packing in multiply injured patients with pelvic ring disruption. *J Orthop Trauma* 2001;15:468-474.

44. Smith WR, Moore EE, Osborn P et al. Retroperitoneal packing as a resuscitation technique for hemodynamically unstable patients with pelvic fractures: Report of two representative cases and a description of technique. *J Trauma* 2005;59:1510-1514.

45. AL Jones, Powell JN, Kellam JF et al. Open pelvic fractures: a multicenter retrospective analysis. *Orthop Clin North Am* 1997;28:345-349.

46. Brenneman FD, Kaytal D, Boulannger BR, et al. Long term outcome in open pelvic fractures. *J Trauma* 1997;42:773-777.

47. Dente CJ, Feliciano DV, Rozycki GS, et al. The outcome of pelvic fractures in the modern era. *Am J Surg* 2005;190(6):830-835.

48. Kudsk KA, Hanna MK. Management of complex perineal injuries. *World J Surg* 2003;27:895-900.

49. Gosselin R, Roberts I, Gillespie W. Antibiotics for preventing infection in open limb fractures. *Cochrane database Syst rev* 2004;1:CD003764.

50. Raffa J, Christensen NM. Compound fractures of the pelvis. *Am J Surg* 1976;132:282-286.

51. Pell M, Flynn WJ, Seibel RW. Is colostomy always necessary in the treatment of open pelvic fractures? *J Trauma* 1998;45:371-373.

52. Woods RK, O'Keefe G, Rhee P et al. Open pelvic fractures and fecal diversion. *Arch Surg* 1998;133:281-286.

53. Faringer PD, Mullins RJ, Feliciano PD et al. Arch Surg 1994;129(9):958-963 discussion 963-964.

54. Lunsjo K, Abu-Zidan FM. Does colostomy prevent infection in open blunt pelvic fractures? A systematic review. *J Trauma* 2006;60:1145-1148.

55. Ferrera PC, Hill DA. Good outcomes of open pelvic fractures. *Injury* 1999;30:187-190.

56. Hughes TM, Perez JV. A case of rectal infarction after sigmoid colectomy for traumatic perforation in a patient with major pelvic fracture. *J Trauma* 1996;40(2):302-303.

57. Demetriades D, Murray JA, Chan L, et al. Penetrating colon injuries requiring resection: diversion or primary anastamosis? An AAST prospective multicenter study. *J Trauma* 2001;50(5):765-775.

58. Sasaki LS, Allaben R, Golwala R et al. Primary repair of colon injuries: a prospective randomized study. *J Trauma* 1995;39(5):895-901.

59. Gonzalez RP, Merlotti GJ, Holevar MR.Colostomy in penetrating colon injury: is it necessary? *J Trauma* 1996;41(2):271-275.

60. Weinberg JA, Fabian TC, Magnotti LJ et al. Penetrating rectal trauma: Management by anatomic distinction improves outcome. *J Trauma* 2006;60:508-514.

61. Aihara R, Blansfield JS, Millham FH et al. Fracture locations influence the likelihood of rectal and lower urinary tract injuries in patients sustaining pelvic fractures. *J Trauma* 2002;52(2):205-208.

62. Avery G, Blackmore CC, Wessells H, et al. Radiographic and clinical predictors of bladder rupture in blunt trauma patients with pelvic fractures. *Acad Radiol* 2006;13(5): 573-579.

63. Morey AF, Iverson AJ, Swan A et al. Bladder rupture after blunt trauma: guidelines for diagnostic imaging. *J Trauma* 2001;51(4):683-686.

64. Quagliano PV, Delair SM, Malhotra AK. Diagnosis of blunt bladder injury: A prospective comparative study of Computed Tomography Cystography and conventional retrograde cystography. *J Trauma* 2006;61(2): 410-422.

65. Deck AJ, Shaves S, Talner L et al. Computerized tomography cystography for the detection of bladder rupture. *J Urol* 2000;164(1):43-46.

66. Richardson J, Leadbetter G. Nonoperative treatment of the ruptured bladder. *J Urol* 1975;114:213-216.

67. Cass AS, Luxemberg M. management of extraperitoneal ruptures of bladder caused by external trauma. *Urology* 1989;33:179-183.

68. Peters PC. Intraperitoneal rupture of the bladder. *Urol Clin N Amer* 1989;16(2):279-282.

69. Parry NG, Rozycki GS, Feliciano DV, et al. Traumatic rupture of the urinary bladder: Is the suprapubic tube necessary? *J Trauma* 2003;54:431-436.

70. Weinberg JA, Fabian TC, Magnotti LJ et al. Penetrating rectal trauma: Management by anatomic distinction improves outcome. *J Trauma* 2006;60: 508-514.

71. Volpe M, Pachter E, Scalea TM, et al. Is there a difference in outcome when treating traumatic intraperitoneal bladder rupture with or without a suprapubic tube? *J Urol* 1999;161:1103-1105.

72. Thomas KR, Kilambi NK, Poole GV. Method of urinary diversion in non-urethral bladder injuries: retrospective analysis of 70 cases. *Am Surg* 1998;64: 77-81.

73. Margolin DJ, Gonzalez RP. Retrospective analysis of traumatic bladder injury: Does suprapubic catheterization alter outcome of healing? *Am Surg* 2004;70(12): 1057-1059.

74. Ziran BH, Chamberlain E, Shuler FD, et al. Delays and difficulties in the diagnosis of lower urologic injuries in the context of pelvic fractures. *J Trauma* 2005;58(3): 533-537.

75. Koraitim MM, Marzouk ME, Atta MA, et al. Risk factors and mechanisms of urethral injury in pelvic fractures. *Br J Urol* 1996;7:876-880.

76. Lowe MA, Mason JT, Luna GK, et al. Risk factors for urethral injuries in men with traumatic pelvic fractures. *J Urol* 1988;140:506-507.

77. Morehouse DD, Belitsky P, Mackinnon KJ. Rupture of the posterior urethra. *J Urol* 1972;107:255-260.

78. Koraitim MM. Pelvic fracture urethral injuries: the unresolved controversy. *J Urol* 1999;161:1433-1441.

79. Zinke H, Furlowe WH. Long term results with transpubic urethroplasty *J Urol* 1985;133:605-606.

80. Moudouni SM, Patard JJ, Manunta A, et al. Early endoscopic realignment of post-traumatic posterior urethral disruption. *Urology* 2001;57:628-632.

81. Porter JR, Takayama TK, Defalco AJ. Traumatic posterior urethral injury and early realignment using magnetic urethral catheters. *J Urol* 1997;158:425-430.

82. Routt ML, Simonian PT, Defalco AJ, et al. Internal fixation in pelvic fractures and primary repairs of associated genitourinary disruptions: a team approach. *J Trauma* 1996;40(5):784-790.

83. Huittinen VM, Slatis P. Nerve injury in double vertical pelvic fractures. *Acta Chir Scand* 1972;138: 571-575.

84. Majeed SA. Neurologic deficits in major pelvic injuries. *Clin Orthop* 1992;282:222-228.

85. Reilly MC, Zinar DM, Matta JM. Neurologic injuries in pelvic ring fractures. *Clin Orthop* 1996;329:28-36.

86. Denis F, Davis S, Comfort T. Sacral fractures: An important problem. Retrospective analysis of 236 cases. *Clin Orthop* 1988;227:67-81.

87. Shenfeld OZ, Kiselgorf D, Gofrit ON, et al. The incidence and causes of erectile dysfunction after pelvic fractures associated with posterior urethral disruption. *J Urol* 2003;169:2173-2176.

88. Harwood PJ, Grotz M, Eardley I, et al. Erectile dysfunction after fracture of the pelvis. *J Bone Joint Surg Br* 2005;87-B:281-290.

89. Wright JL, Nathens AB, Rivara FP, et al. Specific configurations predict sexual and excretory dysfunction in men and women 1 year after pelvic fracture. *J Urol* 2006;176:1540-1545.

90. Spiguel L, Glynn L, Liu D, et al. Pediatric pelvic fractures: A marker for injury severity. *Am Surg* 2006;72: 481-484.

91. Demetriades D, Karaiskakis M, Velmahos GC, et al. Pelvic fractures in pediatric and adult trauma patients: are they different injuries? *J Trauma* 2003;54(6): 1146-1151.

92. Tarman GJU, Kaplan GW, Lerman SL, et al. Lower genitourinary injury and pelvic fractures in pediatric patients. *Urology* 2002;59(1):123-126.

93. Signorino PR, Densmore J, Werner M, et al. Pediatric pelvic injury functional outcome at 6 month follow-up. *J Ped Surg* 2005;40(1):107-112 discussion 112-113.

94. O'Brien DP, Luchette FA, Pereira SJ, et al. Pelvic fracture in the elderly is associated with increased mortality. *Surgery* 2002;132:710-715.

95. Kimbrell BJ, Velmahos GC, Chan LS, et al. Angiographic embolization for pelvic fractures in older patients. *Arch Surg* 2004;139:728-733.

96. Henry SM, Pollack AN, Jones AL, et al. Pelvic fracture in geriatric patients: A distinct clinical entity. *J Trauma* 2002;53:15-20.

97. Leung WY, Ban CM, Lam JJ, et al. Prognosis of acute pelvic fractures in elderly patients: retrospective study. *Hong Kong Med J* 2001;7(2):139-145.

98. Leggon RE, Wood GC, Indeck MC. Pelvic fractures in pregnancy: factors influencing maternal and fetal outcomes. *J Trauma* 2002;53(4):796-804.

99. Curet MJ, Schermer CR, Cemarest GB, Bieneik EJ, Curet LB. Predictors of outcome in trauma during pregnancy: identification of patients who can be monitored for less than 6 hours. *J Trauma.* 2000;49:18-24.

100. Morris JA, Rosenbower TJ, Jurkovich GJ, et al. Infant survival after cesarean section for trauma. *Ann Surg.* 1996;5:481-491.

101. Pohlemann T, Gansslen A, Schellwald O, et al. Outcome after pelvic ring injuries. *Injury* 1996;27:B31-B38.

102. Dujardin FH, Hossenbaccus M, Duparc F, et al, Long term functional prognosis of posterior injuries in high energy pelvic disruption. *J Orthop Trauma* 1998;12(3): 145-150.

103. Kabak S, Halici M, Tuncel M, et al. Funcitonal outcome of open reduction and internal fixation for completely unstable pelvic ring fractures: a report of 40 cases. *J Orthop Trauma* 2003;17(8):555-562.

104. Gruen GS, Leit ME, Gruen RJ, et al. Functional outcome of patients with unstable pelvic ring fractures stabilized with open reduction and internal fixation. *J Trauma* 1995;39(5):838-845.

Chapter **31**

SPINAL CORD INJURY

Kimball I. Maull, MD, and Peter Letarte, MD

INTRODUCTION

There is no greater example in acute care surgery where the expression "First do no harm" is more applicable than in the patient with potential spinal cord injury.[1] The inherent risk to the patient and the practitioner alike make protecting the patient from further injury the overriding concern. Although the primary injury usually determines the ultimate neurologic fate of the patient, it is estimated that 2%-10% of patients with cervical spine injuries suffer additional neurologic injury despite adequate precautions. In certain subgroups of patients, aggravation of the initial injury appears unavoidable and is related to secondary mechanisms such as bleeding into or around the spinal cord, ischemia-reperfusion injury, and the consequences of the inflammatory cascade. Failure to recognize spinal instability jeopardizes patient outcome, however. In a recent multicenter study of the problem, insufficient imaging studies, misreads, and poor quality radiographs were cited as contributing factors.[2]

Spinal cord injuries most commonly occur following motor vehicle crashes, involving both occupants and pedestrians; falls; sports-related injuries, including water sports and diving; and penetrating wounds. Both spinal column and spinal cord injury can follow relatively trivial injury mechanisms, especially in the elderly.[3] Approximately 15% of spinal column injuries involve the spinal cord. Of these, 40% occur in the cervical region, 15% in the thorax, 35% at the thoracolumbar area, and 5% in the lumbar region. Involvement of two noncontiguous areas occurs in 5% of cases. In this chapter, the emphasis on initial management, assessment of spinal stability, and the prevention of complications are intended to optimize outcomes in the group of critically injured patients.

ANATOMIC CONSIDERATIONS

The spinal cord is typically divided into cervical, thoracic, lumbar, and sacral segments. From an injury mechanism perspective, which relates to points of both motion and fixation and facet joint relationships within the spinal column, it is more pertinent to divide the spinal anatomy into five segments: (1) the proximal cervical spine from occiput to the second cervical vertebra, (2) the remaining cervical spine from the third through the seventh cervical vertebra, (3) the thoracic spine from the first through the eleventh thoracic vertebra, (4) the thoracolumbar junction, which includes the twelfth thoracic vertebra and first lumbar vertebra, and (5) the lumbosacral spine from the second lumbar vertebra through the sacrum. The spinal cord is well protected through its course in the spinal column by a series of articulating vertebrae, supported by a complex series of ligaments and muscles that maintain the precise configuration of the spinal cord and spinal nerve roots. In the cervical region, movement of the spine is facilitated by obliquely oriented facet joints, whereas in the thoracic region, the facet joints are more coronally oriented, which allow rotation but limit other motion. In the lumbar spine, the facets are sagitally aligned to facilitate flexion, extension, and lateral bending. Be mindful that the spinal canal is relatively spacious in the high cervical areas and is more limited in the thoracic region.

The blood supply to the spinal cord is from the anterior spinal artery and paired posterior spinal arteries that descend from the intracranial portion of the vertebral arteries and are reinforced by branches from the ascending cervical, cervical portion of the vertebrals, intercostals, and lumbar arteries. The anterior spinal artery supplies the anterior white matter and central gray matter and is interrupted in the lower thoracic spine in 30% of individuals. The posterior spinal arteries supply the posterior and posterolateral white matter of the spinal cord.

BIOMECHANICS AND PATHOPHYSIOLOGY OF INJURY

Injuries to the spinal cord are directly related to injuries of the spinal column. Compression, hyperextension, hyperflexion, and distraction are the principal mechanisms of injury to the spinal column. If the spine is rotated at the moment the force is applied, a combination of these injury mechanisms may be produced. These may lead to spinal cord impact with persistent compression, impact alone with only transient compression, transaction, and/or stretching. Because of its mobility and relative exposure compared with other portions of the spine, the cervical spine is most vulnerable to injury. It is in particular danger from axial loading, which may cause burst fracture through the body of the first cervical vertebra (Jefferson fracture). Hyperextension at the second cervical vertebra from deceleration forces applied to the upper face may lead to odontoid fracture or, in severe circumstances, bilateral fractures of the second cervical ring (hangman fracture) (Fig. 31-1).

Hyperflexion injuries predominate at the lower cervical spine, which may lead to both fractures and dislocations, most commonly at the fifth and sixth cervical vertebrae. Disruption or transposition of the facet joints may occur, leading to instability of the spinal column. Distraction causes traumatic stretching of the spinal cord, often without radiographic evidence of spinal fracture, and is believed to contribute to the spinal cord injury without radiologic abnormality (SCIWORA) commonly seen in children. The underdeveloped vertebral column and hyperelasticity of tissues found in children contribute to this phenomenon.

The thoracic spine is most commonly injured by a direct blow or a hyperflexion. Compression forces also may affect the thoracic spine if the individual sustains axial loading while the thoracic spine is held in flexion (Fig. 31-2). At the thoracolumbar junction, hyperflexion injuries predominate with likely risk from axial loading which may lead to burst fractures. These are often accompanied by significant ligamentous injury

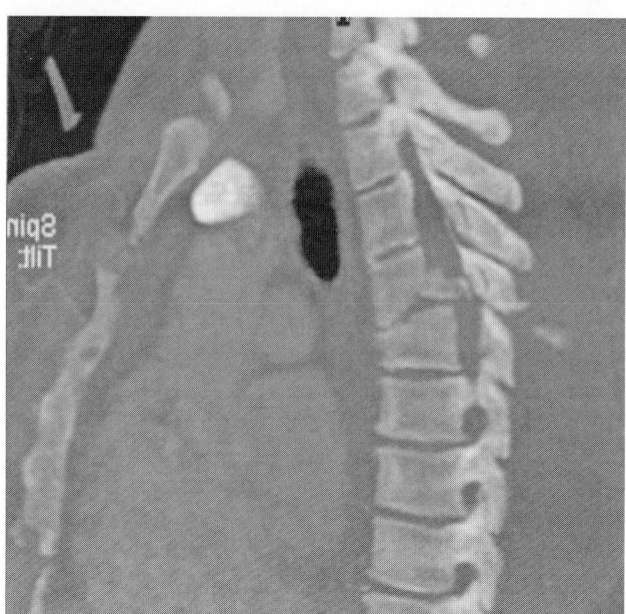

Figure 31-2 *CT showing midthoracic fracture with extrusion of bony fragment into spinal canal.*

and extrusion of bone into the spinal canal. Lumbar fractures usually are caused by hyperflexion, which favors compression fractures.

Complete transaction of the spinal cord is uncommon. Total interruption of spinal cord function occurs in the absence of anatomic transaction, however. This "disconnect" between the brain and effector organs is most often caused by vascular compromise to the spinal cord, which leads to cord ischemia and hemorrhagic necrosis. These vascular changes begin in the gray matter and coalesce to involve the peripheral white matter. The extent of the involvement is most closely related to the initial (primary) injury. Usually by 72 hours postinjury, the full extent of cord compromise is realized and may spread as much as two spinal segments proximal. Autoregulation at the site of injury is lost, and local perfusion of the cord becomes dependent on the systemic arterial blood pressure. Interruption of neuronal conduction through the injured cord is probably related to a combination of mechanical disruption, ischemia, and cord edema, which occurs soon after injury. This vasogenic edema causes cellular swelling, exacerbation of neural deformities, and compromise of local capillary circulation.

More recently, the inflammatory response following spinal cord injury has been implicated as major contributor to secondary injury. Based primarily on aberrations in the arachidonic acid pathway with the conversion of arachidonic acid to prostanoids, local vasoconstriction and lipid peroxidation lead to apoptosis and up-regulation and excitotoxicity. Current research focuses on blocking the arachidonic acid conversion to temper this inflammatory response and on COX-2 inhibition to reduce further spinal cord injury.

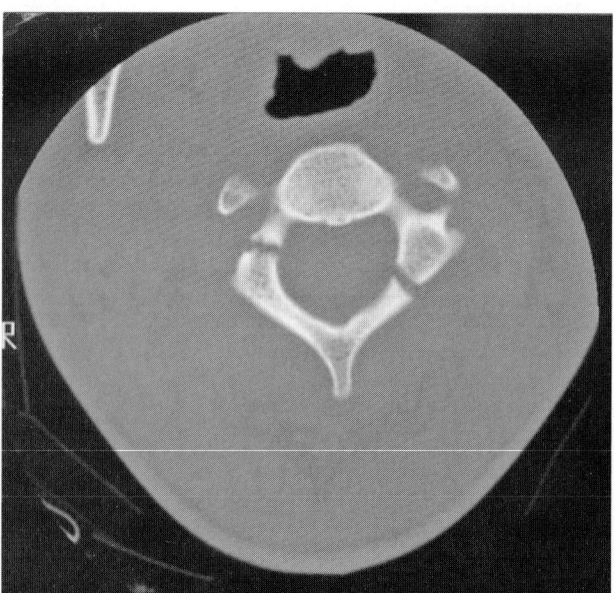

Figure 31-1 *CT showing fracture through right pedicle and left pars of 2nd cervical vertebra (hangman fracture)*

INITIAL MANAGEMENT

IMMOBILIZATION, EXTRICATION, AND TRANSPORT

During the past three decades, the frequency of spinal injuries in patients arriving at the hospital has declined. In part, this is related to improved prehospital care and retrieval technology and the awareness of the importance of immediate spinal immobilization and maintenance of immobilization until clearance is obtained. Early immobilization of the patient, optimally while the patient is still in the vehicle, is recommended to avoid mechanical damage to the spinal cord during extrication. All victims of blunt trauma must be considered at risk and "guilty of spinal injury until proven innocent" by appropriate clinical and radiologic examinations. Conventional thinking adheres to the principles that the vehicle should be removed from the patient, not vice versa. This is not always possible, however, and limitation of spinal motion is critical. Therefore, motor vehicle occupants should be placed in a stiff cervical collar and a short spine board where the cervical collar is maintained and further movement is restricted by taping the head and shoulders to the spine board. These measures allow the patient to be transported in the supine position and permit the patient to be rotated en bloc to the lateral position to prevent aspiration in the event of vomiting. For this reason, sandbags alone are contraindicated. These precautions are based on the recognition that neurologic function can be further compromised by undue motion of an unstable spine.

Spinal immobilization is not innocuous. Skin breakdown, as well as unsafe positioning, are time-dependent complications. Conventional wisdom calls for early assessment of the spine to exclude unstable injuries. Spinal immobilization also restricts access to the patient, makes airway insertion more difficult, and compromises nursing care. Use of a protocol for removing the patient from the spine board can significantly reduce spine board immobilization times.[4] The cervical collar may hide potential neck injuries. It is important to remove the anterior portion of the immobilization collar to examine the neck for external signs of trauma, deformity, swelling, tracheal position, and the presence and audible sounds of the carotid pulses. An assistant should maintain the neck in neutral position during this examination. The cervical collar also elevates intracranial pressure, an unwanted side effect in the head-injured patient. If the spine is "cleared," the patient can be safely removed from both the spine board and the cervical collar.

AIRWAY MANAGEMENT

Prevention of hypoxia is critical to avoiding secondary insults to the spinal cord. Unstable injuries to the cervical spine place the patient requiring an emergency airway at added risk. Although all patients with blunt trauma should be considered at risk, the overall incidence of cervical spine injury is approximately 2%.[5] The presence of coma, focal deficit, or the existence of a spinal injury elsewhere signal an increased likelihood of cervical spine injury. Adequate radiographic assessment of the cervical spine is not always possible prior to the need for airway placement, and an approach that allows for smooth uninterrupted ventilation and the accurate and atraumatic insertion of a definitive airway without jeopardizing the spinal cord clearly benefits the patient. Therefore, some form of immobilization during airway management is imperative. All airway techniques, including bag-valve-mask ventilation and laryngeal mask airway (LMA), produce some element of cervical spine motion.[5] These movements are small and restricted by in-line immobilization, but they are not eliminated completely.

No Class I data exist that advocate one technique over another or confirm a greater risk of neurologic injury using one specific technique versus another. Most anesthesiologists favor bronchoscopic-assisted endotracheal tube insertion, preferable with the patient awake. It is clear that not all circumstances afford these controlled conditions for intubation. In the unconscious patient, most surgeons and emergency physicians favor orotracheal intubation with in-line immobilization maintained by an assistant.[6] In the awake patient, the same technique is favored, supplemented by rapid sequence induction. Nasotracheal intubation, once preferred in terms of restricting cervical motion, has been shown to cause similar cervical spine motion and has its own set of complications if the airway is left in place for long periods. This form of intubation remains an option in the nonapneic patient, however. Cricothyroidotomy is an appropriate alternative if oral or nasal intubations are unsuccessful and is considered safe in terms of preventing cervical motion. Gerling et al[7] recently studied the technique in cadavers undergoing cricothyroidotomy and demonstrated small but reproducible cervical spine displacements.

Current thinking regarding airway management in the patient either at increased risk for or with documented unstable cervical spine injury includes the range of options described above but requires continued spine immobilization in all instances.

RESUSCITATION AND INITIAL ASSESSMENT

Avoiding further injury by proper spinal immobilization and establishment of a definitive airway and ventilation constitute the first steps in resuscitation. Otherwise, the approach to the injured patient with cervical spine injury differs little from other multisystem injured patients. The patient's hemodynamic status is quickly assessed. Two large-bore intravenous cannulas are placed and volume replenishment is begun. Evaluation should proceed in an orderly manner consistent with conventional protocols of primary and secondary clinical assessments. Fractures of the thoracic and lumbar spine often indicate significant acceleration or deceleration and increase the probability of associated injuries. These must be suspected, sought, and dealt with as appropriate. Shock in the spinal cord–injured patient is especially deleterious. Although hypovolemic shock is common in the multisystem-injured patient, it is usually accompanied by tachycardia and an identifiable source of bleeding.

The finding of hypotension and bradycardia should raise suspicions for neurogenic shock and also alert the clinician to the presence of cervical or high thoracic spinal cord injury, if not already diagnosed. Treatment consists of aggressive volume replacement to refill the intravascular compartment, which is dilated from the loss of sympathetic tone. An indwelling urinary catheter allows measurement of urine output. Response to infusions may be further aided by placement of a central venous catheter. Failure to maintain an adequate blood pressure or recurrent transient responses, which are infusion dependent, require pressors to reestablish intravascular tone and avoid deleterious third spacing. Dopamine in therapeutic doses and neosynephrine are favored in this setting and can be tapered over time. It is wise to remember that hemorrhagic shock and neurogenic shock can coexist and, although volume replacement is therapeutic in both instances, ongoing bleeding must be recognized and controlled surgically, if necessary, to optimize outcome.

The complete secondary survey includes the neurologic examination, which is of obvious relevance in the spinal cord-injured patient. In the awake patient, inability to move the extremities and detection of a sensory level are reliable indicators of spine injury. Flaccidity, loss of tendon reflexes, loss of rectal tone, and priapism, are other findings on examination, which support the diagnosis of spinal cord injury. Incomplete deficits are especially important to detect, document, and time. Progression of an incomplete deficit is considered an emergency and may mandate intervention, including surgery.

RADIOGRAPHIC EVALUATION

Recent advances in imaging technology have altered the approach to visualization of the spine and spinal cord in the acutely injured patient.[8] (Figs. 31-3 and 31-4). Rapid, multislice computed tomographic (CT) scanners and magnetic resonance imaging (MRI) allow high-resolution of skeletal (with CT) and soft-tissue (with MRI) detail, including the spinal cord and supporting ligaments.[9,10] Immediate three-dimensional (3-D) CT reconstruction of bony structures provides real-time and precise anatomic detail of skeletal fractures, subluxations, and dislocations (Figs. 31-5 and 31-6). Three-dimensional CT reconstruction can be used without plain radiographs to evaluate these features of the cervical, thoracic, and lumbosacral spine.[11] As these technologies become more widely available,

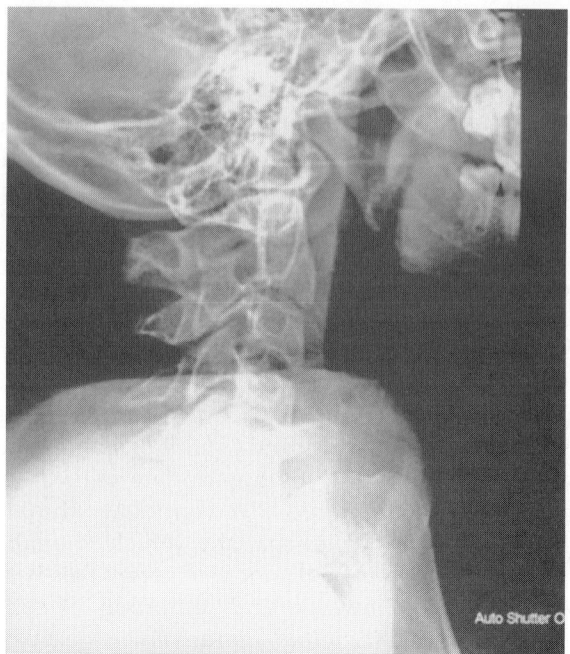

Figure 31-3 *Inadequate lateral cervical spine radiograph showing only first four vertebra. No fracture evident.*

radiologic assessment of the spine and spinal cord will likely involved the routine use of both of these modalities. Access to these technologies is still limited, and, in many areas, plan radiographs remain the "workhorse" for the diagnosis of spine trauma.

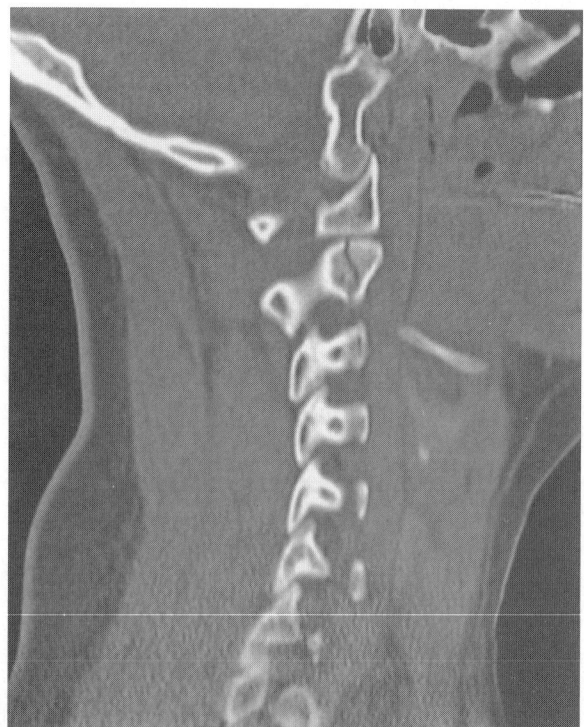

Figure 31-4 *High-resolution CT in same patient as in Fig. 31.3. Fracture clearly visible through body of second cervical vertebra.*

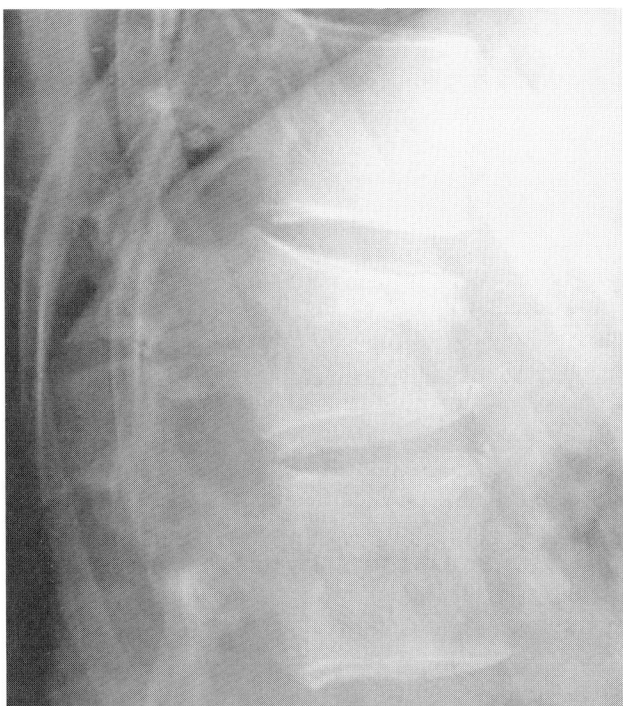

Figure 31-5 *Plain radiograph of first lumbar vertebra showing compression fracture with extension to posterior elements.*

Standard radiographic screening of the acutely injured patient includes a supine anterior-posterior (A-P) chest film, a lateral view of the cervical spine, and an A-P view of the pelvis. Recently, the routine use of plain films of the cervical spine has been challenged.[13]

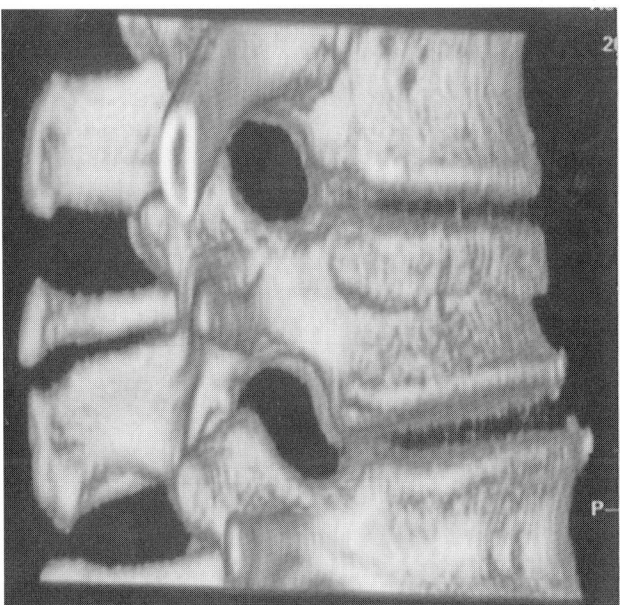

Figure 31-6 *Three-dimensional CT reconstruction at same level (first lumbar vertebra) showing extent of injury in greater detail.*

Based on the facts that the vast majority of patients with blunt injury do not have cervical spine injuries and that enormous resources are wasted evaluating patients with a low likelihood of injury, the necessity for radiographic assessment of the spine in the patient with blunt trauma has been studied independently by two groups.[14,15] In both studies, criteria apply only if the patient is alert, is stable, and has no neurologic deficit.

The National Emergency X-Ray Utilization Study (NEXUS) established low-risk criteria for spinal cord injury (Table 31-1). According to this criteria, distracting injuries were defined as any injury that could impair the patient's ability to react during the clinical assessment, including long-bone fractures, torso trauma requiring surgery, and major soft-tissue injuries, such as crush injuries, burns, and degloving injuries. The decision instrument was applied in the evaluation of over 34,000 patients with a negative predictive value of 99.8%. More recently, the NEXUS decision instrument also was shown to perform well in children.[16] The Canadian C-Spine Decision Rules, which use similar criteria but have more restrictive definitions for intoxication and distraction injuries, also resulted in a high degree of safety when their criteria were applied in the clinical setting.[17] Despite both studies outperforming unstructured physician decision making, the authors caution against using the criteria as the sole determinant of whether to image the cervical spine.[18] It is clear that the clinician must balance clinical judgment with any criteria used to reduce the use of radiographic studies.

Assessment of spine trauma requires A-P and lateral views of the cervical, thoracic, and lumbar spines. An open-mouth odontoid view is part of the initial radiographic assessment of the cervical spine. On the lateral view, the spine must be clearly visualized from the occiput through the top of the first thoracic vertebra. Although an adequate lateral cervical spine film will detect > 80% of cervical spine injuries, it can miss unstable and potentially life-threatening injuries (Figs. 31-7 and 31-8). Lack of visualization of the cervicothoracic junction can be addressed by a "swimmer's view," but this approach has largely been abandoned because of poor image quality and clearer delineation afforded by CT. Oblique views of the cervical spine, although still part of the standard protocol at some

Table 31-1 NEXUS Low-risk Criteria for Spinal Radiography
No neck pain
No posterior midline neck tenderness
No focal neurologic deficit
Absence of intoxication
No distracting injuries

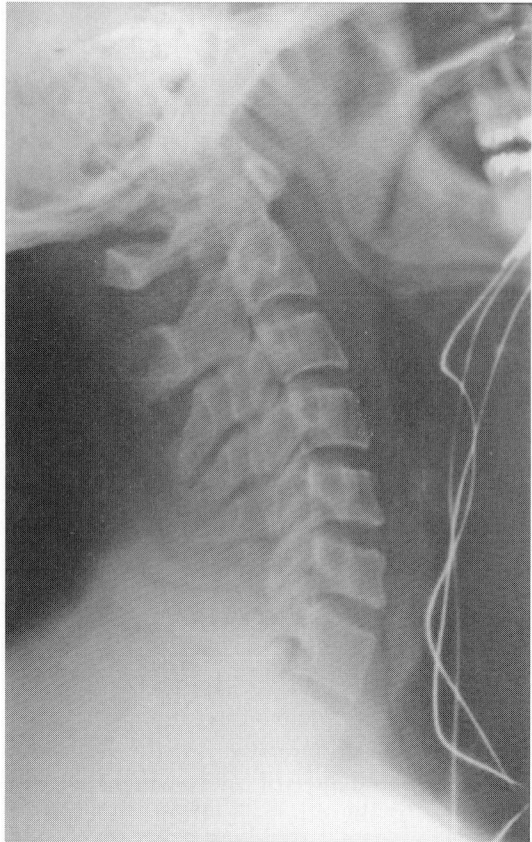

Figure 31-7   *Admission lateral cervical spine radiograph read as normal. Patient heavily intoxicated but asymptomatic.*

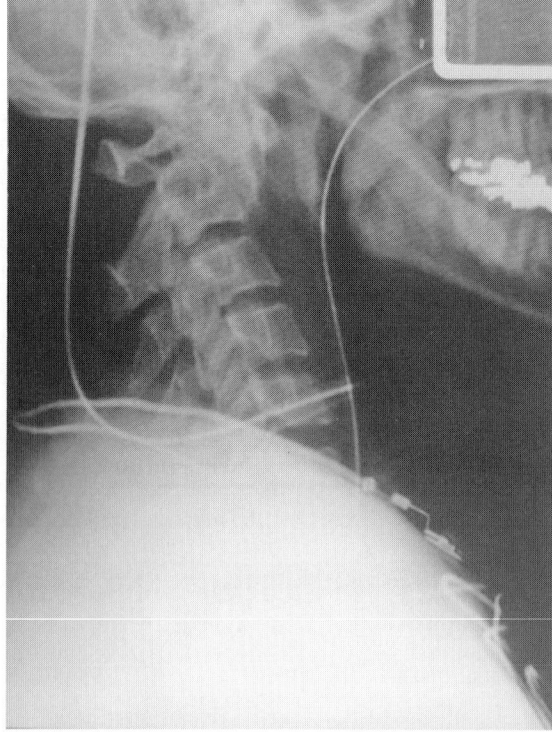

Figure 31-8   *Lateral cervical spine radiograph in same patient as shown in Fig. 31.7 showing highly unstable injury at second cervical vertebra.*

institutions, add little to the overall accuracy of radiographic assessment and are considered by most to be superfluous.[19]

Any fracture or questionable abnormality on plain radiographs should be studied with thin-cut CT imaging. Any focal neurologic deficit or unexplained neck pain should be evaluated through an MRI study, even if the CT image is normal. MRI has the added advantage of demonstrating soft-tissue detail, including the spinal cord, the supporting ligaments, intervertebral disc anatomy, and adjacent edema. MRI is very sensitive but is also nonspecific. Many of the "bright spots" seen on MRI turn out to be of little or no clinical significance. For this reason, MRI was not included in early spine clearance protocols. Its use is now permitted when the MRI is obtained within the first 48 hours postinjury and where the findings are specific enough to be useful. Under these circumstances, MRI can be used to ascertain ligamentous stability, and can replace flexion-extension views.[20,21]

The approach to "clearing the C-spine" has been exhaustively studied. There is a clear distinction between the patient who is awake and alert and the patient who is unresponsive. Clinical Practice Guidelines from the Eastern Association for the Surgery of Trauma (EAST) are one of several approaches currently used to diagnose cervical spine injury and determine the need for continued cervical spine immobilization in the obtunded patient.[22,23] In a clinical reassessment of the EAST guidelines in 124 patients, Ghanta et al[24] concluded that the guidelines were reliable in detecting bony injury in the obtunded patient but were not sensitive enough to diagnose ligamentous injuries or disc herniations. These concerns were amplified by Barrett et al[25] who discovered that over 30% of patients with a cervical spine injury detected by plain films harbored additional spinal injuries and 25% of these injuries were noncontiguous.[25] These authors recommended complete cervical spine CT in this setting.

Basic and advanced algorithms for clearing the cervical spine are presented in Figs. 31-9 and 31-10. The basic algorithm relies almost exclusively on plain radiography and assumes limited CT availability with no access to advanced CT technology or MRI, whereas the advanced algorithm assumes access to both of these advanced imaging modalities. Note that swimmers views and flexion-extension films are no longer considered necessary for clearing the cervical spine if the advanced imaging modalities are available. The clinician should integrate these two algorithms based on imaging availability and the patient's clinical status.

In the absence of an MRI, there will be a small subgroup of patients who lack definitive clearance because of the inability of the practitioner to visualize the entire cervical spine under fluoroscopy. Clinical judgment must be used to determine when and whether to remove cervical immobilization in these patients. It

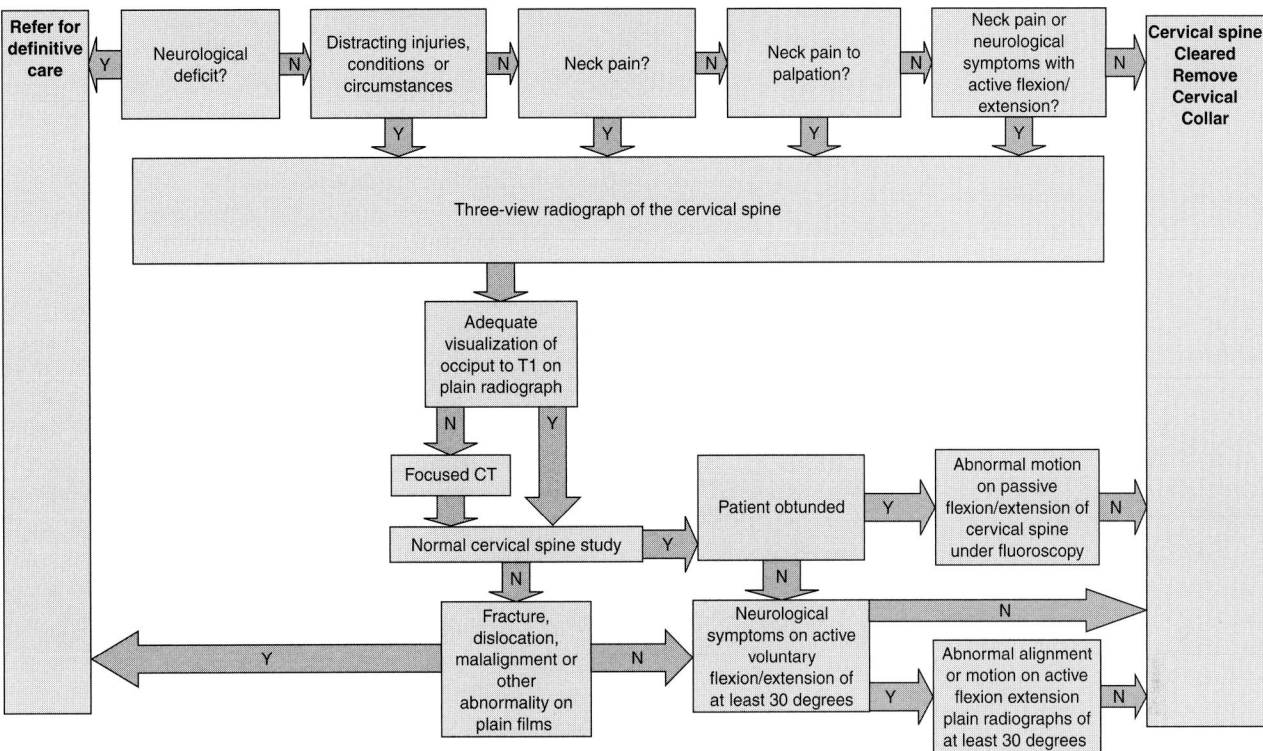

Figure 31-9 *Basic algorithm for clearing the cervical spine following blunt injury in setting without high-resolution CT and MRI.*

also must be emphasized that the finding of a spinal injury at any level mandates radiologic evaluation of the entire vertebral column. Although there is no need to rush the removal of cervical collars, long-term use of these devices limits patient's access, compromises nursing care, and may cause pressure necrosis. In certain critically injured patients who cannot tolerate MRI, a neurosurgical consultation is recommended.

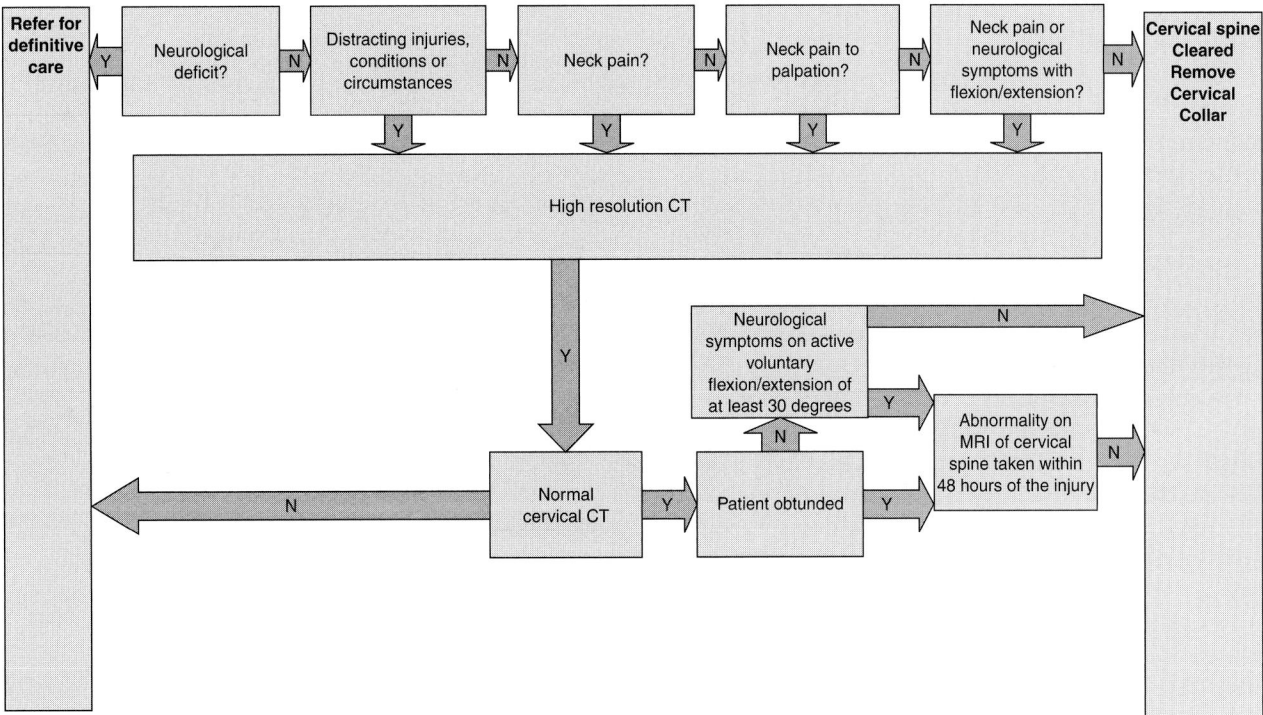

Figure 31-10 *Advanced algorithm for clearing the cervical spine following blunt injury using high-resolution CT and MRI.*

EMERGENCY TREATMENT

PHARMACOLOGIC THERAPY

If a patient shows any signs of a spinal cord injury, complete or incomplete, high-dose methylprednisolone is considered the standard of care.[26] The loading dose should be given as soon as possible but within the first 8 hours postinjury. A dose of 30 mg/kg is given intravenously over the first hour, followed by 5.4 mg/kg/h as an infusion over the next 23 hours. The National Spinal Cord Injury Study: Part III recommends that the infusion be continued for 48 hours if the initial bolus infusion is administered between 3 and 8 hours postinjury. The unopposed parasympathetic effects on the stomach cause gastric hypersecretion, and gastritis/stress ulcer prophylaxis is indicated in the presence of high-dose corticosteroids. The benefit of methylprednisolone on spinal cord injury caused by penetrating wounds has not been demonstrated, and some data show increased complications associated with its use in this context.[27,28] Its use under these circumstances should be avoided.

CERVICAL TRACTION

When a fracture or dislocation of the cervical spine is identified radiographically, traction with MRI-compatible Gardner–Wells tongs is indicated. The tongs are applied to the skull slightly posterior to the external auditory canal to provide a slight bit of extension to the axial traction. Initially, 3 pounds per interspace is applied with follow-up lateral radiographs to determine appropriate alignment and identify any overdistraction after each increment. Additional weight can be added up to 10 pounds per interspace. Although no clear upper limit of weight is described in the literature, the least amount of weight needed to achieve reduction should be used, and patients require careful, frequent imaging to guard against overdistraction and further injury. Local practice may establish limits to guard against such mishaps. Traction is not recommended if a second rostral injury is present or if there is injury at C2. Care should be exercised in patients with ankylosing spondylitis because very little weight may be needed to reduce these patients. with ankylosing spondylosis

Patients who cannot be examined while traction is applied should have an MRI prior to traction placement. The presence of a herniated disc on MRI may indicate that the disc should be removed prior to the placement of traction. Widening of the disc space or insterspinous distance suggests that further traction may be hazardous. Reduction is facilitated by judicious doses of morphine and muscle relaxants. If reduction cannot be achieved, and the patient is not on a ventilator, the patient may be carefully intubated and administered paralytics. Manual reduction with fluoroscopy is usually successful under these circumstances.

After the fracture or dislocation is reduced, the traction weight also should be reduced to the minimum required to maintain the spine in alignment. Patients whose dislocation is not reduced should undergo MRI.

Cervical traction is not without risk. In young patients with ligamentous laxity, stretching of the cord may occur from overdistraction. Fractures are usually complete, occur most commonly through the intervertebral disc, and disrupt the ligamentous support.[29] Neurologic complications are found in more than 15% of these patients. The preexisting deformity can lead to further cord compression if cervical traction is applied too vigorously. Manipulation of the spine must be done with great care in these patients. Occasionally, cervical traction will unintentionally facilitate protrusion of the disc material leading to cord compression. This finding must be recognized immediately and be addressed as a surgical emergency.

EMERGENCY OPERATION

The timing of operative intervention remains a subject of great debate.[30] Supporters of early operation believe that early decompression of the spinal cord may improve return of neurologic function and that early stabilization may prevent secondary mechanical damage to the cord. Patients undergoing early operation also can be mobilized sooner, thereby reducing pulmonary complications, skin breakdown, and other morbidities related to prolonged immobilization. Opponents of early operation cite the effectiveness of traction in reducing skeletal abnormalities and maintaining spinal column stability and the lack of data supporting improved outcome from early operation. There is agreement that early operation should be performed for CSF leak, for failed reduction following closed manipulation or traction methods, and for conus medullaris lesions. Emergency operation is indicated for worsening neurologic deficit, especially in the presence of bone fragments in the canal. If there is no apparent anatomic basis for neurologic deterioration based on plain films or CT, and emergency MRI should be performed to detect the etiology of cord compression. In certain cases, no surgically remediable cause is detected, and T2-weighted MRI images may show high-density signal in the central cord with cephalad extension from the site of injury. This finding most likely represents cord edema, and an emergency operation is unlikely to offer much benefit.

NEUROLOGIC INJURY PATTERNS

COMPLETE VERSUS INCOMPLETE CORD INJURY

Spinal cord injury is defined in terms of the level affected and the completeness of the neurologic deficit. Every effort should be made to determine as soon as possible whether the injury is complete or incomplete. The best time to make this assessment is immediately after the injury and before progression of the spinal contusion. Spinal shock is a physiologic block to nerve conduction that occurs in the absence of structural damage to the spinal cord. It is not to be confused with neurogenic shock, which refers to the hemodynamic changes caused by the interruption of sympathetic pathways that lead to hypotension and slowing of the heart. During the period of spinal shock, certain reflex arcs, which can function without the input of higher centers, are knocked out. For example, the anal wink and bulbocavernous reflex are lost but typically return within 24 hours, an important prognostic sign. Sacral sparing should be determined because intact sacral sensation confirms an incomplete lesion. Sacral sparing is thought to be due to the peripheral location of the sacral neurons, the portion of the spinal cord most resistant to injury.

A complete cord injury means the total loss of neurologic function below the level of the injury. The spinal level is identified by the most distant spinal segment that is still intact. For example, sensation absent below the nipples indicates a T4-level injury. The presence of any motor or sensory function below the level of the injury defines an incomplete cord injury. Knowledge of segmental innervation is useful in determining cord injury level and symmetry of the deficit (Table 31-2). Motor function can be assessed by grading muscle strength and applying an impairment scale

according to the American Spinal Injury Association (ASIA) (Tables 31-3 and 31-4). This provides a uniform method for assessing postinjury motor and sensory status. It further classifies patients according to injury severity, providing a useful decision-making and prognostic tool. By standardizing the assessment, reliable comparisons can be made by members of the health care team as the patient moves through the trauma care continuum from emergency department to rehabilitation. Progress can be monitored and declines can be identified more rapidly.

ANTERIOR CORD SYNDROME

Anterior cord syndrome is caused by interruption of the blood supply to the anterior spinal cord or to direct

Table 31-3   ASIA Assessment of Muscle Strength

Finding	Grade
Total paralysis	0
Palpable or visible contractions	1
Active movement, full range of motion—not against gravity	2
Active movement, full range of motion—against gravity	3
Active movement, full range of motion—against gravity and provides some resistance	4
Active movement, full range of motion—against gravity and provides normal resistance	5

NT = not testable due to factors such as immbolization, pain, or contracture
International Standards for Neurological Classification of SCI published by The American Spinal Injury Association. (ASIA,)

Table 31-2   Relationship of Spinal Segmental Levels to Muscle Function

Level affected	Muscles affected
C3/4/5	Diaphragm
C5	Biceps
C6	Wrist extensors
C7	Triceps/wrist flexors
C8	Finger flexors
T1	Hand intrinsics
T2-T9	Intercostals
T10-T12	Abdominals
T12-L1	Cremasterics
L2	Ilipsoas
L3	Quadriceps
L4	Tibialis anterior
L5	Extensor hallucis
S1	Gastrocnemius
S2	Bladder sphincter
S3	Anal sphincter
S4	Bulbocavernosis

Table 31-4   ASIA Impairment Scale

Finding	Grade
No motor or sensory function and none preserved in sacral segments S4-S5	A = Complete
Sensory, but not motor function, preserved below injury level, including S4-S5	B = Incomplete
Motor function preserved below injury level; > 50% of muscles < grade 3	C = Incomplete
Motor function preserved below injury level; > 50% of muscles > grade 3	D = Incomplete
Motor and sensory functions are normal	E = Normal

International Standards for Neurological Classification of SCI published by The American Spinal Injury Association (ASIA).

trauma limited to the anterior portion of the cord. This type of spinal cord injury is seen following thoracic aorta replacement and is related to a discontinuous anterior spinal artery, which is present in 30% of the population. Injury to the anterior spinal cord causes loss of motor function, pain, and temperature sensation below the level of injury. Proprioception and deep pressure sensation are unaffected. In the usual circumstance where the loss of anterior cord function is complete, prognosis is poor for return of any meaningful function.

CENTRAL CORD SYNDROME

Central cord syndrome tends to occur in patients with preexisting cervical stenosis where space limitations favor the distribution of forces directly to the center of the cord, sparing the periphery. This is reflected in patients over 60 years of age having a poorer prognosis.[31] The etiology of central cord syndrome has been classically described as being based on contusion of the central part of the cord. Recent MRI studies, however, failed to show a correlation between the clinical findings and the anatomy of the cord injury.[32] Because the tracts carrying motor and sensory function to the lower extremities are located laterally, neurologic function to the legs is preserved while the upper extremities may be severely affected. This syndrome carries a more favorable prognosis than the anterior cord syndrome, although residual deficits, especially in the hands, are common.

BROWN–SÉQUARD SYNDROME

Brown–Séquard syndrome is caused by an interruption in the lateral half of the spinal cord and is most commonly seen following penetrating trauma. In complete lesions, there is ipsilateral loss of motor function, proprioception, and deep sensation, as well as contralateral loss of pain and temperature. Incomplete lesions have a more favorable outlook for return of function.

CONUS MEDULARIS INJURIES

Injuries at the lowest portion of the spinal cord usually cause symmetrical lower extremity deficits and may affect the bowel and bladder. Radicular pain is usually absent. Diagnosis rests on confirmation via CT or MRI testing or compression on the conus medularis. If present, this type of injury constitutes a valid indication for early operative decompression to avoid permanent bowel and bladder dysfunction.

CAUDA EQUINA INJURIES

Injuries to the cauda equina cause asymmetrical lower extremity deficits and are commonly accompanied by radicular pain or dysethesias. As opposed to other spinal cord lesions, these present with lower motor neuron findings—hyporeflexia and sensory loss in various nerve root distributions. The function of the bowel and bladder may be retained. Operative

intervention for decompression may be indicated, but it is not as urgent as with conus injuries.

ACCESSING SPINAL STABILITY

The diagnosis of spinal column injury and determination of whether the injury is stable or unstable have obvious implications for both treatment and outcome. Stability is defined as the ability of the spine to limits its displacement and, under physiologic conditions, protect the underlying spinal cord and spinal nerve roots from injury. Unstable injuries are those whereby, under the same conditions, the spine cannot prevent further injury to the spinal cord or spinal nerve roots.

Assessment of spinal stability can be difficult. The three-column concept embraces the importance of an intact posterior ligament complex in maintaining spinal stability. This complex includes the interspinous and supraspinous ligaments, capsules of the facet joints, and ligamentum flavum. The middle column consists of the posterior one-third of the vertebral bodies and discs with the attached posterior longitudinal ligament. The anterior column consists of the anterior two thirds of the vertebral bodies and discs with the attached anterior longitudinal ligaments (Fig. 31-11).

Instability results when there is disruption of two of the columns. Fracture-dislocation results from a combination of forces, including compression, flexion

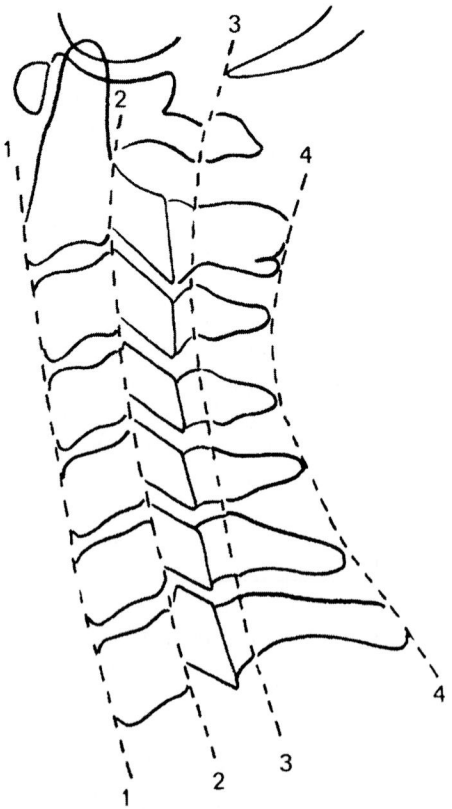

Figure 31-11 *Diagram of the normal anatomy of the cervical spine illustrating the four contour lines: 1. anterior vertebral body line, 2. posterior vertebral body line, 3. spinolaminar line, 4. spinous process line.*

or extension, and rotation. With fracture-dislocation, all three columns may be affected. These are highly unstable injuries; associated complete spinal cord injury occurs in as many as 80% of thoracic spine fracture dislocations. Dislocation without fracture also may occur and be unstable. This is the most dangerous setting for causing further injury because of the failure to recognize the nature of the problem. The plain radiograph may be normal or show only subtle findings, yet the ligaments of all three columns may be torn.

The diagnosis of an unstable injury rests on complete clinical and radiographic assessment of the entire spinal column. Noncontiguous unstable injuries of the spine are not common but do occur. In a recent study of over 1000 patients with spinal fractures, noncontiguous fractures occurred in 3.7%.[33] Diagnosis of the second injury was delayed in 23% of these patients. There is recent evidence to suggest that MRI studies are the investigation of choice in the unconscious patient to detect both instability and noncontiguous injury provided the technique involves sagittal sequencing of the entire vertebral column.[34]

DEFINITIVE MANAGEMENT

The goals of definitive management are to reverse or to limit neurologic injury where possible, to restore spinal stability if needed, and to reestablish the best possible biomechanics to the injured zone.

SPINAL DECOMPRESSION

The reversal or limitation of neurological injury is achieved by decompression of the spinal cord and spinal roots. The utility of spinal cord decompression in any patient with neurological deficits must be given careful consideration. The principal consideration in planning spinal cord decompression is the timing of surgery. Many spine surgeons suggest that ongoing spinal cord ischemia and compression from a compressive spinal injury continue to injure the spinal cord as long as the compression continues. This paradigm, similar to the approach to space-occupying lesions in the head, would argue for rapid decompression of the spinal cord. In fact, although there are studies in progress to assess the impact of rapid decompression on outcome from spinal cord injury, the value of rapid decompression has never been definitively demonstrated.

Timing of spinal decompression, therefore, becomes problematic. There are studies to suggest that outcomes can be improved with decompression within 8, 24, 48, or 72 hours; so far, no studies have argued persuasively enough to establish a standard. This benefit is postulated to exist for patients with incomplete lesions. Patients with complete lesions are believed to have much less chance for recovery of function and decompression; in these patients decompression is believed to be less urgent. For this reason, establishing whether a patient is complete or incomplete is essential in determining the timing and pace of the workup.

The issue of operative timing has impacted the approach to the presurgical workup. As a rule, operative planning requires plain spinal radiographs to rapidly assess the alignment of the spine and the nature of any misalignment or fractures. Plain radiographs also are useful as a baseline to compare postoperative films if the patient cannot be imaged for several days after surgery. CT also will provide this information as well as a detailed look at the bony anatomy that is essential for planning the extent of bony decompression as well as assessment of which vertebrae will allow placement of instrumentation and provide good screw placement.

MRI serves a different role in preoperative planning, defining the extent of spinal cord contusion and posttraumatic intervertebral disc herniations and spinal canal hematomas that may be compressing the spinal cord and that require decompression. These herniations and hematomas are not visible on plan film studies and are difficult to visualize on CT.

Obtaining all of these studies, especially MRI, is time consuming. This is especially true in the context of a busy trauma resuscitation. As a result, even with the intent of rapid decompression of the spinal cord, surgery can be delayed for many hours while these studies are obtained and the patient is stabilized. Because of this, a goal of decompression within 8 hours is, in most cases, not practical. A tension is therefore created between the need for speed in decompression and the need for adequate predecompression studies. This tension is best demonstrated in the argument over whether MRI should be obtained prior to placing patients in cervical traction. Many surgeons believe that early spinal traction can provide early realignment and decompression of the spinal cord while resuscitation and preoperative planning are completed. Others believe that obtaining operative decompression as soon as possible is the best approach, and they do not think that the few extra hours of decompression obtained by spinal traction are worthwhile. Controversy has arisen over whether MRI studies should be obtained prior to placing a patient in cervical traction. Those who advocate cervical traction argue that the goal of cervical traction is rapid decompression of the spinal cord and that MRI unduly delays this goal. Those who argue for MRI studies indicate that as many as 15% of patients will have a posttraumatic herniated cervical disc.

Patients with these types of discs can have the spinal cord compression exacerbated by realignment of the spine with traction, resulting in additional and more severe spinal cord injury. Some surgeons believe that this risk warrants an MRI study prior to placement of cervical traction. It is clear that by the time an MRI has been obtained, enough data have often been obtained to proceed with surgery, and, if the patient has been hemodynamically stabilized, to conclude that proceeding straight to surgery in lieu of instituting spinal traction is the best option. The resolution of this argument lies in knowing the risks to the patient of delaying surgery versus the risks of a posttraumatic herniated disc. Because the risks involved in the timing or delay of surgery are unknown, this controversy remains unresolved.

Spinal cord injury patients often develop complications from their injuries. Most pertinent to operative decision making are pulmonary edema and infections that can manifest starting 2-3 days after the injury. Once these complications arise, the patients become poor operative risks with their surgery being subsequently delayed sometimes for weeks. These delays in turn lead to further complications from immobility such as skin breakdown and venous thromboembolism. Many of these complications can be avoided or diminished if the patient is decompressed and stabilized early. These factors, along with our hypothesis that early decompression may be of benefit to neurologic recovery, argue for surgical intervention early in the patient's course—at least prior to the onset of other postinjury complications.

SPINAL STABILIZATION

Stabilization is the second goal of definitive management for spinal cord injury. The sooner an unstable spine is secured, the sooner the patient can be mobilized, avoiding the complications of immobility. Medicine has progressed from the days of full-body casts and extended periods of immobilization as treatment for spinal cord injury. The morbidity and mortality associated with these approaches were high, with mortality rates as high as 60%. The advent of spinal instrumentation revolutionized the treatment of spinal cord injury with its principal benefit being the ability to rapidly mobilize these patients. A key goal of treatment is to maximize this benefit to our patients with expeditious stabilization and fusion.

Planning for spinal stabilization begins with understanding any instability the patient might have. If the posterior column is disrupted via facet fractures and dislocations, then once the dislocation is realigned, principal stabilization can be achieved by posterior stabilization, probably by posterior fusion via facet screws of other techniques. If the anterior column is compromised via a compression, then once the canal is decompressed via corpectomy, stabilization would occur via interbody fusion and plating, reconstructing the anterior column and relying on the still-intact posterior column to provide support.

It is important to assure that all columns are reconstructed. This sometimes requires stabilization from both anterior and posterior to reconstruct both the anterior and posterior columns. This is essential for injuries such as bilateral facet dislocations, which often involve three column injuries. In such cases,

anterior and posterior surgery (or "360 degree surgery") is required.

RESTORING BIOMECHANICS

The third goal of definitive treatment of spinal cord injury is to leave the patient with acceptable biomechanics. This means attempting to leave the spine in its natural alignment. This can mitigate postinjury pain syndromes, which can result from the cervical spine being left in kyphosis or the lumbar spine being fused without its natural lordosis. Acceptable biomechanics are achieved by ensuring that adequate reduction of injuries, if at all possible, is achieved prior to fusion and fashioning constructs to recreate the previous curvature of the spine.

OPERATIVE APPROACH

The rule of thumb in spinal surgery is to decompress on the same approach as the compression. For example, a compression fracture of the cervical spine that is compressing the anterior cervical spinal cord is best decompressed from the front via a corpectomy. Although it would also decompress the spinal cord, a laminectomy is not considered a good choice because it would leave the spinal cord draped over the compressing defect. Second, any disrupted spinal column must be reconstructed. In most cases, the disrupted spinal column will be on the same aspect of the spine as the compression lesion, but this is not always the case, and care must be taken to be sure each factor has been independently assessed during operative planning. In some cases, decompression must occur from one approach to allow stabilization and realignment to be accomplished safely from another approach. An example would be a violation of the posterior column with an associated kyphosis and posttraumatic herniated disc. In this case, an anterior diskectomy must be completed to allow the spine to be safely realigned and fused posteriorly. In the case of three-column injury, a third anterior fusion might then need to be performed. Operative planning must take all of these factors into account. This is achieved by making an inventory of the operative goals, prioritizing them, and then sequencing the procedures based on this analysis.

Once the plan for definitive spinal surgery has been made, it must be integrated with and at times modified by the ongoing resuscitation. As described previously, these procedures can rapidly become complex and lengthy. Patients may not be stable enough to endure all that needs to be done operatively. These factors must be weighed against the imperatives to rapidly decompress and stabilize the spinal injury. In these cases, a good sense of the goals and priorities of the treatment plan is invaluable. Marginally stable patients may be able to have the urgent pieces of their procedure completed and combined with temporizing measures to allow less critical procedures to be delayed. Often, patients who require multiple approaches for stabilization can be decompressed and stabilized from one approach and placed in a halo for further stabilization, allowing their second stabilization procedures to be delayed.

Fixation by halo remains an important treatment approach. It is the most rigid form of external fixation and can be used as a primary treatment or as an adjunct to internal fixation. It is most commonly employed for the treatment of upper and midcervical fractures and dislocations.[35] The halo device promotes early patient mobilization and reduces hospital confinement compared with supine traction techniques; it is not without complications, however, ranging from pin loosening and superficial pressure sores to pin infection with osteomyelitis, overdistraction, and recurrent instability.[36] In a recent report, Tashjian et al[37] reported a 42% mortality and complications in 66% of elderly patients treated with halo vest immobilization for odontoid fractures. Cardiopulmonary difficulties, including a cardiac arrest rate of 26%, were most striking and significantly higher than in patients treated with other modalities. Despite these drawbacks, halo vest immobilization is an important modality in the overall approach to treating spinal cord injuries. Good team coordination will allow the setting and prioritization of the goals of definitive management and their efficient integration into the total resuscitation plan.

COMPLICATIONS OF SPINAL CORD INJURIES

The difficulties encountered by patients after spinal cord injury range from acute life-threatening problems related to sudden denervation to long-term issues related to immobility. Virtually all patients suffer psychologic issues related to functional loss.

CARDIOVASCULAR INJURIES

Injuries above the second thoracic vertebra may disrupt sympathetic outflow, leading to hypotension and bradycardia. The bradycardia is usually self-limited and gradually improves over time. If the patient is symptomatic, small doses of atropine (0.5-1 mg) may be administered. Rarely, a pacemaker may be required. Because there is unopposed parasympathetic stimulation of the heart, maneuvers that augment parasympathetic activity (intubation, suctioning, passing nasogastric tube) may endanger the patient, and asystole has been reported.

Hypotension is the rule rather than the exception following high thoracic or cervical cord injury. Loss of sympathetic innervation leads to systemic vasodilation and profoundly enlarges the intravascular compartment. Both preload and afterload are adversely affected. Volume replenishment is indicated under close monitoring with a central venous catheter and an arterial line. Blood pressure should be augmented to the 90-100 mm Hg range to preserve perfusion to the spinal cord. Allowing systolic blood pressure to fall below 90 mm Hg in these patients is thought to reduce the quality of patient outcome. Excessive fluid administration should be avoided, however, because of the potential to retain extravascular lung water and develop pulmonary edema. In such cases, infusions of pressors such as dopamine or neosynephrine may restore vascular tone and enhance tissue perfusion. In patients over 40 years of age, and in any patient with a cardiac history, a baseline electrocardiogram and cardiac enzyme tests are indicated.

PULMONARY

Ventilatory difficulties are common, especially in patients with high thoracic or cervical cord compromise. Cord injuries at or above the fifth cervical vertebra are particularly problematic because of the potential for loss of diaphragmatic function. High thoracic or cervical injuries cause loss of the intercostal muscles, which normally increase the A-P diameter of the thorax. Accessory muscles, such as the scalenes, trapezius, and sternocleidomastoid, may be intact but only enhance motion of the upper chest. Inward motion of the abdomen during inspiration suggests loss of the diaphragmatic component. These patients are at risk for acute respiratory failure, and early intubation may be life saving. Over time, with good pulmonary toilet and rotary positioning, patients may become ventilator independent, but they are still at risk for mucous plugging from retained secretions. Patients who do not initially require ventilator support must be observed closely for delayed pulmonary compromise from extension of cord involvement.[38] This is particularly applicable to patients with low to midcervical deficits where ascending cord compromise can result in apnea.

GASTROINTESTINAL

Ileus is a frequent occurrence in the spinal cord–injured patient, which increases the potential for vomiting and aspiration. Nasogastric decompression is indicated in all patients at risk. Standard protocols require high-dose corticosteroid infusions, and, in the presence of unopposed parasympathetic stimulation, the likelihood of gastritis or stress ulcerations is greatly enhanced. Prophylaxis with H2 blockers is indicated. Nutritional requirements are increased to 150% of normal, and early intravenous feedings should be instituted and converted to oral or tube feedings as soon as gastrointestinal function returns. Compared with intragastric feedings, jejunostomy feedings offer added protection from aspiration. Nonetheless, when tube feedings are needed long term, percutaneous gastrostomy is most commonly used.

Constipation follows the loss of sensation to defecate and relaxation of the anal sphincter. Bowel training to avoid impaction should be introduced early and includes the use of stool softeners, suppositories, and enemas.

One of the dangers faced by the spinal cord–injured patient, both short term and over time, is that the lack of innervation prevents timely recognition of acute abdominal diseases. Pancreatitis, cholecystitis, and appendicitis are examples of inflammatory processes that may initially go unrecognized in this patient population, leading to delay in diagnosis and in appropriate therapy. Other intra-abdominal afflictions may be lethal and ultimately be diagnosed only by the pathologist. Unexplained fever, leukocytosis, or elevation of amylase in the spinal cord–injured patient should prompt aggressive workup for intra-abdominal disease.

GENITOURINARY
An indwelling catheter is initially indicated and should be placed in all patients to avoid bladder distention. Allowing the bladder to become distended can greatly complicate subsequent bladder training. Urinary catheters should be removed as soon as the patient is stable to avoid infection, but bladder distention must be scrupulously avoided. Most patients cannot void spontaneously, and the patient should be instructed on sterile in-and-out self-catheterization. This is performed every 4-6 hours and is associated with a lower risk of urinary tract infection.

Sexual function in men with spinal cord injuries varies. Erection may occur and may be augmented by a venous constrictor band or the use of such agents as sildenafil, but ejaculation, which depends on sympathetic innervation, is lost. In some male patients, penile vibratory stimulation may lead to ejaculation. Recent data show a decline in spermatogenesis and sperm motility within a few weeks of spinal injury.[39] Women with spinal cord injuries usually undergo a temporary interruption in menses. Women can become pregnant and bear children, however.

THROMBOEMBOLISM
Prevention of deep venous thrombosis (DVT) is an ongoing challenge in the spinal cord–injured patient. The incidence of DVT varies by report from 9-90%, and pulmonary embolism has been reported in up to 10% of cases. Multiple prophylactic regimens have been recommended; most include some combination of anticoagulation, pneumatic compression, and/or gradient elastic stockings. Aito et al[40] showed a 2% incidence of DVT and no pulmonary embolism in the treatment arm of their prospective clinical trial using color Doppler ultrasonography for baseline and follow-up diagnosis. These authors recommended low-molecular-weight heparin, early mobilization, gradient elastic stockings, and external sequential pneumatic compression during the first 30 days postinjury. Some evidence-based guidelines recommend 90 days of treatment and caution against using only low-molecular-weight heparin. Others have attained satisfactory results with passive range of motion exercises, leg elevation, or pneumatic compression alone.[41]

MUSCULOSKELETAL
The onset of muscle spasticity reflects the loss of central inhibitory stimulation and the emergence of local reflex arcs. Spasticity can develop and progress days to months following injury. Spasticity interferes with nursing care, positioning of the patient, and efforts at rehabilitation. Range of motion exercises and stretching can reduce the phenomenon. Pharmacologic agents may be required. Baclofen, beginning at 20 mg/d, may be increased incrementally up to a dose of 80 mg/d or until the desired effect is achieved. Diazepam also may be of benefit.

Heterotopic ossification is a common complication and occurs in voluntary muscles below the level of cord injury. This inflammatory process leads to calcium deposition in the muscles, restriction of motion, and interference with rehabilitation efforts. Surgical resection may be necessary in extreme cases. Radiotherapy has been effective as a preventive measure when fractures coexist.

Loss of movement also may lead to joint contractures which can affect all joints. Ligamentous shortening and changes in elastic properties surrounding joints contribute to this condition, which further limits patient mobility. Prevention of contractures requires dedicated physical therapy and is an important part of any rehabilitation program.

SKIN
The prevention of skin breakdown is critical to maximizing recovery following spinal cord injury, and effective interventions are nicely summarized in a recent comprehensive review by Reddy et al[42] This is the most common preventable complication following spinal cord injury and is usually caused by a lack of proper nursing care or to ill-fitting equipment. Loss of sensation leads to the failure to discern skin ischemia. Failure to turn and shift pressure off an affected area rapidly leads to skin breakdown. Once a pressure sore has occurred, additional immobilization is required to treat the problem, further interfering with rehabilitation progress. Pressure sores occur most commonly over the sacrum (40%), heels (15%), and ischium (10%). Deep ischial ulcers can cause sepsis and death. Large lesions require extensive debridement and flap closure.

PSYCHIATRIC COMPLICATIONS
Spinal cord injury causes depression, anger, and withdrawal, which may last, in some combination, for up to 2 years or longer following injury. Intentional self-neglect is a manifestation of these feelings of loss, and up to 10% of patients attempt suicide. Psychological counseling is an important part of any rehabilitation program and should be provided in all cases.

SPECIAL PROBLEMS

SPINAL CORD INJURY IN CHILDREN
Children present unique challenges to the clinician both in terms of diagnosis and treatment of spinal

cord injury. Injury mechanisms vary by age and site. The cervical spine is most commonly involved, followed by the thoracic spine.[43] In young children, injuries from motor vehicle crashes and pedestrian impacts predominate, whereas sporting mishaps are the most common cause of spinal cord injuries in adolescents. SCIWORA accounts for 75% of sports-related injuries, and child abuse must be assumed if SCIWORA occurs in infants.[44] According to Hernandez's[45] study of young children, CT did not appear to offer a diagnostic advantage over plain films. In another study, however, a diagnostic error rate of 24% was attributed to unfamiliarity with pediatric spine anatomy and failure to recognize normal variants.[46] Most patients with cervical spine injury can be treated conservatively with either a rigid cervical collar or halo vest. Anterior and posterior operative approaches may be used in selected cases.

PENETRATING TRAUMA TO THE SPINE

Gunshot wounds are the third overall cause of spinal cord injuries but account for the most common etiology in certain high-risk populations. Injury to the cord can be produced either by direct injury or by the concussive effect of a near-miss injury.[47] The thoracic spine is most commonly affected, followed by the lumbar and cervical spine. The spinal column is generally considered stable following penetrating missile injury. If the bullet passes transversely through the spinal canal and fractures pedicles and facets, there is a potential for instability. Spinal cord injury is present in all such instances.

Medzon et al[48] reported three of five cases who required operation for cervical spine instability. The spine was stable in 43 or 49 cases reported by Le Roux and Dunn,[49] and operation was required in six cases. Although there is no consensus regarding the necessity to remove bullets, bullets were removed from the canal in 11 additional patients. Others believe that bullet removal is indicated only if it is at a low thoracic level or below. Associated injuries are common and often dictate survival. Transgastrointestinal spinal injuries have a higher incidence of both spine and wound infection. The role of antibiotics and early operative debridement remain controversial.[50] As we previously noted, methylprednisolone should not be used in the management of penetrating spinal cord injury.

As with other etiologies, penetrating injury is characterized by level of involvement and completeness of neurologic deficit. Patients with incomplete deficits and involvement of the thoracolumbar spine have the best chance of meaningful recovery. Impairment from penetrating wounds of the spine may be profound.[51,52] Aryan et al[53] reported a mean acute care hospitalization of 21 days and mean rehabilitation stay of 86 days for 60 adolescents with gunshot wounds of the spine.

VERTEBRAL ARTERY INJURY

Facet joint dislocations and fractures extending through the transverse foramina of the midcervical spine place the vertebral arteries at greatest risk. Injury mechanisms include compression injuries and distraction injuries, either with the spine in flexion or extension or with lateral flexion, which causes stretching or impingement of the artery, leading to an intimal flap and/or thrombosis.[54] The incidence was 17% in a recent series of patients with cervical spine fractures and dislocations.[55] In most cases, the patient remains asymptomatic because of the collateral circulation from the intact opposite vertebral or the circle of Willis. Ischemic infarction of the cerebellum or the brain stem may occur and be lethal, however. Diagnosis requires recognition of the patient at risk, digital subtraction angiography, or MR angiography. Anticoagulation has been recommended, but the risk/benefit must be weighed in the setting of other injuries, most particularly the spinal injury itself.

REFERENCES

1. Maull KI, Sachatello CR. Avoiding a pitfall in resuscitation: the painless cervical fracture. *South Med J* 1977; 70:477.

2. Levi AD, Hurlbert RJ, Anderson P, et al. Neurologic deterioration secondary to unrecognized spinal instability following trauma—a multicenter study. *Spine* 2006;31:451.

3. Velmahos GC, Jindal A, Chan LS, et al. "Insignificant" mechanism of injury: not to be taken lightly. *J Am Coll Surg* 2001;192:147.

4. Yeung JH, Cheung NK, Graham CA, et al. Reduced time on the spinal board—effects of guidelines and education for emergency department staff. *Injury* 2006; 37:53.

5. Crosby ET. Airway management in adults after cervical spine trauma. *Anesthesiology* 2006;104:1293.

6. Patterson H. Emergency department intubation of trauma patients with undiagnosed cervical spine injury. *Emerg Med J* 2004;21:302.

7. Gerling MC, Davis DP, Hamilton RS, et al. Effect of surgical cricothyrotomy on the unstable spine in a cadaver model of intubation. *J Emerg Med* 2001; 20:1.

8. Bagley LJ. Imaging of spinal trauma. *Radiol Clin North Am* 2006;44:1.

9. Gong JS, Xu JM. Value of multidetector spiral CT in diagnosis of acute thoracolumbar spinal fractures and fracture-dislocation. *Chin J Traumatol* 2004;7:289.

10. Geck MJ, Yoo S, Wang JC. Assessment of cervical ligamentous injury in trauma patients using MRI. *J Spinal Disord* 2001;14:371.

11. McCulloch PT, France J, Jones DL, et al. Helical computed tomography alone compared with plain radiographs with adjunct computed tomography to evaluate the cervical spine after high-energy trauma. *J Bone Joint Surg Am* 2005;87:2388.

12. Richards PJ. Cervical spine clearance: a review. *Injury* 36:248;2005.

13. Stiell IG, Wells GA, Vandemheen KL, et al. The Canadian C-spine rule for radiography in alert and stable trauma patients. *JAMA* 2001;286:1841.

14. Panacek EA, Mower WR, Hoffman JR, et al. Test performance of the individual NEXUS low-risk screening criteria for cervical spine injury. *Ann Emerg Med* 2001;38:22.

15. Viccellio P, Simon H, Pressman BD, et al. A prospective multicenter study of cervical spine injury in children. *Pediatrics* 2001;108:E20.

16. Knopp R. Comparing NEXUS and Canadian C-spine decision rule for determining the need for cervical spine radiography. *Ann Emerg Med* 2004;43:518.

17. Bandiera G, Stiell IG, Wells GA, et al. The Canadian C-spine rule performs better than unstructured physician judgment. *Ann Emerg Med* 2003;42:395.

18. Diaz JJ, Gillman C, Morris JA, et al. Are five-year plain films of the cervical spine unreliable? A prospective evaluation in blunt trauma patients with altered mental status. *J Trauma* 2003;55:658.

19. Bolinger B, Shartz M, Marion D. Bedside fluoroscopic flexion and extension cervical spine radiographs for clearance of the cervical spine in comatose patients. *J Trauma* 2004;56:132.

20. Anglen J, Metzler M, Bunn P, et al. Flexion and extension views are not cost-effective in a cervical spine clearance protocol for obtunded trauma patients. *J Trauma* 2002;52:54

21. Graham AW, Swank ML, Kinard RE, et al. Radiographic assessment of the cervical spine in symptomatic trauma patients. *Neurosurgery* 2002(Suppl);50:3.

22. Pasquale M. Practice management guidelines for trauma: EAST ad hoc committee on guideline development: identifying cervical spine instability after trauma. *J Trauma* 1998;44:945.

23. Chiu WC, Haan JM, Cushing BM, et al. Ligamentous injuries of the cervical spine in unreliable blunt trauma patients: incidence, evaluation, and outcome. *J Trauma* 2001;50:457.

24. Ghanta MK, Smith LM, Polin RS, et al. An analysis of Eastern Association for the Surgery of Trauma practice guidelines for cervical spine evaluation in a series of patients with multiple imaging techniques. *Ann Surg* 2002;68:563.

25. Barrett TW, Mower WR, Zucker MR, et al. Injuries missed by limited computed tomographic imaging of patients with cervical spine injuries. *Ann Emerg Med* 2006;47:129.

26. Lee TT, Green BA. Advances in the management of acute spinal cord injury. *Orthop Clin North Am* 2002; 33:311.

27. Heary RF, Vaccaro AR, Mesa JJ, et al. Steroids and gunshot wounds to the spine. *Neurosurgery* 1997; 41:576.

28. Levy ML, Gans W, Wijesinghe HS, et al. Use of methylprednisolone as an adjunct in the management of patients with penetrating spinal cord injury: outcome analysis. *Neurosurgery* 1996;39:1141.

29. Shen FH, Samartzis D. Cervical spine fracture on the ankylosing spondylitis patient. *J Am Coll Surg* 2005; 200:632.

30. Koivikko MP, Myllynen P, Santavirta S. Fracture dislocations of the cervical spine: a review of 106

31. conservatively and operatively treated patients. *Eur Spine J* 2004;13:610.

31. Dai LY. Acute central cervical cord injury: the effects of age upon prognosis. *Injury* 2001;32:195.

32. Collignon F, Martin D, Lenelle K, et al. Acute traumatic central cord syndrome: Magnetic resonance imaging and clinical observations. *J Neurosurg* 2002;96:29.

33. Wittenberg RH, Hargus S, Steffen R, et al. Noncontiguous unstable spine fractures. *Spine* 2002; 27:254.

34. Vaccaro AR, Madigan L, Schweitzer ME, et al. Magnetic resonance imaging analysis of soft-tissue disruption after flexion-distraction injuries of the subaxial cervical spine. *Spine* 2001;26:1866.

35. Vieweg U, Schultheiss R. A review of halo vest treatment of upper cervical spine injuries. *Arch Orthop Trauma Surg* 2001;121:50.

36. Hayes VM, Silber JS, Siddiqi FN, et al. Complications of halo fixation of the cervical spine. *Am J Orthop* 2005; 34:271.

37. Tashjian RZ, Majercik S, Biffl WL, et al. Halo vest immobilization increases early morbidity and mortality in elderly odontoid fractures. *J Trauma* 2006;60:199.

38. Urdenata F, Layon AJ. Respiratory complications in patients with traumatic cervical spine injuries. *J Clin Anesth* 2003;15:398.

39. Biering-Sorenson F, Sonksen J. Sexual function in spinal cord lesioned men. *Spinal Cord* 2001;39:455.

40. Aito S, Pieri A, D'Andrea M, et al. Primary prevention of deep venous thrombosis and pulmonary embolism in acute spinal cord injured patients. *Spinal Cord* 2002; 40:300.

41. Kurtoglu M, Yanar H, Bilsel Y, et al. Venous thromboembolism prophylaxis after head and spinal trauma: intermitten pneumatic compression devices versus low molecular weight heparin. *World J Surg* 2004;28:807.

42. Reddy M, Gill SS, Rochon PA. Preventing pressure ulcers: a systematic review. *JAMA* 2006;296:974.

43. Reddy SP, Junewick JJ, Backstrom JW. Distribution of spinal fractures in children: does age, mechanism of injury, or gender play a significant role? *Pediatr Radiol* 2003;33:776.

44. Brown RL, Brunn MA, Garcia VF. Cervical spine injuries in children: a review of 103 patients treated consecutively at a level 1 pediatric trauma center. *J Pediatr Surg* 2001;36:1107.

45. Hernandez JA, Chupik C, Swischuk LE. Cervical spine trauma in children under 5 years: productivity of CT. *Emerg Radiol* 2004;10:176.

46. Avellino AM, Mann FA, Grady MS, et al. The misdiagnosis of acute cervical spine injuries and fractures in infants and children: the 12 year experience of a level 1 pediatric and adult trauma center. *Childs Nerv Syst* 2005;21:122.

47. Mirovsky Y, Shalmon E, Blankstein A, et al. Complete paraplegia following gunshot injury without direct trauma to the cord. *Spine* 2005;30:2436.

48. Medzon R, Rothenhaus T, Bono CM, et al. Stability of cervical spine fractures after gunshot wounds to the head and neck. *Spine* 2005;30:2274.

49. Le Roux JC, Dunn RN. Gunshot injuries of the spine— a review of 49 cases managed at the Groote Shuur

Acute Spinal Cord Injury Center. *S Afr J Surg* 2005; 43:165.

50. Quigley KJ, Place HM. The role of debridement and antibiotics in gunshot wounds of the spine. *J Trauma* 2006;60:814.

51. Putzke JD, Richard JS, DeVivo MJ. Quality of life after spinal cord injury caused by gunshot. *Arch Phys Med Rehabil* 2001;82:949.

52. Putzke JD, Richard JS, DeVivo MJ. Gunshot versus nongunshot spinal cord injury: acute care and rehabilitation outcomes. *Am J Phys Med Rehabil* 200180:366.

53. Aryan HE, Amar AP, Ozguar BM, et al. Gunshot wounds of the spine in adolescents. *Neurosurgery* 2005; 57:748.

54. Inamasu J, Guiot BH. Vertebral artery injury after blunt cervical trauma: an update. *Surg Neurol* 2006;65:238.

55. Taneichi H, Suda K, Kajino T, et al. Traumatically induced vertebral artery occlusion associated with cervical spine injuries: prospective study using magnetic resonance angiography. *Spine* 2005;30:1955.

Chapter 32

THE INITIAL CARE OF THE BURN PATIENT

Frederick W. Endorf, MD, Richard L. Gamelli, MD, and Frederick A. Luchette, MD

INTRODUCTION

The initial care of the burned patient presents unique challenges to even experienced acute care surgeons. Hemodynamic instability, hypoxia secondary to inhalation injury, and prodigious fluid needs are but a few of the obstacles encountered in the early care of these severely injured patients. Technological advances and rapid progression in our understanding of burn physiology have led to great strides in improving outcomes. A fundamental grasp of the principles of burn resuscitation is essential to the armamentarium of the acute care surgeon.

PREDICTORS OF MORTALITY AND CRITERIA FOR TRANSFER

A commonly used formula for predicting mortality in burns in the past was percent mortality equals patient age in years plus percent total body surface area (%TBSA).[1] Over the past 30 years, advancements in burn care have resulted in an overall mortality for all burn injuries that has been reported to be as low as 4%, rendering this formula of historic interest only. However, certain risk factors still play a large role in determining a smaller subset of burned patients that will have significant mortality. Ryan et al[2] performed a retrospective review of 1665 burned patients and developed a mortality formula based on three risk factors: age greater than 60 years, greater than 40% TBSA burned, and presence of concomitant inhalation injury. Their formula predicts 0.3%, 3%, 33%, or 90% mortality for 0, 1, 2, or 3 risk factors, respectively. A prospective test of the formula yielded similar results.[2] Age as a single variable in a predictive mortality equation was validated by Moreau et al.[3] in a retrospective review of over 6000 burn patients.

Improvements in mortality have come in part from the development of specialized burn units, and patients with severe burns are more frequently being transferred to regional burn centers for comprehensive multidisciplinary care. This prompted the American Burn Association to develop guidelines for transfer to a verified burn center (Table 32-1). These guidelines include: second- and third-degree burns on >10% TBSA in patients under 10 years or over 50 years old, or greater than 20% TBSA in other age groups. This also includes third-degree burns of > 5% in any age group, or any burns involving difficult areas such as the face, hands, feet, genitalia, or perineum. They also recommend transfer for electrical or chemical burns, and in those patients with inhalation injury. Pediatric patients and patients with complicated preexisting disorders are also recommended for transfer to centers with specific capabilities for their needs. Patients with concurrent trauma, in which their traumatic injuries are a greater immediate threat, should be stabilized at an appropriate trauma center prior to transfer.[4]

INITIAL PREOPERATIVE EVALUATION

The primary survey of the burned patient should follow the guidelines described as a part of the Advanced Trauma Life Support Course (ATLS) (Fig. 32-1). In particular, airway management in the burned patient may be especially challenging. Direct thermal injury to the upper airways or smoke inhalation may cause the rapid onset of airway edema, which may be severe in nature. The aspiration of hot liquids may result in a condition not unlike epiglottitis and will require immediate intubation.[5] Warning signs seen on physical examination may include facial or perioral burns, burned nasal hair, voice hoarseness, or outright wheezing and even stridor. Even mild suspicion should prompt elective endotracheal intubation. If available, an awake fiberoptic technique may lessen the risk of airway compromise seen with rapid sequence intubation. Nasotracheal intubation may be required in the presence of concurrent oral

A burn unit may treat adults or children or both. Burn injuries that should be referred to a burn unit include the following:

1. Partial thickness burns greater than 10% total body surface area (TBSA).
2. Burns that involve the face, hands, feet, genitalia, perineum, or major joints.
3. Third-degree burns in any age group.
4. Electrical burns, including lightning injury.
5. Chemical burns.
6. Inhalation injury.
7. Burn injury in patients with preexisting medical disorders-that could complicate management, prolong recovery, or affect mortality.
8. Any patients with burns and concomitant trauma (such as fractures) in which the burn injury poses the greatest risk of morbidity or mortality. In such cases, if the trauma poses the greater immediate risk, the patient may be initially stabilized in a trauma center before being transferred to a burn unit. Physician judgment will be necessary in such situations and should be in concert with the regional medical control plan and triage protocols.
9. Burned children in hospitals without qualified personnel or equipment for the care of children.
10. Burn injury in patients who will require special social, emotional, or long-term rehabilitative intervention.

trauma. Care should be taken while securing the endotracheal tube in place, as progression of edema will make reintubation more difficult.[4]

As part of the primary survey, intravenous access should be rapidly obtained. Two large-caliber peripheral intravenous lines should be placed through non-burned skin if possible. Central lines may be necessary if access is difficult and will often be needed long term in severely burned patients for multiple infusions and hemodynamic monitoring. Intraosseous lines are effective in pediatric patients with difficult venous access, and in extreme cases sternal intraosseous access has been used in adult burn patients.[6] Unexpected changes in hemodynamic status during the primary survey may be an indication of other occult injuries and should prompt appropriate further radiologic evaluation.

The secondary survey, in addition to excluding concurrent traumatic injuries, may be tailored to specific concerns for the burned patient. Unexplained neurologic changes in the absence of intracranial injury may be sequelae of inhaled toxins such as carbon monoxide, which will be discussed in greater detail later in this chapter. Air swallowing with respiratory distress may lead to acute gastric dilation and

can be treated with a nasogastric tube. An indwelling urinary catheter is essential in the evaluation of resuscitation, and rarely one must divide a severely burned foreskin to permit access the urethral meatus.[4] Determining peripheral perfusion is important in circumferential burns and will be described in the section Operative Management on escharotomy.

Formulas determining resuscitation volumes for burned patients typically rely on %TBSA. Thus, it is important to make a quick but accurate assessment of burn size. The so-called "rule of nines" is an effective way to roughly estimate burn size. In adults, the anterior and posterior trunk each make up 18%, each of the lower extremities is 18%, each of the upper extremities is 9%, and the head is 9%, although the head in children consumes more of the body surface area. The Lund and Browder diagram is commonly used, and is an easy and accurate way to determine burn size.[7]

ASSESSMENT OF BURN DEPTH

Burn depth is commonly stratified to four degrees based on their clinical severity, and clinical signs and symptoms vary for each degree. First-degree or superficial burns are typically described in severe sunburn. These burns are painful but do not blister acutely. Second-degree or partial thickness burns are further subdivided into superficial partial thickness or deep partial thickness, which is determined by the depth of dermis involved. This becomes an important distinction because superficial partial thickness burns will usually heal with local wound care, while most deep partial thickness burns require excision and skin grafting. Second-degree burns are extremely painful and are characterized by blistering and associated serous fluid drainage. Third-degree or full thickness burns involve the entire dermis and are typically firm, painless to touch, and nonblanching. Fourth-degree burns involve underlying adipose tissue, tendon, muscle, or bone.

Despite years of experience, burn surgeons can err in predicting the healing of partial thickness burns. Hoping to improve on clinical judgment alone, multiple new technologies have been applied in the search for a better assessment. Full-thickness biopsy is the most accurate method for determining burn depth. Unfortunately, histologic diagnosis comes at the price of a painful and time-consuming procedure, and a dedicated skin histopathologist is needed to confirm the diagnosis, which is not available at certain times.[8] Immunofluorescent staining of frozen sections is a quick and easy technique, but use thus far has been restricted to in vitro laboratory studies.[9] Noncontact ultrasonography is a repeatable and relatively painless modality that may aid in predicting nonhealing partial thickness burns.[10] Laser Doppler imaging is a burgeoning area of study in which Doppler measurements of skin perfusion are correlated with burn depth and

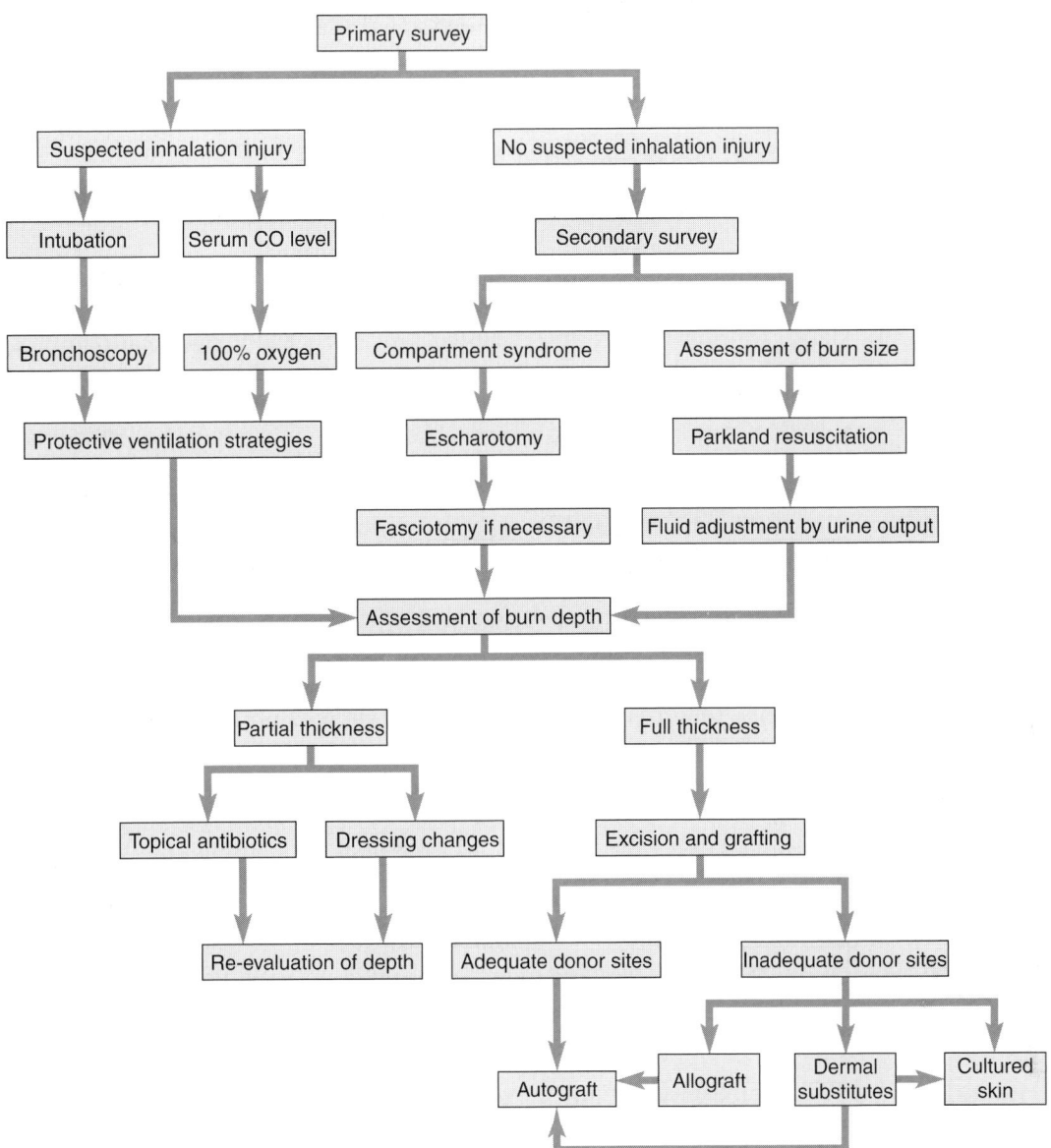

Figure 32-1 *Algorithm for the primary survey of burn patient.*

subsequent healing.[11] A multicenter trial found that serial laser Doppler measurements can result in as high as 81% specificity and 81% positive predictive value in the early identification of nonhealing wounds.[12] Fiberoptic confocal imaging,[13] indocyanine green angiography,[14] and polarization-sensitive optical coherence tomography[15] have performed well on the benchtop but have been relegated to the laboratory primarily due to cost and difficulty of use. It is well established that burn wound depth may convert from superficial partial thickness to deep partial thickness over time. The primary culprit in this progression is typically invasive burn wound infection. However, microvascular analysis of burn depth in a rat model has shown that inadequate resuscitation can lead to conversion of burn depth as well.[16] Laboratory investigation has shown that IL-8 is released from injured

skin with a resultant influx of neutrophils. This neutrophil aggregation may worsen tissue injury with a progression of burn depth.[17]

RESUSCITATION

The severely burned patient requires massive fluid resuscitation unlike that seen in any other patient population. Burn wounds precipitate an early release of cytokines and inflammatory mediators that, in turn, cause generation of oxygen-free radicals with a resultant systemic capillary leak.[4] Many fluid resuscitation formulas have been developed to predict fluid needs in the acute resuscitative period, but none will be perfect for each individual patient. The most commonly used of these is the Parkland or Baxter formula, in which a total of 4 ml/kg/%TBSA burn of lactated Ringer solution is predicted to be given over 24 hours, half of that in the first 8 hours, and half in the subsequent 16 hours postinjury. Fluid administration is adjusted to ensure a urine output of 0.5 ml/kg/h in adults or 1 ml/kg/h in children. Other formulas may be better for pediatric patients, as children also need maintenance fluids in addition to resuscitative fluid, and infants require glucose supplementation also due to low glycogen reserves. The Galveston group uses lactated Ringer at 5000 ml/m² BSA burn/d + 2000 ml/m² BSA burn/d for their large pediatric burns.[7]

Unfortunately, the Parkland formula tends to underestimate fluid volumes given in actual practice.[18] In Baxter's original work, he showed that 12% of patients would require greater than 4 ml/kg/%TBSA burn, but a recent multicenter survey reported that 58% of patients were requiring fluid volumes above what was predicted by the Parkland formula.[19] Friedrich et al[20] in Seattle compared current patients with matched historical controls and found that this "fluid creep" is a relatively recent occurrence. In a follow-up study from Seattle, Sullivan et al[21] noted that the use of opioid analgesics had increased over a similar time period. These authors theorized that increased opioid use may cause hemodynamic changes and a subsequent need for increased resuscitative fluid volumes. Investigators at the U.S. Army Institute of Surgical Research examined predictive factors for higher-than-expected fluid requirements. They found that increasing burn size and body weight were associated with higher fluid volumes in the first 24 hours and that after 24 hours mechanical ventilation became an additional risk factor for increased fluid needs. In this particular study, higher resuscitative volumes were not associated with higher mortality.[22] Another report by the same group looked at admission data and injury severity in an attempt to predict those patients that would fail resuscitation. Despite including a wide range of admission variables, only the classic variables of burn size and inhalation injury correlated with resuscitative failure.[23] Inhalation injury is well known to cause increased fluid requirements in the acute period. A landmark study by Navar et al[24] compared burn patients with inhalation injury to burn patients without inhalation injury. In their cohort, burn patients without inhalation injury needed 3.98 ml/kg/%TBSA burn, which correlated extremely well with the Parkland data. However, in patients with a burn and inhalation injury, the average fluid acquired from resuscitation was 5.76 ml/kg/%TBSA burn. These patients also had significantly increased sodium requirements in the acute resuscitation period.[24] Even centers using less than the predicted Parkland formulas have found marked increases in fluid needs with concomitant inhalation injury.[25]

Baxter's original formula called for the addition of colloid to the resuscitative fluids after the first 24 hours. It is believed that capillary integrity returns at 24 hours and thus colloid may be more likely to remain in the intravascular space after the first day.[4] The use of colloid has been advocated in several other formulas as well, including the Brooke and Evans formulas, as well as the Demling formula incorporating dextran.[7] The shared rationale is to minimize large-volume crystalloid solution, which may be associated with untoward side effects such as pulmonary edema, peripheral edema, and abdominal compartment syndrome.[26] A notable decrease in overall fluid volumes has been noted with the addition of colloid, but no study has shown any statistically significant improvement in long-term outcomes.[7] Albumin use in particular has been a frequent point of contention. In an ovine model, albumin use increased colloid osmotic pressure with an associated decrease in edema and restoration of cardiac output.[27] However, the use of albumin may actually worsen the buildup of lung water as a result of reabsorption of edema fluid.[28] Albumin administration may also cause inhibition of gut barrier function, but this insult may be prevented by inhibition of inducible nitric oxide synthase.[29] A Cochrane review of the use of albumin in a mixed critically ill patient population showed no benefit in the acute resuscitation of burn patients. In fact, their data suggested that albumin may actually increase mortality in critically ill patients.[30]

In the search for techniques to minimize crystalloid volumes during resuscitation, hypertonic solutions have been examined as well. Hypertonic solutions do indeed decrease initial resuscitation volumes, but it appears to only be a short-term effect.[31] Some groups have found that outcomes are actually worse with hypertonic saline,[32] and at the very least they tend to cause a hyperchloremic acidosis.[33] Gut barrier function may also be compromised by the use of hypertonic solutions, although this is also ameliorated by inhibition of inducible nitric oxide synthase.[34]

Other interesting pharmacologic manipulations have been attempted during the resuscitation period. High-volume hyperdynamic resuscitation with the use of inotropes showed no benefit in a sheep model compared to resuscitation with the Parkland formula alone.[35] High doses of ascorbic acid (vitamin C) may reduce volume requirements and burn wound edema and may help prevent pulmonary compromise.[36]

ENDPOINTS OF RESUSCITATION AND MONITORING

Classically, a combination of appropriate vital signs and urine output has guided resuscitation of burn patients. These relatively primitive values maintain much of their clinical effectiveness today. However, the high prevalence of confounding comorbidities such as congestive heart failure, hypertension, and chronic renal insufficiency may cloud the clinical picture. Investigation continues into other effective measures of the success of burn resuscitation. Even with adequate urinary output, an average base deficit of less than −6 on the first hospital day may correlate with the development of acute respiratory distress syndrome (ARDS) and a higher incidence of organ failure,[37] although some authors advocate the use of serum lactate rather than base deficit.[38] Gastric mucosal perfusion may be poor in severely burned patients even with adequate arterial pH and lactate levels,[39] and may be related to overall mortality.[40] More invasive monitoring has had mixed results. A trial comparing resuscitation guided by pulmonary artery catheters to resuscitation with Parkland formula alone showed that the catheter group received more fluid overall but did not have significant improvements in filling pressures or cardiac output.[41] The calculation of intrathoracic blood volume may help guide resuscitation and in one study resulted in improved cardiac index and oxygen delivery.[26] Holm et al showed that oxygen consumption was reliant on oxygen delivery in the initial resuscitation, and they found that the correlation was stronger in survivors.[42] Invasive techniques often have prohibitive risks and costs, and they have yet to prove superior to the old standards of vital signs and urine output.

THERMAL INJURY

OPERATIVE MANAGEMENT

The most immediate surgical intervention in burned patients is escharotomy. The nearly rigid eschar of severely burned skin acts as a binder around compartments that are undergoing continued massive swelling. When the pressure in the compartment increases, it will impinge on venous drainage and eventually arterial perfusion of the affected area. This is most commonly, but not exclusively, seen in circumferential burns. In the chest, this is manifested by hypoventilation and increased peak airway pressures. In the abdomen, an abdominal compartment syndrome may occur with decreased urine output, hypotension, and also may contribute to high airway pressures. In the extremities, one may see pain or numbness, delayed capillary refill, or even loss of peripheral pulses. Serial examinations and clinical suspicion are the most important diagnostic modalities in determining the need for escharotomy, but adjuncts may include bladder pressures for suspected abdominal compartment syndrome.[43] Percutaneous invasive pressure monitoring in the extremities may need to pass through contaminated wounds and adds little to the clinical diagnosis.[44]

Escharotomies can typically be performed at the bedside using electrocautery (Fig. 32-2). Properly done escharotomies will result in a visible release of underlying subcutaneous tissue with separation of the incision edges. Care must be taken to avoid escharotomies that are too deep, particularly in the areas of the upper arm (brachial artery), elbow (ulnar nerve), and knee (peroneal nerve).[4] Thoracic escharotomies are often

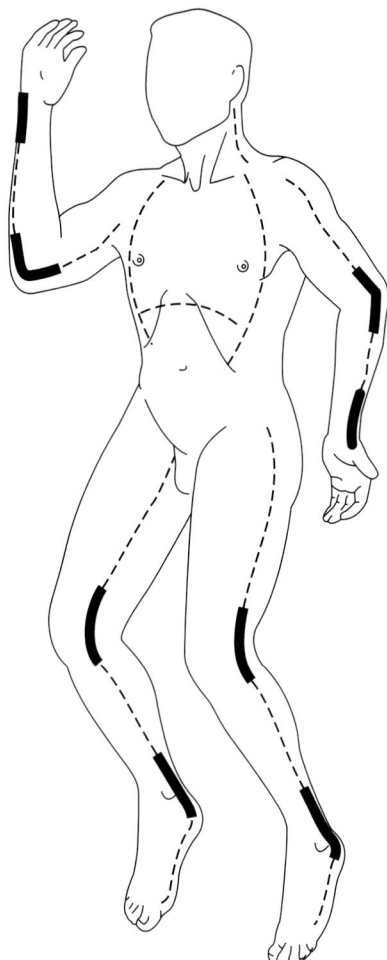

Figure 32-2 *Common areas for escharotomies.*

made over the midline sternum and are extended in a bilateral subcostal fashion.[45] In children, axial flank incisions connected across the anterior midline may also be effective.[4] Confirmation of complete release can be rapidly made by measuring peak airway pressures. Lateral abdominal incisions are usually sufficient to release the abdomen and may be carried down to the lateral lower extremities if necessary. Extremity escharotomies are typically in a longitudinal direction on the medial and lateral sides. If the hand is involved, incisions can be extended to the thenar and hypothenar eminences, and digit escharotomies should be placed on the dorsolateral aspects.[45] Incomplete response of signs and symptoms after sufficiently generous escharotomies may signal the need for fasciotomies, which are typically performed in an operating room setting.[4] Investigation has been made into enzymatic agents for escharotomy for remote settings such as the battlefield. Unfortunately, these agents take as long as 30 minutes to work and thus are not well suited for hospital practice.[46]

After the initial resuscitation of the burned patient, planning must be initiated for definitive treatment of the burn wounds. Historically, burns were treated conservatively until the eschar was lifted off, and only then was skin grafting begun. Janzekovic first described early excision and skin grafting in 1970,[47] and in the 1980s this philosophy became widely accepted as repeated studies showed better survival and fewer hospital days in patients with very large burns.[48-50] These still were staged excisions, limited primarily by blood loss and shortage of donor sites. Blood loss and transfusion needs have subsequently decreased by as much as ten times,[51] using adjuncts such as tourniquets, epinephrine clysis,[52] and topical thrombin.[7] Thus, investigators have been pushing the envelope of earlier excision in massive burns. The Galveston group has found that delaying complete excision beyond 48 hours may result in delayed wound closure, increased wound infections, and more hospital days.[53] Early excision may also abrogate the inflammatory and hypermetabolic responses in children with large burns.[54] This policy of early complete excision necessitates the use of cadaveric allograft or synthetic skin substitutes for coverage due to the lack of useful donor sites.[7]

Repeat tangential excision using Weck or Goulian blades removes the burn eschar while preserving maximal healthy subcutaneous tissue. A pressurized water dissector is useful on difficult areas such as the face and hands.[55] Healthy dermis has a shiny whitish appearance with miliary punctate bleeding. Excision may need to be carried to fat or fascia in deep burns, although burned tendon and bone should not be debrided due to a tendency to granulate over time with subsequent flap or skin coverage. An air-powered dermatome is used to harvest split-thickness donor skin, and this skin may be meshed to cover larger areas of excised burn. Meshing has the additional benefit of allowing drainage and preventing hematoma or seroma formation under grafts, both of which are known to compromise the adherence of the graft. Staples or absorbable sutures are used to secure the grafts, although fibrin and cyanoacrylic glues have been used as adjuncts to ensure graft adherence.[51]

POSTOPERATIVE WOUND CARE

Open burn wounds are extremely painful and are subject to large amounts of insensible fluid losses. Burn wounds also are very susceptible to infection, and invasive infection can convert superficial partial thickness burns to deep partial thickness burns requiring grafting. A wide variety of topical agents and dressings are currently used to prevent these untoward outcomes. Silver-containing topicals and dressings are the mainstay of initial wound care. Silver sulfadiazine is a white cream that is relatively painless to apply, has a broad antibiotic effect, and has no metabolic side effects. Unfortunately, it does not penetrate well through thick eschar. It can be

easily applied to gauze dressings that are in turn applied to areas of burn. Silver nitrate solution is also an effective topical antimicrobial but may cause staining and also hyponatremia.[4] Acticoat (Westaim Biomedical Inc.) is a silver-impregnated cloth dressing that has the advantage of only needing dressing changes every 2-3 days rather than the twice-daily regimen of other topical antibiotics. Mafenide acetate solution is another broad-spectrum antibiotic with good penetration but is somewhat painful on application to initial burn wounds. However, it is a translucent nonviscous solution and therefore is well suited for dressings over fresh skin grafts. Mafenide acetate is a carbonic anhydrase inhibitor so patients with large surface areas treated with this solution must be monitored for metabolic disturbances. Other specific topicals may be tailored to culture-proven invasive wound infections. For instance, gentamicin cream may be used in gram-negative infections, and vancomycin solution or mupirocin cream for methicillin-resistant staphylococcus.

Second-degree burns are typically treated with dressing changes and expectant management, but patients may have large areas of second-degree burns. Several methods have been tried to accelerate healing of second-degree wounds and decrease the discomfort associated with serial dressing changes. Occlusive dressings such as Biobrane (Mylan Bertex Pharmaceuticals), silver-impregnated hydrofiber dressings (Aquacel Ag, Convatec), and even bioengineered skin substitutes (TransCyte, Smith and Nephew) have been used with good results. Some groups advocate debridement and homograft application for massive second-degree burns (> 40% TBSA) and have shown that it reduces length of hospital stay compared to topical antibiotic dressings.[56]

Massive full-thickness burns require skin grafting for definitive coverage. Unfortunately, the sites available for donor skin may be limited. Cadaveric skin and synthetic or bioengineered skin substitutes have all been incorporated in the treatment of these large burns. Integra (Integra Life Sciences Corporation) is a bilayer dermal substitute with a collagen-based artificial dermis as the inner layer and a silastic outer layer. The outer layer acts as a barrier to prevent moisture loss and infection for approximately 2 weeks, at which time the underlying dermis becomes vascularized. The outer layer is then removed and autograft applied to the area. Some groups have reported fewer donor site complications, less hypertrophic scarring, and ease of use across joints. Alloderm (LifeCell Corporation) is an acellular human dermis that also may be used in combination with skin grafting to cover large areas of burned skin.[57,58]

Cultured epithelial autografts can be made from a biopsy of the patient's own skin but require a long time period for an adequate size graft to mature and are very fragile and difficult to handle intraoperatively. A major recent development has been the synthesis of a cultured skin substitute made up of a collagen-glycosaminoglycan substrate with autologous keratinocytes and fibroblasts. Used in combination with Integra, this technique is fairly rapid, markedly decreases donor site need, and has good surgical and cosmetic outcomes.[59-61]

ANESTHESIA AND ANALGESIA

Burned patients may require multiple trips to the operating room to have their wounds definitively closed. Anesthesiologists can be invaluable allies in optimizing these procedures and preventing regression in the condition of these critically ill patients. Early, detailed preoperative communication between the surgical team and anesthesiologists should reduce hurdles such as vascular access and invasive monitoring. The need for blood and blood products should be anticipated and the blood bank notified early. Patient positioning may often be unconventional during burn procedures, so the anesthesiologist must be aware of any plans so that they may better anticipate any obstacles from an anesthesia standpoint. Enteral feeds may be continued throughout surgery in intubated patients or those patients with a tracheostomy, but enteral feedings should be held 4 hours in advance of surgery for nonintubated patients to minimize the risk of aspiration.[62] Succinylcholine is not used for induction in burn patients because of the risk of hyperkalemia, and rocuronium has been championed as a better paralytic for burned patients.[63] Propofol, etomidate, and thiopental are all appropriate for use in burned patients, and ketamine is especially effective in pediatric patients. The volatile anesthetics do not seem to vary in their effects on burned patients.[62] Topical lidocaine applied to donor sites at the time of harvest reduces perioperative narcotic use.[64]

Opioids are still the most commonly used analgesics in burned patients. Frequent dressing changes, particularly in children, may cause anxiety that can be relieved with ketamine or intravenous or intranasal benzodiazepines. Adjuncts such as music and behavioral therapy, hypnosis, and computer games or virtual reality may be of some use in ameliorating burn pain.[62] A profound ileus may result from chronic narcotic use, so an aggressive bowel motility regimen should be used. Oral naloxone may reduce ileus without sacrificing pain relief.

INHALATION INJURY

PREOPERATIVE MANAGEMENT

Associated smoke inhalation injury is common in burned patients and is the leading immediate cause of burn mortality. The U.S. Army Institute of Surgical Research treated 1256 burn patients from 1985 to 1990, of which 330 (26%) had concomitant inhalation injury. Of those 330, 97 (29.4%) died of their injuries.[65]

The University of North Carolina-Chapel Hill studied 1447 patients with burns and found a 20% incidence of inhalation injury, with 31% mortality.[66] Shirani et al[67] showed that inhalation injury, together with burns, increased mortality by up to 20% over burns alone. Inhalation injury in conjunction with pneumonia increased mortality by up to 60% over burns alone. Patients with burns, inhalation injury, and ARDS in combination may have mortality as high as 66%.[68] Inhalation injury in combination with burns is associated with up to three times the hospital length of stay when compared to burns alone.[69]

OPERATIVE MANAGEMENT

Confirmation of the clinical suspicion of inhalation injury is typically made by fiberoptic bronchoscopy. Common findings include erythema, carbonaceous deposits, edema, bronchorrhea, and friability, rarely progressing to hemorrhage. Severe injury can result in sloughing of mucosa with subsequent endoluminal obliteration.[70] Chest X-ray is not sensitive in acute injury unless the injury is massive. Thoracic CT scan was used in one study to successfully identify inhalation injury in 8 of 10 patients by the appearance of upper airway edema. Unfortunately, CT scan in the unstable patient is not always logistically possible and may limit this approach, unless the patient is already undergoing CT scanning for concomitant trauma.[71] 99-Technetium scanning, xenon scanning, endobronchial biopsy, and tracheobronchial cytology all are more useful for confirmatory studies and for logistical reasons are not useful on initial evaluation of the patient with suspected inhalation injury.[72]

POSTOPERATIVE MANAGEMENT

Treatment of inhalation injury remains mostly supportive at this time. Airway edema can improve with simple measures such as elevating the head of the bed and judicious use of fluids after the initial resuscitation.[4] Beta-agonists are useful in the presence of bronchospasm, and interest has been keen in finding other helpful nebulized agents. Acetylcysteine is a free-radical scavenger that in its nebulized form may lessen the harmful effects of high levels of inhaled oxygen. Aerosolized heparin helps to prevent formation of fibrin plugs and may decrease the buildup of obstructive casts in the airways. These adjuncts may transiently improve pulmonary parameters and decrease reintubation rates but have not decreased mortality.[7] Steroids have no proven benefit on morbidity and mortality after inhalation injury and may actually be associated with more infectious complications. They should be reserved for patients with bronchospasm unresponsive to other therapies, or patients that were steroid dependent prior to injury.[73] Intrabronchial surfactant[74] and inhaled nitric oxide[75] have been used in burn patients with inhalation injuries with some early promising results. Aerosolized tissue plasminogen activator[76] and recombinant human antithrombin[77] have shown some success in sheep models of inhalation injury.

Avoidance of high peak airway pressures is important in these patients, and protective lung ventilation should be used when possible. Permissive hypercapnia that still maintains a pH greater than 7.2 has resulted in improved outcomes in burned children.[78] High-frequency percussive ventilation (HFPV) has shown promise in children with inhalation injury refractory to conventional modes of ventilation. The Shriner Hospital in Galveston in a small study of 13 children compared with historical controls showed less pneumonia, better PaO_2:FiO_2 ratios, lower peak pressures, and less work of breathing with HFPV.[79] High-frequency oscillator ventilation (HFOV) has also been successful in children and may also show short-term benefits in oxygenation of adult patients with inhalation injury and ARDS. Long-term outcomes benefits in adults are not yet clear.[80] In one case report, extracorporeal membrane oxygenation (ECMO) was used in two adult patients with severe inhalation injury who failed maximum conventional ventilation. Both patients survived after 300 and 288 hours of ECMO, but the authors cautioned that this tactic should only be considered in the face of imminent respiratory death.[81] New frontiers are emerging in the care of patients with inhalation injury. Ongoing trials of an arteriovenous carbon dioxide removal device have been successful in sheep with smoke inhalation and burn-induced ARDS. The device uncouples carbon dioxide removal and oxygen transfer, with carbon dioxide transferred across a membrane and oxygen diffused across native lungs with low-frequency positive-pressure ventilation.[82] The device is commercially available in Europe but has not been approved as of yet for clinical use in the United States.

Most severe burns will require tracheostomy for their prolonged hospital course, and this may improve patient comfort and security of the airway. However, Saffle et al.[83] found that early tracheostomy at an average of 4 days postburn did not reduce ventilator days or overall mortality when compared with a group undergoing tracheostomy at 14 days postburn.

Fluid resuscitation needs are clearly elevated in patients with burns and inhalation injury in combination.[24,25] The severity of injury by bronchoscopy may not necessarily predict increased fluid requirements, but the ratio of partial pressure of arterial oxygen to the inhaled fraction of oxygen (P:F ratio) may help to delineate which patients will have volume needs above those predicted by the Parkland formula.[70] In a sheep model, the degree of airway inflammation correlated with increased fluid needs, rather than alveolar dysfunction alone.[84] Smoke inhalation may also predispose patients to late infectious complications by increasing alveolar leukocyte recruitment in the presence of endotoxin.[85]

Another feared complication of inhalation injury is carbon monoxide (CO) poisoning, one of the most common causes of immediate death after inhalation injury. Inhalation of a 0.1% CO mixture may cause carboxyhemoglobin level as high as 50%, and CO has an affinity for hemoglobin 200-250 times greater than that of oxygen. This decreases oxyhemoglobin and leads to the often-rapid onset of anoxia and death.[86] The diagnosis may be suspected in patients with unexplained neurologic symptoms or the classic "cherry red" appearance of the skin. An arterial carboxyhemoglobin level is essential because pulse oximetry is known to be falsely elevated in patients with CO poisoning. Administration of 100% oxygen via mechanical ventilation is the standard method of eliminating carbon monoxide from the bloodstream. The half-life of CO is 250 minutes in room air but is reduced to 40-60 minutes in a patient on 100% oxygen.[87] Hyperbaric oxygen therapy is cumbersome to use in critically ill patients, and it is not clear whether any neuroprotective benefits are derived with its use.[51]

Hydrogen cyanide may also be produced in fires that burn nitrogen-containing polymers. Prehospital personnel may notice a "bitter almond" odor, and these patients may have a nonresponsive lactic acidosis or S-T elevation on ECG that may mimic myocardial infarction.[88] Toxicity results from inhibition of cytochrome oxidase by cyanide, which in turn causes inhibition of cellular oxygenation.[89] Treatment involves IV sodium thiosulfate (125-250 mg/kg) and hydroxocobalamin (4 g), and 100% oxygen. Sodium thiosulfate changes cyanide to a nontoxic thiocyanate, but onset is slow. Hydroxocobalamin is a chelating agent that rapidly forms a complex with cyanide and increases renal excretion and is the immediate treatment of choice.[86]

Electrical injury is a less common but potentially severe form of thermal injury. In addition to standard care for burn injuries, special attention should be directed to characteristic injuries associated with high-voltage exposures. Most cardiac arrhythmias occur in the acute period, so these patients should have an electrocardiogram performed and be placed on cardiac monitors. If these are normal, prolonged monitoring greater than a few hours is unnecessary.[90,91] Compartment syndrome requiring fasciotomy is not uncommon in electrical injury, even in patients with little to no exterior evidence of burns. These patients must also undergo evaluation for rhabdomyolysis and myoglobinuria. Ophthalmologic and otoscopic examination is also important, particularly in lightning injuries.[92]

Chemical burns are another etiology of burns with a separate set of issues specific to their care. Great care should be taken in ensuring that the agent has been completely removed from the patient and the area copiously irrigated for at least 30 minutes. One of the most common agents causing chemical burns is hydrofluoric acid due to its inclusion in industrial cleansers.

Treatment, after initial irrigation, consists of neutralization with calcium. Calcium gluconate in dimethyl sulfoxide may be applied directly to small wounds, or subcutaneous or intravenous infiltration of calcium gluconate may be required.[93,94] An intra-arterial infusion of calcium gluconate has been used in hydrofluoric acid burns to the face.[95] A rapidly growing number of burns are associated with accidents during the illegal manufacture of methamphetamines. These are typically young males with burns to the face and hands and a vague or uncertain history of what led to the injury. These patients often require higher than predicted fluid resuscitation volumes, and diligent surveillance for signs of withdrawal is essential.[96,97]

Deep vein thrombosis (DVT) has classically been believed to be rare in burned patients, and due to their large open wounds many clinicians have been reticent to use heparin prophylaxis in this patient population. However, a recent study of 148 burn patients who were hospitalized more than three days revealed that 9 (6%) of those patients had a DVT and two suffered a documented pulmonary embolus, one that was fatal.[98] In a retrospective study of 4102 burn patients, Fecher et al[99] found DVT in only 0.25% of patients. However, this group routinely used subcutaneous heparin prophylaxis in their patients and saw no bleeding complications.

CONCLUSION

Burn care is one of the most rapidly evolving fields in medicine today. There is an ongoing shortage of dedicated burn surgeons currently in training,[100] so it is clear that the acute care surgeon will be at the forefront of continuing progress in the field. A clear understanding of the principles of burn resuscitation will be invaluable to the acute care surgeon of the future.

REFERENCES

1. Zawacki BE, Azen SP, Imbus SH, Chang YT. Multifactorial probit analysis of mortality in burn patients. *Ann Surg* 1979;189:1-5.
2. Ryan CM, Schoenfeld DA, Thorpe WP, et al. Objective estimates of the probability of death from burn injuries. *N Engl J Med* 1998;362-366.
3. Moreau AR, Westfall PH, Cancio LC, Mason AD Jr. Development and validation of an age-risk score for mortality prediction after thermal injury. *J Trauma* 2005;58(5):967-972.
4. Sheridan RL. Burns. *Crit Care Med* 2002;30(11): S500-S514.
5. Sheridan RL. Recognition and management of hot liquid aspiration in children. *Ann Emerg Med* 1996;27:89-91.
6. Frascone R, Kaye K, Dries D, Solem L. Successful placement of an adult sternal intraosseous line through burned skin. *J Burn Care Rehabil* 2003;24(5):306-308.
7. Ramzy PI, Barret JP, Herndon DN. Thermal Injury. *Crit Care Clin* 1999;15(2):333-352.
8. Watts AM, Tyler MP, Perry ME, et al. Burn depth and its histological measurement. *Burns* 2001;27(2):154-160.
9. Ho-Asjoe M, Chronnell CM, Frame JD, et al. Immunohistochemical analysis of burn depth. *J Burn Care Rehabil* 1999;20(3):207-211.
10. Iraniha S, Cinat ME, VanderKam VM, et al. Determination of burn depth with noncontact ultrasonography. *J Burn Care Rehabil* 2000;21(4):333-338.
11. Bray R, Forrester K, Leonard C, et al. Laser Doppler imaging of burn scars: a comparison of wavelength and scanning methods. *Burns* 2003;29(3):199-206.
12. Mileski WJ, Atiles L, Purdue G, et al. Serial measurements increase the accuracy of laser Doppler assessment of burn wounds. *J Burn Care Rehabil* 2003;24:187-191.
13. Vo LT, Anikijenko P, McLaren WJ, et al. Autofluorescence of skin burns detected by fiber-optic confocal imaging: evidence that cool water treatment limits progressive thermal damage in anesthetized hairless mice. *J Trauma* 2001;51(1):98-104.
14. Kamolz LP, Andel H, Haslik W, et al. Indocyanine green video angiographies help to identify burns requiring operation. *Burns* 2003;29(8):785-791.
15. Srinivas SM, de Boer JF, Park H, et al. Determination of burn depth by polarization-sensitive optical coherence tomography. *J Biomed Opt* 2004;9(1):207-212.
16. Kim DE, Phillips TM, Jeng JC, et al. Microvascular assessment of burn depth conversion during varying resuscitation conditions. *J Burn Care Rehabil* 2001;22(6):406-416.
17. Garner WL, Rodriguez JL, Miller CG, et al. Acute skin injury releases neutrophil chemoattractants. *Surgery* 1994;116(1):42-48.
18. Cartotto RC, Innes M, Musgrave MA, et al. How well does the Parkland formula estimate actual fluid resuscitation volumes? *J Burn Care Rehabil* 2002;23(4): 258-265.
19. Engrav LH, Colescott PL, Kemalyan N, et al. A biopsy of the use of the Baxter formula to resuscitate burns or do we do it like Charlie did it? *J Burn Care Rehabil* 2000;21(2):91-95.
20. Friedrich JB, Sullivan SR, Engrav LH, et al. Is supra-Baxter resuscitation in burn patients a new phenomenon? *Burns* 2004;30(5):464-466.
21. Sullivan SR, Friedrich JB, Engrav LH, et al. "Opioid creep" is real and may be the cause of "fluid creep." *Burns* 2004;30(6):583-590.
22. Cancio LC, Chavez S, Alvarado-Ortega M, et al. Predicting increased fluid requirements during the resuscitation of thermally injured patients. *J Trauma* 2004;56(2):404-414.
23. Cancio LC, Reifenberg L, Barillo DJ, et al. Standard variables fail to identify patients who will not respond to fluid resuscitation following thermal injury: brief report. *Burns* 2005;31(3):358-365.
24. Navar PD, Saffle JR, Warden GD. Effect of inhalation injury on fluid resuscitation requirements after thermal injury. *Am J Surg* 1985;150(6):716-720.

25. Dai NT, Chen TM, Cheng TY, et al. The comparison of early fluid therapy in extensive flame burns between inhalation and noninhalation injuries. *Burns* 24(7):671-675.

26. O'Mara MS, Slater H, Goldfarb IW, Caushaj PF. A prospective, randomized evaluation of intra-abdominal pressures with crystalloid and colloid resuscitation in burn patients. *J Trauma* 2005;58(5):1011-1018.

27. Carvajal HF, Parks DH. Optimal composition of burn resuscitation fluids. *Crit Care Med* 1988;16:695-700.

28. Goodwin CW, Dorethy J, Lam V, Pruitt BA. Randomized trial of efficacy of crystalloid and colloid resuscitation on hemodynamic response and lung water following thermal injury. *Ann Surg* 1983;197:520-531.

29. Chen L-W, Wang J-S, Hwang B, et al. Reversal of the effect of albumin on gut barrier function in burn by the inhibition of inducible isoform of nitric oxide synthase. *Arch Surg* 2003;138(11):1219-1225.

30. Cochrane Injuries Group Albumin Reviewers. Human albumin administration in critically ill patients: Systematic review of randomized controlled trials. *BMJ* 1998;317:235-240.

31. Kinsky MP, Milner SM, Button B, et al. Resuscitation of severe thermal injury with hypertonic saline dextran: effects on peripheral and visceral edema in sheep. *J Trauma* 2000;49(5):844-853.

32. Huang PP, Stucky FS, Dimick AR, et al. Hypertonic sodium resuscitation is associated with renal failure and death. *Ann Surg* 1995;221:543-554.

33. Berger MM, Pictet A, Revelly JP, et al. Impact of a bicarbonated saline solution on early resuscitation after major burns. *Intensive Care Med* 2000;26:1382-1385.

34. Chen L-W, Hwang B, Wang J-S, et al. Hypertonic saline-enhanced postburn gut barrier failure is reversed by inducible nitric oxide synthase inhibition. *Crit Care Med* 2004;32(12):2476-2484.

35. Shah A, Connolly CM, Kirschner RA, et al. Evaluation of hyperdynamic resuscitation in 60% TBSA burn-injured sheep. *Shock* 2004;21(1):86-92.

36. Tanaka H, Matsuda T, Miyagantani Y, et al. Reduction of resuscitation fluid volumes in severely burned patients using ascorbic acid administration: a randomized, prospective study. *Arch Surg* 2000;135(3):326-331.

37. Cartotto R, Choi J, Gomez M, Cooper A. A prospective study on the implications of a base deficit during fluid resuscitation. *J Burn Care Rehabil* 2003;24(2):75-84.

38. Jeng JC, Jablonski K, Bridgeman A, Jordan MH. Serum lactate, not base deficit, rapidly predicts survival after major burns. *Burns* 2002;28(2):161-166.

39. Venkatesh B, Meacher R, Muller MJ, et al. Monitoring tissue oxygenation during resuscitation of major burns. *J Trauma* 2001;50(3):485-494.

40. Lorente JA, Ezpleta A, Esteban A, et al. Systemic hemodynamics, gastric intramucosal PCO_2 changes, and outcome in critically ill burn patients. *Crit Care Med* 2000;28(6):1728-1735.

41. Holm C, Mayr M, Tegeler J, et al. A clinical randomized study on the effects of invasive monitoring on burn shock resuscitation. *Burns* 2004;30(8):798-807.

42. Holm C, Melcer B, Horbrand F, et al. The relationship between oxygen delivery and oxygen consumption during fluid resuscitation of burn-related shock. *J Burn Care Rehabil* 2000;21(2):147-154.

43. Tsoutsos D, Rodopoulou S, Keramidas E, et al. Early escharotomy as a measure to reduce intraabdominal hypertension in full-thickness burns of the thoracic and abdominal area. *World J Surg* 2003;27(12):1323-1328.

44. Sheridan RL, Tompkins RG, McManus WF, et al. Intracompartmental sepsis in burn patients. *J Trauma* 1994;36:301-305.

45. Wolf SE, Herndon DN. Burns. In: Townsend MD, ed. *Sabiston Textbook of Surgery*, 17th ed. Philadelphia, PA: Elsevier-Saunders;2004:578.

46. Krieger Y, Rosenberg L, Lapid O, et al. Escharotomy using an enzymatic debridement agent for treating experimental burn-induced compartment syndrome in an animal model. *J Trauma* 2005;58(6):1259-1264.

47. Janzekovic Z. A new concept in the early excision and immediate grafting of burns. *J Trauma* 1970;10(12):1103-1108.

48. Demling RH. Improved survival after massive burns. *J Trauma* 1983;23(3):179-184.

49. Deitch EA. A policy of early excision and grafting in elderly burn patients shortens the hospital stay and improves survival. *Burns Incl Therm Inj* 1985;12:109-114.

50. Thompson P, Herndon DN, Abston S, Rutan T. Effect of early excision on patients with major thermal injury. *J Trauma* 1987;27(2): 205-207.

51. Sheridan RL, Tompkins RG. What's new in burns and metabolism. *J Am Coll Surg* 2004;198(2):243-263.

52. Sheridan RL, Szyfelbein SK. Staged high dose epinephrine clysis in pediatric burn excisions: Proceedings of the American Burn Association. *J Burn Care Rehabil* 1998;19:S199.

53. Xiao-Wu W, Herndon DN, Spies M, et al. Effects of delayed wound excision and grafting in severely burned children. *Arch Surg* 2002;137:1049-1054.

54. Barret JP, Herndon DN. Modulation of inflammatory and catabolic responses in severely burned children by early burn wound excision in the first 24 hours. *Arch Surg* 2003;138:127-132.

55. Klein MB, Hunter S, Heimbach DM, et al. The Versajet water dissector: a new tool for tangential excision. *J Burn Care Rehabil* 2005;26(6):483-487.

56. Naoum JJ, Roehl KR, Wolf SE, Herndon DN. The use of homograft compared to topical antimicrobial therapy in the treatment of second-degree burns of more than 40% total body surface area. *Burns* 2004;30(6):548-551.

57. Jones I, Currie L, Martin R. A guide to biological skin substitutes. *Br J Plast Surg* 2002;55(3):185-193.

58. Kearney JN. Clinical evaluation of skin substitutes. *Burns* 2001;27(5):545-551.

59. Boyce ST, Warden GD. Principles and practices for treatment of cutaneous wounds with cultured skin substitutes. *Am J Surg* 2002;183(4):445-456.

60. Boyce ST, Kagan RJ, Yakuboff KP, et al. Cultured skin substitutes reduce donor skin harvesting for closure of excised, full-thickness burns. *Ann Surg* 2002;235(2):269-479.

60. Boyce ST, Kagan RJ, Meyer NA, et al. The 1999 clinical research award. Cultured skin substitutes combined with Integra Artificial Skin to replace native skin autograft and allograft for the closure of excised full-thickness burns. *J Burn Care Rehabil* 1999;20(6): 453-461.

62. MacLennan N, Heimbach DM, Cullen BF. Anesthesia for major thermal injury. *Anesthesiology* 1998;89(3): 749-770.

63. Han T, Kim H, Bae J, et al. Neuromuscular pharmacodynamics of rocuronium in patients with major burns. *Anesth Analg* 2004;99(2):386-392.

64. Jellish WS, Gamelli RL, Furry PA, et al. Effect of topical local anesthetic application to skin harvest sites for pain management in burn patients undergoing skin-grafting procedures. *Ann Surg* 1999;229(1):115-120.

65. Rue LW III, Cioffi WG Jr, Mason AD Jr, et al. Improved survival of burned patients with inhalation injury. *Arch Surg* 1993;128:772-780.

66. Smith DL, Cairns BA, Ramadan F, et al. Effect of inhalation injury, burn size, and age on mortality: a study of 1447 consecutive burn patients. *J Trauma* 1994;37: 655-659.

67. Shirani KZ, Pruitt BA, Mason AD. The influence of inhalation injury and pneumonia on burn mortality. *Ann Surg* 1987;205(1):82-87.

68. Darling GE, Keresteci MA, Ibanez D, et al. Pulmonary complications in inhalation injuries with associated cutaneous burn. *J Trauma* 1996;40(1):83-89.

69. Tredget EE, Shankowsky HA, Taerum TV, et al. The role of inhalation injury in burn trauma. A Canadian experience. *Ann Surg* 1990;212(6):720-727.

70. Endorf F, Gamelli RL. Inhalation injury, pulmonary perturbations, and correlation with acute fluid resuscitation requirements. *J Burn Care Rehabil* 2007;28(1): 80-3.

71. Gore MA, Joshi AR, Nagarajan G, et al. Virtual bronchoscopy for diagnosis of inhalation injury in burnt patients. *Burns* 2004;30:165-168.

72. Evidence-based surgery. *J Am Coll Surg* 2003;196(2): 308-312.

73. Moylan JA, Alexander LG Jr. Diagnosis and treatment of inhalation injury. *World J Surg* 1978;2:185-191.

74. Pallua N, Warbanow K, Noah EM, et al. Intrabronchial surfactant application in cases of inhalation injury: first results from patients with severe burns and ARDS. *Burns* 1998;24(3):197-206.

75. Sheridan RL, Hurford WE, Kacmarek RM, et al. Inhaled nitric oxide in burn patients with respiratory failure. *J Trauma* 1997;42:629-634.

76. Enkhbaatar P, Murakami K, Cox R, et al. Aerosolized tissue plasminogen inhibitor improves pulmonary function in sheep with burn and smoke inhalation. *Shock* 2004;22(1):70-75.

77. Murakami K, McGuire R, Cox RA, et al. Recombinant antithrombin attenuates pulmonary inflammation following smoke inhalation and pneumonia in sheep. *Crit Care Med* 2003;31(2):577-583.

78. Sheridan RL, Kacmarek RM, McEttrick MM, et al. Permissive hypercapnia as a ventilator strategy in burned children: Effect on barotraumas, pneumonia, and mortality. *J Trauma* 1995;39:854-859.

79. Cortiella J, Mlcak R, Herndon D. High frequency percussive ventilation in pediatric patients with inhalation injury. *J Burn Care Rehabil* 1999;20(3): 232-235.

80. Cartotto R, Ellis S, Gomez M, Cooper A, Smith T. High frequency oscillatory ventilation in burn patients with the acute respiratory distress syndrome. *Burns* 2004;30: 453-463.

81. Thompson JT, Molnar JA, Hines MH, et al. Successful management of adult smoke inhalation with extracorporeal membrane oxygenation. *J Burn Care Rehabil* 2005;26(1):62-66.

82. Vertrees RA, Nason R, Hold MD, et al. Smoke/burn injury-induced respiratory failure elicits apoptosis in ovine lungs and cultured lung cells, ameliorated with arteriovenous CO_2 removal. *Chest* 2004;125(4): 1472-1482.

83. Saffle JR, Morris SE, Edelman L. Early tracheostomy does not improve outcome in burn patients. *J Burn Care Rehabil* 2002;23:431-438.

84. Demling R, Lalonde C, Youn YK, Picard L. Effect of graded increases in smoke inhalation injury on the early systemic response to a body burn. *Crit Care Med* 1995;23(1):171-178.

85. Wright MJ, Murphy JT. Smoke inhalation enhances early alveolar leukocyte responsiveness to endotoxin. *J Trauma* 2005;59(1):64-70.

86. Prien T, Traber DL. Toxic smoke compounds and inhalation injury—a review. *Burns Incl Therm Inj* 1988;14:451-460.

87. Crapo RO. Smoke-inhalation injuries. *JAMA* 1981;246: 1694-1696.

88. Becker CE. The role of cyanide in fires. *Vet Hum Toxicol* 1985;27:487-490.

89. Charnock EL, Meehan JJ. Postburn respiratory injuries in children. *Pediatr Clin North Am* 1980;27: 661-676.

90. Cunningham PA. The need for cardiac monitoring after electrical injury. *Med J Aust* 1991;154:765-766.

91. Fish RM. Electrical injury: Part III: cardiac monitoring indications, the pregnant patient, and lightning. *J Emerg Med* 2000;18:181-187.

92. Koumbourlis AC. Electrical injuries, *Crit Care Med* 2002;30(11):S424-S430.

93. Hatzifotis M, Williams A, Muller M, Pegg S. Hydrofluoric acid burns. *Burns* 2004;30(2):156-159.

94. Dunser MW, Ohlbauer M, Rieder J, et al. Critical care management of major hydrofluoric acid burns: a case report, review of the literature, and recommendations for therapy. *Burns* 2004;30(4):391-398.

95. Nguyen LT, Mohr WJ 3rd, Ahrenholz DH, Solem LD. Treatment of hydrofluoric acid burn to the face by carotid artery infusion of calcium gluconate. *J Burn Care Rehabil* 2004;25(5):421-424.

96. Danks RR, Wibbenmeyer LA, Faucher LD, et al. Methamphetamine-associated burn injuries: a retrospective analysis. *J Burn Care Rehabil* 2004;25(5): 425-429.

97. Warner P, Connolly JP, Gibran NS, et al. The methamphetamine burn patient. *J Burn Care Rehabil* 2003;24(5):275-278.

98. Wibbenmeyer LA, Hoballah JJ, Amelon MJ, et al. The prevalence of venous thromboembolism of the lower extremity among thermally injured patients determined by duplex sonography. *J Trauma* 2003;55: 1162-1167.

99. Fecher AM, O'Mara MS, Goldfarb IW, et al. Analysis of deep vein thrombosis in burn patients. *Burns* 2004;30(6):591-593.

100. Faucher LD. Are we headed for a shortage of burn surgeons? *J Burn Care Rehabil* 2004;25(6):464-467.

INDEX

Note: Page numbers followed by *f* and *t* indicate figures and tables, respectively.